PLASTIC SURGERY

Editor

JOSEPH G. McCARTHY, M.D.

Lawrence D. Bell Professor of Plastic Surgery and
Director of the Institute of Reconstructive Plastic Surgery
New York University Medical Center
New York, New York

Editors, Hand Surgery Volumes

JAMES W. MAY, JR., M.D.

Director of Plastic Surgery and Hand Surgery Service
Massachusetts General Hospital
Associate Clinical Professor of Surgery
Harvard Medical School
Boston, Massachusetts

J. WILLIAM LITTLER, M.D.

Past Professor of Clinical Surgery
College of Physicians and Surgeons
Columbia University, New York
Senior Attending Surgeon
The St. Luke's–Roosevelt Hospital Center
New York, New York

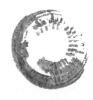

PLASTIC SURGERY

VOLUME 5

TUMORS OF THE HEAD & NECK
AND SKIN

W.B. SAUNDERS COMPANY
A Division of Harcourt Brace & Company
Philadelphia ▪ London ▪ Toronto
Montreal ▪ Sydney ▪ Tokyo

W.B. SAUNDERS COMPANY
A Division of
Harcourt Brace & Company

The Curtis Center
Independence Square West
Philadelphia, PA 19106

Library of Congress Cataloging-in-Publication Data

Plastic surgery.
     Contents: v. 1. General principles—v. 2–3.
The face—v. 4. Cleft lip & palate and craniofacial
anomalies—[etc.]
     1. Surgery, Plastic.   I. McCarthy, Joseph G., 1938–
[DNLM: 1. Surgery, Plastic. WO 600 P7122]

RD118.P536   1990   617′.95   87–9809

ISBN 0–7216–1514–7   (set)

25/7/94

Editor: W. B. Saunders Staff
Designer: W. B. Saunders Staff
Production Manager: Frank Polizzano
Manuscript Editor: David Harvey
Illustration Coordinator: Lisa Lambert
Indexer: Kathleen Garcia
Cover Designer: Ellen Bodner

Volume 1 0–7216–2542–8
Volume 2 0–7216–2543–6
Volume 3 0–7216–2544–4
Volume 4 0–7216–2545–2
Volume 5 0–7216–2546–0
Volume 6 0–7216–2547–9
Volume 7 0–7216–2548–7
Volume 8 0–7216–2549–5
8 Volume Set 0–7216–1514–7

Plastic Surgery

Printed in the United States of America.

Last digit is the print number: 9   8   7   6   5   4   3

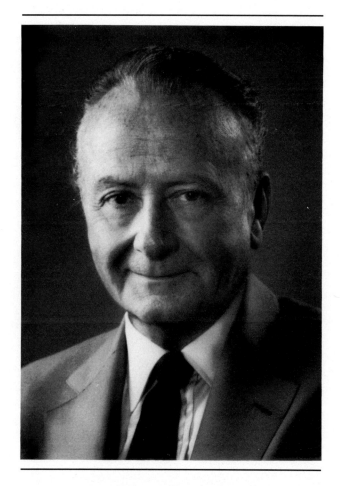

John Marquis Converse
(1909–1981)

This book is dedicated to John Marquis Converse. His enthusiasm for plastic surgery was unrivaled and his contributions to the field were legendary. Through his many writings he not only educated and inspired the plastic surgeon in the era after World War II, but also helped to define modern plastic surgery. This book is a testimony to his professional accomplishments.

Contributors

DAVID B. APFELBERG, M.D.
Assistant Clinical Professor of Plastic Surgery, Stanford University School of Medicine; Director, Comprehensive Laser Center, Palo Alto Medical Foundation, Palo Alto, California.

STEPHAN ARIYAN, M.D.
Professor of Surgery and Chief of Plastic and Reconstructive Surgery, Yale University School of Medicine; Chief of Plastic Surgery, Yale–New Haven Hospital, New Haven; Consultant in Plastic Surgery, Veterans Administration Hospital, West Haven, Connecticut.

VAHRAM Y. BAKAMJIAN, M.D.
Clinical Associate Professor of Surgery (Plastic Surgery), University of Rochester School of Medicine and Dentistry and Stanford University School of Medicine; Associate Chief, Department of Head and Neck Surgery and Oncology, Roswell Park Memorial Institute, Buffalo, New York.

DANIEL C. BAKER, M.D.
Associate Professor of Surgery (Plastic Surgery), New York University School of Medicine; Attending Surgeon, University Hospital, Bellevue Hospital Center, Manhattan Eye, Ear & Throat Hospital, and Manhattan Veterans Administration Hospital, New York, New York.

PHILIP BONANNO, M.D.
Clinical Professor of Surgery, New York Medical College; Associate Clinical Professor of Plastic Surgery, New York University Medical Center; Attending Surgeon, Bellevue Hospital, New York, Westchester Medical Center, Valhalla, and Northern Westchester Hospital Center, Mount Kisco, New York.

PHILLIP R. CASSON, M.B., F.R.C.S.
New York University School of Medicine; Attending Surgeon, University Hospital, Bellevue Hospital Center, Manhattan Veterans Administration Hospital, and New York Eye & Ear Infirmary, New York, New York.

ZENO N. CHICARILLI, M.D.
Assistant Clinical Professor of Surgery (Plastic Surgery), Yale University School of Medicine; Attending Surgeon, Yale–New Haven Hospital and Hospital of St. Raphael, New Haven, Connecticut.

JOSEPH FISCHER, M.D.
Attending Surgeon, Community General Hospital, Syracuse, New York.

WILLIAM Y. HOFFMAN, M.D.
Assistant Professor of Surgery, Division of Plastic and Reconstructive Surgery, University of California, San Francisco, School of Medicine; Chief, Division of Plastic and Reconstructive Surgery, San Francisco General Hospital, San Francisco, California.

IAN T. JACKSON, M.B., Cн.B., F.R.C.S., F.A.C.S.
Director, Institute for Craniofacial and Reconstructive Surgery, Providence Hospital, Southfield, Michigan.

MORTON R. MASER, M.D.
Assistant Clinical Professor of Plastic Surgery, Stanford University Medical Center; Attending Surgeon, Stanford University Hospital, Palo Alto, California.

JOHN B. MULLIKEN, M.D.
Associate Professor of Surgery, Harvard Medical School; Director, Craniofacial Center, Division of Plastic Surgery, Children's Hospital Medical Center and Brigham and Women's Hospital, Boston, Massachusetts.

IRVING M. POLAYES, M.D., D.D.S.
Clinical Professor of Plastic and Reconstructive Surgery, Yale University School of Medicine; Associate Section Chief, Plastic and Reconstructive Surgery, Yale–New Haven Hospital, New Haven, Connecticut.

GEORGE L. POPKIN, M.D.
Professor of Clinical Dermatology, New York University School of Medicine; Attending Physician, University Hospital, New York, New York.

PERRY ROBINS, M.D.
Associate Professor of Clinical Dermatology, New York University School of Medicine; Attending Physician, University Hospital, Bellevue Hospital, and Veterans Administration Hospital, New York, New York.

KEVIN SHAW, M.D.
Head, Section of Plastic Surgery, Mayo Clinic, Jacksonville, Florida.

AUGUSTUS J. VALAURI, D.D.S.
Professor of Surgery (Maxillofacial Prosthetics), New York University School of Medicine; Clinical Professor of Removable Prosthodontics and Occlusion, New York University School of Dentistry; Chief of the Maxillofacial Prosthetics Service, Institute of Reconstructive Plastic Surgery, New York University Medical Center, New York, New York.

Preface

Where does a book begin? Initially, I think of a warm September afternoon in a hotel in Madrid when I first organized an outline of the chapters while waiting for an international surgery meeting to begin. However, a scientific book is only an extension of earlier publications. This text is descended from *Reconstructive Plastic Surgery*, edited in 1964 by my predecessor John Marquis Converse, and reedited in 1977. I had been Assistant Editor of the latter. Many of the ideas and principles, if not the exact words, that were integral to the teaching and writing of Dr. Converse live on in the present volumes. *Reconstructive Plastic Surgery* in turn was derived from his earlier collaboration with V. H. Kazanjian, *The Surgical Treament of Facial Injuries*, published in 1949, 1959, and 1974.

Earlier textbooks by Nélaton and Ombrédanne (1904), Davis (1919), Gillies (1920), and Fomon (1939) had played a germinal role in the development of modern plastic surgery. However, even these books represented only a continuum of publications extending back over the centuries to Tagliacozzi and Sushruta. Indeed, there are also the many surgeons who never published but who by their teachings contributed greatly to the body of knowledge that is represented in the present publication. Their concepts, too, have found their way into the plastic surgery literature for the edification of another generation of students.

My own career has been greatly influenced by my teachers, and their spirit has remained an integral part of my personal and professional life. This heritage of the plastic surgeon–teacher represents the spirit of this book.

The title defines the subject—*Plastic Surgery*. Adjectives such as *reconstructive* or *esthetic* are misleading and redundant and represent artificial divisions of this surgical specialty. The parents of the infant undergoing cleft lip repair are more interested in the *esthetic* aspects of the procedure, which traditionally has been regarded as *reconstructive*. The contemporary face lift, long perceived as an *esthetic* operation, represents a surgical reconstruction of the multiple layers of the soft tissues of the face. Plastic surgery, a term first popularized by Zeis in 1838, is preferred.

With the deliberate exception of parts of Chapters 1 and 35, originally written by Dr. Converse and revised through subsequent editions of various books, few paragraphs in these volumes remain unchanged from the 1977 edition. Many of the authors, however, have used material from the previous editions. Line drawings prepared for these editions by Daisy Stillwell have been reproduced again where appropriate. With the death of Ms. Stillwell, I was fortunate to recruit yet another outstanding medical artist, Craig Luce, to draw hundreds of new illustrations to reflect the continuing developments in this specialty.

The purpose of this book is to define the specialty of plastic surgery. To accomplish this goal, contributions have been sought from the acknowledged leaders of this discipline in all of its ramifications. The clinical applications of plastic surgery, practiced over the whole of the human anatomy, range from skin grafting to the management of uncommon craniofacial clefts, to replantation of the lower extremity. Its practice varies from uncomplicated procedures to sophisticated multistage reconstructions that ally the plastic surgeon with other specialists. The chapters that follow vary in the same way from the short and direct to the lengthy and complex. More than any other, this type of surgery strives for the restoration or improvement of form as well as the restoration of function. The teaching of plastic surgery thus lends itself to illustration. The contributors to this book have been encouraged to use drawings and photographs liberally as an enhancement of the principles and techniques described in the text. Special attention has been given to the sizing and placement of more than 5000 illustrations submitted in accordance with this plan. The contributors and publisher have also made every effort to acknowledge and cite the work of other authors. In a text of this magnitude any omission, while understandable, is regrettable.

In Volume 1 will be found discussions of the essential principles basic to all plastic surgery: wound healing, circulation of the skin, microneurovascular repairs, skin expansion, and grafting of tendons, nerves, and bone, as well as their associated methods of repair. This is the largest of the volumes and testifies to the broadening scope of the field. Much of what is now fundamental to the training of a plastic surgeon was only imagined a generation ago.

After the discussion of general principles in Volume 1, the organization of the text is by anatomic regions. Volumes 2 and 3 are devoted to the face; here, as throughout the book, each chapter draws upon the expertise of acknowledged master surgeons particularly experienced in the subjects on which they have written.

Clefts of the lip and palate as well as severe craniofacial anomalies make up Volume 4. In addition to plastic surgery, these chapters incorporate contributions from the allied fields of embryology, craniofacial growth and development, orthodontics, prosthodontics, speech pathology, and neurosurgery.

Volume 5 covers tumors of the skin and head and neck and Volume 6 the trunk, lower extremity, and genitourinary system. Of particular note, the text details recent advances in reconstruction that involve newly developed flaps of ingenious design and considerable sophistication.

The application of plastic surgical principles and techniques of the upper extremity are discussed in Volumes 7 and 8 under the editorship of Drs. James W. May, Jr., and J. William Littler. The latter, one of the most esteemed and influential hand surgeons of the modern era, edited the upper extremity section in 1964 and 1977. He has been joined in this edition by Dr. May, who is qualified in both hand surgery and microsurgical reconstruction. Both, who are my personal friends, brought their usual enthusiasm, experience, and equanimity to bear on this project. Because surgery of the upper extremity is practiced so extensively, ample space has been afforded for the comprehensive description of the reconstructive procedures specifically designed for the restoration of injured parts. Much of the current progress in plastic surgery of the upper extremity has been made possible by the gradual perfection of microvascular techniques, and these newer developments have been incorporated into the text.

Continuing change, the hallmark of all medical and surgical practice, dictates the need for a reference book such as this and makes its accomplishment a challenging task for everyone involved. With the writing of these words the lengthy process of revising, updating, and improving is ended. The book is committed to the press with the promise that it is both complete and current, in the belief that readers will find it an invaluable resource, and with the hope that it makes a contribution to the body of plastic surgery knowledge and to the education of tomorrow's plastic surgeon.

JOSEPH G. McCARTHY, M.D.

Acknowledgments

The authors or contributors, all with heavy clinical responsibilities and demands, have contributed greatly and are responsible for this text. In addition to outlining their personal views, they have conducted exhaustive literature searches and have organized their illustrative material. They represent the heart and soul of the book.

I wish also to acknowledge my fellow faculty members at the Institute of Reconstructive Plastic Surgery, since their work and concepts, as well as their encouragement, have been so important in the development of this text: Sherrell J. Aston, Donald L. Ballantyne, Robert W. Beasley, Phillip R. Casson, David T.W. Chiu, Peter J. Coccaro, Stephen R. Colen, Court B. Cutting, Barry H. Grayson, V. Michael Hogan, Glenn W. Jelks, Frances C. Macgregor, Thomas D. Rees, Blair O. Rogers, William W. Shaw, John W. Siebert, Charles H. M. Thorne, Augustus J. Valauri, Donald Wood-Smith, and Barry M. Zide. Dr. Frank Cole Spencer, George David Stewart Professor of Surgery and Chairman of the Department of Surgery at the New York University Medical Center, has always championed the goals of the Institute and has especially encouraged development in the newer areas of craniofacial surgery and microsurgery.

I should also pay tribute to Ms. Karen Singer, who did so much of the bibliographic study, and Wayne Pearson and Harry Weissfisch, who provided photographic support. I must also acknowledge my associates at the Institute, Robert E. Bochat, Linda Gerson, Donna O'Brien, Caren Crane, Marilyn Deaton, Margy Maroutsis, Marjorie Huggins, and others for acts of kindness and support during the years of preparation of this book.

Mr. Albert Meier, Senior Editor at Saunders, had a major share in the organization and editing of this book. A friend and colleague since 1974 when we began the Second Edition, I have benefited immensely from his advice and counsel. He has also shown an unusual sense of understanding throughout this project. Special thanks are also due to David Harvey, Frank Polizzano, and Richard Zorab of the W. B. Saunders Company for their support.

I am also grateful to the residents and fellows at the Institute of Reconstructive Plastic Surgery, whose boundless enthusiasm is ever encouraging and who have given generously of their time to proofread manuscripts and galleys: Christopher Attinger, Constance Barone, Richard Bartlett, P. Craig Hobar, William Hoffman, Armen Kasabian, Gregory LaTrenta, George Peck, Rosa Razaboni, Gregory Ruff, John Siebert, R. Kendrick Slate, Henry Spinelli, Michael Stevens, Charles Thorne, and Douglas Wagner.

Special thanks are also due to my colleagues and friends at the National Foundation for Facial Reconstruction, whose support and encouragement have provided a unique environment at the Institute that is conducive to writing and research.

Finally, I want to thank my family, Karlan, Cara, and Stephen, for their love and understanding during the demanding years of this project, especially those times spent at a desk when I may have appeared distracted or lost in thought. They remain my main support and life focus.

I also want to thank my friends, especially Charles and Heather Garbaccio, who had the ability to offer those special moments of lightheartedness, good cheer, and camaraderie.

JGM

Contents

Volume 5

Tumors of the Head & Neck and Skin

PLASTIC SURGERY

65

William Y. Hoffman
Daniel C. Baker

Pediatric Tumors of the Head and Neck

The presence of a mass in an infant or child causes great consternation in both physicians and parents. It is important for the surgeon to have a complete understanding of the differential diagnosis in order to reassure the family and to carry out an adequate diagnostic work-up. Although the vast majority of head and neck masses in children are benign (and most of these are inflammatory), malignancies can be devastating, and must be ruled out by appropriate examination and diagnostic studies.

Approximately one-quarter of childhood malignancies are found in the head and neck. The incidence appears to drop slightly with increasing age, being 20 per 100,000 population before the age of 5 years and 10 per 100,000 population in the following ten years.

PREOPERATIVE EVALUATION

Completion of the history taking and physical examination should lead to a diagnosis in most cases. The presence of a mass since birth suggests a benign process, usually of mesodermal origin. A recent respiratory tract infection suggests an inflammatory origin. The rate and duration of growth should also be ascertained.

The age of the patient provides some clues to the diagnosis. Benign mesodermal anomalies—hemangiomas and cystic hygromas—are the most common lesions of the head and neck at birth and in the first year of life. Teratomas and dermoid cysts are also seen in the first year of life, although they are less frequent in the head and neck region than in other anatomic areas. Branchial cleft sinuses may be noted at birth, but cysts of branchial cleft origin, although presumably present at birth, may not present until adolescence. Malignancies are rarely seen in the first year; at this age, leukemias, retinoblastomas, and brain tumors are most common, with lymphomas and sarcomas predominating after age 5 years. Salivary gland tumors are generally seen after age 10 years.

The physical examination also aids in the differentiation of benign and malignant masses. The findings common to any physical examination should be noted, e.g., size, location, mobility, tenderness, and quality of the overlying skin. The location of a mass is frequently characteristic in certain lesions (these are discussed under the specific lesions below). Transillumination may distinguish between a cystic and a solid mass; the former is almost always benign. Movement of a mass during swallowing may suggest attachment to the thyroid gland or the hyoid bone. Characteristic locations for certain lesions— teratomas in the midline anterior neck, rhabdomyosarcomas in the orbit, ear, or nasopharynx—may suggest a diagnosis.

A careful examination should include direct inspection of the oropharynx, hypopharynx, and nasopharynx. Extremely small caliber endoscopes are available for examination and biopsy of previously inaccessible areas such as the posterior nasopharynx and the larynx. The use of these instruments in smaller children may require general anesthesia. In the presence of lymph node enlargement, axillary and inguinal nodes should also be examined; the abdomen should be examined for masses that might be the primary foci for metastatic nodes.

Biopsy should be considered whenever there is a doubt regarding the possibility of malignancy, as well as in certain benign conditions such as neurofibromatosis or fibrous dysplasia. In addition to standard incisional or excisional biopsies, fine needle aspiration cytology has become established as a minimally invasive technique with high sensitivity and specificity in a variety of lesions. If a malignant tumor is considered a possibility, communication with the pathologist before the biopsy ensures adequate-sized samples and fixation of the specimen (Larson, Robbins, and Butler, 1984). Electron microscopy may be useful in the diagnosis of sarcomas; this study requires glutaraldehyde fixation and should be considered before the time of biopsy (Feldman, 1982).

RADIOGRAPHIC IMAGING

Plain films of the neck and sinuses are particularly useful to visualize the air-filled spaces of the head and neck region. Soft tissue or bony masses may be difficult to interpret on plain films because of the overlying shadows of the craniofacial skeleton. Ultrasound should be considered as a means of differentiating cystic from solid masses. With newer ultrasonographic methods, excellent anatomic definition can also be obtained (Ward-Booth and associates, 1984; Sherman and associates, 1985; Kraus and associates, 1986).

Substantial improvements in the quality of computed tomography (CT) have revolutionized the diagnostic approaches to head and neck masses in children (Russell, 1985). Axial slices can provide information regarding the cystic or solid nature of the mass, the extent of deep involvement or extension, the bony erosion, and the anatomic location of the mass in relation to other structures (Silverman, Korobkin, and Moore, 1983). A high degree of diagnostic accuracy has been reported for CT scanning in cervical infections (Nyberg and associates, 1985), branchial cleft cysts (Salazar, Duke, and Ellis, 1985), salivary gland tumors (Bryan and associates, 1982; Golding, 1982), and other malignancies of the head and neck (Krol and Strong, 1986). Three-dimensional reconstruction of the CT images can be performed; these are quite accurate for examination of skeletal changes, but are less so for soft tissue masses because of the fairly narrow band of CT numbers describing most soft tissue (Fig. 65–1).

Magnetic resonance imaging (MRI) is a new modality that is particularly useful in the definition of soft tissue masses. It does not image bone well, largely because of the decreased blood flow through bone. The indications for MRI as opposed to CT scans are still being defined at this time.

INFLAMMATORY MASSES

Lymphadenopathy

Neck masses of lymphoid origin are a frequent occurrence following upper respiratory tract infections. Although these most commonly result from *Staphylococcus aureus* or beta-hemolytic *Streptococcus* species (80 to 90 per cent), numerous other etiologic agents have been described, including a full spectrum of bacterial and viral organisms (Bedros and Mann, 1981). Most bacterial adenopathy presents with tenderness on palpation but without evidence of overlying skin involvement. If a patient does not respond rapidly to penicillin or first-generation cephalosporin therapy, additional antibiotics should be

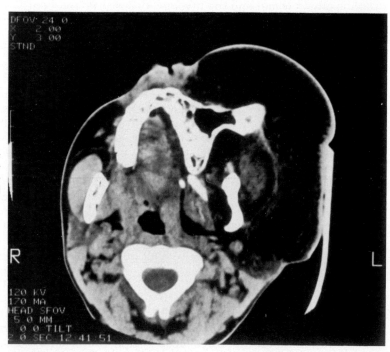

Figure 65–1. Axial CT scan demonstrating an extensive neurofibroma with displacement and hypertrophy of the craniofacial skeleton.

added to treat gram-negative and anaerobic organisms.

Needle aspiration may provide culture material and may also be curative for small abscesses. Ultrasound and computed tomography have both been used to delineate the origin and extent of lymphoid masses, as well as to localize abscess cavities when present.

Excisional biopsy of an enlarged lymph node should be performed when the usual diagnostic maneuvers have been carried out without yield. The reported results of cervical lymph node biopsies in children show that approximately 80 per cent are hyperplastic or granulomatous, 18 per cent represent a lymphoma or other lymphoreticular malignancy, and only 2 per cent are involved with metastatic or primary head and neck disease.

Chronic Cervical Lymphadenitis

Mycobacteria, both tuberculous and atypical, are the most common etiologic agents for chronic suppuration in cervical lymph nodes. Hippocrates mentioned drainage of suppurative neck nodes, and in the Middle Ages scrofula was known as the "King's evil" after several reigning sovereigns claimed to effect cures by touching the patients. In recent years there has been an increased incidence of this relatively unusual disease, with the influx of immigrants from endemic areas in Asia and South America. Chronic granulomatous disease in the neck typically presents in children under 6 years old, with painless progressive enlargement of nodes that ultimately form "cold" abscesses, which may mimic neoplasms (Levin-Epstein and Lucente, 1982).

Tuberculous cervical adenitis (scrofula) occurs in approximately 5 per cent of all cases of tuberculosis, but in up to two-thirds of cases of extrapulmonary disease (Cantrell, Jensen, and Reid, 1975). Pathologic study reveals a range of findings from simple hyperplasia to caseating necrosis, and organisms are seen in most cases. Approximately one-half of patients with tuberculous neck nodes have systemic symptoms, although the chest radiograph and sputum smear may be negative. Skin tests are diagnostic in virtually all cases. Treatment should consist of surgical excision of the involved nodes, as simple incision and drainage frequently results in draining fistulas; patients should concomitantly receive long-term antituberculous chemotherapy (Appling and Miller, 1981; Castro, Hoover, and Zuckerbraun, 1985).

Atypical mycobacteria may present more diagnostic difficulty, because the chest radiograph is often normal and the involved nodes usually unilateral. The most common organisms isolated in large series are *M. scrofulaceum* and *M. avium-intracellulare* (Saitz, 1981). Specific skin tests for these organisms exist but are difficult to obtain; patients may be weakly positive to tuberculin testing. Schaad and associates (1979) reviewed 380 cases of atypical mycobacterial lymphadenitis and found that surgical excision of nodes alone was curative in over 90 per cent, in contradistinction to incision and drainage, which was effective in only 16 per cent. Medical management alone effected no cures. Other pathologic states that have been described as causing similar presentations include cat scratch disease, actinomycosis, tularemia, and sarcoidosis (Lane, Keane, and Potsic, 1980).

Lateral Pharyngeal Abscesses

Suppuration of an untreated deep lymph node or extension of a peritonsillar abscess may lead to the development of a lateral pharyngeal abscess, which may represent a surgical emergency. The abscesses present as fullness in the lateral cervical region, with tenderness and dysphagia as early signs. Progression of the infectious process may lead to trismus, hoarseness, cough, and dyspnea; in the advanced stage, there may be progression to sepsis, airway obstruction, and possible carotid artery erosion.

A plain lateral radiograph of the neck may demonstrate soft tissue swelling in the posterior pharyngeal space. As noted above, ultrasound and computed tomography further delineate the abscess cavity, and may guide percutaneous drainage if the cavity is accessible. Wide surgical drainage is mandatory if the later complications of sepsis or airway obstruction have occurred; tracheotomy may also be required.

Sialadenitis

Inflammation accounts for more than one-third of the pathologic conditions of the salivary glands in the pediatric patient. Regardless of whether the submaxillary or parotid gland is affected, the clinical presentation is similar, with a tender, swollen gland. Acute parotitis is seen most commonly in premature infants and children with systemic illness; it is frequently associated with dehydration, fever, or immunosuppression. Postoperative parotitis is rarely seen in children, although it is probably the most common form of salivary gland inflammation seen in adults. Possible causes include inspissation of mucus and retrograde infection, as well as congenital sialoangiectasis. *S. aureus* is the most common organism found. Therapy consists of antibiotics and hydration.

Recurrent parotitis is primarily a disease of childhood, seen most frequently in the preadolescent years. The etiology may be related to sialoangiectasis, which was found in 11 of 16 patients in one series (David and O'Connel, 1970). *Streptococcus* is the most common offending organism. Most cases resolve spontaneously in the teenage years; hence, therapy is generally symptomatic, consisting of hydration, antibiotics, and occasionally duct dilation and drainage. Parotidectomy is rarely required.

Chronic parotitis is similar to the recurrent form of the disease in its periodic presentation, but does not display clinical signs of infection. Autoimmune disease and allergy have been implicated as etiologic factors. Symptomatic therapy consists of local heat and massage, as well as control of any underlying systemic disease.

Unlike inflammation of the parotid, acute submaxillary gland infection is associated with stones or congenital strictures. Generally, removal of the calculi is inadequate and resection of the involved gland is required (Kaban, Mulliken, and Murray, 1978).

DEVELOPMENTAL ANOMALIES

Branchial Cleft Anomalies

Branchial cleft anomalies include branchiogenic sinuses, cartilaginous rests, fistulas, and cervical cysts. Between the third and sixth weeks of embryonic development, the neck develops four clefts and four corresponding pharyngeal pouches, which are separated by a membrane, the branchial plate (see Chaps. 46 and 62). Fistulas form when the branchial clefts fail to close completely, with rupture of the branchial plate (Fig. 65–2). A complete fistulous tract may form, one end may close with the formation of a blind sinus tract, or both ends may close with a cyst resulting from the preservation of a central cellular rest. The sinuses and cysts that re-

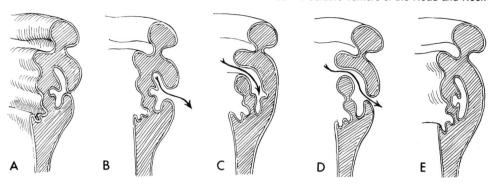

Figure 65–2. Series of diagrams to show how several kinds of tracts and cysts may arise through faulty development of the pharyngeal wall. *A,* Normal pharynx showing closure of the cervical sinus. *B,* Incomplete closure of the cervical sinus forming the basis for a tract opening externally upon the surface of the neck. *C,* Rupture of the closing membrane leaving a permanent opening into the position of the second pouch. *D,* Branchial fistula resulting from a combination of the conditions in *B* and *C. E,* Cystic remnant of the cervical sinus. (Adapted with permission from Ward, G. E., and Hendrick, J. W.: Diagnosis and Treatment of Tumors of the Head and Neck. Copyright 1950. The Williams & Wilkins Company, Baltimore.)

main in communication with the pharynx are particularly prone to infection and may present with cellulitis and abscess formation.

Branchial cleft cysts typically present as a smooth, nontender mass, lying along the anterior border of the sternocleidomastoid muscle between the external auditory canal and the clavicle. There is frequently a history of waxing and waning size associated with upper respiratory infections. Fistulas, in contrast, are usually palpable as fibrous cords; the external opening may be extremely small and may be associated with skin tags or cartilaginous remnants. The cutaneous orifice of the fistula retracts with swallowing because of the connection to the pharyngeal wall.

First branchial cleft anomalies are uncommon. They are always above the level of the hyoid bone; the external orifice is usually found in the vicinity of the auricle or beneath the mandibular ramus. The fistulas may traverse the parotid gland and are variably situated in relationship to the branches of the facial nerve (Olsen, Maragos, and Weiland, 1980; Liston, 1982; Al Fallouji and Butler, 1983).

Second branchial cleft anomalies are the most common (Fig. 65–3), and are usually found near the junction of the middle and lower thirds of the sternocleidomastoid muscle. Fistulas characteristically follow the carotid sheath, crossing the hypoglossal nerve and passing between the internal and external carotid arteries (near the bifurcation of the common carotid artery) to reach the tonsillar fossa (Salazar, Duke, and Ellis, 1985).

Third branchial cleft anomalies are rare. The external orifice may be located in a similar manner to the second branchial cleft fistulas, along the anterior border of the lower half of the sternocleidomastoid muscle; the

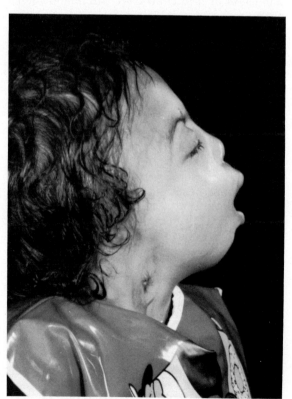

Figure 65–3. Branchial cleft (second) cyst. Note the external orifice along the anterior aspect of the sternocleidomastoid muscle.

fistula passes behind the internal carotid artery and ends at the piriform sinus.

Fourth branchial cleft anomalies have not been clinically demonstrated, despite a theoretical basis for their existence.

Branchial cleft cysts and fistulas are generally lined by squamous epithelium; 10 per cent of cases have ciliated columnar epithelium. Keratin, hair follicles, sweat glands, and sebaceous glands may be present. There may be a prominent lymphocytic reaction, with germinal centers present in the walls that react to upper respiratory tract infections. Fine needle aspiration cytology has been reported as a means of diagnosis of branchial cleft cysts (Ramos-Gabatin and Watzinger, 1984). Ultrasound and CT scanning may also be of assistance (Byrd and associates, 1983; Salazar, Duke, and Ellis, 1985).

The variable age at onset mandates a thorough work-up of presumed branchial cleft anomalies. Cinberg and associates (1982) reported that four of 18 adult patients, ranging in age from 37 to 74 years and diagnosed as having simple cysts, proved to have metastatic carcinoma with unknown primaries. A few cases of branchial cleft carcinoma have been reported (Jablokow, Kathuria, and Wang, 1982; Shreedhar and Tooley, 1984), since Martin's initial report (Martin, Morfit, and Ehrlich, 1950) and the establishment of criteria for the diagnosis of branchiogenic carcinoma.

Therapy consists of total surgical extirpation of the entire fistulous tract and any coexistent cyst. Superficial skin tags and cartilaginous rests can be removed easily under local anesthesia in the older child. Removal of a branchial cleft cyst and/or fistula requires general anesthesia, with preparation for significant dissection of the facial nerve in first branchial cleft anomalies, and of the neck vessels in second and third branchial cleft anomalies.

Thyroglossal Duct Remnants

The thyroid gland develops from the thyroglossal duct, extending from the foramen cecum in the posterior midline of the tongue through the hyoid bone to the midline of the lower neck (Fig. 65–4). Persistence of the thyroglossal duct may result in cysts, fistulas, and thyroid gland remnants along its course.

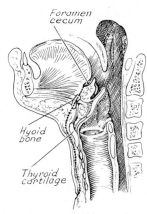

Figure 65–4. Thyroglossal duct sinus and/or fistula. The dotted line traces the pathway from the foramen cecum at the tongue through the hyoid bone, in front of the thyroid cartilage, and onto the skin in the midline of the neck. (Adapted from Marcus, E., and Zimmerman, L. M.: Principles of Surgical Practice. Copyright © 1960 by McGraw-Hill Book Company, Inc.)

Clinical presentation usually consists of a round cystic mass just below the hyoid bone in the midline of the neck. The lesions are usually asymptomatic despite their fairly large sizes. The cysts move with swallowing. Small cysts without infection may be observed; larger cysts, which cause cosmetic deformity or chronic drainage, should be excised. Extirpation includes the cyst, the body of the hyoid bone, and the fistulous tract up to the foramen cecum (Fig. 65–5).

Laryngocele

A laryngocele is an air-filled cyst arising from the laryngeal ventricle between the true and false vocal cords. If confined to the larynx, it is known as an internal laryngocele and may cause stridor and a weakened voice; an external laryngocele extends through the thyrohyoid membrane to present as a nontender, compressible mass that increases in size with a Valsalva maneuver. An air-filled sac may be demonstrated on lateral radiography or CT scan. A laryngocele presenting near the sternocleidomastoid muscle may be confused with a branchial cleft cyst, but the association with the thyrohyoid membrane and the absence of fistulous tract confirm the diagnosis. Surgical excision of the lesion is the only therapy for larger, symptomatic lesions; a lateral cervical approach is recommended. Smaller lesions may be observed (Baker, Baker, and McClatchey, 1982).

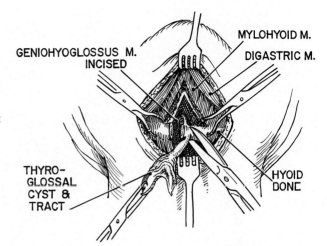

GENIOHYOGLOSSUS M. INCISED

MYLOHYOID M.

DIGASTRIC M.

THYRO- GLOSSAL CYST & TRACT

HYOID BONE

Figure 65–5. Dissection of the thyroglossal cyst and tract.

Teratomas and Dermoids

Teratomas are rare congenital tumors that occur in one in 4000 births. There is a male-to-female ratio of 1:6. The tumors are most commonly in the sacrococcygeal area and the ovaries. Less than 10 per cent are found in the head and neck region; one review found only 14 head and neck teratomas out of a total series of 245 (Tapper and Lack, 1983).

Teratomas contain elements from all three germ cell layers, often in different stages of maturation. Rudimentary organ formation may be seen. Head and neck teratomas (Fig. 65–6) have a preponderance of neurogenic tissue (Batsakis, 1984). Although these are generally tumors of newborns, teratomas may also occur in older patients and are associated with a higher incidence of malignancy with increasing age. In one series, six of nine patients over 15 years of age with teratomas showed evidence of malignant degeneration (Watanatittan, Othersen, and Hughson, 1981). Survival is directly related to the ability to extirpate the tumor in the first six months of life (Stone, Henderson, and Guidio, 1967; Tapper and Lack, 1983).

In the neck, teratomas often arise within or adjacent to the thyroid gland and cause compression of neck structures. Polyhydramnios may be noted, owing to the inability of the fetus to swallow amniotic fluid; this finding is associated with an increased incidence of stillbirth and premature births (Hajdu and associates, 1966). Neck teratomas frequently present with respiratory distress at birth; the mortality rate in unoperated cases may be as high as 80 per cent (Stone, Henderson, and Guidio, 1967). Early surgery has reduced the

mortality rate to 15 per cent (Abemayor and associates, 1984; Gundry and associates, 1983). Other head and neck sites include the orbit, the midline of the nose, and the sinuses. Teratoid tumors, or hairy polyps, are most commonly found in the nasopharynx as polyps with a long, relatively avascular stalk; they are easily snared for diagnosis and cure.

Dermoid cysts contain epithelium and adnexal structures. They are typically found in the lateral brow and in the midline of the nose (Fig. 65–7) or neck. Large lesions with intraorbital extension may cause exophthalmos. Midline nasal dermoids may present as a small pit near the radix but may extend into the septum, cribriform plate, and dura, and should therefore be investigated with CT scanning before surgery. Dermoid cysts of the neck have presented with large masses causing respiratory obstruction soon after birth, requiring early surgical intervention. Extirpation of the lesions may require a craniofacial approach in order to remove the skeletal extension of the cysts.

BENIGN TUMORS

Neurofibromas and Related Tumors

Neurofibromas are benign growths of multiple cellular elements of peripheral nerves. They may occur in isolation in the head and neck, or as multiple lesions, as in von Recklinghausen's disease (neurofibromatosis). The latter is seen more commonly in children; isolated tumors occur more often in adults.

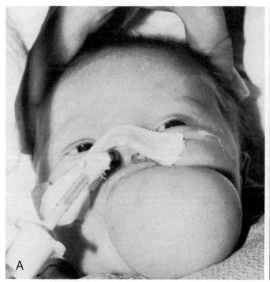
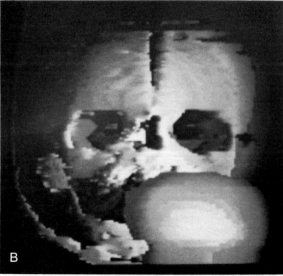

Figure 65–6. Teratoma arising from the palate (extracranial) in a newborn. *A,* Preoperative view. *B,* Three-dimensional CT scan showing that the lesion is extracranial. (Patient of Dr. Joseph G. McCarthy, New York University.)

Von Recklinghausen's (1882) disease is an autosomal dominant disorder of unknown etiology characterized by multiple neural sheath tumors (Fig. 65–8), café au lait spots, and bone lesions. Griffith and associates (1972) reviewed 50 cases of neurofibromatosis and found that 92 per cent of patients had tumors, 68 per cent café au lait spots, and 46 per cent a positive family history. Thirty-three per cent had bony abnormalities, including 25 per cent with scoliosis; 42 per cent had intracranial anomalies, and 16 per cent were mentally retarded. Skull and facial bone deformities may be seen on plain films or on CT scan, with osteolytic lesions observed in the mandible and skull even in the absence of tumor. An associated anomaly of the facial skeleton is aplasia of the greater wing of the sphenoid bone (Fig. 65–9), leading to pulsatile exophthalmos; this may occur in the absence of tumor (Gupta and associates, 1979).

Neurofibromatosis follows a characteristic course of steady growth in childhood, with the appearance of multiple subcutaneous and cutaneous nodules; Maceri and Saxon (1984) found that somewhat more than one-third of patients had head and neck involvement. Plexiform lesions are locally invasive in soft tissue and may cause significant deformity (Crikelair and Cosman, 1968). Malignant degeneration of tumors occurs in 5 to 15 per cent of patients, manifested by symptoms of sudden increase in tumor size and severe localized pain.

Treatment consists of surgical resection, either total or subtotal, and depends on the age of the patient, the location and growth rate of the tumor, and the degree of functional or cosmetic deformity. Multiple staged debulking procedures are commonly performed, usually with limited success. The tumors tend to be unencapsulated, and dissection can be hampered by an intimate association of the

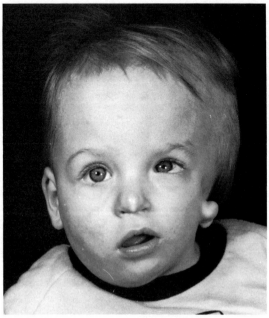

Figure 65–7. Dermoid of the midline of the nasal tip. (Patient of Dr. Joseph G. McCarthy, New York University.)

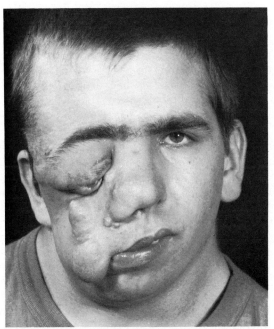

Figure 65–8. Von Recklinghausen's disease in an adolescent male characterized by multiple neural sheath tumors and pachydermatous involvement of the orbital, nasal, and cheek structures. He also has café au lait spots.

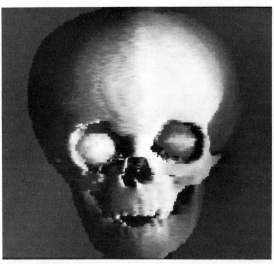

Figure 65–9. Three-dimensional CT scan demonstrating aplasia of the greater wing of the sphenoid bone with exophthalmos and displacement of the globe in a patient with neurofibromatosis. (Courtesy of Dr. Joseph G. McCarthy, New York University.)

tumor with the facial nerves and muscles. In severe deformities, consideration may be given to radical resection of all involved skin and subcutaneous tissue, and resurfacing with a skin graft or thin cutaneous free tissue transfer (Adekeye, Abiose, and Ord, 1984). The typical orbital deformity is treated by a craniofacial surgical approach, with a subtotal tumor resection and bone grafting of the roof of the orbit, and expansion of the orbital volume to accommodate the tumor mass (Marchac, 1984) (see Chap. 33).

Benign Lipomatous Tumors

Infantile Lipoblastomatosis (Chung and Enzinger, 1973). Lipoblastomatosis refers to tumors made up of immature or embryonal fat cells. The myxoid stroma seen histologically may be confused with myxoid or well-differentiated liposarcoma; the benign tumor has few mitoses and no evidence of atypia. Most are well-circumscribed growths resem-

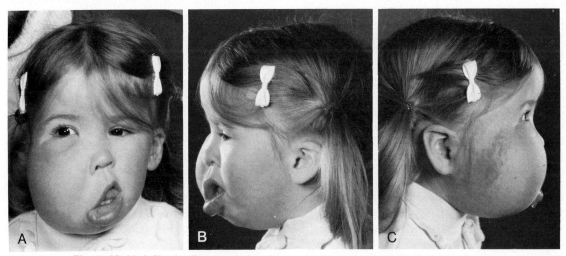

Figure 65–10. Infiltrating lipomatosis in a 4 year old girl. *A,* Frontal view. *B, C,* lateral views.

3184 Tumors of the Head and Neck

bling lipomas, occurring primarily in children under 10 years of age. The diffuse form, seen in approximately one-third of patients, is locally invasive and is associated with a somewhat higher recurrence rate. In one series, four of 35 cases occurred in the head and neck region; there was a 14 per cent recurrence rate overall. Surgical excision is the only therapy for these lesions (Chung and Enzinger, 1973).

Congenital Infiltrating Lipomatosis. This is a rare clinicopathologic entity (Fig. 65–10) that is distinct from common lipomata in that it is unencapsulated and tends to infiltrate local tissue. Histologic study demonstrates mature lipocytes that do not display the proliferative changes, pleomorphism, and mitoses of liposarcoma. They may mimic neurofibromatosis or lymphangiomas. Treatment consists of aggressive early surgical excision; as with neurofibromas, subtotal resection may be the only alternative in the attempt to balance preservation of function and cosmesis (Mattel and Persky, 1983; Slavin and associates, 1983).

Angiofibromas

Angiofibromas are benign vascular tumors that most commonly present in the nasopharynx in adolescent males. Three-quarters of patients present with severe or recurrent epistaxis; two-thirds have nasal obstruction. The tumors tend to invade locally, growing into the pterygomaxillary fossa and the paranasal sinuses. CT scanning is useful in defining the extent of the lesion. Arteriography confirms the diagnosis and identifies the blood supply; embolization may also be performed to reduce intraoperative blood loss. There have been case reports of malignant transformation to fibrosarcoma (Witt, Shah, and Sternberg, 1983).

Surgical resection is the treatment of choice, since natural regression of these neoplasms has not been demonstrated. A lateral rhinotomy or transpalatine approach has been recommended. Twenty per cent of the tumors have intracranial extensions and require a combined neurosurgical and craniofacial approach for resection. Operative blood loss may be considerable, averaging over 2500 ml in one series (Witt, Shah, and Sternberg, 1983). Surgery is effective in eradicating the tumor in 80 to 85 per cent of cases. Similar results are reported for radiation

therapy (Cummings and associates, 1984), but the possible sequelae of radiation must be considered, especially in younger patients. In general, radiation therapy is reserved for recurrences or for tumors in which total resection is not possible because of functional or cosmetic impairment.

Nodular Fasciitis

This pseudosarcomatous proliferation of soft tissue is of importance because of its frequent confusion with fibrosarcoma. In the head and neck region, nodular fasciitis most commonly occurs deep in the soft tissue, in close proximity to the mandible and along the sternocleidomastoid muscle. It may represent an anomalous reparative process after injury. Surgical excision of the tumors with minimal margins and without other therapy has been curative in most cases (Dahl and Jarlstedt, 1980).

Infantile Myofibromatosis

This form of myofibromatosis occurs almost exclusively in children under 2 years of age; 60 per cent of cases are noted in the first month. Its name derives from the histologic findings of cells that have an appearance between fibroblasts and smooth muscle. Three-quarters are solitary tumors, and 69 per cent occur in males; a multicentric type is also described, which may involve bone and viscera as well as soft tissue. The latter carries a 20 per cent mortality rate from visceral (pulmonary) involvement; the solitary type generally does well after only limited surgical excision (Chung and Enzinger, 1981).

MALIGNANT TUMORS

Malignant tumors are rare in children. The incidence of various tumors changes with the age of the population. The first year of life is associated with a particularly low incidence of malignant neoplasms. In the first five years, leukemia, retinoblastoma, and central nervous system tumors predominate. As children progress toward adolescence, lymphomas and soft tissue sarcomas are the more common malignant tumors and, in fact, represent the most common head and neck malignancies in childhood (Jaffe and Jaffe, 1973; Raney and associates, 1981).

Management of these tumors requires a multidisciplinary approach, as in adults. The addition of radiotherapy and chemotherapy has markedly improved the survival rate with specific tumors. Surgical removal of tumors in the head and neck may require resection and reconstruction of the craniofacial skeleton as well as the soft tissue; CT scans are extremely useful in the diagnosis of the lesion and planning of the surgical approach. The specific therapeutic regimen for each tumor type is discussed below.

Lymphomas

Lymphoid tumors are the most common childhood malignancies in the head and neck, making up over 50 per cent of head and neck tumors in one series (Jaffe and Jaffe, 1973). Non-Hodgkin's lymphoma is more common in children under 15 years of age; Hodgkin's lymphoma predominates in older patients. The typical presentation is that of a nontender cervical mass, but lymphomas may occur primarily in the posterior pharynx or tonsils as well as in the cervical nodes (Larson, Robbins, and Butler, 1984). In the absence of other adenopathy, the work-up of a solitary enlarged neck node should include a thorough search for a primary tumor. In patients under 20 years of age, however, only 2 per cent of lymph nodes biopsied reveal carcinoma; 80 per cent reveal benign lesions and 18 per cent lymphomas (Lee, Terry, and Lukes, 1980; Bedros and Mann, 1981; Raney and associates, 1981).

Hodgkin's disease is more likely to occur as an isolated node, approximately 80 per cent of patients presenting with cervical adenopathy. A biopsy of the involved node is necessary for diagnosis. Histologic subtypes include lymphocyte predominance, nodular sclerosis, mixed cellularity, and lymphocyte depletion, in order of worsening prognosis. The stage of disease, reflecting the extent of involvement, outweighs the histologic findings for establishing the prognosis. Staging laparotomy, with liver biopsy, splenectomy, and sampling of multiple abdominal nodes, has been challenged by computed tomography, which can reveal almost the same information without operative intervention.

The accepted staging classification for Hodgkin's and non-Hodgkin's lymphomas is as follows:

I. Involvement of a single lymph node region (I) or of a single extralymphatic organ or site (IE).

II. Involvement of two or more lymph node regions on the same side of the diaphragm (II), or localized involvement of an extralymphatic organ or site and of one or more lymph node regions on the same side of the diaphragm (IIE).

III. Involvement of lymph node regions on both sides of the diaphragm (III); there may be splenic involvement (IIIS), extralymphatic organ or site (IIIE) involvement, or both (IIISE).

III1. Involvement limited to the lymphatic structures of the upper abdomen (spleen; splenic, celiac, or hepatic portal nodes).

III2. Lower abdominal nodes (para-aortic, iliac, or mesenteric nodes).

IV. Diffuse or disseminated involvement of one or more extralymphatic organs or tissue, regardless of lymph node involvement.

"S" indicates the presence of symptoms, e.g., night sweats, pruritus, fever, or weight loss.

Stages I and II Hodgkin's disease are curable diseases today, more than 90 per cent of the patients being free of disease after radiotherapy. Treatment of more advanced stages is also extremely successful today, either extensive radiotherapy or chemotherapy being utilized initially, and chemotherapy being used for salvage of patients who fail radiotherapy (Handler and Raney, 1981).

Non-Hodgkin's lymphoma includes a variety of tumors with a common lymphoid origin. In children, non-Hodgkin's lymphoma is more common than Hodgkin's disease; because of the high incidence of head and neck involvement by Hodgkin's lymphoma, the chances of a malignant neck mass being one or the other are approximately equal. These are more aggressive tumors, and generalized lymph node involvement and extranodal sites are more common than in Hodgkin's disease. The solitary neck mass is an unusual presentation in non-Hodgkin's lymphoma. As in Hodgkin's disease, treatment is by radiotherapy of the involved areas for Stages I and II, and chemotherapy or combinations of radiation and chemotherapy for more advanced stages (Brecher and associates, 1978; Handler and Raney, 1981).

Sarcomas

Soft tissue sarcomas occur with approximately half the frequency of lymphomas, representing 6 per cent of all malignancies in children under 15 years old. The various sarcomatous tumors have a common origin from mesenchymal tissue, but their biologic behavior is extremely varied. Therapy must be individualized and based on the histologic stage, the age of the patient, and the location of the tumor (Miser and Pizzo, 1985). Multimodal therapy has markedly improved survival from most types of soft tissue sarcomas (Farr, 1981).

Rhabdomyosarcomas. Rhabdomyosarcoma represents 5 to 15 per cent of childhood neoplasms and over 50 per cent of all childhood sarcomas. The overall rarity of the tumor led in 1972 to the formation of the Intergroup Rhabdomyosarcoma Study, which has produced intensive study of the tumor, its manifestations, and the responses to various therapeutic interventions in over 700 patients (Gaiger, Soule, and Newton, 1981).

The incidence of rhabdomyosarcoma follows a bimodal pattern, the early peak occurring in children 2 to 6 years of age (most commonly in the head and neck). The later peak in adolescence is seen most commonly in the male genitourinary tract. More than one-half of rhabdomyosarcomas occur in the head and neck (Soule and associates, 1968); in this region, one-half are parameningeal, one-quarter in the orbit, and one-quarter in other sites. Orbital tumors cause early symptoms and signs (pain and proptosis). For this reason they are generally diagnosed and treated earlier than tumors in other anatomic locations (90 per cent carry a three year survival rate). This is in contrast to tumors of the middle ear or nasopharynx, where metastases either by direct extension or by hematogenous spread have frequently occurred at the time of diagnosis (Feldman, 1982). Overall, 10 to 20 per cent of patients have distant metastatic disease at the time of initial diagnosis, the most common sites being lung, bone, and bone marrow (Sutow and associates, 1982).

Histologic examination of the tumors reveals three major types: embryonal (accounting for almost 80 per cent of head and neck rhabdomyosarcomas), alveolar (10 per cent), and pleomorphic (10 per cent). The alveolar type is found more frequently in the extremities and carries a somewhat worse prognosis than the others (Gaiger, Soule, and Newton, 1981). A publication by the Intergroup Rhabdomyosarcoma Study found a significant difference in survival between groups with "favorable" histology and those with "unfavorable" findings, specifically anaplastic cytology and monomorphous round cells. Of the 405 patients studied, 81 per cent fortunately demonstrated favorable histologic findings (Wharam and associates, 1984).

The therapy for rhabdomyosarcoma has historically been frustrating, with frequent recurrences and poor long-term survival. The addition of new radiotherapy and chemotherapy regimens has markedly enhanced survival. Total surgical extirpation of the tumor is performed whenever possible; when this cannot be achieved, as is often the case in head and neck sites, biopsy and/or debulking set the stage for therapeutic radiation and chemotherapy, usually with a combination of vincristine, dactinomycin, and cyclophosphamide (Exelby, 1981). The two year survival rate is higher than 80 per cent in patients with localized disease.

Orbital tumors are most commonly treated with biopsy followed by radiation and chemotherapy, with excellent results, as noted above. Parameningeal tumors have a much greater tendency to early metastasis to the adjacent central nervous system, and results of therapy have improved with inclusion of these adjacent regions in the radiation ports (Raney and associates, 1981).

Fibrosarcomas. Fibrosarcomas make up 11 per cent of soft tissue sarcomas in childhood. The pathologic findings tend to be similar to those seen in adults, but there are fewer mature cellular elements and increased round cell infiltrates. Soule and Pritchard (1977) reviewed 110 cases of fibrosarcoma in the pediatric population; only 20 per cent occurred in the head and neck. Children under 5 years of age have an improved prognosis, demonstrating better than 80 per cent five year survival with local control of disease (Chung and Enzinger, 1976); adjuvant therapy appears to be of no benefit in this population. In older children or adolescents, as in adults, prognosis is related to the histologic grade, with 60 per cent overall five year survival. These data correspond to the rate of distant metastases, which is less than 10 per cent in children under 5 years of age, and 50 per cent in those over 10 years of age (Soule and Pritchard, 1977). The role of radiation and chemotherapy in the older age group is still under investigation; these modalities are presently reserved for cases of local recurrence or metastatic disease.

Other Sarcomas. Most histologic types of

sarcomas have been reported in the pediatric population. They have in common similar treatment protocols, surgical resection being preferred whenever possible, radiation for control of local disease, and chemotherapy for distant metastases. Liposarcomas make up only 4 per cent of childhood soft tissue sarcomas, in contrast to adults, in whom they account for 15 to 20 per cent (Kaplan and associates, 1981). Local invasion is common, although less than 5 per cent have distant metastases; radiation has been used to control local disease (Castleberry and associates, 1984). Hemangiopericytoma, an unusual tumor in both the pediatric and the adult populations, occurs more frequently in the head and neck and carries a high incidence of metastatic disease. The tumor is highly sensitive to chemotherapy; five year survival is as high as 70 per cent. An infantile form of this tumor has been described that, like infantile fibrosarcoma, follows a more benign course than in older patients, and it can be treated by surgical excision only. Neurofibrosarcoma occurs in association with von Recklinghausen's disease, although only 5 to 15 per cent of patients with neurofibromatosis develop malignancies (meningiomas and other neuroectodermal tumors may also be seen in this syndrome). As with other sarcomas, multimodal therapy appears to yield the best results (Miser and Pizzo, 1985).

Salivary Gland Tumors

Tumors of the salivary glands (see Chap. 67) are rare in children (Table 65–1). Sixty per cent of the salivary gland neoplasms seen in the pediatric age groups are vascular malformations, hemangiomas of the parotid gland being the most common (see Chap. 66).

Solid tumors are even more uncommon, constituting only 3 to 5 per cent of all salivary gland tumors in large series (Krolls, Trodahl, and Boyers, 1972; Schuller and McCabe, 1977). Approximately two-thirds of the solid salivary gland tumors in children are benign, pleomorphic adenoma accounting for the majority. The distribution of histologic types of malignant tumors differs from that in adults in that mucoepidermoid carcinoma is the most common; one study found adenoid cystic carcinoma in five of 16 cases (Baker and Malone, 1985). Treatment is similar to that for adults, with conservative excision of benign tumors and aggressive resection of malignant tumors. Conley and Tinsley (1985) reported 15 mucoepidermoid cancers in children, 70 per cent of whom underwent facial nerve resection and 50 per cent regional nodal dissection; all patients were alive at 10 years of age.

Other Tumors

Squamous cell carcinoma of the oropharynx and nasopharynx is rarely seen in children; when it occurs, it is treated much as adult tumors of the same histologic type, with surgical resection when possible, supplemented by radiation therapy and adjuvant chemotherapy (Deutsch, Mercado, and Parsons, 1978).

Cancer of the thyroid gland may also be seen, particularly in patients exposed to earlier radiation for dermatologic or other disorders. Medullary carcinoma of the thyroid, a particularly malignant lesion, is seen in

Table 65–1. Salivary Gland Neoplasms in Children (428)

Benign		Malignant	
Hemangioma	111	Mucoepidermoid carcinoma	73
Mixed tumor	94	Acinous cell carcinoma	18
"Vascular proliferative"	40	Undifferentiated carcinoma	14
Lymphangioma	18	Undifferentiated sarcoma	9
Lymphoepithelial tumor	3	Malignant mixed tumor	9
Cystadenoma	3	Adenocarcinoma	11
Warthin's tumor	3	Adenoid cystic carcinoma	6
Plexiform neurofibroma	2	Squamous cell carcinoma	3
Xanthoma	2	Mesenchymal sarcoma	2
Neurilemoma	1	Rhabdomyosarcoma	2
Adenoma	1	Malignant epithelial tumor	1
Lipoma	1	Ganglioneuroblastoma	1
Total	279	Total	149

Adapted from Schuller, D. E., and McCabe, B. F.: Salivary gland neoplasms in children. Otolaryngol. Clin. North Am., 10:399, 1977.

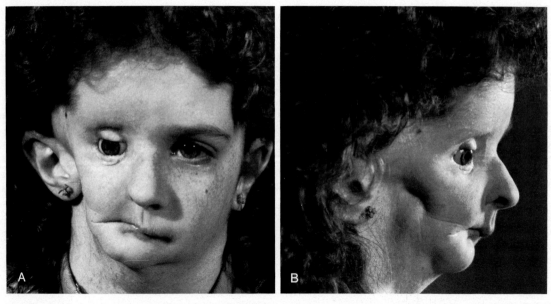

Figure 65–11. A 15 year old girl after radiation and chemotherapy at age 2 years for rhabdomyosarcoma that resulted in severe underdevelopment of the craniofacial skeleton and soft tissue. She is wearing an ocular shell. *A,* Frontal view. *B,* Profile.

multiple endocrine adenomas Type IIB, in association with neurofibromas, pheochromocytomas, and parathyroid adenomas (Herzog, 1983; Joppich and associates, 1983).

LATE SEQUELAE OF CANCER THERAPY

The essential biologic basis of adjuvant chemotherapy and radiotherapy in the treatment of malignancies is the preferential effect on actively growing cells. In the pediatric population, while these forms of therapy have greatly enhanced survival, long-term effects on normal growing structures are also seen. Radiation, in particular, may arrest growth of the teeth and of the craniofacial skeleton (Fig. 65–11); in a large study (Jaffe and associates, 1984), 82 per cent of radiated patients had dental or maxillofacial abnormalities. Dental abnormalities after radiation include delayed or arrested development, incomplete calcification, and caries; chemotherapy may have similar effects, but to a lesser degree. Other late sequelae of radiation include xerophthalmia, cataracts, hypopituitarism, and hearing loss, among others (Fromm and associates, 1986). The complications are related to the dosage and the location of the radiation fields, as well as to the age of the patient; they mandate close

follow-up of these patients by an interdisciplinary team, including the appropriate specialists.

REFERENCES

Abemayor, E., Newman, A., Bergstrom, L., Dudley, J., Magidson, J. G., and Llung, B. M.: Teratomas of the head and neck in childhood. Laryngoscope, *94*:1489, 1984.

Adekeye, E. O., Abiose, A., and Ord, R. A.: Neurofibromatosis of the head and neck: clinical presentation and treatment. J. Maxillofac. Surg., *12*:78, 1984.

Al Fallouji, M. A., and Butler, M. F.: First branchial cleft anomaly. Postgrad. Med. J., *59*:447, 1983.

Appling, D., and Miller, R. H.: Mycobacterium cervical lymphadenopathy: 1981 update. Laryngoscope, *91*:1259, 1981.

Atkinson, J. B., Mahour, G. H., Isaacs, H., Jr., and Ortega, J. A.: Hemangiopericytoma in infants and children: a report of six patients. Am. J. Surg., *148*:372, 1984.

Baker, H. L., Baker, S. R., and McClatchey, K. D.: Manifestations and management of laryngoceles. Head Neck Surg., *4*:450, 1982.

Baker, S. R., and Malone, B.: Salivary gland malignancies in children. Cancer, *55*:1730, 1985.

Batsakis, J. G. (Ed.): Tumors of the Head and Neck. 2nd Ed. Baltimore, Williams & Wilkins Company, 1979.

Batsakis, J. G.: Pathology consultation. Nomenclature of the developmental tumors. Ann. Otol. Rhinol. Laryngol., *93*:98, 1984.

Bedros, A. A., and Mann, J. P.: Lymphadenopathy in children. Adv. Pediatr., *28*:341, 1981.

Belin, R. P., Richardson, J. D., Richardson, D. L., Vandiviere, M. H., Wheeler, W. E., and Jona, J. Z.: Diagnosis and management of scrofula in children. J. Pediatr. Surg., 9:103, 1974.

Brecher, M. L., Sinks, L. F., Thomas, R. R., and Freeman, A. I.: Non-Hodgkin's lymphoma in children. Cancer, 41:1997, 1978.

Bryan, R. N., Miller, R. H., Ferreyro, R. I., and Sessions, R. B.: Computed tomography of the major salivary glands. AJR, 139:547, 1982.

Byrd, S. E., Richardson, M., Gill, G., and Lee, A. M.: Computer-tomographic appearance of branchial cleft and thyroglossal duct cysts of the neck. Diagn. Imaging, 52:301, 1983.

Cantrell, R. W., Jensen, J. H., and Reid, D.: Diagnosis and management of tuberculous cervical adenitis. Arch. Otolaryngol., 101:53, 1975.

Castleberry, R. P., Kelly, D. R., Wilson, E. R., Cain, W. S., and Salter, M. R.: Childhood liposarcoma: report of a case and review of the literature. Cancer, 54:579, 1984.

Castro, D. J., Hoover, L., and Zuckerbraun, L.: Cervical mycobacterial lymphadenitis. Medical vs. surgical management. Arch. Otolaryngol., 111:816, 1985.

Chung, E. B., and Enzinger, F. M.: Benign lipoblastomatosis: an analysis of 35 cases. Cancer, 32:482, 1973.

Chung, E. B., and Enzinger, F. M.: Infantile fibrosarcoma. Cancer, 38:729, 1976.

Chung, E. B., and Enzinger, F. M.: Infantile myofibromatosis. Cancer, 48:1807, 1981.

Cinberg, J. Z., Silver, C. E., Molnar, J. J., and Vogl, S. E.: Cervical cysts: cancer until proven otherwise? Laryngoscope, 92:27, 1982.

Conley, J., and Baker, D. C.: Cancer of the salivary glands. In Suen, J. Y., and Myers, E. N. (Eds.): Cancer of the Head and Neck. London, Churchill Livingstone, 1981.

Conley, J., and Tinsley, P. P., Jr.: Treatment and prognosis of mucoepidermoid carcinoma in the pediatric age group. Arch. Otolaryngol., 111:322, 1985.

Crikelair, G. F., and Cosman, B.: Histologically benign, clinically malignant lesions of the head and neck. Plast. Reconstr. Surg., 42:343, 1968.

Cummings, B. J., Blend, R., Keane, T., Fitzpatrick, P., Beale, F., et al.: Primary radiation therapy for juvenile nasopharyngeal angiofibroma. Laryngoscope, 94:1599, 1984.

Dahl, I., and Jarlstedt, J.: Nodular fasciitis in the head and neck. A clinicopathological study of 18 cases. Acta Otolaryngol. (Stockh.), 90:152, 1980.

David, R. B., and O'Connel, E. J.: Suppurative parotitis in children. Am. J. Dis. Child., 119:332, 1970.

Deutsch, M., Mercado, R., Jr., and Parsons, J. A.: Cancer of the nasopharynx in children. Cancer, 41:1128, 1978.

Ducatman, B. S., Scheithauer, B. W., Piepgras, D. G., Reiman, H. M., and Ilstrup, D. M.: Malignant peripheral nerve sheath tumors. A clinicopathologic study of 120 cases. Cancer, 57:2006, 1986.

Evans, M. E., Gregory, D. W., Schaffner, W., and McGee, Z. A.: Tularemia: a 30-year experience with 88 cases. Medicine, 64:251, 1985.

Exelby, P. R.: Surgery of soft tissue sarcomas in children. Natl. Cancer Inst. Monogr., 56:153, 1981.

Farr, H. W.: Soft part sarcomas of the head and neck. Semin. Oncol., 8:185, 1981.

Feldman, B. A.: Rhabdomyosarcoma of the head and neck. Laryngoscope, 92:424, 1982.

Fromm, M., Littman, P., Raney, R. B., Nelson, L., Handler, S., et al.: Late effects after treatment of twenty children with soft tissue sarcomas of the head and neck. Experience at a single institution with a review of the literature. Cancer, 57:2070, 1986.

Gaiger, A. M., Soule, E. H., and Newton, W. A., Jr.: Pathology of rhabdomyosarcoma: experience of the Intergroup Rhabdomyosarcoma Study, 1972–78. Natl. Cancer Inst. Monogr., 56:19, 1981.

Golding, S.: Computed tomography in the diagnosis of parotid gland tumours. Br. J. Radiol., 55:182, 1982.

Griffith, B. H., McKinney, P., Monroe, C. W., and Howell, A.: Von Recklinghausen's disease in children. Plast. Reconstr. Surg., 49:647, 1972.

Gundry, S. R., Wesley, J. R., Klein, M. D., Barr, M., and Coran, A. G.: Cervical teratomas in the newborn. J. Pediatr. Surg., 18:382, 1983.

Gupta, S. K., Nema, H. V., Bhatia, P. L., Sasibabu, K., and Kesharwani, R.: The radiological features of craniofacial neurofibromatosis. Clin. Radiol., 30:553, 1979.

Hajdu, S. I., Faruque, A. A., Hajdu, E. O., and Morgan, W. S.: Teratomas of the neck in infants. Am. J. Dis. Child., 111:412, 1966.

Handler, S. D., and Raney, R. B.: Management of neoplasms of the head and neck in children. 1. Benign tumors. Head Neck Surg., 3:395, 1981.

Hays, D. M.: Malignant solid tumors of childhood. Curr. Probl. Surg., 23:161, 1986.

Herzog, B.: Thyroid gland diseases and tumours: surgical aspects. Prog. Pediatr. Surg., 16:15, 1983.

Jablokow, V. R., Kathuria, S., and Wang, T.: Squamous cell carcinoma arising in branchiogenic cyst: branchial cleft carcinoma. J. Surg. Oncol., 20:201, 1982.

Jaffe, B. F., and Jaffe, N.: Head and neck tumors in children. Pediatrics, 51:731, 1973.

Jaffe, N., Toth, B. B., Hoar, R. E., Ried, H. L., Sullivan, M. P., and McNeese, M. D.: Dental and maxillofacial abnormalities in long-term survivors of childhood cancer: effects of treatment with chemotherapy and radiation to the head and neck. Pediatrics, 73:816, 1984.

Joppich, I., Roher, H. D., Hecker, W. C., Knorr, D., and Daum, R.: Thyroid carcinoma in childhood. Prog. Pediatr. Surg., 16:23, 1983.

Kaban, L. B., Mulliken, J. B., and Murray, J. E.: Sialadenitis in childhood. Am. J. Surg., 135:570, 1978.

Kaplan, R., Bratcher, G. O., Freeman, D., Seid, A. B., and Cotton, R.: Liposarcoma of the neck: report of a case. Laryngoscope, 91:1375, 1981.

Kraus, R., Han, B. K., Babcock, D. S., and Oestreich, A. E.: Sonography of neck masses in children. AJR, 146:609, 1986.

Krol, G., and Strong, E.: Computed tomography of head and neck malignancies. Clin. Plast. Surg., 13:475, 1986.

Krolls, S. O., Trodahl, J. N., and Boyers, R. C.: Salivary gland tumors in children. A survey of 430 cases. Cancer, 30:459, 1972.

Lane, R. J., Keane, W. M., and Potsic, W. P.: Pediatric infectious cervical lymphadenitis. Otolaryngol. Head Neck Surg., 88:332, 1980.

Larson, D. L., Robbins, K. T., and Butler, J. J.: Lymphoma of the head and neck: a diagnostic dilemma. Am. J. Surg., 148:433, 1984.

Lee, Y., Terry, R., and Lukes, R. J.: Lymph node biopsy for diagnosis: a statistical study. J. Surg. Oncol., 14:53, 1980.

Levin-Epstein, A. A., and Lucente, F. E.: Scrofula—the dangerous masquerader. Laryngoscope, 92:938, 1982.

Liston, S. L.: The relationship of the facial nerve and first branchial cleft anomalies—embryologic considerations. Laryngoscope, 92:1308, 1982.

Maceri, D. R., and Saxon, K. G.: Neurofibromatosis of the head and neck. Head Neck Surg., 6:842, 1984.

Malone, B., and Baker, S. R.: Benign pleomorphic adenomas in children. Ann. Otol. Rhinol. Laryngol., 93:210, 1984.

Marchac, D.: Intracranial enlargement of the orbital cavity and palpebral remodeling for orbitopalpebral neurofibromatosis. Plast. Reconstr. Surg., 73:534, 1984.

Martin, H., Morfit, H. M., and Ehrlich, H.: The case for branchiogenic cancer (malignant branchioma). Ann. Surg., 132:867, 1950.

Mattel, S. F., and Persky, M. S.: Infiltrating lipoma of the sternocleidomastoid muscle. Laryngoscope, 93:205, 1983.

Maurer, H. M.: Current concepts in cancer. Solid tumors in children. N. Engl. J. Med., 299:1345, 1978.

Miser, J. S., and Pizzo, P. A.: Soft tissue sarcomas in childhood. Pediatr. Clin. North Am., 32:779, 1985.

National Cancer Institute Monograph No. 56: Symposium on soft tissue sarcomas in children, April, 1981.

Nyberg, D. A., Jeffrey, R. B., Brant-Zawadzki, M., Federle, M., and Dillon, W.: Computed tomography of cervical infections. J. Comput. Assist. Tomogr., 9:288, 1985.

Olsen, K. D., Maragos, N. E., and Weiland, L. H.: First branchial cleft anomalies. Laryngoscope, 90:423, 1980.

Ramos-Gabatin, A., and Watzinger, W.: Fine needle aspiration and cytology in the preoperative diagnosis of branchial cyst. South. Med. J., 77:1187, 1984.

Raney, R. B., Jr., Donaldson, M. H., Sutow, W. W., Lindberg, R. D., Maurer, H. M., and Tefft, M.: Special considerations related to primary site in rhabdomyosarcoma: experience of the Intergroup Rhabdomyosarcoma Study, 1972–76. Natl. Cancer Inst. Monogr., 56:69, 1981.

Raney, R. B., Jr., and Handler, S. D.: Management of neoplasms of the head and neck in children. II. Malignant tumors. Head Neck Surg., 1:334, 1979.

Russell, E. J.: The radiologic approach to malignant tumors of the head and neck, with emphasis on computed tomography. Clin. Plast. Surg., 12:343, 1985.

Saitz, E. W.: Cervical lymphadenitis caused by atypical mycobacteria. Pediatr. Clin. North Am., 28:823, 1981.

Salazar, J. E., Duke, R. A., and Ellis, J. V.: Second branchial cleft cyst: unusual location and a new CT diagnostic sign. AJR, 145:965, 1985.

Schaad, U. B., Votteler, T. P., McCracken, G. H., Jr., and Nelson, J. D.: Management of atypical mycobacterial lymphadenitis in childhood: a review based on 380 cases. J. Pediatr., 95:356, 1979.

Schramm, V. L., Jr.: Inflammatory and neoplastic masses of the nose and paranasal sinuses in children. Laryngoscope, 89:1887, 1979.

Schuller, D. E., and McCabe, B. F.: Salivary gland neoplasms in children. Otolaryngol. Clin. North Am., 10:399, 1977.

Sessions, R. B., Zarin, D. P., and Bryan, R. N.: Juvenile

nasopharyngeal angiofibroma. Am. J. Dis. Child., 135:535, 1981.

Sherman, N. H., Rosenberg, H. K., Heyman, S., and Templeton, J.: Ultrasound evaluation of neck masses in children. J. Ultrasound Med., 4:127, 1985.

Shreedhar, R., and Tooley, A. H.: Carcinoma arising in a branchial cyst. Br. J. Surg., 71:115, 1984.

Silverman, P. M., Korobkin, M., and Moore, A. V.: Computed tomography of cystic neck masses. J. Comput. Assist. Tomogr., 7:498, 1983.

Slavin, S. A., Baker, D. C., McCarthy, J. G., and Mufarrij, A.: Congenital infiltrating lipomatosis of the face: clinicopathologic evaluation and management. Plast. Reconstr. Surg., 72:158, 1983.

Soule, E. H., Mahour, G. H., Mills, S. D., and Lynn, B.: Soft tissue sarcomas of infants and children: a clinicopathologic study of 135 cases. Mayo Clin. Proc., 43:313, 1968.

Soule, E. H., and Pritchard, D. J.: Fibrosarcoma in infants and children: a review of 110 cases. Cancer, 40:1711, 1977.

Stone, H. H., Henderson, W. D., and Guidio, F. A.: Teratomas of the neck. Am. J. Dis. Child., 113:222, 1967.

Sutow, W. W., Lindberg, R. D., Gehan, E. A., Ragab, A. H., Raney, R. B., Jr., et al.: Three-year relapse-free survival rates in childhood rhabdomyosarcoma of the head and neck. Cancer, 49:2217, 1982.

Tapper, D., and Lack, E. E.: Teratomas in infancy and childhood. A 54-year experience at the Children's Hospital Medical Center. Ann. Surg., 198:398, 1983.

von Recklinghausen, F.: Ueber die multiplen Fibrome der Haut und ihre Beziehung zu den multiplen Neuromen (1882), translated by Crump, T. Adv. Neurol., 29:259, 1981.

Ward-Booth, R. P., Williams, E. D., Faulkner, T. P., and Earl, P. D.: Ultrasound: a simple noninvasive examination of cervical swellings. Plast. Reconstr. Surg., 73:577, 1984.

Watanatittan, S., Othersen, H. B., Jr., and Hughson, M. D.: Cervical teratoma in children. Prog. Pediatr. Surg., 14:225, 1981.

Wharam, M. D., Jr., Foulkes, M. A., Lawrence, W., Jr., Lindberg, R. D., Maurer, H. M., et al.: Soft tissue sarcoma of the head and neck in childhood: nonorbital and nonparameningeal sites. A report of the Intergroup Rhabdomyosarcoma Study (IRS). I. Cancer, 53:1016, 1984.

Witt, T. R., Shah, J. P., and Sternberg, S. S.: Juvenile nasopharyngeal angiofibroma: a 30-year clinical review. Am. J. Surg., 146:521, 1983.

Zitelli, B. J.: Neck masses in children: adenopathy and malignant disease. Pediatr. Clin. North Am., 28:813, 1981.

66

John B. Mulliken

Cutaneous Vascular Anomalies

CLASSIFICATION

HEMANGIOMAS
  Pathogenesis
  Diagnosis and Natural History
  Complications in the Proliferation Phase
  The Involution Phase
  History of Treatment
  Current Management

VASCULAR MALFORMATIONS
  Pathogenesis

LOW FLOW VASCULAR MALFORMATIONS
  Capillary Malformations (CM)
  Hyperkeratotic Vascular Stains
  Telangiectasias
  Lymphatic Malformations (LM)
  Venous Malformations (VM)

HIGH FLOW VASCULAR MALFORMATIONS
  Arteriovenous Malformations (AVM)

COMBINED VASCULAR MALFORMATIONS AND
      HYPERTROPHY SYNDROMES
  Klippel-Trenaunay Syndrome
  Parkes Weber Syndrome
  Maffucci's Syndrome
  Multiple Dysplasia Syndromes

Words have been stumbling blocks on the road to an understanding of vascular anomalies. Bewildering nosologic systems have evolved offering an array of admixed histologic and descriptive terms. The same word is often applied to entirely disparate vascular lesions. For example, "hemangioma" is commonly used in a generic sense to describe a variety of vascular lesions, both congenital and acquired, of differing etiologies and natural histories. This confusing nomenclature has been largely responsible for illogical treatment of cutaneous vascular lesions.

The term "anomalies," as used in the title, signifies any deviation in normal cutaneous vasculature, be it congenital or acquired. On the basis of clinical and cellular studies, the vascular anomalies of infancy and childhood are divided into two major categories: *hemangiomas* and *malformations* (Mulliken and Glowacki, 1982). A consistent nomenclature is used throughout this chapter, and every attempt has been made to relate this nosologic system to terms found elsewhere in the literature. This field is replete with syndromic designations, usually prefixed with personal names; whenever possible, these eponyms are defined in anatomic terms. The presentation of cutaneous vascular anomalies in an understandable terminology permits accurate diagnosis and prognosis and proper treatment, and also stimulates studies of pathogenesis.

CLASSIFICATION

Descriptive Classification

The earliest descriptions of vascular birthmarks were derived from the concept of *maternal impressions*—that if a woman's emotions were sufficiently affected during pregnancy, the fetus might feel the shock and register it as a skin blemish (Mulliken and Young, 1988). Thus, the birthmark resembled the object or circumstance that produced the mother's emotional state. The mother who had longed for strawberries, raspberries, or cherries, or who in some cultures refused these fruits, might find her baby indelibly marked. The fact that vascular anomalies are

3191

so commonly found on the face and scalp was attributed to the pregnant woman's tendency to touch these locations in a gesture of fright when alarmed by the sight of blood. Nosology, based on brightly colored edibles, continues in the present day, e.g., "strawberry hemangioma," "cherry angioma," "port-wine stain," and "salmon patch."

The mother was indicted by the Latin terms for vascular anomalies, such as *macula materna, naevus maternus*, or *stigma metrocelis* (Hooper, 1838). Bell (1815) accurately described arteriovenous malformation, calling it "aneurysm by anastomosis," and realized that this is a separate entity from the common *naevus maternus* of infancy. Other observant surgeons noted the benign nature of *naevi materni* in comparison with the more dangerous "aneurysm by anastomosis," also known as "cirsoid aneurysm," "pulsatile fungus hematode," or "erectile tumor." Nevertheless, any classification of vascular anomalies, based on descriptive terminology, is predisposed to inaccuracy and confusion because lesions that look similar may have quite different etiologies and behavior.

Anatomicopathologic Classification

Virchow (1863) examined vascular anomalies with a microscope and devised a category based on channel architecture: (1) *angioma simplex*, a lesion composed of capillaries; (2) *angioma cavernosum*, a replacement of normal vasculature with large channels; and (3) *angioma racemosum*, in which the tissue consisted of markedly dilated interconnected vessels.

Virchow's former student Wegner (1876–1877) proposed a similar histomorphic division of lymphatic swellings: *lymphangioma simplex, lymphangioma cavernosum*, and *lymphangioma cystoides*. Virchow's *angioma simplex* became synonymous with "strawberry mark" or "capillary hemangioma"; the latter term was subsequently misapplied to port-wine stain with its capillary-sized channels. The microscopic designation "cavernous" hemangioma came to be indiscriminately assigned to vascular lesions that involute (Lampe and Latourette, 1956; Simpson, 1959), to those that never involute (Costello, 1949; MacCollum and Martin, 1956; Andrews and associates, 1957), and to those that seem to regress occasionally (Matthews,

1968). The conceptual confusion was further aggravated by the introduction of a new word "hamartoma" to designate a developmental anomaly, but one with the capacity for benign cellular proliferation (Albrecht, 1907). The term "hamartoma" is still indiscriminately applied to diverse soft tissue lesions such as neurofibroma, lymphatic malformation, port-wine stain, and the common hemangioma of infancy.

Contemporary pathologists continue to prefer the word "hemangioma" in its broadest sense. The Stout-Lattes system (Stout and Lattes, 1967) and the classification of vascular anomalies by Enzinger and Weiss (1983) list benign and malignant vascular tumors alongside vascular malformations and acquired lesions.

Any strictly histopathologic classification, without clinical correlation, has not proved to be useful in the diagnosis and management of vascular anomalies.

Embryologic Classification

At the beginning of the century, there was an intense interest in cardiovascular embryology (Sabin, 1902; Lewis, 1905–1906; Woollard, 1922). Rienhoff (1924) studied vascular development in chicken and pig embryos and concluded that vascular anomalies were the result of faulty embryogenesis, either arterial, venous, or combined arteriovenous in type. Limb vascular anomalies were easily explained as arrests at various stages of channel development (deTakats, 1932; Malan, 1974; Szilagyi and associates, 1976). It was hypothesized that the common hemangiomas of childhood were embryonic rests of angioblastic cells (Malan, 1974).

These attempts at an embryologic classification, albeit fanciful, are conceptually appealing and superficially logical. However, when put to the trial of clinical usefulness, embryologic classifications fail to guide the management of the wide variety of vascular birthmarks.

Biologic Classification

In 1975 a prospective study was undertaken by the author to define the cellular features of various anomalies, seen in infancy and childhood, and to correlate the findings with the physical examination and natural history. These investigations showed that, on the basis of cell kinetics, there are two major types of vascular anomalies: *hemangiomas*, lesions demonstrating endothelial hyperplasia; and *malformations*, lesions with normal endothelial turnover (Mulliken and Glowacki, 1982).

HEMANGIOMAS

The Greek noun suffix *-oma* denotes a swelling or tumor; in modern usage, a tumor is characterized by cellular hyperplasia. Therefore, the unmodified noun *hemangioma* should be restricted to a vascular tumor that grows by cellular proliferation. Hemangioma is the most common tumor of infancy; it is synonymous with older terms, e.g., "capillary," "hypertrophic," or "juvenile" hemangioma or "benign hemangioendothelioma." Endothelial cells normally show few, if any, mitotic figures and very long doubling times. Thymidine incorporation studies of hemangiomas documented increased endothelial cell turnover (Mulliken and Glowacki, 1982). The rapidly growing hemangioma necessitates pari passu the dilatation and formation of new feeding and draining vascular channels, subordinate vessels, within and around the perimeter of the tumor. The hemangioma of infancy is in a *proliferating phase* for the first year of life, then enters an *involuting phase*, lasting several years (Table 66–1).

The term "hemangioma" also applies to hypercellular tumors of vascular origin seen in adults; e.g., there are rare examples of "hemangioma of muscle," as well as other benign synovial and neural hemangiomas (Allen and Enzinger, 1972; Enzinger and

Table 66–1. Biologic Classification of Vascular Birthmarks

Hemangiomas	Malformations
Proliferating phase	Capillary (CM)
Involuting phase	Lymphatic (LM)
	Venous (VM)
	Arterial (AM)
	Combined:
	arteriovenous (AVM)
	capillary-lymphatic (CLM)
	capillary-venous (CVM)
	lymphatico-venous (LVM)
	capillary-lymphatico-venous (CLVM)

Based on Mulliken, J. B., and Glowacki, J.: Hemangiomas and vascular malformations in infants and children: a classification based on endothelial characteristics. Plast. Reconstr. Surg., *69*:412, 1982.

Weiss, 1983). There is another rare tumor of adulthood of borderline malignancy called "epithelioid hemangioma" (angiolymphoid hyperplasia with eosinophilia, histocytoid hemangioma, Kimura's disease) (Rosai, Gold, and Landy, 1979; Enzinger and Weiss, 1983).

VASCULAR MALFORMATIONS

The other major category of vascular anomalies are properly designated *malformations*. These are structural anomalies, inborn errors of vascular morphogenesis. They exhibit a normal rate of endothelial cell turnover throughout their natural history. It is clinically important to separate the vascular malformations into "low flow" (either capillary, venous, lymphatic, or combined forms) or "high flow" (arteriovenous) categories. Although a single type of channel anomaly may predominate, there often are combined channel anomalies (Table 66–1).

CHARACTERISTICS THAT DISTINGUISH HEMANGIOMA FROM VASCULAR MALFORMATION

Clinical Differences. The clinical criteria are by far the most important for a proper diagnosis. A hemangioma usually is not seen in the newborn nursery; approximately one-third present as a small, macular red spot. Rarely, a fully grown hemangioma is seen at birth. Hemangioma is characterized by rapid postnatal growth and very slow involution. Females are more commonly affected; the gender ratio is 3:1 (Mulliken and Glowacki, 1982).

Cutaneous vascular malformations, by definition, are present at birth. Most of them are clearly seen. However, lymphatic, venous, and arteriovenous anomalies often appear later in childhood or in early adulthood. A vascular malformation grows proportionately with the child; it may expand secondary to sepsis, trauma, or hormonal changes. Vascular malformations have no gender predilection.

Cellular Differences. The rapidly growing hemangioma is composed of plump, rapidly dividing endothelial cells. In addition, mast cells, known to play a role in neoangiogenesis, increase during the proliferating phase (Glowacki and Mulliken, 1982). The mast cells fall to normal levels as involution is concluded. Ultrastructural studies of involuting phase hemangiomas reveal multilamination of the basement membrane and interactions between mast cells and local macrophages, fibroblasts, and multinucleated giant cells (Dethlefsen, Mulliken, and Glowacki, 1986).

Tissue specimens of enlarging vascular malformations show no evidence of cellular hyperplasia, but rather a progressive ectasia of structurally abnormal vessels. The malformed channels are lined by flat, quiescent endothelium, lying on a thin basal lamina. Mast cells are not increased on histologic examination of resected vascular malformations.

Tissue culture studies also demonstrate behavioral differences between hemangiomas and vascular malformations. Capillary endothelium, derived from infant hemangiomas, forms capillary tubules in vitro, whereas capillary endothelium from vascular malformations is difficult to culture (Mulliken, Zetter, and Folkman, 1982).

Hematologic Differences. A large hemangioma can cause platelet trapping, a shortened platelet half-life, and profound thrombocytopenia (the Kasabach-Merritt syndrome). A hemangioma may also evidence consumptive coagulopathy, but this is probably a secondary phenomenon.

Vascular malformations, particularly the venous type, cause a true intravascular coagulation defect with only mild thrombocytopenia and slightly decreased platelet survival.

Radiographic Differences. Angiographic study shows hemangioma as a well-circumscribed mass with intense, prolonged tissue staining that is usually organized in a lobular pattern. Feeding arteries may form an equatorial network at the periphery of the tumor (Burrows and associates, 1983).

Vascular malformations are diffuse lesions consisting entirely of vessels without intervening parenchymal staining. The angiographic pattern depends on the predominant channel type, i.e., capillary, venous, arterial, or a combination.

Skeletal Differences. Skeletal changes associated with vascular anomalies also reveal a dichotomy between hemangioma and vascular malformation (Boyd and associates, 1984). Proliferating hemangioma rarely causes bony or cartilaginous distortion or hypertrophy. Macrotia or maxillary and mandibular overgrowth may occur, presumably secondary to increased blood flow during proliferation. Hemangiomas may also produce a mass effect, e.g., depression of the outer cal-varia, shift of the nasal skeleton, or secondary enlargement of the orbit. In contrast, low flow vascular malformations are frequently associated with diffuse skeletal hypertrophy, distortion, or elongation. The high flow arteriovenous malformations often cause destructive interosseous changes (Boyd and associates, 1984).

A classification of disease is successful only if it has diagnostic applicability, helps in planning therapy, and guides studies of pathogenesis. This simplified classification of vascular anomalies can be called "biologic" because it combines cellular features with clinical behavior. It is a practical system—one that *does not* necessitate complicated diagnostic studies, and biopsy is not usually a requisite. An accurate medical history, a physical examination, and (if necessary) repeated clinical evaluation permit accurate classification of cutaneous vascular anomalies in the vast majority of patients (Finn, Glowacki, and Mulliken, 1983).

HEMANGIOMAS

Pathogenesis

EARLY INTUITIVE THEORIES

The critical question is: When does a hemangioma begin? Is hemangioma a growth of sequestrated vasoformative cells or does it arise de novo as a postembryonic tumor (neoangiogenesis)? Virchow (1863) speculated that the mechanism was a progressive irritation of tissue, particularly likely to occur about the margins of fetal clefts that are well supplied with blood vessels. Laidlaw and Murray (1933) suggested that hemangiomas are phylogenetic remnants of vascular tufts that served as accessory lungs in the skin of primitive amphibia. Malan (1974) proposed that "dormant angioblasts" become activated to form hemangiomas—a delayed expression of genetically programmed growth and involution of the embryonic capillary network. Kaplan (1983) stated that hemangioma is a failure of normal morphogenesis from the embryonic stage of undifferentiated capillary network.

ANIMAL MODELS

Studies of the pathogenesis of human hemangioma have been handicapped by the failure to develop a suitable model in lower animals. Most vascular lesions in animals, e.g., swine, chickens, and dogs, are developmental abnormalities that remain unchanged during the life of the animal (Munro and Munro, 1982; Wells and Morgan, 1980). Malignant vascular neoplasms are also seen in animals (Waller and Rubarth, 1967) and in young chickens (Monlux and Delaplane, 1952; Darcel and Franks, 1953).

Repeated topical methylcholanthrene application to the skin of white Peking ducks produces hemangiomatous tumors, and some of these spontaneously regress (Rigdon, 1954, 1955; Rigdon, Walker, and Teddlie, 1956). Other carcinogens, benzanthracene (Howell, 1963), nitrosamine (Toth, Magee, and Shubik, 1964), and dimethylhydrazine (Toth and Wilson, 1971), induce both benign and malignant vascular tumors within the soft tissue and liver of rodents. Some induced tumors regress, but most metastasize as sarcomas and kill the host.

Until an appropriate animal model is forthcoming, investigation into the pathogenesis of hemangiomas must rely on analysis of available tissue specimens and studies of the biologic phenomenon of vascular neogenesis.

PROLIFERATION: LIGHT MICROSCOPY

The hallmark of the immature hemangioma is proliferation of endothelial cells, forming syncytial masses, with and without lumens (Fig. 66–1A). Later in the proliferative phase, the vascular channels are not so compressed and capillary-sized lumens can be seen, lined by plump endothelial cells. Reticulin stain confirms that the proliferating endothelial cells lie within a limiting reticulin sheath, and periodic acid–Schiff (PAS) stain demonstrates the thickened basement lamina (Fig. 66–1B). The more mature hemangioma is organized into lobular compartments, separated by fibrous septa that contain large caliber feeding and draining vessels (Fig. 66–1C).

Autoradiography demonstrates incorpora-

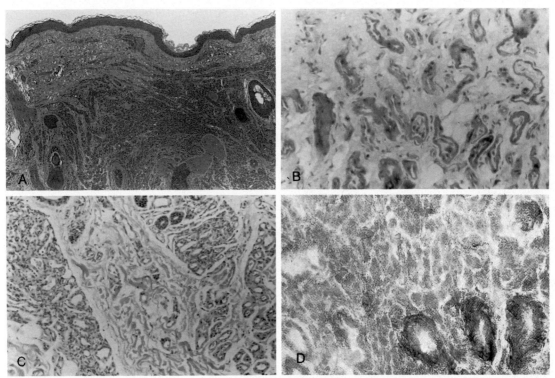

Figure 66–1. Hemangioma histology: proliferating phase. *A,* Endothelial hyperplasia within the papillary and reticular dermis; four month specimen (H & E, × 16). *B,* Periodic acid–Schiff stain demonstrates thickened basement membranes surrounding the lumens (PAS, × 82). *C,* Lobule formation is more obvious in this hemangioma from a 2 year old child. The vascular channels are larger; there are still foci of endothelial proliferation. Feeding-draining vessels are seen in the fibrous interlobular septa (H & E, × 40). *D,* Autoradiograph of a two year hemangioma showing persistent foci of endothelial turnover (× 100). (From Mulliken, J. B., and Young, A. E.: Vascular Birthmarks: Hemangiomas and Malformations. Philadelphia, W. B. Saunders Company, 1988.)

tion of tritiated thymidine into replicating endothelial DNA (Fig. 66–1*D*). The endothelium is differentiated to the extent that alkaline phosphatase can be demonstrated within cytoplasmic granules and also Factor VIII production, as shown by both peroxidase and fluorescent antibody techniques (Mulliken and Glowacki, 1982).

Mast cells are conspicuous in hemangioma tissue stained with safranin O or toluidine blue (Fig. 66–2*A*). There is a 30- to 40-fold increase in the number of mast cells aligned along hemangioma vessels compared with normal tissues, age and site matched. Specimens of involuted hemangioma show a normal level of mast cells (Fig. 66–2*B*) (Glowacki and Mulliken, 1982). Pasyk and associates (1984) also noted increased mast cells in the fibrous regions of hemangiomas and suggested that these cells are implicated in the involution process. The role of mast cells in the evolution of hemangiomas is not yet fully understood. Mast cell granules contain amines, such as serotonin, and other vasoactive substances, such as prostaglandins and leukotrienes, as well as acid hydrolases and neutral proteases. Mast cells also produce heparin, a highly sulfated glycosaminoglycan. Laboratory studies suggest that mast cells play an intermediary role in vasoproliferation during tissue repair and during tumor neovascularization (Kessler and associates, 1976). Mast cell–conditioned medium stimulates the in vitro migration, but not the proliferation, of capillary endothelial cells (Azizkhan and associates, 1980). Mast cells produce heparin, known to be a potent stimulus for migration of cultured capillary endothelium (Azizkhan and associates, 1980), and heparin potentiates the proliferation of endothelium by endothelial cell growth factor (ECGF) (Thornton, Mueller, and Levine, 1983). Thus, the evidence suggests that, although mast cells are probably not the direct cause of endothelial proliferation in hemangioma, the cells play a central role in the growth and involution of these tumors.

PROLIFERATION: ELECTRON MICROSCOPY

Electron micrographs show that a proliferating hemangioma is comprised of plump endothelium that demonstrate characteristics

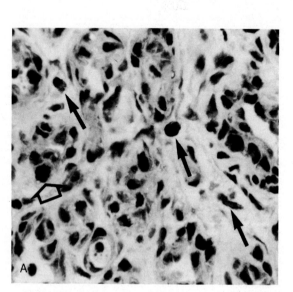

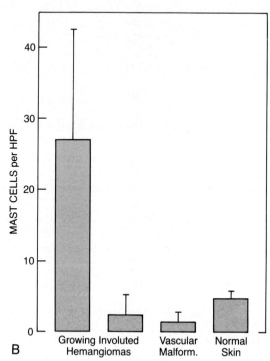

Figure 66–2. Mast cells in hemangioma. *A,* Mast cells (*thin arrows*) in a four month hemangioma specimen; note the cell in mitosis (*open arrow*) (toluidine blue, × 856). *B,* Mast cell counts per high power field in growing and involuted hemangiomas, vascular malformations, and normal skin specimens. Values expressed as means ± SD. (*B,* from Mulliken, J. B., and Young, A. E.: Vascular Birthmarks: Hemangiomas and Malformations. Philadelphia, W. B. Saunders Company, 1988.)

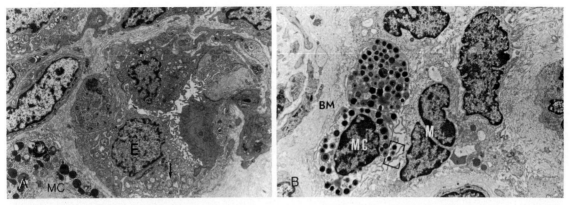

Figure 66–3. Hemangioma proliferation: electron microscopy. *A,* Eight month hemangioma exhibiting plump endothelium (E) with signs of intracellular activity: convoluted nuclear membranes, swollen mitochondria (*arrow*), rough endoplasmic reticulum, and free ribosomes. Note the mast cell (MC) aligned along the multilaminated basement membrane that surrounds the vessel (× 7700). *B,* Two mast cells (MC), lined along a thickened basement membrane (BM), are interacting with a macrophage (M). Brackets indicate detachment of mast cell granules from the cell surface (× 5200). (From Dethlefsen, S. M., Mulliken, J. B., and Glowacki, J.: An ultrastructural study of mast cell interactions in hemangiomas. Ultrastruct. Pathol., *10*:175, 1986. By permission of Hemisphere Publishing Corporation, New York, NY.)

of intracellular activity: convoluted nuclear membrane, swollen mitochondria, membranes of rough endoplasmic reticulum, and clusters of free ribosomes (Höpfel-Kreiner, 1980). Multilamination of the basement membrane is a pathologic hallmark of the proliferative phase hemangioma (Fig. 66–3*A*) (Höpfel-Kreiner, 1980; Iwamoto and Jakobiec, 1979; Mulliken and Glowacki, 1982). It is proposed that cyclical endothelial proliferation and death cause multilamination of the basal membrane (Vracko and Benditt, 1970).

Mast cells are seen with their long microvillous projections aligned along the vessel walls and parallel to the laminations of the basement membrane (Dethlefsen, Mulliken, and Glowacki, 1986). During proliferation and early involution, the mast cells appear to interact with macrophages and fibroblasts (Fig. 66–3*B*). There is ultrastructural evidence of the release of mast cell material and subsequent uptake by adjacent cells: macrophages and fibroblasts lie in close contact with mast cells, cytoplasmic bridges are seen between mast cells and fibroblasts, and there are pinocytic vesicles along the periphery of opposing cells (Dethlefsen, Mulliken, and Glowacki, 1986).

INVOLUTION: LIGHT AND ELECTRON MICROSCOPY

Natural regression is the most intriguing biologic characteristic of the common hemangioma of childhood. Some investigators have assumed a priori that involution is the result of thrombosis and infarction (Watson and McCarthy, 1940; MacCollum and Martin, 1956; Matthews, 1968). There is, however, no microscopic evidence of such a mechanism. Proliferation and involution occur concurrently after the first year, i.e., even when involution is well under way there are scattered proliferative foci (Mulliken and Glowacki, 1982). In hemangioma specimens of children 2 to 5 years of age there are fewer cells, while individual vascular channels become more prominent as the lining endothelial cells flatten. At the same time there is progressive deposition of perivascular, inter- and intralobular fibrous tissue (Fig. 66–4*A*). The involuted hemangioma exhibits a "cavernous" appearance, which can be histologically confused with a venous malformation (Fig. 66–4*B*).

With the electron microscope, tissue from an involuting hemangioma reveals signs of endothelial discontinuity and vessel degradation. The lumens contain endothelial cell debris (Fig. 66–5*A*). The prominent cellular interactions, seen in the proliferative phase, are no longer obvious. The end stage involuted hemangioma is composed of thin-walled vessels that resemble normal capillaries. The basement membrane remains multilaminated and there are islands of fat and dense collagen deposited in the perivascular areas (Fig. 66–5*B*) (Dethlefsen, Mulliken, and Glowacki, 1986).

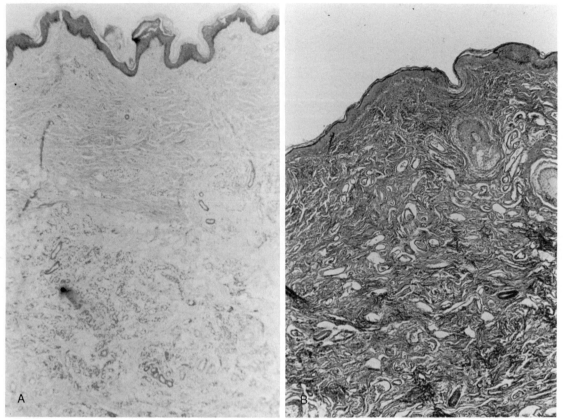

Figure 66–4. Hemangioma involution: light microscopy. *A,* Hemangioma from a 2 year old child showing inter- and intralobular fibrosis and dilated channels (H & E, × 25). *B,* The final stage of regression: the large, thin-walled remaining channels in the dermis have a "cavernous" appearance, not to be confused with venous malformation (H & E × 16). (From Mulliken, J. B., and Young, A. E.: Vascular Birthmarks: Hemangiomas and Malformations. Philadelphia, W. B. Saunders Company, 1988.)

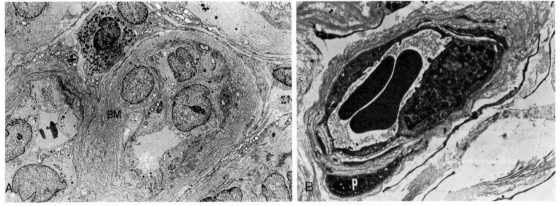

Figure 66–5. Hemangioma involution: electron microscopy. *A,* In this three year hemangioma specimen, the endothelial lining is disrupted and degenerating endothelial cells partially obstruct the vessel lumen. The basement membrane (BM) is still multilayered and contains cellular debris and pericytic processes (× 2800). *B,* In this fully involuted hemangioma, the vessel has reverted to a more normal architecture, resembling a dilated capillary. The wall is lined by a single endothelial cell and is surrounded by a pericyte (P). The multilaminated basement membrane is thinner and disorganized; interstitial collagen fibers are seen (× 9180). (From Mulliken, J. B., and Young, A. E.: Vascular Birthmarks: Hemangiomas and Malformations. Philadelphia, W. B. Saunders Company, 1988.)

HEMANGIOMAS: POSSIBLE HORMONAL EFFECT

Endogenous hormones may be important in the growth and involution of hemangioma. Sasaki, Pang, and Wittliff (1984) hypothesized that hemangiomas contain steroid hormone receptors that mediate cellular proliferation. Serum estradiol 17-β levels in infants with proliferating hemangiomas were four times higher than in control samples or serum from patients with vascular malformations. Using a receptor assay, they also found that biopsy specimens exhibited abnormally high levels of specific estradiol 17-β binding sites, compared with normal skin and vascular malformation tissue. In vitro estrogen binding capacity of hemangioma explants was inhibited by both high and low doses of cortisone. Furthermore, the serum estradiol levels diminished in infants in whom the hemangioma began to regress with systemic prednisone (Sasaki, Pang, and Wittliff, 1984).

HEMANGIOMA: AN ANGIOGENIC DISEASE

The concept that tumors are *angiogenesis dependent* provides new insights into the pathogenesis of hemangioma (Folkman, 1974, 1976). Under normal conditions, endothelium has an exceedingly low mitotic rate that can be measured only in years (Denekamp, 1984). Capillaries are normally prevented from growing by physiologic regulation of the local angiogenic factors. Several angiogenic factors have been purified, their amino acid sequences determined, and their gene structure known (Folkman and Klagsbrun, 1987). The angiogenic factors appear to fall into two main groups: (1) those that act directly on vascular endothelium to stimulate mitosis or migration and (2) those that act indirectly by mobilizing host helper cells (e.g., macrophages and mast cells) to release endothelial growth factors. Thus, a nascent hemangioma may result from endothelial proliferation secondary to increased levels of stimulatory angiogenic factors or a decreased level of normally present growth-inhibitory factors. Further studies from Folkman's laboratory suggest that helper cells may be important in hemangiomatous proliferation. A likely candidate is the mast cell. There is a 40-fold increase in mast cells prior to ingrowth of new capillaries using the chick chorioallantoic membrane model (Kessler and associates, 1976). Zetter (1980) showed that mast cell–conditioned medium or tumor-conditioned medium stimulates migration of cultured capillary endothelia. The mast cell product heparin is known to bind to endothelium and to enhance migration; protamine selectively blocks migration (Zetter, 1980; Taylor and Folkman, 1982). Other investigators reported that mast cell granules cause proliferation of cultured human endothelial cells (Thornton, Mueller, and Levine, 1983; Marks and associates, 1986). These findings offer an intriguing explanation for the increased numbers of mast cells seen in proliferating hemangiomas (Glowacki and Mulliken, 1982).

If, indeed, hemangioma is an angiogenic disease, a logical therapeutic approach would be pharmacologic control with angiogenesis inhibitors. It is known that prednisone accelerates involution in some rapidly growing hemangiomas. Cortisone and hydrocortisone, but not dexamethasone, are antiangiogenic in the presence of heparin and heparin fragments (Folkman and associates, 1983). Certain tetrahydrocortisone analogues, which lack glucocorticoid and mineralocorticoid activity, are more potent "angiostatic" drugs than the parent hormone hydrocortisone (Crum, Szabo, and Folkman, 1985). Perhaps specific angiostatic drugs may soon be available to treat the infant with a destructive hemangioma.

Diagnosis and Natural History

INCIDENCE

Hemangioma is the most common tumor of infancy. The frequency in newborn infants, in the first few days of life, is 1.1 to 2.6 per cent (Pratt, 1967; Jacobs and Walton, 1976). Most hemangiomas appear postnatally, so that by 1 year of age the frequency is 10 to 12 per cent in Caucasian children (Holmdahl, 1955; Jacobs, 1957). In the author's institution, hemangiomas are uncommon in black children; however, Pratt (1967) reported an incidence of 1.4 per cent at examination during the first week of life. Hemangiomas are more common in females than in males, in a 3:1 ratio (Bowers, Graham, and Tomlinson, 1960; Finn, Glowacki, and Mulliken, 1983). The early studies of preterm infants (birth weights in the 1500 to 2500 gm range) showed an equal frequency of hemangioma compared with full-term infants (Greenhouse, 1955; Holmdahl, 1955). However, in premature infants with low birth weight (below 1000 gm), hemangioma occurs more frequently (22.9 per cent) during the first year of life (Amir and associates, 1986).

FIRST SIGNS

Occasionally a fully grown hemangioma is seen at birth; however, most are manifest during the first to fourth weeks of life. The initial sign of a nascent hemangioma is either an erythematous macular patch, a blanched spot, or a localized telangiectasia, surrounded by a pale halo (Fig. 66–6A) (Payne and associates, 1966; Hidano and Nakajima, 1972). A hemangioma may grow as a single localized tumor or may simultaneously proliferate in multiple sites anywhere in the body. Approximately 80 per cent of hemangiomas present as a single lesion; 20 per cent of affected infants have more than one hemangioma (Margileth and Museles, 1965).

The hallmark of the hemangioma is rapid neonatal growth (Fig. 66–6B). If cellular proliferation begins in the superficial dermis, the skin becomes raised and finely bosselated with a vivid crimson color. If a hemangioma proliferates in the lower dermis and subcutaneous layer, without involving the papillary dermis, the lesion may appear slightly raised with a bluish hue or the overlying skin can be smooth, with normal color, or may exhibit faint telangiectatic vessels (Fig. 66–7A). The deep hemangiomas were once labeled "cavernous" or, if the lesion involved both deep and superficial skin layers, the old term was "mixed, capillary-cavernous" hemangioma. These microscopic adjectives, "capillary" and "cavernous," are clinically confusing and should be avoided. It is best to refer to a bright red hemangioma as "superficial" and to call the lesion with normal skin a "deep" hemangioma. Often, hemangiomas present with both deep and superficial proliferation.

MULTIPLE HEMANGIOMAS

Hemangiomas occur most frequently in the head and neck region (60 per cent), followed in frequency by the trunk (25 per cent) and the extremities (15 per cent) (Finn, Glowacki, and Mulliken, 1983). Hemangiomas can also

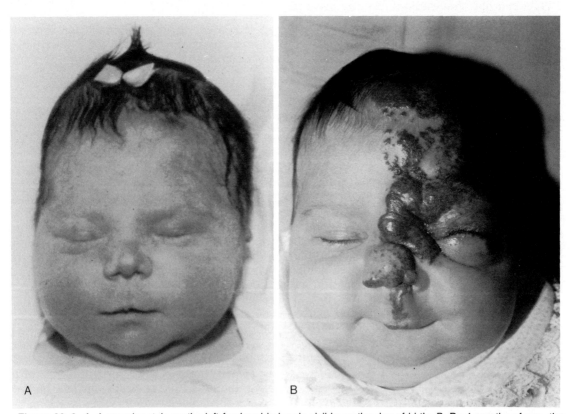

A

B

Figure 66–6. *A,* A macular stain on the left forehead is barely visible on the day of birth. *B,* By 4 months of age, the child in *A* has a large hemangioma infiltrating the face and obstructing the left eye. (From Mulliken, J. B., and Young, A. E.: Vascular Birthmarks: Hemangiomas and Malformations. Philadelphia, W. B. Saunders Company, 1988.)

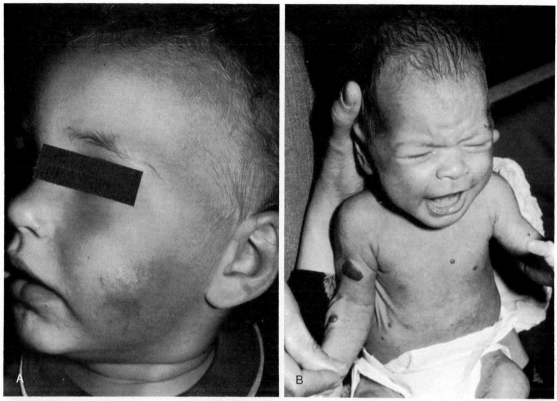

Figure 66–7. *A,* A tumor in the cheek appeared at 1 month of age; the skin has a bluish hue with fine telangiectasia. The diagnosis is hemangioma (deep). *B,* Multiple cutaneous hemangiomas, characteristically dome shaped. (From Mulliken, J. B., and Young, A. E.: Vascular Birthmarks: Hemangiomas and Malformations. Philadelphia, W. B. Saunders Company, 1988.)

be found in lymph nodes, spleen, liver, thymus, gastrointestinal tract, lung, urinary bladder, gallbladder, pancreas, and adrenal glands (Cooper and Bolande, 1965; Burman, Mansell, and Warin, 1967; Holden and Alexander, 1970). It is rare for an infant with visceral hemangiomatosis not to have cutaneous involvement, or to manifest only a few lesions. The corollary statement is also true, namely that some infants with multiple cutaneous lesions do not have associated hemangiomas of internal organs (Fig. 66–7*B*). There are also reported cases of hemangiomas in the meninges, brain, and spinal cord (Burke, Winkelmann, and Strickland, 1964; Burman, Mansell, and Warin, 1967; Cooper and Bolande, 1965).

CLINICAL DIFFERENTIAL DIAGNOSIS

The patient's *history* is the most critical determinant in differentiating a hemangioma from a malformation. The hemangioma grows rapidly, beginning in the first weeks after birth, at a rate beyond that of the infant. Vascular malformations, however, may or may not be noted at birth; once detected, they expand commensurately with the child. *Color* can be a useful clue. A superficial hemangioma has a bright scarlet color that gradually deepens during the first year of life. Malformations have a persistent vascular hue, depending on the components, capillary, lymphatic, venous, or arterial. Two axioms help to distinguish hemangioma from vascular malformation. The first is that *not all hemangiomas look like a strawberry.* The skin overlying a deep hemangioma may be of normal color, a bluish tint, or (in rare instances) a pale shade with scattered telangiectasia (Fig. 66–8). The corollary axiom is that *not all strawberry-like vascular lesions are hemangiomas.* A cutaneous capillary-venous, lymphaticovenous, or pure venous malformation can look remarkably similar to a hemangioma (Fig. 66–9).

Palpation is also helpful in differentiating vascular lesions. In so doing, one can imagine

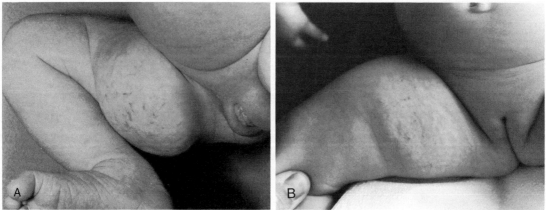

Figure 66–8. *A,* A 1 month old girl with vascular tumor of the right medial thigh, present at birth. The skin is raised and pale, and contains tiny serpiginous vessels. (From Mulliken, J. B., and Young, A. E.: Vascular Birthmarks: Hemangiomas and Malformations. Philadelphia, W. B. Saunders Company, 1988.) *B,* The hemangioma rapidly regressed over one year.

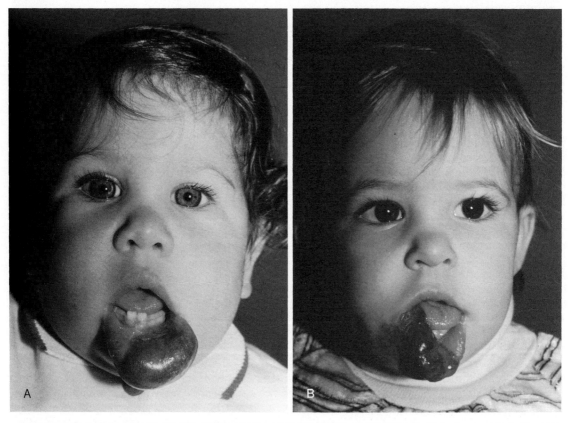

Figure 66–9. *A,* A 1 year old girl with rapidly growing vascular lesions of the lower lip that appeared just after birth. They have a doughy consistency and cannot be completely compressed. Diagnosis: hemangioma. Prognosis: involution. *B,* A 1 year old girl with vascular lesion of lip, present since birth and growing proportionately. It is easily compressible and thrombi can be palpated. Diagnosis: venous malformation. Prognosis: continued commensurate growth with likely expansion and dentoalveolar distortion. (From Mulliken, J. B., and Young, A. E.: Vascular Birthmarks: Hemangiomas and Malformations. Philadelphia, W. B. Saunders Company, 1988.)

the differences in microscopic appearance: hemangioma is a dense cellular tumor whereas a vascular malformation is composed of dilated channels and sparse parenchyma. A hemangioma feels firm and rubbery, and the blood contained within the tumor cannot be evacuated by pressure. In contrast, most vascular malformations are soft, easily compressible, and rapidly emptied of blood by digital pressure.

In most instances, a hemangioma can be differentiated from a vascular malformation without the need for complicated or invasive diagnostic techniques (Finn, Glowacki, and Mulliken, 1983; Mulliken, 1984). Granted, in some instances the physician must honestly admit to the parents that another examination in several months may be necessary before their infant's vascular birthmark can be accurately diagnosed. Usually, parents accept a clear explanation of the most likely diagnoses and the fact that, in most cases, immediate therapy is not necessary.

However, one must always be wary when an infant presents with a rapidly growing soft tissue mass that feels unusually firm; sarcoma is the differential diagnosis. Radiographic study, particularly computed tomography, may be useful and biopsy may be indicated.

RADIOGRAPHIC DIFFERENTIAL DIAGNOSIS

In certain locations, for example, the pre-auricular cheek area or cervical region, it may be difficult to differentiate a deep hemangioma, without its telltale cutaneous signs, from a lymphatic or venous malformation. Computed tomography, with dye injection, highlights a proliferative phase hemangioma as a well-circumscribed tumor with homogeneous density and enhancement (Fig. 66–10). Hemangioma in its involuting phase shows a more variegated density and distinct lobular architecture. On the other hand, computed tomographic studies of vascular malformations characteristically demonstrate tissue heterogeneity. Venous anomalies occasionally have calcifications with heterogeneous density. Pure lymphatic anomalies are seen as multilocular cysts that may show enhancement in the septa with intravenous contrast injection (Fig. 66–11). Skeletal deformation rarely occurs with hemangioma; bone hypertrophy and distortion are more typical of an adjacent lymphatic or venous malformation.

Arteriography is rarely indicated in the evaluation of cutaneous hemangiomas. It may be necessary when embolization is contemplated for an infant with a giant heman-

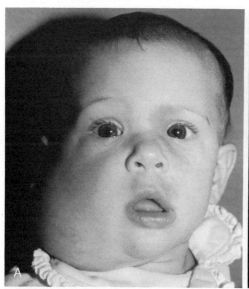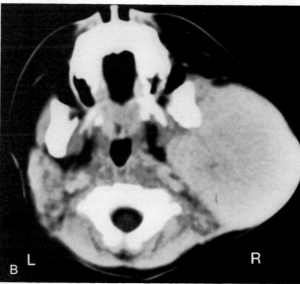

Figure 66–10. *A,* A 1 year old child with a port-wine stain of the left face and a large subcutaneous mass in the right cheek. Differential diagnosis: deep hemangioma versus lymphatic malformation. *B,* CT study demonstrates homogeneous dye enhancement, confirming the clinical diagnosis of hemangioma. Since this is the most common tumor of childhood, it is not surprising that it could occur coincidentally with a vascular malformation (port-wine stain). (From Mulliken, J. B., and Young, A. E.: Vascular Birthmarks: Hemangiomas and Malformations. Philadelphia, W. B. Saunders Company, 1988.)

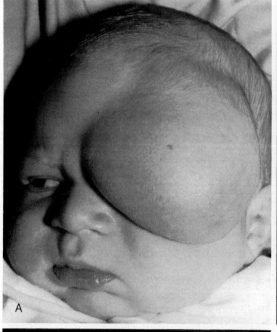

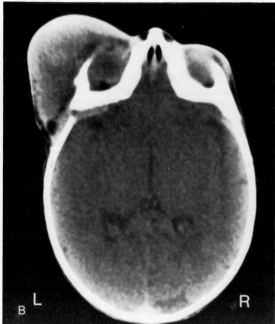

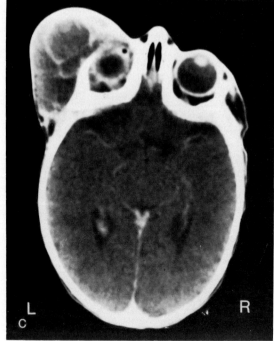

Figure 66–11. *A,* Cystic mass of the forehead and eyelid, present at birth and enlarging with the child. Differential diagnosis: lymphatic (LM) versus lymphaticovenous malformation (LVM). *B,* CT study of the child in *A,* showing homogeneous low density mass within the orbit and frontal region. *C,* Axial CT study, after dye injection, showing nonenhanced, honeycombed configuration of the lesion with a few septal vessels, extending into the retrobulbar cone. This is the typical CT appearance of a lymphatic malformation (LM). (From Mulliken, J. B., and Young, A. E.: Vascular Birthmarks: Hemangiomas and Malformations. Philadelphia, W. B. Saunders Company, 1988.)

gioma or visceral hemangiomatosis that causes platelet trapping and/or congestive heart failure. The angiographic characteristics useful in differentiating cutaneous hemangioma from a vascular malformation have been described by Burrows and associates (1983).

PYOGENIC GRANULOMA

Pyogenic granuloma ("lobular capillary hemangioma") is a proliferative vascular lesion, often clinically confused with hemangioma; unfortunately, both share the histologic designation "capillary hemangioma." A pyogenic granuloma appears suddenly. A history of trauma to the area is rarely elicited from the parents. Usually the patient is an older infant or young child, although the lesions also occur in adults. Cheek, eyelids, and extremities are the typical location for pyogenic granuloma. It also presents on the lips, oral mucosa, tongue, and nasal cavity (Mills, Cooper, and Fechner, 1980). A curious and not infrequent occurrence is a pyogenic granuloma within a port-wine vascular birthmark, either intra- or extraorally (Fig. 66–12A).

An early pyogenic granuloma, with its epidermis intact, bears some resemblance to a tiny hemangioma (Fig. 66–12B). The pyogenic lesion usually has a pedunculated shape with a tiny stalk. In time, this growing vascular lesion loses its epidermal mantle, and is covered by a brown-black crust or bright red granular surface. A pyogenic granuloma may grow to 1 cm in diameter.

The term "pyogenic granuloma" implies an infectious cause, but scientific evidence for this theory is lacking. Although they can occur within small wounds or after repeated irritation, most pyogenic granulomas appear without a history of skin trauma. The common presenting tale is one of repeated episodes of bleeding, often refractory to pressure and repeated application of caustics.

Proliferating vascular cells are seen on histologic examination, admixed in an edematous stroma filled with a variable number of inflammatory cells. The characteristic "epidermal collarette" is located where the epithelial covering at the base of the lesion meets the surrounding normal skin (Davies and Marks, 1978). A deep-seated lobule of capillaries is the main histologic identifying feature of this entity, rather than secondary changes in the superficial tissue, e.g., edema, inflammation, collarette formation, or epidermal ulceration (Mills, Cooper, and Fechner, 1980). The pathologist often designates the lesion a "capillary hemangioma, granuloma type" or "lobular capillary hemangioma." It may be difficult to make a light microscopic differentiation between a true hemangioma of infancy and a pyogenic granuloma. However, pyogenic granuloma exhibits immunocytochemical and ultrastructural differences: it is predominantly perithelial, rather than an endothelial tumor (Padilla, Orkin, and Rosai, 1987).

A pyogenic granuloma rarely shows necrosis and the site heals without medical min-

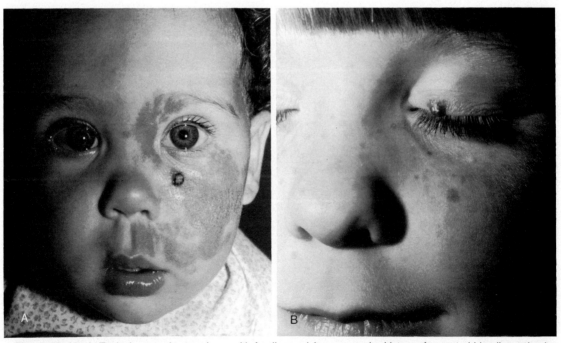

Figure 66–12. A, Typical pyogenic granuloma with fragile overlying scar and a history of repeated bleeding episodes. These lesions often appear in port-wine stained skin. (From Mulliken, J. B., and Young, A. E.: Vascular Birthmarks: Hemangiomas and Malformations. Philadelphia, W. B. Saunders Company, 1988.) B, A pyogenic granuloma that suddenly appeared in the upper eyelid of a 4 year old girl.

istrations; it is repeated bleeding that necessitates therapy. Recurrence usually follows cauterization with a silver nitrate stick, because the lesion extends into the deep dermis. Electrocoagulation or laser coagulation gives more predictable results. If these measures fail, or as primary therapy, excision and linear closure are recommended.

Complications in the Proliferation Phase

ULCERATION

Less than 5 per cent of hemangiomas ulcerate (Margileth and Museles, 1965), the result of tumor proliferation through the epidermal basement membrane. Occasionally, ulceration is noted in a hemangioma at birth; it usually occurs at the height of the proliferative phase, in tense, distended lesions (Fig. 66–13*A*) (Bowers, Graham, and Tomlinson, 1960). Ulceration is more common in hemangiomas located in the lips and anogenital areas. Secondary infection invariably accompanies ulceration; there are patients in whom ulceration and infection cause extensive destruction of the facial soft tissues (the so-called "wildfire hemangioma") (Fig. 66–13*B*).

OBSTRUCTION

Visual. Obstruction of the visual axis, causing deprivation amblyopia and failure to develop binocular vision, is the best known example of a hemangioma impinging on a critical anatomic location (Fig. 66–13*B*) (Robb, 1977; Stigmar and associates, 1978; Thomson and associates, 1979; Haik and associates, 1979). An upper eyelid hemangioma can also cause anisometropia, resulting in amblyopia, even though the child's vision is not apparently occluded. The mass effect of a periorbital hemangioma can distort the growing cornea, producing refractive errors, both astigmatic and myopic (Robb, 1977). Another ophthalmologic complication of hemangioma is strabismus; this may be either paralytic (resulting from hemangiomatous infiltration of the extraocular muscles) or secondary to the amblyopia (Stigmar and associates, 1978).

Any periorbital hemangioma, particularly in the upper eyelid, should be refracted, using retinoscopy with cycloplegia. Serial refraction is mandatory to demonstrate the onset and possible worsening of visual changes. Even large hemangiomas of the lower eyelid and cheek region are unlikely to cause visual disturbances.

Late complications of periorbital and ad-

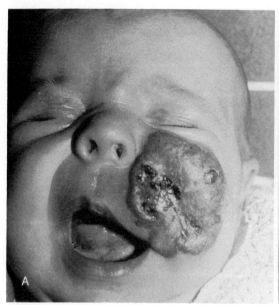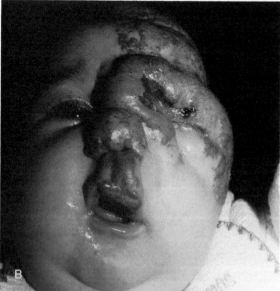

Figure 66–13. *A,* Spontaneous ulceration in a bosselated hemangioma in a 3 month old child. *B,* Hemangioma obstructing the left eye in a 5 month old child with ulceration and secondary infection causing destruction of the medial canthal tissue (see Fig. 66–6 for earlier photographs). (From Mulliken, J. B., and Young, A. E.: Vascular Birthmarks: Hemangiomas and Malformations. Philadelphia, W. B. Saunders Company, 1988.)

nexal hemangiomas include asymmetric refractive error, globe proptosis, blepharoptosis, and optic atrophy (Robb, 1977; Stigmar and associates, 1978).

Respiratory. A hemangioma growing within the nasal tip may block the vestibular passages during the first three months of life, when the infant is an obligatory nose breather. However, there usually is unilateral obstruction of the nasal airway, or the narrowing occurs slowly so that the infant adapts and breathes orally.

Hemangiomatous proliferation in the subglottic airway is insidious and potentially life threatening. Characteristically, the infants are asymptomatic at birth, but within six to eight weeks develop biphasic stridor, accompanied by respiratory distress. The typical clinical presentation is either a protracted episode of laryngotracheitis or recurrent bouts of "croup" (Healy and associates, 1980). Approximately one-half of infants with subglottal hemangioma have associated cutaneous hemangiomas, usually in the cervicofacial region.

In any infant suspected of having laryngeal hemangioma, anterioposterior and lateral radiographs should be taken to detect eccentric subglottal swelling. Direct laryngoscopy confirms the diagnosis; the typical finding is a smooth, compressible mass in the posterior subglottal area, which often extends around either lateral wall (Fig. 66–14A). The mucosal surface may exhibit a few telangiectatic vessels or may be stained bright red by the submucosal hemangioma. Subglottic hemangioma rarely spreads circumferentially or encroaches the trachea or the true vocal cords (Fig. 66–14B) (Healy and associates, 1980).

Auditory. A hemangioma of the parotid region may obstruct the external auditory canal, causing a mild to moderate conductive hearing loss. The blockage is relieved with regression of the tumor. This is a potential problem if there is bilateral obstruction, persisting beyond 1 year of age, when auditory conduction is necessary for normal speech development.

BLEEDING

Spontaneous bleeding from a punctate area within a florid superficial hemangioma is an unusual occurrence; occasionally there is associated skin ulceration. More worrisome is the possibility of a generalized clotting disorder, first described in 1940 by Kasabach and Merritt and manifest with petechiae, ecchymoses, or internal bleeding. The term "Kasabach-Merritt syndrome" should be reserved for a bleeding disorder that results from a profound thrombocytopenia (as low as 2000 to 40,000 per cu mm) that is associated with either a large hemangioma or extensive hemangiomatosis. It is not known what mass of hemangioma tissue can trigger this bleeding complication; there is one case of intrauterine and perinatal bleeding in an infant with a 5 × 7 cm hemangioma (Bowles, Kostopoulos-Farri, and Papageorgiou, 1981). Ra-

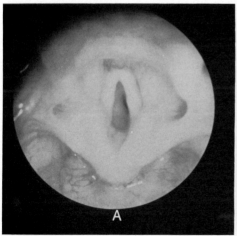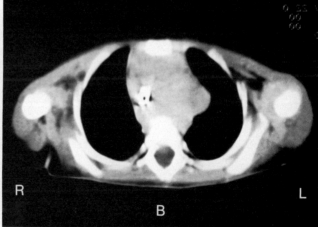

Figure 66–14. *A,* Laryngoscopic view showing a left subglottic hemangioma in a 2 month old infant admitted with biphasic stridor. (Courtesy of Trevor McGill.) *B,* Enhanced axial CT scan through the upper chest in a 7 month old child who required tracheostomy for a circumferential subglottic hemangioma. Note the extension around the trachea and upper mediastinum with dislocation of the tracheostomy tube. (From Mulliken, J. B., and Young, A. E.: Vascular Birthmarks: Hemangiomas and Malformations. Philadelphia, W. B. Saunders Company, 1988.)

diolabeled platelets have a shortened survival in patients with extensive hemangiomas (Ardissone, Pecco, and Italiano, 1980; Bona and associates, 1980; Koerper and associates, 1983; Sondel and associates, 1984). Scintillation counting, after infusion of radioactive chromium–labeled platelets, demonstrates maximal activity over the hemangioma, as well as the spleen, suggesting sequestration of platelets in this organ (Kontras and associates, 1963). Platelet thrombi are seen in microscopic sections of excised hemangiomas (Good, Carnazzo, and Good, 1955; Hill and Longino, 1962; Kontras and associates, 1963). Consumption coagulopathy may also occur with hemangiomas; it is more likely when infection complicates the clinical presentation (Ardissone, Pecco and Italiano, 1980; Cartwright and Van Coller, 1981; Esterly,

1983; Koerper and associates, 1983; David, Evans, and Stevens, 1983).

The Kasabach-Merritt syndrome classically occurs during the early postnatal period of rapid hemangiomatous growth. The danger signs are the onset of acute hemorrhage (gastrointestinal, pleural, peritoneal, or central nervous system) or a rapid increase in the size of the hemangioma secondary to intralesional bleeding into the tumor. Petechiae and ecchymoses are initially seen overlying and adjacent to the hemangioma; later, other skin areas are involved. The hemangioma may become tense and the overlying skin may be shiny and discolored, findings suggesting cellulitis.

A complete blood count, with a review of the peripheral blood smear for evidence of microangiopathy, and a platelet count should

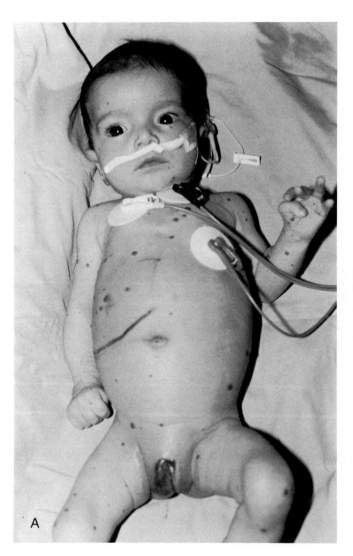

Figure 66–15. *A,* A 3 month old girl with multiple cutaneous hemangiomas, hepatomegaly, anemia, and congestive heart failure.

A

be taken in high risk infants; these include a child with a hemangioma greater than 5 cm in diameter, with multiple hemangiomas, or with signs suggesting a bleeding tendency, e.g., petechiae, bruising, gastrointestinal bleeding, or unexpected anemia. If there is thrombocytopenia or if an operative procedure is planned (whether related to the hemangioma or not), additional studies should be performed for evidence of consumptive coagulopathy: prothrombin time (PT), activated partial thromboplastin time (aPTT), fibrinogen, fibrin degradation products, and fibrinopeptide A.

CONGESTIVE HEART FAILURE: MULTIPLE CUTANEOUS AND HEPATIC HEMANGIOMAS

Patients with multiple neonatal hemangiomas present another potentially lethal complication. These infants can show at 2 to 8 weeks of life the triad of congestive heart failure, hepatomegaly, and anemia (Touloukian, 1970; McLean and associates, 1972). There usually are multiple hemangiomas of the skin; they are often quite small (5 to 10 mm in diameter) and hemispherical (Fig. 66–15A). The most common sites of visceral involvement are, in descending order, the liver, lungs, and gastrointestinal tract. High output cardiac failure can also occur with large cutaneous hemangiomas in the absence of visceral hemangiomas (Stern, Wolf, and Jarratt, 1981). Hepatic hemangiomas occur more commonly in female infants, as do cutaneous

lesions, with a reported 2:1 ratio (deLorimier, 1977).

The hepatomegaly is often out of proportion to the degree of congestive heart failure; frequently a systolic bruit is heard over the enlarged liver. Less common presenting features are transient obstructive jaundice (Wishnick, 1978), intestinal obstruction, and portal hypertension (Larcher, Howard, and Mowat, 1981). There are also cases of rupture in the newborn producing massive intra-abdominal hemorrhage (Stone and Nielson, 1965). A platelet-trapping coagulopathy (Kasabach-Merritt syndrome) may also complicate hepatic hemangiomas and may manifest with alimentary tract hemorrhage (Albert and Benisch, 1970).

Hepatic hemangiomas can be documented and followed during therapy by radiographic means: ultrasonography, computed tomography, or radionucleotide scanning. In preparation for embolization or operative therapy, selective celiac angiography or digital angiography is particularly valuable in determining the configuration, size, and blood supply of the lesions. In immature lesions, the veins fill rapidly, indicating shunting through the hemangiomatous tissue. In older lesions, in infants over 2 months of age, the hypervascular nodules are clearly seen in the venous phase (Fig. 66–15B,C).

Histologic diagnosis is rarely necessary to exclude hepatoblastoma, and percutaneous needle biopsy also carries a high risk of intraperitoneal hemorrhage. The clinical triad of hepatomegaly, congestive heart failure (in

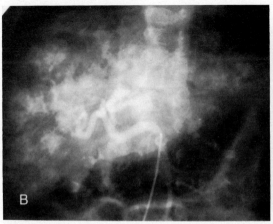
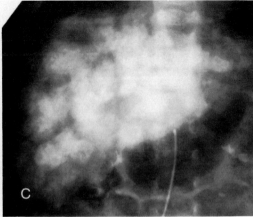

Figure 66–15 *Continued B,* Selective hepatic arteriogram (arterial phase) shows an enlarged common hepatic artery and its branches supplying densely staining tumors throughout the liver. *C,* The venous phase demonstrates persistent homogeneous staining and discrete tumor margins, typical of a hemangioma. (From Mulliken, J. B., and Young, A. E.: Vascular Birthmarks: Hemangiomas and Malformations. Philadelphia, W. B. Saunders Company, 1988.)

the absence of congenital cardiac disease), and cutaneous hemangiomas, in conjunction with positive radiographic data, is sufficient evidence that treatment is required (Touloukian, 1970).

Although spontaneous regression is expected with visceral and hepatic hemangiomas, the overall mortality rate is as high as 54 per cent (Berman and Lim, 1978). Death is usually the result of congestive heart failure, infection, or hemorrhage. The mortality data may be distorted because of past failure to differentiate liver hemangioma from arteriovenous malformation (Mulliken, 1988a).

SKELETAL DISTORTION

Skeletal changes secondary to hemangioma are unusual, e.g., deviation of the nasal pyramid, minor indentation of the calvaria, and orbital enlargement (Williams, 1979; Boyd and associates, 1984). The mechanism is presumed to be a mass effect of the hemangioma on the adjacent bone. There are also rare instances of hypertrophy of the auricular cartilage or facial bones in children with a large unilateral hemangioma.

The Involution Phase

After a period of rapid growth, the hemangioma seems to stabilize for a time, growing at the same rate as the child. This usually becomes evident between 6 and 10 months of age. It is important to reiterate that proliferation and involution are not distinct phases in the life cycle of hemangioma. Proliferation slowly abates while involution begins to predominate. One of the first signs of regression is fading of the shiny crimson surface to a dull purple hue. In time, the surface assumes a mottled grayish mantle that seems to spread centrifugally toward the periphery of the lesion.

It soon becomes obvious that the child is growing disproportionately to the hemangioma. The lesion is less tense to palpation. The parents may remark that the child is not so fussy or that, when the child cries, the hemangioma does not swell as much as it did at an earlier time.

By age 5 years, the last traces of color are usually fading. The skin left behind after regression exhibits mild atrophy; has a wrinkled quality, perhaps with a few telangiectatic vessels; and is slightly more pale than the surrounding normal skin. Some hemangiomas cause tissue expansion of the overlying skin that persists after involution is complete. In other instances, the involuted hemangioma remains as a fibrofatty residuum. If ulceration complicated the proliferative phase, the healed area is evidenced by a central yellow-white patch. This type of scarred skin will never have the quality that results from involution without intercedent ulceration.

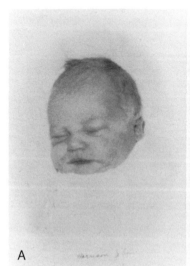 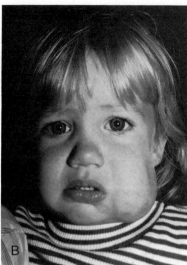 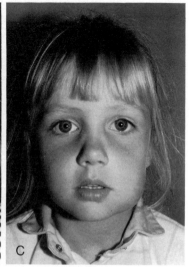

Figure 66–16. Involution of a deep hemangioma. *A,* Nursery photograph of an apparently normal infant. *B,* At age 1½ years the child has a deep hemangioma of the cheek. *C,* At age 5 years the hemangioma is regressing. (From Mulliken, J. B., and Young, A. E.: Vascular Birthmarks: Hemangiomas and Malformations. Philadelphia, W. B. Saunders Company, 1988.)

Clinical studies confirm that complete resolution of hemangioma occurs in over 50 per cent of children by age 5 years, and in 70 per cent by age 7 years, with continued improvement in the remaining children until ages 10 to 12 years (Lister, 1938; Simpson, 1959; Bowers, Graham, and Tomlinson, 1960; Pratt,

1967). Neither sex, race, site, size, presence at birth, duration of proliferative phase, nor clinical appearance of the hemangioma appear to influence the course of involution (Simpson, 1959; Bowers, Graham, and Tomlinson, 1960; Finn, Glowacki, and Mulliken, 1983). Involution proceeds at the same rate

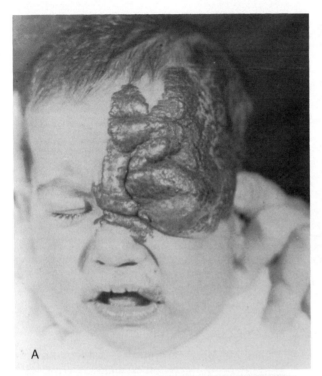

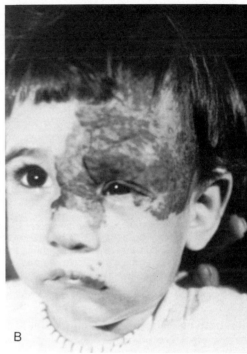

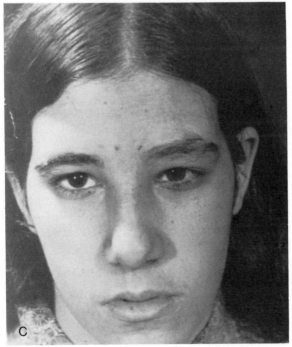

Figure 66–17. Involution of a superficial hemangioma. *A,* A newborn with an extensive hemangioma of the face. *B,* At age 4 years the hemangioma is in its involuting phase. *C,* At age 14 years involution is complete. There is expansion of the eyebrow; skin texture is excellent. (From Mulliken, J. B., and Young, A. E.: Vascular Birthmarks: Hemangiomas and Malformations. Philadelphia, W. B. Saunders Company, 1988.)

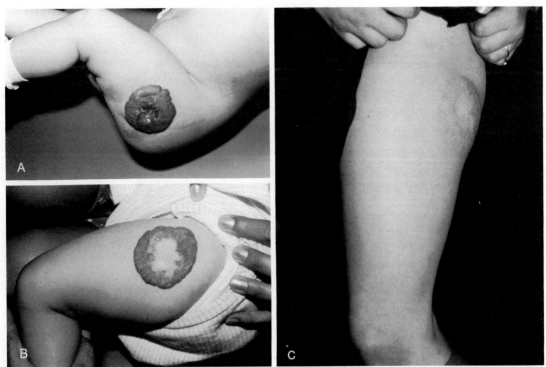

Figure 66–18. Spontaneous ulceration during the proliferative phase. *A,* A deep ulcer in a florid hemangioma of the thigh. *B,* Healing by epithelization leaves a pale central scar. *C,* Involution at age 7 years; note the remarkable shrinkage of skin once filled with hemangioma. (From Mulliken, J. B., and Young, A. E.: Vascular Birthmarks: Hemangiomas and Malformations. Philadelphia, W. B. Saunders Company, 1988.)

for both deep and superficial hemangiomas (Figs. 66–16 to 66–18).

History of Treatment

Over the centuries, physicians have been remarkably resourceful in their attempts to treat hemangiomas *(naevi materni).*

LIGATION AND EXCISION

In his 1714 treatise, Turner favored surgical resection, ligation, and caustics for vascular birthmarks. During the nineteenth century, surgeons devised ingenious methods of interrupting the vascular supply to a hemangioma using figure-of-eight, spiral, or interlocking subcutaneous sutures of catgut, wire, or silk (Curling, 1850; Murray, 1864; Bobbs, 1870–1871).

Until the natural involution of hemangiomas was fully appreciated in the second quarter of the twentieth century, surgical excision continued to be a primary mode of therapy (Davis and Wilgis, 1934; Matthews, 1954; Modlin, 1955).

ARTIFICIAL ULCERATION

The old observation that a hemangioma that ulcerates goes on to heal, leaving skin of a pale color, suggested that artificially induced ulceration would work as well. To this end, a variety of astringents and caustics have been applied to superficial hemangiomas, including potash and lime, fuming nitric acid, liquor arsenical, and croton oil (Gross, 1859; Kingston, 1862; Blair, 1884). Marshall (1830) described piercing a hemangioma with a lancet daubed in "vaccine lymph" to incite vesiculation, crusting, and eventual healing. Efforts to freeze hemangiomas became popular early in the current century (Pusey, 1907; Bunch, 1911). Carbon dioxide slush or solid CO_2 crayon techniques were once commonly employed (Semon, 1934; MacCollum, 1935).

ELECTROLYSIS AND THERMOCAUTERY

Hemangiomas were not overlooked in the rush to find medical applications for galvanic electricity during the Victorian era. A hot wire of silver or platinum was placed on the hemangioma, or needles were inserted subcutaneously prior to activation of a number of batteries to adjust the voltage (Knott, 1875; Coombs, 1881).

Modern thermocautery units, with a needlepoint attachment, were used to puncture deep hemangiomas, a technique called "endothermy coagulation" (MacCollum, 1935), or to cause surface coagulation (Matthews, 1954, 1968). This modality is the antecedent of today's sophisticated laser technology as a source of thermal energy to destroy hemangiomas (Apfelberg and associates, 1981; Hobby, 1983) (see Chap. 75).

SCLEROSANT THERAPY

Injection of "stimulating solutions" for treatment of hemangiomas had its shadowy beginnings in the nineteenth century: ergot (Hammond, 1876), tannic acid, carbonic acid (Bradley, 1876), iron perchloride (Hodges, 1864), and 95 per cent alcohol (Holgate, 1889). In the twentieth century, sclerosant therapy continued with 5 per cent sodium morrhuate (Watson and McCarthy, 1940), quinine hydrochloride, hypertonic saline (Andrews and Kelly, 1932), ethamolin (Matthews, 1954), and sodium tetradecyl sulfate (Walsh and Tompkins, 1956).

RADIATION

Radiation for hemangiomas was remarkably successful, reaching its heyday in the 1930 to 1950 era. Several modalities were used: thorium-X varnish (Bowers, 1951), interstitial gamma irradiation (Brown and Byars, 1938), radon brass plaques (Watson and McCarthy, 1940), and external beam irradiation (Paterson and Tod, 1939; Dana and Beyer, 1966). Long-term follow-up analysis of children given radiation for hemangiomas (300 to 600 rads) showed that, up to 20 years later, the rate of tumor incidence was no greater than that for sarcoma in the general population (Li, Cassady, and Barnett, 1974).

It is difficult to correct the late skin changes that follow irradiation for hemangioma, e.g., atrophy, contracture, pigmentation, and telangiectasia. More important, there are many well-documented cases of sarcoma developing 20 to 30 years after small radiation doses for hemangioma (Ward and Buchanan, 1977; Bennett, Keller, and Ditty, 1978). Patients treated with even low dosage radiation to the neck region have a cumulative risk of developing carcinoma of the thyroid, parathyroid dysfunction, and salivary gland tumors. Mammary hypoplasia is a disturbing problem for the young woman treated with irradiation in infancy for breast hemangioma (Skalkeas, Gogas, and Pavlatos, 1972). There are also cases of radiation-induced internal carotid artery occlusion, resulting from therapy for facial hemangioma during infancy (Wright and Bresnan, 1976).

The advent of steroid therapy for hemangiomas now limits the need for radiation therapy. Some investigators maintain that the risk-to-benefit ratio is sufficiently low for judicious irradiation to remain an alternative form of treatment for hepatic hemangiomas that are unresponsive to steroids, or for lesions that interfere with vision or obstruct vital structures, e.g., the subglottic airway (Order, 1979).

COMPRESSION

Compression therapy for hemangioma can be traced to the early nineteenth century (Abernethy, 1811; Boyer, 1815). Pressure also was advocated by Forster (1860); for an infant with a scalp hemangioma he used a lead plate, plaster of Paris, and elastic bands, applied for six to eight weeks. There are contemporary reports of success from use of compressive elastic garments for hemangiomas of the extremities (Moore, 1964; Mangus, 1972; Miller, Smith, and Shochat, 1976). In view of the predictable regression of a hemangioma, it is difficult to document the efficacy of any proposed remedy. To date, there are no controlled prospective studies to confirm the value of compression therapy.

Current Management

PRIMUM NON NOCERE

Descriptions of spontaneous involution of *naevi materni* can be found scattered throughout nineteenth century medical literature (Abernethy, 1811; Wardrop, 1818; Warren, 1837; Bobbs, 1870–1871; Duncan, 1870; Patterson, 1894). Nonetheless, confusion over the natural history of hemangiomas continued until 1938, when Lister published his prospective study. From 1931 to 1938 he observed 93 hemangiomas in 77 children and concluded: "no exception has been found to the rule that naevi which grow rapidly during the early months of life subsequently retrogress and disappear of their own accord, on the average about the fifth year of life" (Lister, 1938). Lister's findings were subsequently confirmed by others (Anderson, 1944; Brain and Calnan, 1952; Wallace, 1953; Walter, 1953; Ronchese, 1953; Blackfield and associates, 1957; Simpson, 1959; Bowers, Graham, and Tomlinson, 1960; Margileth and Museles, 1965).

Thus, for the vast majority of hemangiomas, nothing need be done; however, this does not mean that nothing *should* be done. The physician must fully appreciate the parents' anguish, since their child, who was normal at birth, now has a rapidly growing tumor. Time is well spent giving the parents a thorough explanation about the natural history of hemangioma. They will want to know what caused the growth; the mother, especially, may feel that she is at fault. Conflicting ideas from other physicians and relatives must be resolved. Photographs and measurements should be taken during the initial visit so that subsequent changes in the lesion can be documented. Textbook illustrations, showing the course of involution and late skin change of a similar hemangioma and location, are a welcome relief to the parents.

An infant with a proliferating hemangioma should be seen as often as necessary to monitor the growth and reassure the parents. More frequent visits are necessary when there is a large or ulcerated hemangioma, or when the lesion is in a critical area such as the upper eyelid or upper airway. By 6 to 8 months of age, when growth begins to plateau and early signs of regression are seen, the parents welcome comparison with earlier measurements and pictures.

LOCAL COMPLICATIONS: BLEEDING AND ULCERATION

Bleeding from a punctate area of a florid hemangioma can be a frightening problem. Parents should be instructed to press a clean pad on the bleeding point for ten minutes while watching the clock. Repeated bleeding episodes may require placement of a mattress suture. Local bleeding may also be a manifestation of systemic coagulopathy.

Ulceration is another local problem often seen in the proliferative stage. Treatment consists of cleansing, dressing changes as necessary, and daily application of a topical antibiotic ointment. If there is diffuse ulceration and cellulitis, systemic antibiotics are indicated. It often takes several weeks for an ulcerated hemangioma to heal by epithelization. Recurrent ulceration, after healing, is extremely rare.

STEROID THERAPY

In 1963 a serendipitous discovery was made at the Johns Hopkins Hospital when a large facial hemangioma began to shrink coincidentally with steroid administration for thrombocytopenia (Zarem and Edgerton, 1967). Subsequent investigators confirmed that prednisone may hasten the onset and rate of involution of hemangiomas (Fost and Esterly, 1968; Brown, Neerhout, and Fonkalsrud, 1972). The response is reported to be in the range of 30 (Bartoshesky, Bull, and Feingold, 1978) to 90 per cent (Edgerton, 1976).

Systemic steroids should be used only in selected infants with hemangioma, those with (1) a cervicofacial lesion, causing distortion of features; (2) a large lesion especially with recurrent bleeding, ulceration, and/or infection; (3) a lesion that interferes with physiologic function (breathing, vision, hearing, eating); (4) a lesion complicated by platelet depletion coagulopathy (the Kasabach-Merritt syndrome); or (5) a lesion complicated by high output cardiac failure (Fig. 66–19).

An immature (proliferating phase) hemangioma is far more responsive to steroid therapy than a mature (involuting phase) lesion in a child over 1 year of age (Edgerton, 1976). Prednisone is administered orally, 2 to 3 mg per kg per day for two to three weeks. A sensitive hemangioma shows signs of responsiveness within seven to ten days: softening, lightening of color, and diminished growth rate. If there is no effect, the steroid should be discontinued. If the hemangioma responds to steroid therapy, the dose can be lowered to 1 mg per kg per day, or the infant can be given an alternate-day regimen, with further reduction of the dose to 0.75 mg per kg per day. The steroid dosage should be tapered as soon as possible, this decision being based on the tumor's sensitivity, location, and maturity. Usually, prednisone is given for a cycle of four to six weeks followed by a rest period. A judgment to repeat the course of steroid is made based on the age, location, and initial response of the lesion. There is no reason to continue steroids after the hemangioma has entered the involuting phase. Rebound growth may occur at reduced steroid dosage in proliferating phase lesions; an additional

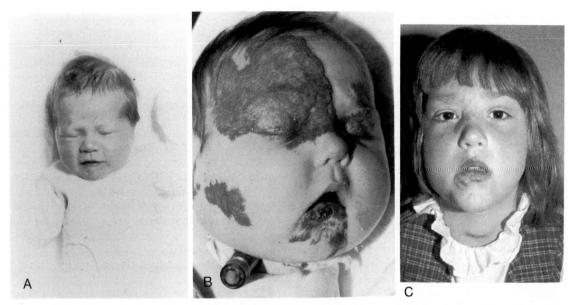

Figure 66–19. Systemic steroid therapy for an extensive hemangioma with complications. *A,* A healthy newborn girl. *B,* At age 5 months, a cervicofacial hemangioma obstructed the upper airway, necessitating tracheostomy. The patient was given systemic steroid therapy because of distortion of the facial structures, obstruction of the right eye, and lip ulceration. There is early "graying" of the hemangioma. *C,* Regression at age 5 years; additional improvement is expected. (From Mulliken, J. B., and Young, A. E.: Vascular Birthmarks: Hemangiomas and Malformations. Philadelphia, W. B. Saunders Company, 1988.)

two to three week cycle of prednisone may have to be reinstituted at a dosage of 1 mg per kg per day or on alternate days.

Few complications are seen with short-term, high dose prednisone. Infants on this regimen often evidence decreased appetite and a temporary retardation of growth. Transient facial edema also may occur, but there is no evidence of significant hypertension or salt and water retention. There are studies to document that even two doses of hydrocortisone given to a neonate may depress T-cell function and cause immunologic abnormalities (Gunn and associates, 1981). Perhaps for this reason, infants on prednisone are at increased risk of otitis media, pneumonia, and possible overwhelming sepsis. Thus, it is advisable to use the lowest effective dose of prednisone for the shortest time, until the hemangioma begins to regress.

The mechanism by which corticosteroid accelerates involution of hemangiomas is not known. There are two hypotheses. Cortisone is known to cause vasconstriction, in the presence of adrenal insufficiency, in the hamster (Wyman, Fulton, and Shulman, 1953) and the rat (Zweifach, Shor, and Black, 1953). On the basis of these studies, Edgerton (1976) proposed that the channels and sinusoids of proliferating hemangioma are sensitive

to steroids and undergo vasoconstrictive changes resulting in shrinkage of the capillaries.

Another theory is that steroids modulate control of endothelial proliferation. Folkman and associates (1983) showed that certain cortisone analogues inhibit angiogenesis in the presence of heparin and heparin fragments (Crum, Szabo, and Folkman, 1985). Sasaki, Pang, and Wittliff (1984) demonstrated that hormone receptors are important in mediating the action of glucocorticoids on proliferating hemangiomas. Using a receptor assay system, these investigators showed that hemangiomas contain increased specific estradiol 17-β binding sites, and furthermore that both low and high doses of cortisone inhibit estrogen binding to hemangioma tissue explants. They also documented that infants with hemangiomas that respond to prednisone show decreased levels of serum estradiol during therapy, compared with infants with nonresponsive hemangiomas.

CHEMOTHERAPY

There are isolated accounts of the efficacy of chemotherapeutic agents in treating hemangiomas. In the pre-steroid era, Rush (1966) used intra-arterial nitrogen mustard for a large facial hemangioma. The alkylating agent was administered when the child was 8 months old and when the lesion had reached a plateau in its growth curve. Cyclophosphamide has been used successfully in three infants with life-threatening pleuropericardial and liver hemangiomas that failed to respond to either systemic steroids or radiation therapy (Hurvitz and associates, 1986).

EMERGENT PROBLEMS IN THE PROLIFERATION PHASE

Upper Eyelid Hemangioma and Intralesional Steroids. Steroid administration is the treatment of choice if the hemangioma occludes the visual axis or causes astigmatism, strabismus, or anisometropia. *Intralesional* steroid injection for hemangiomas was introduced as a way to minimize the systemic effects of oral administration. This approach was first reported in a series of 115 children by Azzolini and Nouvenne (1970). Although periorbital hemangiomas respond to oral prednisone (De Venecia and Lobeck, 1970), the intralesional route has special application for lesions in this location (Zak and Morin, 1981; Kushner, 1979, 1985; Brown and Huffaker, 1982). The dosage is calculated on the basis of the child's weight and the size of the hemangioma. Kushner (1985) recommended that each treatment should not exceed the injection of more than 40 mg triamcinolone acetate and 6 mg betamethasone. The infant is usually placed under light general anesthesia. A 27 gauge needle is used and multiple punctures are necessary to distribute the steroid throughout the lesion. The response rate is in the 60 to 80 per cent range, although a second injection six to eight weeks later is usually necessary (Fig. 66–20) (Kushner, 1985). Local injection of steroids commonly results in cholestin plaque deposits and soft tissue atrophy; however, both problems are temporary (Kushner, 1985). Patching the noninvolved eye forces the use of the affected eye and minimizes the development of amblyopia and strabismus.

Intralesional steroid injection for eyelid hemangiomas carries an attendant risk of hemorrhage or hematoma in the retrobulbar space, both a threat to vision. Occlusion of the central retinal artery and damage to the optic nerve can occur after retrobulbar injection of corticosteroid (Ellis, 1978). There is also the danger of accidental intraocular injection of depot steroid (Zinn, 1981). Because of these potential complications, one should hesitate before using intralesional injection for a hemangioma that extends posteriorly into the orbital cone. Alternatively, systemic steroids should be considered when there is periorbital hemangiomatous infiltration and ocular proptosis.

In rare instances, surgical excision, total or subtotal, can be employed for a localized hemangioma of the upper eyelid (Azzolini and associates, 1983). Embolization has also been utilized when there is partial or complete ocular occlusion (Burrows and associates, 1987). In the past, radiation therapy was commonplace for palpebral hemangioma. However, this modality carries a risk of causing a cataract (Bek and Zahn, 1960) and it has been superseded by steroid therapy.

Subglottic Hemangioma. Any infant with a cutaneous hemangioma, particularly if in the cervicofacial region, and who presents with persistent respiratory stridor should be suspected of having a laryngeal hemangioma. The diagnosis is confirmed by endoscopy, and treatment is determined by the size and extent of the subglottic narrowing. The older infant with minimal airway obstruction can be closely observed, because the hemangioma is entering the involution phase. The younger infant whose airway is not severely compromised should be given a trial of oral prednisone, but watched closely (Cohen and Wang, 1972; Overcash and Putney, 1973). An infant who presents with high grade obstruction and recurrent airway problems is a candidate for tracheostomy or CO_2 laser excision. Healy, McGill, and Friedman (1984) reported a high rate of success using the CO_2 laser to excise obstructive subglottic hemangiomas. There is no evidence that laser coagulation accelerates involution. Rather, the airway is physically opened by laser excision and by subsequent scarring of the remaining tissues. The rare circumferential subglottic hemangioma should not be treated by CO_2 laser excision because of the increased likelihood of subglottic stenosis (Healy, McGill, and Friedman, 1984); the laser is also not indicated in cases with diffuse hemangiomatous involvement of the mediastinum.

Tracheostomy may be necessary in cases of extensive airway hemangioma, or in infants who fail to respond to systemic steroids. After the hemangioma is well into its regression phase, with or without the help of steroids, the child can be safely decannulated.

External beam radiation probably no

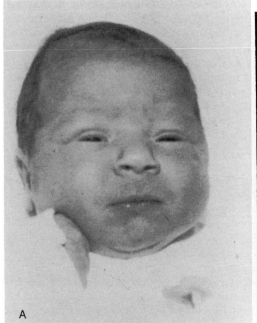

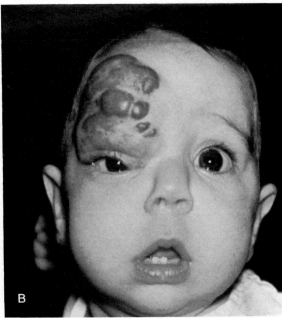

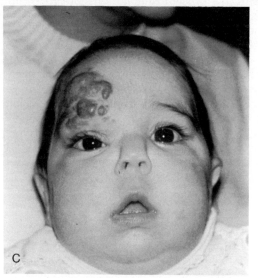

Figure 66–20. Intralesional steroid therapy for an upper eyelid hemangioma causing visual complications. *A,* Appearance at birth. *B,* A 6 month old infant with astigmatism in the right eye secondary to an upper eyelid hemangioma. *C,* Two weeks after a second intralesional injection of triamcinolone (100 mg), there is shrinkage of the eyelid tumor and opening of the palpebral fissure. (From Mulliken, J. B., and Young, A. E.: Vascular Birthmarks: Hemangiomas and Malformations. Philadelphia, W. B. Saunders Company, 1988.)

longer has a role in the management of subglottic hemangioma (Tefft, 1966). Implantation of radioactive gold grains was advocated by Benjamin and Carter (1983). Embolization (with polyvinyl alcohol–calibrated particles) is reportedly useful to treat obstructing subglottic hemangioma (Burrows and associates, 1987).

Cutaneous-Visceral Hemangiomatosis with Congestive Heart Failure. There appears to be a critical mass of hemangiomatous tissue beyond which high output congestive heart failure and systemic clotting changes

are likely to develop. These infants, fortunately rare, usually have combined cutaneous and hepatic hemangiomas, and even less frequently an isolated giant cutaneous hemangioma. There is a high morbidity and mortality rate (approaching 50 per cent) after bleeding and cardiac complications occur (deLorimier and associates, 1967). However, even large asymptomatic liver hemangiomas may resolve spontaneously without the need for therapy (Matolo and Johnson, 1973).

If signs and symptoms of congestive heart failure develop in the presence of a large cutaneous hemangioma or visceral hemangiomas, the following scheme of management is suggested (Larcher, Howard, and Mowat, 1981; Pereyra, Andrassy, and Mahour, 1982). Digoxin and diuretics and fluid restriction are instituted along with prednisone, at an initial dose of 2 mg per kg per day. Cutaneous hemangiomas are observed for signs of early "graying" and softening, as a simple way to judge the response to steroids. Serial determination of cardiac output by echocardiography may be needed to monitor the effectiveness of steroids. Ultrasonography and/or computed tomography can be repeated to document shrinkage of liver hemangiomas during the course of steroid therapy. There is diminution of hepatomegaly and control of congestive heart failure in 70 per cent of patients treated medically (Rocchini and associates, 1976; Clemmensen, 1979; Pereyra, Andrassy, and Mahour, 1982).

If medical management fails, i.e., if there is no improvement in the infant's condition after a 10 to 14 day trial of systemic steroids, angiography should be performed in preparation for either embolic therapy or surgical intervention. Digital subtraction radiography clearly demonstrates the rapid flow into liver hemangiomas, with typically enlarged hepatic arteries and other dilated intercostal and subphrenic vessels (Fig. 66–21*A*).

Embolization with Gelfoam has been tried for hepatic hemangioma; however, renal infarction is a potential complication (Tegtmeyer and associates, 1977). A remarkable example of the efficacy of Gelfoam pellet embolization for a giant hemangioma of the thigh and pelvis was documented by Argenta and associates (1982). Tiny coils can be used to obliterate the hepatic artery proximal to the hemangiomas, a useful adjunctive method to control congestive heart failure until involution begins (Fig. 66–21*B*).

If embolic therapy is not available or if this approach is unsuccessful in controlling the congestive failure, surgical therapy is necessary. Hepatic artery ligation, first successfully performed by deLorimier and associates (1967), has been repeated by others (Laird and associates, 1976; Keller and Bluhm, 1979; Shannon, Buchanan, and Votteler, 1982). Larcher, Howard, and Mowat (1981) recommended that any infant under 6 weeks of age presenting with intractable cardiac failure should be considered for immediate hepatic artery ligation. Arterial ligation alone, however, may fail to control symptoms, and this procedure is not without its hazards: e.g., liver necrosis and abscess formation have occurred (Pereyra, Andrassy, and Mahour, 1982).

Rupture and/or intraperitoneal hemorrhage from liver hemangiomas may necessitate hepatic resection, but because the liver is usually diffusely involved, hepatic lobectomy may not be effective (Touloukian, 1970). When the hemangioma is localized, liver resection can be performed successfully, but this is not without risk, even in the absence of high output congestive heart failure (Wag-

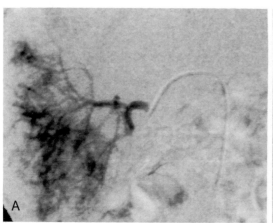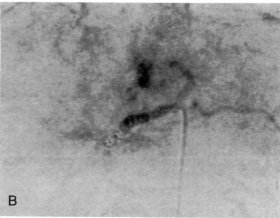

Figure 66–21. Embolization for hepatic hemangioma. *A,* Digital subtraction angiography: selective injection of the right hepatic artery demonstratres enlarged branches feeding a hemangioma of the right lobe (see Fig. 66–15*A*). *B,* Repeat injection into the celiac artery following embolization of the right hepatic artery with three minicoils. Note the absent filling with reflux into the left hepatic and splenic arteries. (Courtesy of K. E. Fellows.) (From Mulliken, J. B., and Young, A. E.: Vascular Birthmarks: Hemangiomas and Malformations. Philadelphia, W. B. Saunders Company, 1988.)

get, Inkster, and Ashcroft, 1969; Matolo and Johnson, 1973).

There is a remarkable case report of a massive pelvic hemangioma, causing intractable congestive heart failure, successfully treated by ligation of the hypogastric arterial supply and subtotal excision (Price and associates, 1972).

Radiotherapy may still play a role in the treatment of hepatic hemangiomas (Park and Phillips, 1970; Dehner and Ishak, 1971; Kagan, Jaffe, and Kennamer, 1971). However, most authors cite the associated increased mortality for irradiation, and suggest that it not be employed unless other forms of therapy are contraindicated or unsuccessful (McLean and associates, 1972; Larcher, Howard, and Mowat, 1981).

Berman and Lim (1978) reviewed the world literature on concurrent cutaneous and hepatic hemangiomas and found the mortality rate to be 81 per cent if no treatment was given, in contrast to 29 per cent for infants who received early aggressive therapy in the form of either steroids, hepatic irradiation, hepatic artery ligation, or lobectomy. The overall mortality rate in 59 cases of combined cutaneous-hepatic hemangiomas was 54 per cent.

Coagulopathy (Kasabach-Merritt Syndrome). Profound thrombocytopenia can occur in the presence of a large cutaneous hemangioma or combined cutaneous-visceral hemangiomatosis. Infants seem to tolerate moderately severe thrombocytopenia without bleeding because of their relative immobility (Esterly, 1983). Therefore, if there is no evidence of bleeding, aggressive therapy to control a low platelet count is not indicated. The Kasabach-Merritt syndrome is a self-limited condition. The platelet level always returns to normal after the hemangioma regresses (Wallerstein, 1961) or is excised (Hill and Longino, 1962).

If there is evidence of thrombocytopenia and bleeding without an associated consumptive coagulopathy, steroid therapy should be considered (Evans and associates, 1975). For an individual infant, the decision to treat must be weighed against the potential hazards of untoward steroid effects. Young infants given prednisone are at increased risk of developing life-threatening sepsis. A two to four week period of prednisone administration, 2 to 4 mg per kg per day, is necessary for an adequate trial (Esterly, 1983).

Cyclophosphamide therapy is another alternative if the hemangioma fails to respond to steroids, and life-threatening bleeding continues (Hurvitz and associates, 1986). For a localized giant hemangioma with coagulopathy, Gelfoam embolization should also be considered (Argenta and associates, 1982).

Another hematologic approach is to remedy the thrombocytopenia. There is no specific platelet count that can be used as a guide for treatment in the absence of bleeding. Platelet transfusions are unlikely to be beneficial since the thrombocytopenia is secondary to increased platelet trapping and destruction. Koerper and associates (1983) reported an increase in platelet counts in infants with platelet trapping syndromes, including hemangiomas, after treatment with double-agent antiplatelet therapy, i.e., aspirin and dipyridamole. However, Sondel and associates (1984) found that there was no benefit from antiplatelet therapy for the Kasabach-Merritt syndrome.

LASER THERAPY

There are publications advocating argon laser treatment of hemangiomas in the proliferative phase (Apfelberg and associates, 1981; Hobby, 1983). Argon laser penetrates the skin, and the blue-green light is absorbed by red cells within the hemangioma and normal vessels in the papillary dermis (see Chap. 75). The absorbed light energy is transformed into heat, causing thrombosis or destruction of the vascular channels and perivascular tissue. Thermal damage within the skin may cause ulceration of the superficial portion of the hemangioma; the end result is scar. Persistence of the deep hemangioma is commonly seen after argon laser therapy. This finding is understandable because currently available argon lasers do not penetrate deeper than 1.5 mm into the skin, a depth hardly sufficient to damage more than the superficial layer of most cutaneous hemangiomas. At the present time, argon laser treatment cannot be recommended for the common cutaneous hemangioma of infancy. Laser is useful in treating capillary dermal malformations (as discussed in Chap. 75).

OPERATIVE THERAPY

If every hemangioma began as a localized nest of cells, the ideal treatment would logically be early excision before the tumor extended into the surrounding dermis (Modlin,

1955; Andrews and associates, 1957). However, there are two flaws in this logic track. First, the hemangioma that is small when first seen may well be destined to remain diminutive. In this instance, lenticular excision may leave a more obvious scar than the skin changes that follow natural involution. Second, a particular hemangioma's size and distribution seem to be predetermined; i.e., it begins as a field transformation that may include skin, the subcutaneous layer, and muscle. Therefore, an extensive nascent lesion is out of bounds for simple excision at the outset. Third, from a practical viewpoint, most infants do not come to medical attention until the hemangioma has reached a size at which excision would be disfiguring.

The great majority of hemangiomas should be left alone, allowing proliferation and involution to run their course. Nevertheless, there are definable stages in the hemangioma life cycle when excision should be considered. The windows for surgical therapy are conveniently divided into (1) infancy, (2) early childhood or preschool years, and (3) late childhood to early adolescence.

During Infancy. There are rare indications for operative therapy in infancy. A possible case in point is the isolated hemangioma of the upper eyelid, causing obstruction of vision or astigmatism (Thomson and associates, 1979). Surgical excision may also be useful for an eyelid hemangioma that fails to respond to steroid therapy, or for a more mature hemangioma that is unlikely to respond (Fig. 66–22). Superficial parotidectomy once was advised for hemangioma, the most common parotid tumor of infancy, but is no longer recommended. There are excellent results following involution of parotid hemangiomas, particularly considering the difficulty of complete removal and the danger of facial nerve damage in infants (Williams, 1975).

During Early Childhood (Preschool). Excision of a hemangioma may be indicated for psychosocial reasons before or at the time of school attendance. A facial hemangioma can seriously interfere with the emerging awareness of body image in a 3 to 5 year old child. A child with a facial hemangioma is usually accepted by nursery school and kindergarden classmates. Psychologic trouble is more likely to develop during the first grade when the child is exposed to older classmates.

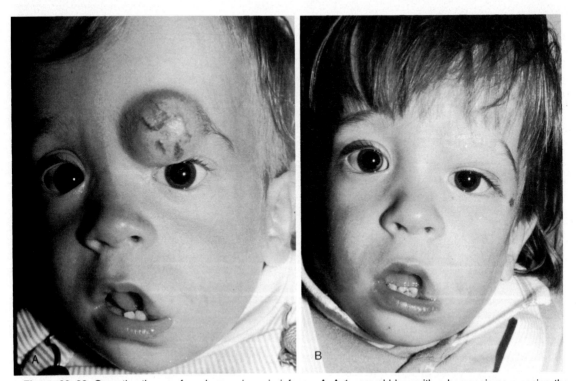

Figure 66–22. Operative therapy for a hemangioma in infancy. *A,* A 1 year old boy with a hemangioma pressing the upper cornea, resulting in 1.5 diopters astigmatism. *B,* No residual astigmatism in the eye nine months after subtotal excision of the hemangioma. (From Mulliken, J. B., and Young, A. E.: Vascular Birthmarks: Hemangiomas and Malformations. Philadelphia, W. B. Saunders Company, 1988.)

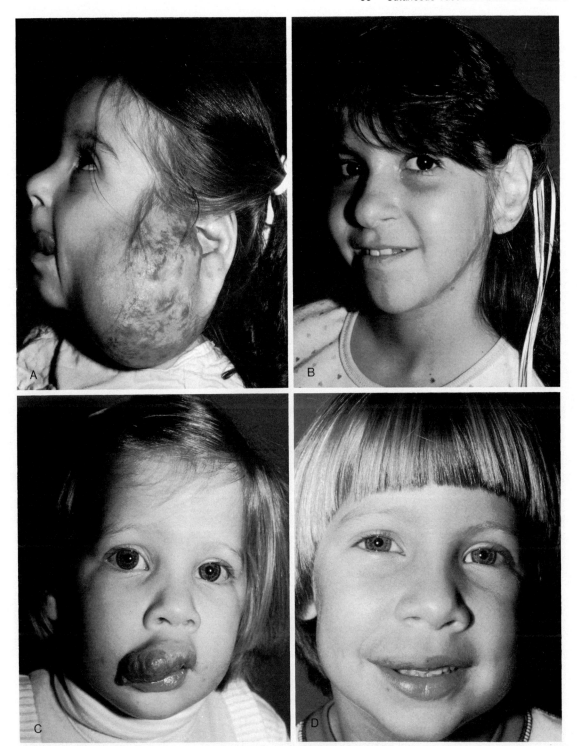

Figure 66–23. Operative therapy for hemangioma in early childhood. *A,* A large facial hemangioma in a 2½ year old girl. *B,* Redundant skin and tumor were excised at age 4 years; dissection was performed superficial to the seventh cranial nerve. Appearance at age 10 years. Note the auricular enlargement, a rare example of skeletal hypertrophy secondary to a hemangioma. *C,* A 5 year old girl with involuting phase hemangioma of the lip. Even with complete regression, excess mucosa and submucosa remain. *D,* One year after contour excision. (From Mulliken, J. B., and Young, A. E.: Vascular Birthmarks: Hemangiomas and Malformations. Philadelphia, W. B. Saunders Company, 1988.)

Thus, excision to improve contour may be undertaken in special circumstances, particularly when it is obvious that skin resection will be necessary in the future, notwithstanding the final result from involution. The skin expansion effect of a large hemangioma may result in redundant skin, after regression. Removing the central section of the lesion improves contour and minimizes the child's body image distortion (Fig. 66–23A,B). A hemangioma of the vermilion mucosa often remains quite bulky and should be considered for contour excision during this time frame (Fig. 66–23C,D). Glabellar and eyebrow lesions, particularly if there is central scarring, should be evaluated for subtotal excision before the child's entry into school. The excisional axis should be placed within the relaxed skin tension lines. Resection should not be overzealous for fear of causing later contour deformity. Residual fibrofatty tissue can always be removed when the child is older.

The nose is a psychologically sensitive focus. Nasal tip hemangiomas are notoriously slow to show regression, and they often leave behind a mass of fibrofatty tissue. Thomson and associates (1979), in a small series of patients, documented that the results without active treatment of nasal tip lesions surpassed those managed by excision (Fig. 66–24). However, in carefully selected children, there is a role for subtotal removal to improve nasal contour. Nasal hemangiomas are usually spheroidal; there is a natural tendency to envision a need for both a transverse and a vertical wedge excision. A useful technique is a low "flying bird" skin excision, in conjunction with subtotal removal of the hemangioma and approximation of the splayed alar cartilages (Fig. 66–25). Care should be taken not to remove too much tissue, which in time, and with continued involution, might produce a blunt nasal tip.

During Late Childhood and Adolescence. It is usually best to wait until the child is 8 to 12 years of age before trimming the residual skin that exists after regression. The skin often looks remarkably normal, particularly if the hemangioma involved only the reticular dermis. More often, the skin is

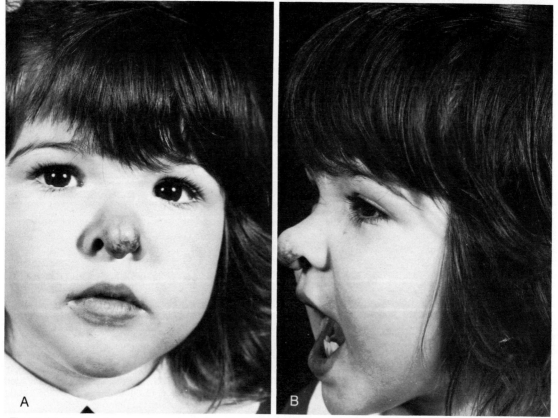

Figure 66–24. Nasal hemangioma: involution. *A,* A 1 year old girl with a nasal hemangioma. *B,* Profile at 1 year of age.

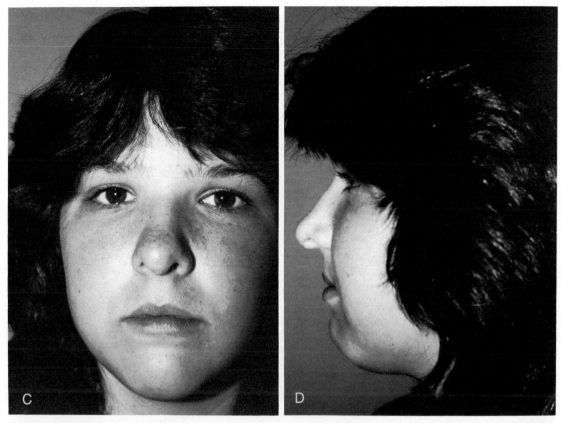

Figure 66–24 *Continued C,* Result of normal involution at age 15. *D,* Profile: note the change in the columellolabial angle.

atrophic and contains tiny telangiectatic vessels. If there was ulceration during the proliferative phase, this area becomes a hypopigmented or yellow-tan scar. There is usually sufficient extra skin remnant after involution for linear closure to be easily accomplished. If there is insufficient normal skin, linear closure can be facilitated by preliminary skin expansion. Staged excision is also useful, particularly for involuted hemangiomas of the lip, cheeks, glabella, and scalp (Fig. 66–26). Blepharoplasty and rhytidoplasty types of excisions are helpful in order to tighten the loose, crepelike skin that may remain after involution of large facial hemangiomas. Ptosis correction and eyelid revision are often necessary after regression of an upper eyelid lesion.

During infancy, facial structures can be destroyed by an ulcerated and secondarily infected hemangioma. Although it is tempting to correct a soft tissue defect with a local flap (e.g., from the cheek or forehead), it is best to use tissue expansion techniques in order to minimize further scarring on a child's face. An anatomic defect can also be reconstructed by using tissue transferred from a distant donor site.

VASCULAR MALFORMATIONS

Pathogenesis

Vascular malformations are structural abnormalities, the result of errors in morphogenic processes that shape the embryonic vascular system between the fourth and tenth weeks of intrauterine life. The anomalies are almost always sporadic, nonfamilial aberrations. There are, by contrast, a few inheritable vascular abnormalities, such as the Rendu-Osler-Weber syndrome, Fabry's disease, and ataxia-telangiectasia. Not all vascular malformations are "congenital," i.e., obvious at birth; many of the abnormalities manifest themselves years or decades postnatally.

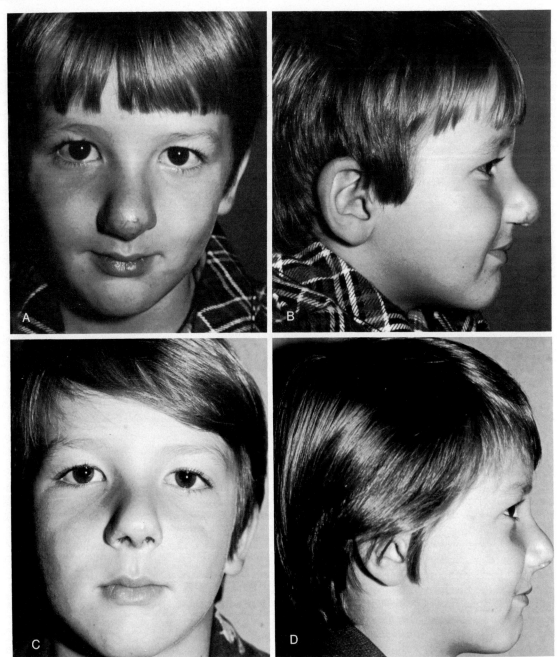

Figure 66–25. Nasal hemangioma: contour excision in childhood. *A,* A 6 year old boy with nasal hemangioma. *B,* Preoperative profile. *C,* Frontal view two years postoperatively. *D,* Lateral view two years postoperatively. (From Mulliken, J. B., and Young, A. E.: Vascular Birthmarks: Hemangiomas and Malformations. Philadelphia, W. B. Saunders Company, 1988.)

EMBRYOLOGY OF THE BLOOD VASCULAR SYSTEM

Current opinion is that the embryonic endothelium of all vascular tissue arises in situ directly from primitive mesenchyme (the "local origin theory"). However, the investing pericytes and smooth muscle cells are derived from neuroectoderm (neural crest) and not from mesoderm (Sabin, 1902, 1920; Woollard, 1922; Woollard and Harpman, 1937).

In the first stage, undifferentiated mesenchymal cells aggregate in islands and cords; cells on the periphery of these structures subsequently develop into definitive angio-

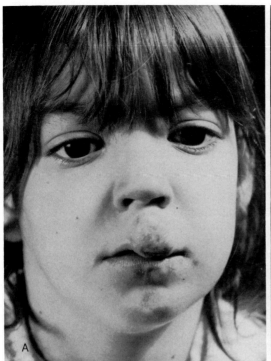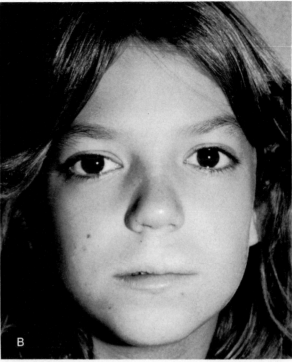

Figure 66–26. Excision of an involuted hemangioma during late childhood. *A,* A 7 year old girl with residual hemangioma of the upper lip (despite 275 rads given during the early proliferative phase). *B,* At age 11 years after two stage excision in the transverse and vertical axes. (From Mulliken, J. B., and Young, A. E.: Vascular Birthmarks: Hemangiomas and Malformations. Philadelphia, W. B. Saunders Company, 1988.)

blasts, forming primal capillary structures. In the next stage, there is coalescence of contiguous capillary channels and the disappearance of others, forming a network of vessels called the *retiform plexus.* The final stage is development of mature vessels. In the upper limb the central artery becomes the subclavian-axillary trunk, whereas below the elbow it persists as a tiny interosseous artery. In the lower limb the axial artery forms the femoropopliteal vessels.

EMBRYOLOGY OF THE LYMPHATIC SYSTEM

The lymphatic system develops later than the blood vascular system and its morphogenesis may be influenced by the blood vascular system. Sabin (1902, 1904, 1905), using India ink injections in pig embryos, showed that lymphatic vessels grow out into the surrounding mesenchyme from lymph sacs that are derived from veins. Lewis (1905–1906) confirmed her findings in the rabbit embryo, and also noted that the lymphatic sacs separate from parent veins and later make new con-

nections. The "centrifugal sprouting theory" of Sabin-Lewis is supported by studies in human embryos (35 to 65 days old) (van der Putte, 1977). The jugular, subclavian, thoracic, retroperitoneal, and ilioinguinal lymph sacs appear between the second and sixth weeks of intrauterine life. From the seventh week onward the jugular channels spread to connect with the subclavian (axillary) lymph sacs. The juguloaxillary complex extends caudally to anastomose with the internal thoracic and ilioinguinal channels (Patten, 1968). By the ninth week the thoracic duct is a continuous channel, opening at its cephalic end into the left jugular sac and draining into the internal jugular-subclavian vein junction. Extensions of the jugular sac channels propagate into the head, neck, and upper limb and connect with lymphatic channels that have sprouted from peripheral veins. In a similar fashion, extensions from the ilioinguinal channels grow outward to join the peripheral lymphatics of the lower limb. All processes are complete by the 12th week, although the system does not have a full set of competent valves until the beginning of the fifth month (Kampmeier, 1969).

MALDEVELOPMENTS

The Woollard drawings of the developing limb bud vasculature have served as inspiration for theories of the pathogenesis of vascular anomalies (Rienhoff, 1924; de-Takats, 1932; Malan, 1974; Szilagyi and associates, 1976; Kaplan, 1983; Mulliken, 1982). These are merely speculations about how an error, at any particular developmental stage, might be expressed as a malformation. During the stage of the undifferentiated capillary network, disorganization in cell movement, patterning, or segregation could cause a vascular abnormality (Mulliken, 1982). Sequestrated and maldeveloped areas, during the retiform plexus stage, could result in either a capillary, venous, or lymphatic malformation or combined low flow malformation. Failure of regression of arteriovenous communications could cause isolated fistulas and other types of high flow anomalies (Fig. 66–27). In the later developmental stages, vascular trunks may form improperly, leaving the deep vessel aplasias and hypoplasias of the Klippel-Trenaunay syndrome in which, in addition, embryonic vessels such as the postaxial vein of the leg may fail to regress (Young, 1988a).

Theories to explain lymphatic anomalies also derive from classical descriptive embryology. It can be envisioned that cystic types of cervicofacial, thoracic, and axillary malformations ("cystic hygromas") are the result of dysmorphogenesis of the primitive jugular, subclavian, and axillary sacs. It is possible that there is a failure to reestablish venous connections (Fig. 66–28). Later in embryogenesis, errors within the developing peripheral lymphatics produce small channel anomalies, in a spectrum ranging from localized "lymphangiomas" to aplasias and hypoplasias, presenting as lymphedema. The cutaneous lymphatic anomalies ("lymphangioma circumscriptum") have been attributed to obstruction of the deep lymph trunks in the embryo, with the obstruction causing back-up of lymph into the cutaneous lym-

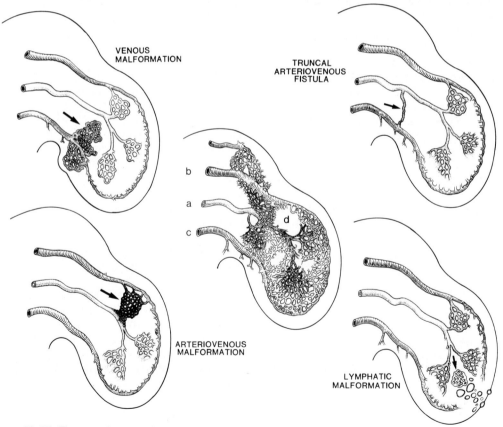

Figure 66–27. The vascular rete of the embryonic anterior limb bud (equivalent to a 6 week human embryo) (after Woollard, H. H., 1922). a = retiform central (axial) artery; b = cephalic vein; c = basilic vein; d = primitive capillary plexus undergoing resorption. Maldevelopment, during this stage, results in low flow or high flow vascular anomalies.

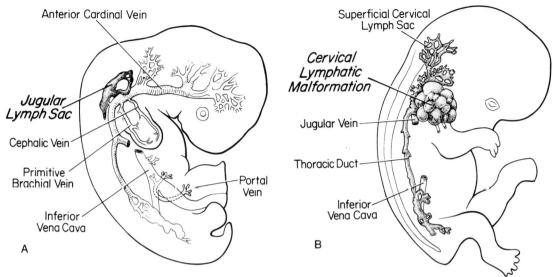

Figure 66–28. Embryology of the cervical lymphatic malformation. *A,* Relationship of the developing jugular lymph sac to the venous system in a 6 week human embryo. *B,* A cystic cervical lymphatic anomaly in a 9 week human embryo, perhaps the result of failure of reconnections between the jugular sac system and the internal jugular vein. (Redrawn after Sabin, F. R. *In* Keibel, F., and Mall, F. P., Eds.: Manual of Human Embryology. Philadelphia, J. B. Lippincott Company, 1910.)

phatic vessels. This hypothesis emanates from the perceived similarity in the clinical appearance of cutaneous lymphatic anomalies and the skin vesicles that occur after lymphatic obstruction secondary to an operation or radiotherapy. An alternative theory is that cutaneous lymph anomalies represent a failure of regression of sequestrated peripheral lymphatic channels (Young, 1988a).

The etiology of lymphedema (see Chap. 83) has been assumed, until recently, to be on the basis of "hypoplasia" of the lymphatic vessels as visualized on lymphography. Studies demonstrate fibrosis in lymph nodes and delayed transit time through nodes, suggesting that the primary fault may not be in the lymphatic vessels but in the nodes themselves, the observed hypoplasia and nonfilling of distal lymphatics being merely the result of secondary obstruction and stagnation (Kinmonth and Eustace, 1976; Kinmonth and Wolfe, 1980).

THEORIES OF MECHANISM

Hemodynamic Theories

Little is known about how, or at exactly which stage, vascular malformations occur. Thoma (1893) was first to propose "laws" that govern how hemodynamics influence vascular morphogenesis: (1) the velocity of blood flow determines vascular caliber, (2) the length of a vessel is determined by the pulling force by surrounding tissues, (3) the thickness of the vessel wall is determined by the pressure exerted by the blood flow, and (4) increased terminal blood pressure results in formation of new capillaries. Factors other than pressure and velocity of blood flow must be important in vascular morphogenesis: for example, biochemical and hormonal factors (Ryan and Barnhill, 1983). However, the inability of known teratogens, toxins, chemicals, or trauma to produce an anomaly resembling a human vascular malformation is remarkable and suggests that simple aberrations in local physiochemical factors may not be responsible (Young, 1988a).

There is evidence that skeletal anomalies, seen in association with vascular anomalies, may be secondary to abnormal blood flow in utero. Studies of fluid dynamics in the developing chicken wing have shown that flow in the peripheral limb mesoderm is subcompartmentalized in an anteroposterior fashion, whereas the limb core has differential flow in a proximodistal direction (Caplan and Koutroupas, 1973; Jargiello and Caplan, 1983). This finding suggests that differential blood flow may affect mesodermal microenvironments, e.g., specific nutrient and oxygen levels, and thus determine limb skeletal morphogenesis.

A hemodynamic explanation has been proposed for the complex pattern of the Klippel-

Trenaunay syndrome (capillary-lymphatic-venous malformation with skeletal overgrowth). Failure of normal regression of embryonic precapillary arteriovenous connections could cause an increase in the size and number of veins and could be responsible for the predictable histologic changes of venous intimal thickening, elastosis, and ectasia (Coget and Merlen, 1980). Increased blood flow and decreased capillary resistance would cause mild venous hypertension, which experimentally can result in increased bone growth and superficial varicosities (Baskerville, Ackroyd, and Browse, 1985).

Further insight into the importance of hemodynamic factors is provided by studies of the process of vascular growth in the presence of tumor (Folkman, 1974; Folkman and Cotran, 1976). Capillary endothelium, derived from fetal and adult tissue, is capable of forming a network of tubules in tissue culture—"angiogenesis in vitro" (Folkman and Haudenschild, 1980). Thus, patterning of embryonic endothelium to form a plexus can also presumably occur in the absence of blood flow.

Theories Relating to the Nervous System

In the first review paper on vascular malformations, Trélat and Monod (1869) espoused the "neurovegetative" theory that the primary fault occurs in the developing autonomic nervous system. This theory is supported by the clinical finding of cutaneous capillary malformations in what appear to be a "metameric" distribution, and the occasional finding of hyperhidrosis over vascular malformations. The geographic patterns seen with port-wine stains, particularly along the trigeminal nerve distribution, also suggest an etiologic relationship to the developing peripheral nervous system. Neuroectoderm is known to contribute the pericytes and smooth muscle cells to vascular walls (Johnston, 1966; Nozue and Tsuzaki, 1974); thus, abnormal development of neuroectodermal elements might be implicated in vascular malformation. The neurogenic hypothesis is supported by the finding of decreased perivascular nerve density in port-wine stains (Smoller and Rosen, 1986).

Genetic Mechanisms

Even familial vascular anomalies are not necessarily "congenital," i.e., observed at birth. In the *Rendu-Osler-Weber syndrome* (hereditary hemorrhagic telangiectasia) the skin and mucosal lesions may appear in early childhood, or more commonly may emerge after puberty. Inherited in an autosomal dominant pattern, the genetic abnormality is revealed as a structural weakness of the walls of small vessels (Jahnke, 1970). *Fabry's disease* ("angiokeratoma corporis diffusum universale") is a rare, sex-linked recessive disorder of sphingolipid metabolism manifested by cutaneous vascular papules and progressive and fatal cardiorenal failure (Desnick and Sweeley, 1987). *Fucosidosis* is another enzymatic deficiency disorder that may present with diffuse keratotic vascular lesions over the trunk and upper legs (Smith and associates, 1977). *Ataxia-telangiectasia* (Louis-Bar syndrome) is transmitted by an autosomal recessive gene and is characterized by cerebellar ataxia, severe immunologic deficiency, and the appearance of cutaneous and ocular telangiectasias during early childhood (Kraemer, 1987).

LOW FLOW VASCULAR MALFORMATIONS

Capillary Malformations (CM)

PORT-WINE STAINS

These birthmarks are often incorrectly categorized as "capillary hemangioma" or by the Latin appellation *nevus (naevus) flammeus*. At a cellular level, these are not proliferative lesions. Port-wine stains and various other telangiectasias belong under the broad heading of low flow vascular malformations (capillary type) (Mulliken and Glowacki, 1982).

Port-wine stains have an equal gender distribution and are seen in 0.3 per cent of newborn infants (Jacobs and Walton, 1976). The skin discoloration is usually, but not always, evident at birth; the stain may be hidden by the erythema of neonatal skin or may not be visible because of neonatal anemia.

Forty-five per cent of facial port-wine stains are restricted to one of the three trigeminal sensory areas (Enjolras, Riché, and Merland, 1985). Conversely, 55 per cent of facial port-wine stains are noted to overlap sensory dermatomes, cross the midline, or occur bilaterally (Fig. 66–29A). The mucous membranes are often involved contiguously with facial

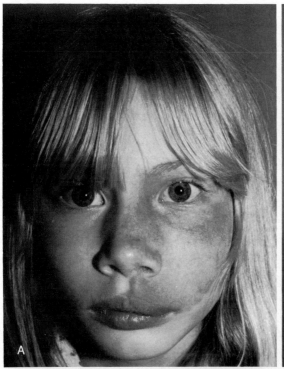
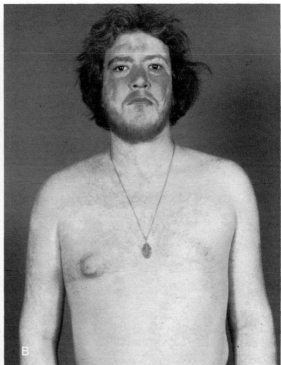
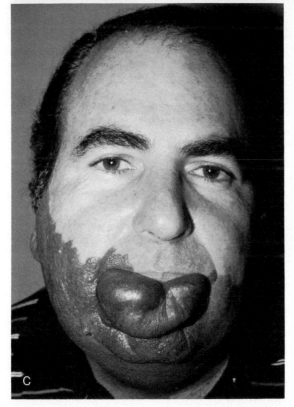

Figure 66–29. Patterns of port-wine stains. *A,* Dermal stain in V1 and entire V2 distribution with slight overgrowth of the lip and maxilla. The brain CT scan and ophthalmologic examinations are normal. *B,* Diffuse staining of the face, the trunk, and all extremities; there is no evidence of central nervous system involvement. Note the breast asymmetry. *C,* V3 port wine stain in a 42 year old male. Note the dark color, soft tissue overgrowth, nodular areas, and venous ectasia of the lower lip. (From Mulliken, J. B., and Young, A. E.: Vascular Birthmarks: Hemangiomas and Malformations. Philadelphia, W. B. Saunders Company, 1988.)

capillary malformations. Diffuse scattered staining, in geographic patterns, may occur over the trunk and extremities, in association with or in the absence of a facial vascular birthmark (Fig. 66–29*B*).

A port-wine stain is flat and sharply demarcated, and grows proportionately with the child. The color ranges from pale pink to deep red, the hue deepening when the child cries, has a fever, or is in a warm environment. The pink flush, characteristic of infancy, gradually darkens to a deep red shade during young adulthood, and to a purple color during middle age. With aging, the surface of the port-wine stain often becomes studded with nodular lesions; in addition, soft tissue and skeletal hypertrophy may become more obvious (Fig. 66–29*C*). Pyogenic granulomas frequently develop within port-wine stained skin; this is particularly common with intraoral stains (Swerlick and Cooper, 1983) (see Fig. 66–12*A*).

On microscopic examination, a port-wine stain is characterized by ectatic capillary to venular sized channels within both the papillary and upper reticular dermis. The vessels are thin walled and lined by flat, mature endothelium with undetectable cellular turnover (Mulliken and Glowacki, 1982). More detailed histologic studies by Barsky and associates (1980) showed that a port-wine stain consists of an increased number of abnormally dilated vessels in the dermis. By using immunoperoxidase staining techniques, a decrease in perivascular nerve density was noted by Smoller and Rosen (1986). The neural deficit may be responsible for altered vascular tone and thus may contribute to the progressive ectasia seen in port-wine stains.

Associated Morphogenetic Deformities

The literature is replete with references to port-wine stains in association with specific malformation syndromes. Most of these, however, are cases of mistaken identity and more accurately refer to the common macular neonatal stain of the glabellofrontal area that predictably fades with time (see *nevus flammeus neonatorum*, p. 3234).

Port-wine marks may occur in conjunction with other vascular anomalies. On the trunk or the extremities, there may be coexistent venous and lymphatic abnormalities (the Klippel-Trenaunay syndrome). A vascular stain may signify a deep arteriovenous malformation anywhere on the body, as mani-

fested by signs of increased circulatory flow, e.g., elevated skin temperature, bruit, and thrill.

Port-wine stains often accompany developmental defects of the central neural axis. A capillary stain on the posterior thorax may indicate an underlying arteriovenous malformation of the spinal cord (Cobb's syndrome) (Cobb, 1915; Doppman and associates, 1969; Jessen, Thompson and Smith, 1977). However, less than one-fourth of spinal vascular malformations have an associated cutaneous stain that may or may not be segmental (Aminoff, 1988). A vascular blemish located over the midline lower lumbar region is also a "red flag" signaling possible underlying spinal dysraphism, lipomeningocele, tethered spinal cord, and diastematomyelia (Fig. 66–30*A,B*). There may be subtle signs of neurogenic bladder dysfunction or lower extremity weakness; careful neurologic examination, spinal radiography, and bladder function studies are indicated (Bauer, 1988). An infant with an occipital dermal stain and abnormal hair tuft may have an underlying meningoencephalocele (Fig. 66–30*C,D*). A facial port-wine stain may be seen with a unilateral arteriovenous malformation of the retina and intracranial optic pathway, an entity known by the syndromic terms Bonnet-Dechaume-Blanc in the French literature (Bonnet, Dechaume, and Blanc, 1937) and Wyburn-Mason in the English literature (Wyburn-Mason, 1943; Théron, Newton and Hoyt, 1974). The Sturge-Weber syndrome is the best known central nervous system vascular malformation associated with port-wine stain.

STURGE-WEBER SYNDROME

In 1879 Sturge described a 6½ year old girl with a capillary stain on her right face, buphthalmos, and focal left-sided seizures. He predicted that the girl should have a "port-wine mark" on the surface of the right brain. In 1897 autopsy on a similar case by Kalischer proved that Sturge was correct. In 1922 Weber described this entity as a syndrome and published a roentgenogram showing the typical intracranial calcifications (Weber, 1922). A strict definition of the Sturge-Weber complex includes vascular anomalies of the upper facial dermis, choroid plexus, and ipsilateral leptomeninges. However, the disorder presents in a spectrum of variable expressivity; various eponyms apply when only one or more of the features are present. The syndrome has

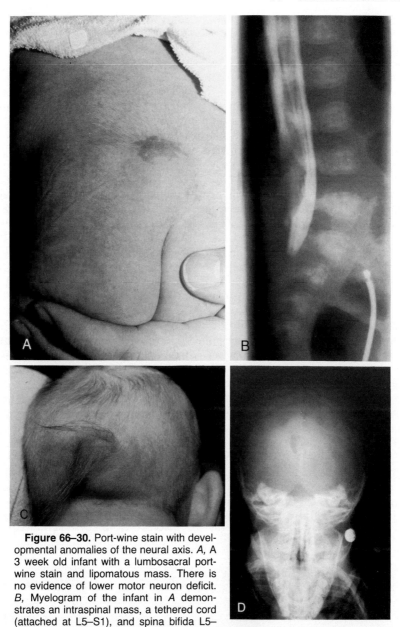

Figure 66–30. Port-wine stain with developmental anomalies of the neural axis. *A,* A 3 week old infant with a lumbosacral port-wine stain and lipomatous mass. There is no evidence of lower motor neuron deficit. *B,* Myelogram of the infant in *A* demonstrates an intraspinal mass, a tethered cord (attached at L5–S1), and spina bifida L5–S1. *C,* A 5 month old infant with an occipital stain and abnormal patch of hair. *D,* Meningoencephalocele defect seen in Towne's view radiograph of the patient in *C.* (From Mulliken, J. B., and Young, A. E.: Vascular Birthmarks: Hemangiomas and Malformations. Philadelphia, W. B. Saunders Company, 1988.)

an equal gender incidence and occurs sporadically. Enjolras, Riché and Merland (1985) proposed that the Sturge-Weber complex represents an error of morphogenesis within a specific region of the cephalic neural crest, giving rise to abnormal vasculature in the upper facial dermis, choroid, and pia-arachnoid.

Studies of facial stains emphasize that only those patients with a port-wine mark within the ophthalmic area alone (V1), or extending into the maxillary (V2) and mandibular (V3) regions, are at high risk of having ocular and intracranial vascular anomalies (Stevenson, Thomson, and Morin, 1974; Enjolras, Riché, and Merland, 1985). Infants with dermal staining of the V2 and/or V3 trigeminal areas only are not at increased risk. The dermal staining in the Sturge-Weber complex also frequently covers the entire face, neck, trunk, and extremities. There may be associated overgrowth of connective tissue and skeleton, producing macrocephaly or midfacial hypertrophy in the area covered by the stain. The skeletal hypertrophy may be noted at birth and is progressive (Fig. 66–31 *A,B*).

Standard radiographs reveal the gyriform ("tramline") intracranial calcification, especially in the parieto-occipital region. Computed tomography is the most sensitive technique for identifying cerebral calcification in early infancy (Fig. 66–31*C*). The mineral deposition is in the cerebral cortex, beneath the leptomeningeal vascular anomaly (Krabbe, 1934). Cerebral angiography, in patients with fully expressed Sturge-Weber syndrome, shows capillary and venous malformations of the leptomeninges, even in the absence of calcification (Poser and Taveras, 1957).

Focal or generalized seizures are common presenting features of neurologic involvement and often commence during infancy. There is a 45 per cent chance of a child having ipsilateral glaucoma if there is a port-wine stain in the area supplied by both the ophthalmic and maxillary divisions of the trigeminal nerve. Staining in either one of the upper fifth nerve divisions is not associated with glaucoma (Stevenson, Thomson, and Morin, 1974). It is critical that the diagnosis of glaucoma be made early in infancy, before irreversible ocular damage occurs. Childhood glaucoma is often difficult to control by medical therapy. An infant with a port-wine stain of the eyelid should be examined by an ophthalmologist every six months until the age of 2 to 3 years, and continue to be seen yearly thereafter.

Treatment of Port-Wine Stains

There is a colorful history of attempts to lighten or expunge port-wine stains. The methodology can be classified as (1) scarification, (2) camouflage, or (3) surgical excision.

Scarification. The concept that scarring the skin would diminish the color of a port-wine mark was applied in several forms: multiple parallel incisions (Squire, 1879), electric current attached to acupuncture needles (galvanopuncture) (Beard, 1877), electrocoagulation (Morton, 1909), ultraviolet lamp (Kromayer, 1910; MacCollum, 1935), radiation therapy (Bowers, 1951), rubbing with sandpaper (Jönsson, 1947), and freezing (Morel-Fatio, 1964; Goldwyn and Rosoff, 1969). None of these methods gave satisfactory results; laser photocoagulation is now used to obliterate dermal vascular anomalies, as discussed in Chapter 75.

Camouflage

Tattooing. The first attempt to tattoo a port-wine stain is credited to Pauli (1835), one century before tattooing was rediscovered (Brown, Cannon, and McDowell, 1946; Conway, 1948; Conway, McKinney, and Climo, 1967). Problems include the transient nature of the coverage, variation in response to pigment deposition, color abnormalities at the treated margin, and raised vascular papules secondary to needle trauma. Even with more

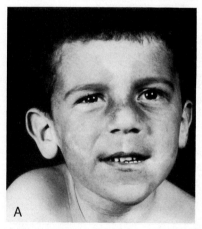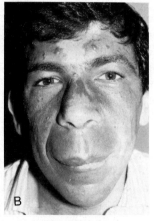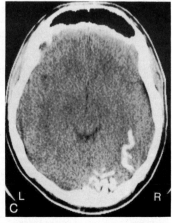

Figure 66–31. Sturge-Weber syndrome. *A,* A 6 year old boy with bilateral V1–V2 dermal staining. *B,* The patient at age 24: note the maxillary overgrowth and elongation of the midface. The patient has glaucoma and presented with bleeding from ectatic vasculature in the maxillary gingiva. *C,* Axial CT scan of the patient demonstrates serpentine calcifications in the right occipital lobe. (From Mulliken, J. B., and Young, A. E.: Vascular Birthmarks: Hemangiomas and Malformations. Philadelphia, W. B. Saunders Company, 1988.)

sophisticated color matching, the results are disappointing (Thomson and Wright, 1971; Grabb, MacCollom, and Tan, 1977). Tattooed skin has an unnatural, fixed, masklike appearance, unalterable by stimuli that normally change facial color. Tattooing is no longer recommended.

Cosmetics. There is still a place for external camouflage with cosmetic creams in the treatment of port-wine stains. The two well-known products are Covermark (Lydia O'Leary) and Dermablend (Flori Roberts). It requires an average of 20 minutes to apply the foundation, additional creams, and setting powder. Daily use of make-up demands a patient's full commitment. Cosmetics may be objectionable to those who need help the most, the children. Teenaged girls and young women are more likely to use make-up since it is socially acceptable. Cosmetics become less satisfactory in the older patient with hypertrophy and skin nodularity. In one survey, only 28 per cent of patients with port-wine stains were consistently using external cosmetic cover (Cosman, 1980).

Surgical Excision. With aging, port-wine stained skin becomes hypertrophic and cob-blestone-like in texture, with a deep purple color. Thicker application of make-up no longer camouflages the patch of pebbled skin. In selected patients, satisfactory results can be obtained with excision and application of thick split-thickness or full-thickness skin grafts, patterned to fit the esthetic facial units (Clodius, 1977, 1986). The grafts should be harvested from color-matched areas, e.g., retro- and/or postauricular regions, supraclavicular areas, or the scalp (Fig. 66–32). For replacement of bearded areas, Clodius recommended that scalp skin from the mastoid region be used, 10 to 14 days after epilation. Plucking causes the follicles to migrate upward into the dermis, thus increasing the hair density within the graft (Clodius and Smahel, 1979).

No matter what the quality of the grafted area, there is always a border effect with normal skin that calls attention to the reconstruction. More serious problems after excision and grafting include (1) scar hypertrophy at the juncture of the graft and normal skin, (2) unpredictable graft pigmentation, and (3) abnormal texture. Skin expansion may be used before excision of a moderate-sized port-

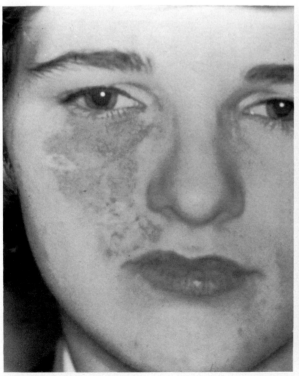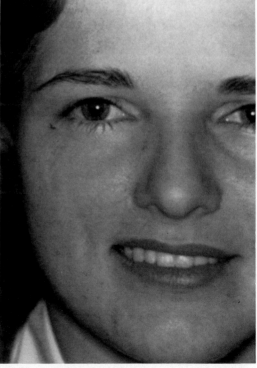

Figure 66–32. Excision of a localized port-wine stain of the right cheek and replacement with a full-thickness retroauricular skin graft. (Courtesy of J. E. Murray.) (From Mulliken, J. B., and Young, A. E.: Vascular Birthmarks: Hemangiomas and Malformations. Philadelphia, W. B. Saunders Company, 1988.)

wine stained area, thus permitting linear closure along the facial unit borders (Argenta, Watanabe, and Grabb, 1983).

NEVUS FLAMMEUS NEONATORUM

Neonatal stains are pink, macular, and irregularly outlined. They blanch completely with pressure and become suffused when the infant cries (Fig. 66–33A). This common entity is often confused with the very uncommon port-wine stain because it shares the same Latin term, *nevus (naevus) flammeus*. Pratt (1967) found that 42 per cent of Caucasian neonates and 31 per cent of black neonates have a *nevus flammeus nuchae*. A lower incidence of nuchal staining (23.4 per cent) was noted in Chinese and Malaysian infants (Tan, 1972). Jacobs and Walton (1976) examined 1058 newborn infants and found that 40.3 per cent had neonatal stains in the following distribution: 81 per cent on the nape of the neck, 45 per cent on the eyelids, and 33 per cent on the glabella.

Nevus flammeus neonatorum ("angel's kiss," "stork bite," "salmon patch") may be more of a physiologic phenomenon than a true dermatopathologic lesion. Histologic ex-amination fails to demonstrate ectasia in infant skin specimens; however, moderate ectasia of the subpapillary vessels is seen in older children with nuchal staining (Schnyder, 1955).

There is a remarkable tendency for these lesions to vanish within the first year of life, leaving no residual evidence. The nuchal patches fade somewhat more slowly than the anterior facial stains (Smith and Manfield, 1962). In a study of Danish schoolchildren between the ages of 6 and 17 years, Øster and Nielsen (1970) noted that the incidence of persistent nuchal staining was 46.2 per cent in females and 35 per cent in males. In addition, they found that interscapular telangiectasia was more common in girls (40 per cent) than in boys (32 per cent). In girls, there was an increased incidence of staining in the 12 to 13 year old group, with a subsequent age-related decrease; the incidence was independent of age for boys. It is possible that hormones, known to modulate vascularity, may influence the dermal microcirculation in these particular anatomic regions. Nuchal staining can persist into adulthood, becoming more obvious with blood pressure elevation, emotional episodes, or physical exertion. A

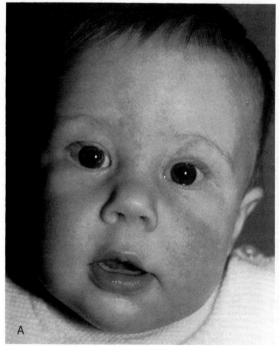 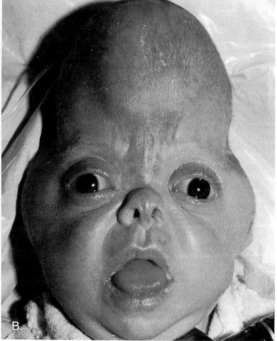

Figure 66–33. Macular staining of infancy. *A,* An infant with common nevus flammeus neonatorum of the glabella and upper eyelids. The stains usually fade within one to two years. *B,* Central forehead dermal stain in an infant with trilobar calvarial deformity (craniosynostosis, Pfeiffer's syndrome.) (From Mulliken, J. B., and Young, A. E.: Vascular Birthmarks: Hemangiomas and Malformations. Philadelphia, W. B. Saunders Company, 1988.)

permanent cervical stain is referred to as "Unna's nevus" or *erythema nuchae* (Øster and Nielsen, 1970). Unna's nevus may have a familial tendency (Merlob and Reisner, 1985), as also seen in forehead capillary stains.

Glabellar and nuchal staining of infancy is often included as a phenotypic finding in a variety of malformation syndromes, including Beckwith-Wiedemann, trisomy 13–15, Brachmann–de Lange, Rubenstein-Taybi, SC-pseudothalidomide-Roberts, and others. A prominent V-shaped stain of the central forehead is also seen in craniofacial synostosis (Figure 66–33B). However, since a forehead stain is so commonly seen in a normal infant, it is arguable whether there is any etiopathologic significance to its presence with a rare dysmorphogenic syndrome.

Hyperkeratotic Vascular Stains

Certain vascular stains have a rough warty surface; in the past, these lesions have been generically called "angiokeratomas." However, on the basis of histopathologic criteria, two separate categories can be differentiated: (1) a congenital telangiectatic abnormality ("hypertrophic nevus flammeus" or "verrucous hemangioma"), characterized by vascular ectasia involving both the dermis and subcutaneous tissue; and (2) "angiokeratoma," a lesion (apparently "acquired") in which ectasia is seen only in the papillary dermis (Imperial and Helwig, 1967b). Endo-

thelial hyperplasia cannot be demonstrated in either category of hyperkeratotic stain, and therefore the terms "verrucous hemangioma" and "angiokeratoma" are, in this sense, both misnomers. It is critical that there not be a precise differentiation between "acquired" and "congenital" vascular anomalies. A vascular malformation may not become clinically apparent until the structural abnormality of the vessel walls is manifest during adolescence or adulthood. There is increasing evidence that the hyperkeratotic vascular stains are true malformations. They are subdivided into (1) capillary-lymphatic malformations (usually seen at birth) and (2) "angiokeratomas" (which appear after birth).

CAPILLARY-LYMPHATIC MALFORMATIONS (CLM)

These combined low flow dermal vascular anomalies (old terms: "hypertrophic nevus flammeus," "verrucous hemangioma," "lymphangioma circumscriptum," "hemangiolymphangioma") are usually obvious at birth. These are light pink to bluish-red in color, well demarcated, and most commonly located on the lower extremities, but they are also seen on the chest, abdomen, and arms (Imperial and Helwig, 1967b). With trauma, altered hemodynamics, or possibly secondary infection, the lesions become more keratotic and wartlike. The color and consistency are determined by the amount of blood within the abnormal dermal channels and by the overlying verrucous changes (Fig. 66–34).

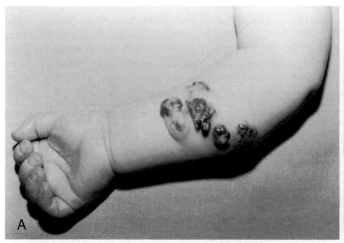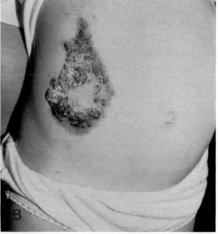

Figure 66–34. Capillary-lymphatic malformation (CLM). *A,* CLM of the distal forearm, present at birth; there are color changes with bleeding into the vascular spaces. *B,* CLM of the abdomen. Note the warty excrescences, typical of the dermal lymphatic anomaly. In the past, this lesion was labeled "angiokeratoma circumscriptum." (*B* from Mulliken, J. B., and Young, A. E.: Vascular Birthmarks: Hemangiomas and Malformations. Philadelphia, W. B. Saunders Company, 1988.)

On histologic examination, the lesions demonstrate dilated capillary to venular sized vessels in the dermis and subcutaneous tissue. The vessels are deficient in elastic fibers. Larger ectatic channels, some with proteinaceous material, are clearly abnormal lymphatic vessels. The epidermal hyperkeratosis and parakeratosis are reactive, rather than primary features (Imperial and Helwig, 1967b).

This lesion is a localized lymphatic malformation combined with abnormal dermal blood vessels. Therapy necessitates wide excision, usually down to fascia. The defect may be closed in a linear fashion; more often a split-thickness skin graft is needed to achieve primary closure.

ANGIOKERATOMAS

The term "angiokeratoma" refers to a group of skin lesions that present as dark-red to black papules 1 to 10 mm in size. As separate dermatologic entities, the angiokeratomas are best remembered by their eponyms and anatomic predilections: (1) *Mibelli* lesions on the hands and feet, (2) *Fordyce* lesions on the perineum, and (3) *Fabry* lesions on the trunk and thighs. It is difficult to differentiate one type of angiokeratoma from another by clinical appearance or by light microscopy. Ultrastructural and three-dimensional reconstructions show a close resemblance between the angiokeratomas of Fabry and Fordyce; they are abnormalities of preexisting microvasculature and not the result of neoangiogenesis (Braverman and Ken-Yen, 1983).

The angiokeratomas may have an underlying genetic basis (Imperial and Helwig, 1967a), and in two types (Fabry's disease and fucosidosis) biochemical abnormalities have been detected.

Treatment of the angiokeratomas is usually symptomatic. Often the lesions bleed easily and weep, either spontaneously or after abrasion. The area should be kept clean and covered with petrolatum-based antibiotic ointment. Electrocoagulation, cryotherapy, or laser therapy may be used to control troublesome bleeding points (Flores and associates, 1984; Pasyk, Argenta, and Schelbert, 1988).

Angiokeratoma of Mibelli

In 1889 Mibelli coined the word "angiokeratoma" to describe warty purplish spots over the bony prominences of the extremities. The lesions typically appear during adolescence, first as telangiectasias that later coalesce, forming tiny hemorrhagic keratotic papules (3 to 5 mm in diameter) on the dorsal and volar surfaces of the hands and feet; the ankles, knees, palms, and elbows may also be involved. The lesion is more commonly seen in females, and the distribution and frequent association with acrocyanosis, chilblain, and frostbite suggest that cold sensitivity is a precipitating factor. Familial occurrence of this condition has been reported, which suggests a dominant mode of inheritance with variable penetrance (Smith, Prior, and Park, 1968).

Angiokeratoma of Fordyce

In 1896 Fordyce described a 60 year old male who had developed warty vascular lesions of the scrotum, similar clinically and histologically to Mibelli's cases, but without the history of chilblain. Fordyce's angiokeratoma is seen most commonly in males over the age of 30 and is located on the genitalia, lower abdomen, and thighs. Similar lesions occur rarely on the labia of older women (Novick, 1985). The angiokeratomas have a linear configuration, and on closer examination are made up of tiny, red, soft, compressible papules (Fig. 66–35A). With advancing age the lesions become larger, darker, more numerous, and keratotic in appearance. Although scrotal angiokeratomas are usually asymptomatic, they can become pruritic and may bleed when traumatized. Some investigators believe that these lesions are vascular ectasias secondary to venous obstruction, increased intravascular pressure, or thrombosis, caused by various genitourinary disorders such as varicocele, hernia, prostatitis, thrombophlebitis, tumor of the epididymis, and lymphogranuloma venereum (Evans, 1962; Imperial and Helwig, 1967c).

Angiokeratoma Circumscriptum

In 1915 Fabry described a localized hyperkeratotic vascular skin disorder, calling it *angiokeratoma circumscriptum* (Fabry, 1915). The condition manifests as unilateral cutaneous purple papules and blood-filled cystic spaces, located over the trunk, lower legs, and thighs. The lesions may be present at birth or may appear in infancy or early childhood; they grow proportionately and enlarge to become several centimeters in diameter.

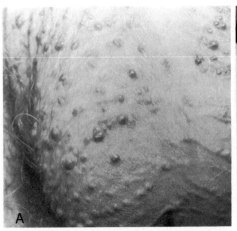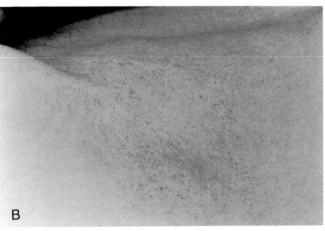

Figure 66–35. The eponymous "angiokeratomas." *A,* Angiokeratoma of Fordyce of the scrotum in a 50 year old patient. (Courtesy of H. A. Haynes.) *B,* Fabry's disease in a 25 year old male with diffuse hemispherical red papules over the flanks and abdomen. (Courtesy of H. A. Haynes.) (From Mulliken, J. B., and Young, A. E.: Vascular Birthmarks: Hemangiomas and Malformations. Philadelphia, W. B. Saunders Company, 1988.)

Females are reportedly affected three times as often as males (Imperial and Helwig, 1967a).

From descriptions in the literature (Sehgal, Ghorpade, and Koranne, 1984; Pasyk, Argenta, and Schelbert, 1988), it is likely that angiokeratoma circumscriptum is indeed a vascular malformation of the capillary-lymphatic type (see Fig. 66–34).

Angiokeratoma Corporis Diffusum Universale (Fabry's Disease)

Described in 1898 by Fabry and independently by Anderson, this is a rare, hereditary, sex-linked recessive disorder of sphingolipid metabolism (alpha-galactosidase A deficiency) (Wallace, 1973). The disease is biochemically characterized by an abnormal glycolipid (ceramide trihexoside) attached to sphingosine and deposited in the cytoplasm of vascular endothelium, pericytes, renal epithelium, neural cells, corneal epithelium, and cardiac muscle fibers. The diagnosis is confirmed by skin biopsy and appropriate histologic stains for glycolipid granules.

The disease presents in homozygous males during childhood or early adolescence, with an intense burning pain in the fingers and toes. Before puberty, vesicles usually appear over the hips, buttocks, and perineum (the bathing trunk area). Although the lesions can occur anywhere, they rarely appear on the face. The cutaneous lesions are minute,

blood-filled, hemispheric, purple or bluish-red papules, often with overlying keratosis (Fig. 66–35*B*). The condition is manifest clinically with fevers, renal dysfunction, peripheral edema, and dyshidrosis. Most men with Fabry's angiokeratoma die in the fourth decade as a result of renal failure or hypertensive cardiovascular disease. There is variable mild expressivity in the heterozygous female; only 26 per cent develop skin lesions.

Fucosidosis

Fucosidosis is another genetic enzymatic deficiency disease that may present with diffuse angiokeratomas. The condition is inherited in an autosomal recessive manner and is characterized by an absence or deficiency of the lysosomal enzyme alpha-L-fucosidase (Durand, Borrone, and Della Cella, 1966). Fucose (containing glycosaminoglycans, glycolipids, and polysaccharides) accumulates in the tissues of affected homozygotic individuals, who evidence varying degrees of mental retardation, spasticity, and skeletal dysplasia (Smith and associates, 1977; Hurwitz and Kerber, 1981). Some affected individuals develop multiple angiokeratomas in early childhood, primarily on the trunk and upper legs and similar in appearance and distribution to those of Fabry's disease. Tissue specimens from patients with fucosidosis do not demonstrate the intracellular lipid inclusions of Fabry's disease (Smith and associates, 1977).

Telangiectasias

CUTIS MARMORATA TELANGIECTATICA CONGENITA (CMTC)

Some children, when placed in a low temperature environment, exhibit a cutaneous mottling that disappears when the child is warmed. This is merely an accentuated pattern of normal cutaneous vascularity called *cutis marmorata* or *livedo reticularis*. The appearance is similar to that of the veins visible in the skin of some delicate, fair-haired Caucasian women.

There is a distinct pathologic entity, first described by van Lohuizen and known by the term *cutis marmorata telangiectatica congenita* (CMTC) (van Lohuizen, 1922). These rare newborn infants have a livid cutaneous marbling, even at normal temperatures, that becomes more pronounced with lower temperature or with crying. The involved skin has a

distinctive deep purple color, it is depressed in a serpiginous reticulated pattern, and ulceration may be present. It occurs in a localized, segmental, or generalized distribution; the trunk and extremities are more commonly involved than the face and scalp (Fig. 66–36A). There are reported examples of CMTC in association with defective long bone growth (Fitzsimmons and Starks, 1970) and with congenital glaucoma and mental retardation (Petrozzi and associates, 1970; South and Jacobs, 1978).

CMTC occurs sporadically in an equal gender distribution (Way and associates, 1974; South and Jacobs, 1978). There are reports suggesting that it may be an autosomal dominant disorder of low penetrance (Andreev and Pramatarov, 1979; Kurczynski, 1982).

Almost all affected infants with CMTC show improvement of the skin changes during the first year of life, continuing into adolescence (Fig. 66–36B). However, skin atrophy

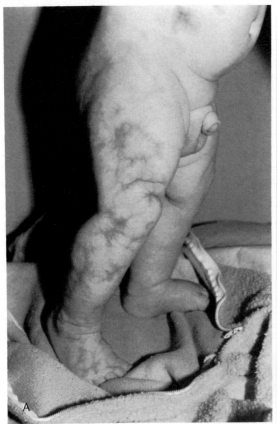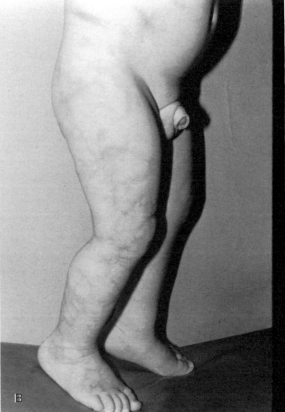

Figure 66–36. Cutis marmorata telangiectatica congenita (CMTC). *A,* CMTC in a 5 month old male. Note the serpiginous and discolored craters of the leg and trunk. *B,* Improvement apparent at 1 year of age. The venous ectasia, skin atrophy, and pigmentation usually persist into adulthood. (From Mulliken, J. B., and Young, A. E.: Vascular Birthmarks: Hemangiomas and Malformations. Philadelphia, W. B. Saunders Company, 1988.)

and pigmentation often persist into adulthood in association with ectasia of the superficial veins in the involved extremities.

RENDU-OSLER-WEBER SYNDROME

This disorder (also known as hereditary hemorrhagic telangiectasia, HHT) was first distinguished from hemophilia by Rendu in 1896. Osler (1901) gave a complete clinical description and established the inherited nature of the disease. Weber (1907a,b) presented another case in 1907 and invited Osler to examine the patient. Hanes (1909) first described the histopathology of the skin lesions and accurately called the disease "hereditary hemorrhagic telangiectasia."

Inherited in an autosomal dominant pattern, the homozygous form of HHT is probably lethal. The incidence is one to two per 100,000 in the European population and considerably less in other races (Martini, 1978).

The characteristic skin lesions are discrete, spider-like, bright red maculopapules, usually 1 to 4 mm in diameter and typically located on the face, tongue, lips, nasal and oral mucous membranes, conjunctiva, palmar aspect of the fingers, and nail beds (Fig. 66–37A). Lesions can occur on other mucosal surfaces, e.g., the gastrointestinal tract, bladder, and bronchial and vaginal linings, and they have also been found in liver, spleen, pancreas, kidney, and brain (Chandler, 1965; Cooke, 1986).

The telangiectatic skin lesions may appear in early childhood, but more commonly they become apparent after puberty (the third to fourth decade) and increase in number with advancing age. The vascular papules are prone to ulceration and bleeding. Hemor-

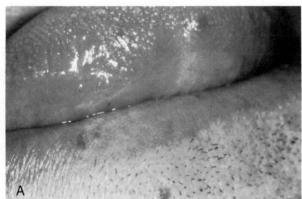
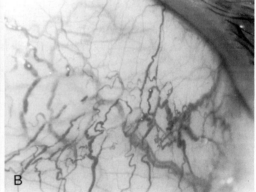
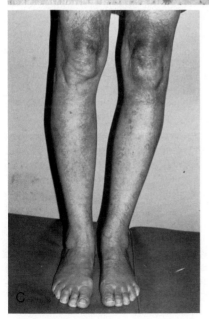

Figure 66–37. Telangiectasias. *A,* Rendu-Osler-Weber syndrome. Typical red maculopapular lesions of the lips and tongue in a 55 year old male. (Courtesy of H. A. Haynes.) *B,* Ataxia-telangiectasia: dilated tortuous vessels in the bulbar conjunctiva of a 17 year old male. (From Donaldson, D. D. *In* Atlas of External Diseases of the Eye. St. Louis, C. V. Mosby Company, 1968, p. 280.) *C,* Generalized essential telangiectasia: gradual onset of linear telangiectasia of the lower extremities in a 60 year old woman. (*A* and *C* from Mulliken, J. B., and Young, A. E.: Vascular Birthmarks: Hemangiomas and Malformations. Philadelphia, W. B. Saunders Company, 1988.)

rhage may present as epistaxis, hematemesis, hematuria, or melena. Bleeding from telangiectasias in the brain or spinal cord can produce neurologic symptoms. There may be pulmonary arteriovenous fistulas and pulmonary hypertension (Trell and associates, 1972), hepatic telangiectasis with a peculiar type of liver cirrhosis ("pseudocirrhosis") (Martini, 1978), and aneurysms of large elastic arteries, including the aorta (Trell and associates, 1972).

The pathogenesis of HHT involves structurally weak vessels that become dilated, elongated, and tortuous. Some studies show that it is the small arteries and arteriolar-precapillary sphincters that lack elastic fibers (Hales, 1956). Other studies show remarkably few changes in the arterioles and suggest that the primary vascular abnormalities lie in the capillaries and small venules (Martini, 1978). Ultrastructural examination of the dilated vessels reveals intact endothelium, continuous basal lamina but no elastic lamina, and inadequate smooth muscle elements (Jahnke, 1970).

The mechanism of bleeding in HHT is a local hemostatic abnormality, perhaps related to increased plasminogen activator content, resulting in elevated fibrinolysis in the pericapillary tissues (Kwaan and Silverman, 1973). Topical treatment of epistaxis is favored, e.g., pressure, packing, and microfibrillar collagen (Avitene). Laser coagulation is another therapeutic option (Shapshay and Oliver, 1984). If there is continued bleeding from a surgically accessible area, a split-thickness skin graft can be used to replace the involved septal mucosa (Saunders, 1960). This technique can be successful in diminishing epistaxis, although there is a tendency toward crusting and fetor (Ulsø, Vase, and Stoksted, 1983). In addition, telangiectasias can reappear within the skin graft (McCabe and Kelly, 1972; Ulsø, Vase, and Stoksted, 1983).

ATAXIA-TELANGIECTASIA

Transmitted by an autosomal gene, this disorder (also known as Louis-Bar syndrome) is characterized by cerebellar ataxia, ocular and cutaneous telangiectasis, and frequent serious respiratory tract and sinus infections. The patients evidence severe immunologic deficiency with diminished levels of immunoglobulins A, G, and E; structural anomalies of the thymus and lymph nodes; and unusual susceptibility to lymphoma and T cell leukemia (Ammann and associates, 1969).

Progressive cerebellar ataxia usually begins during the second or third year of life; the cutaneous and ocular abnormalities occur at 3 to 6 years of age. Symmetric bright red telangiectases are generally first noted in the nasal and temporal areas of the bulbar conjunctiva (Fig. 66–37*B*). Later telangiectasias appear on the eyelids, nasal bridge, cheeks, ears, neck, upper chest, and flexor surfaces of the forearms. Poorly controlled eye movement, called oculomotor dyspraxia, often develops.

The course of the disease is progressive; death typically occurs in the second decade of life from recurrent pulmonary infections and bronchiectasis or from lymphoreticular malignancy (Kraemer, 1987).

GENERALIZED ESSENTIAL TELANGIECTASIA

Hutchinson (1889–1890) described a 15 year old girl who developed "a peculiar form of serpiginous and infective naevoid disease"; soon thereafter, Radcliffe-Crocker (1893) proposed the term "angioma serpiginosum" for the entity. It is now recognized as an acquired idiopathic vascular ectasia and is best known as *generalized essential telangiectasia* (Rook, Wilkinson, and Ebling, 1979).

The disorder occurs almost exclusively in females; the reported cases are sporadic, although there may be a familial incidence (Marriott, Munro, and Ryan, 1975). The onset varies widely; lesions can appear before puberty, although presentation in middle adulthood is more typical.

The primary lesions are pin sized, red to purple vascular puncta, appearing in groups. The lesions extend frighteningly over several years, forming gyrate or serpiginous patterns or extensive sheets of telangiectases. There is often a fiery red erythematous background (Fig. 66–37*C*). The telangiectasia occurs predominantly on the lower extremities, although any body area may be affected except the palms, soles, and mucous membranes. Histologic examination demonstrates thin-walled ectatic vessels in the upper corium with no signs of inflammation or hyperplasia (McGrae and Winkelmann, 1963). Late partial regression has been seen, but is never complete.

VASCULAR SPIDERS AND SIMILAR LESIONS

Acquired vascular marks called "spider nevus," "spider telangiectasis," "nevus araneus," or incorrectly "stellate hemangioma" have been comprehensively studied by Bean (1958). The lesions most commonly occur in the face and over the dorsum of the hands, fingers, and forearms. A spider lesion consists of a central arteriole from which superficial vessels radiate (Fig. 66–38). The blood flow is efferent, and therefore pressure with a tiny blunt instrument over the central vessels causes blanching, and a centrifugal flush when it is released. Diascopy is another diagnostic maneuver; when a glass slide is gently pressed over the lesions, the pulsations of the central vessel are observed.

Spider marks typically appear on children in the preschool and school-age groups. Alderson (1963) found them in 47.5 per cent of healthy English schoolchildren; the highest incidence was between 7 and 10 years of age, with no significant difference between boys and girls. A study of North American children between the ages of 5 and 15 years showed that 37 per cent of boys and 48 per cent of girls had at least one vascular spider (Wenzl

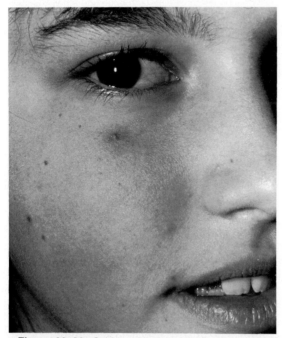

Figure 66–38. Spider mark (telangiectasia) commonly appears in the malar area of healthy children. (From Mulliken, J. B., and Young, A. E.: Vascular Birthmarks: Hemangiomas and Malformations. Philadelphia, W. B. Saunders Company, 1988.)

and Burgert, 1964). Spontaneous disappearance of spider marks occurs after puberty. Bean (1958) noted vascular spiders in 10 to 15 per cent of normal adults.

Similar vascular lesions occur on the skin during pregnancy and have been called "hemangioma" of pregnancy (Barter, Letterman, and Schurter, 1963) or *granuloma gravidarum* when located on the gingiva, palate, or septum. They typically appear during the second to fifth months of gestation, and increase in size and number throughout the pregnancy. By the ninth month, 66 per cent of gestating Caucasian women have vascular spiders. The lesions may reach 5 mm in diameter. They usually disappear during the early puerperium. However, large lesions may persist, and vanished lesions often reappear in the same location with a subsequent pregnancy. The microanatomy is an expansion of a normal dermal end artery, containing glomus cells, which divides into radial vessels with the structure of veins (Bean, 1958).

There is gathering evidence that hormonal modulation of dermal vasculature accounts for the appearance of spider lesions in pregnancy. This theory would also explain spiders in liver failure and palmar erythema, and the increased frequency of spider marks in pubertal females (Wenzl and Burgert, 1964).

Spider lesions can be treated by punctate cautery or laser photocoagulation; however, they tend to recur unless the abnormal vessels are completely obliterated.

Lymphatic Malformations (LM)

TERMINOLOGY

The term "cystic hygroma" was introduced by Wernher in his 1843 monograph to distinguish lymphatic malformation from other cervical anomalies. Wegner (1876–1877) proposed a histomorphologic classification for lymphatic anomalies, called "lymphangiomas," "simplex," "cavernous," and "cystoides." The designation "lymphangioma circumscriptum" was used by Morris in 1889 to describe a localized lymphatic anomaly with vesicular skin lesions.

The term "lymphangioma" is a misnomer because the suffix "-oma" implies a potential for growth by cellular mitosis and invasion (Mulliken and Glowacki, 1982). These lesions are abnormalities of lymphatic development, yet there is a long-standing discussion over whether they have a proliferative capacity (Goetsch, 1938; Harkins and Sabiston, 1960; Broomhead, 1964; Bill and Sumner, 1965). It is more likely that a lymphatic malformation expands secondary to fluid accumulation, cellulitis, or inadequate drainage of the anomalous lymphatic channels (Willis, 1960).

The lymphatic malformations have engendered other semantic problems, e.g., the hybrid terms, "lymphangiohemangioma" and "hemangiolymphangioma." A more precise designation for these is *capillary-lymphatic malformation* (CLM) or *lymphaticovenous malformation* (LVM), combined vascular anomalies containing abnormal lymphatic and blood-filled channels.

HISTOLOGY

The anomalous channels are lined by a single layer of flattened endothelium, whether the specimen be a cystic or diffuse type of lymphatic malformation. The pale yellow fluid found in cystic lesions microscopically appears acidophilic and protein rich. Blood cells within the spaces may indicate recent hemorrhage into the specimen, or the lesion may in fact be a CLM or LVM. Mural thrombi are often noted in combined low flow malformations. Nodular collections of lymphocytes, including follicles with germinal centers, are frequently observed in the connective tissue within a lymphatic malformation. The vessel walls are of variable thickness; some are quite thin; and others contain dense fibromuscular tissue with both striated and smooth muscle elements (Fig. 66–39). Abnormal lymphatic tissue can also be seen within large nerves and the walls of local blood vessels.

CLINICAL FINDINGS

Lymphatic anomalies occur with equal frequency in both sexes and all races (Gross, 1953). The cervicofacial and axillary region is the most common location, followed in frequency by the extremities and trunk (Ninh and Ninh, 1974; Bhattacharyya and associates, 1981). A cystic lymphatic anomaly can be diagnosed in utero by ultrasonography, as early as 12 weeks of gestation (Garden and associates, 1986) (Fig. 66–40). Most lymphatic malformations are first noted in the newborn nursery. In one series, 65 per cent of lymphatic anomalies were seen at birth,

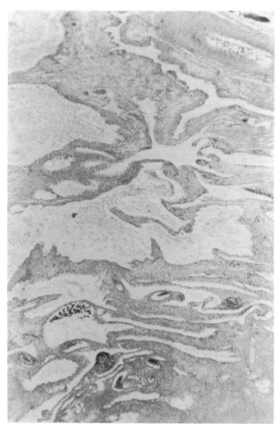

Figure 66–39. Microscopic section of a cervical lymphatic malformation demonstrates both large and small channels with a barely discernible endothelial lining. The fibrous walls of variable thickness contain lymphoid aggregates (H & E, × 10). (From Mulliken, J. B., and Young, A. E.: Vascular Birthmarks: Hemangiomas and Malformations. Philadelphia, W. B. Saunders Company, 1988.)

80 per cent during the first year of life, and 90 per cent by the second year (Gross, 1953). Lymphatic malformations also can emerge in adulthood (Nussbaum and Buchwald, 1981).

Lymphatic vascular anomalies present in diverse forms, ranging from tiny cutaneous or mucosal blebs (likened to frog spawn) to large-channel or multilocular lesions. The various clinical manifestations can be explained by the differences of channel dysmorphology, the depth and extent of primary involvement, and the degree of fibrous tissue reaction. There may be generalized swelling (lymphedema) of the facial region and extremities, or a localized multilocular cystic lesion. The large, cystic-type anomalies are usually translucent. Cystic lymphatic anomalies occasionally manifest after intralesional hemorrhage, presenting as opaque, firm swellings. A true neoplasm must be consid-

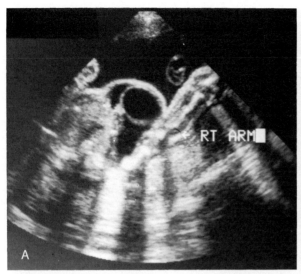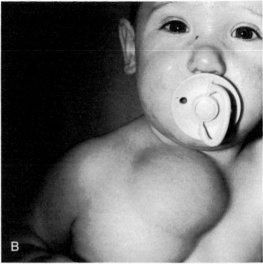

Figure 66–40. Intrauterine diagnosis with ultrasonography. *A,* Sonogram at 15 weeks' gestation reveals a fetus with a multicystic anomaly of the axillary and cervical region. *B,* The child in *A* with a lymphatic malformation within the neck, anterior chest, and brachial plexus. (From Mulliken, J. B., and Young, A. E.: Vascular Birthmarks: Hemangiomas and Malformations. Philadelphia, W. B. Saunders Company, 1988.)

ered as a possible diagnosis if such a mass appears in the parotid region.

The cystic lymphatic malformation, in the past called "cystic hygroma" or "cavernous lymphangioma," most frequently occurs in the anterior cervical triangle (Ninh and Ninh, 1974). Cystic lesions also present in the posterior cervical triangle, shoulder, axilla, lower face, and lateral trunk, in decreasing order of frequency. Approximately 2 per cent of cystic-type anomalies also involve the mediastinum, and radiographic examination may demonstrate displacement of the trachea, esophagus, or pharynx (Ravitch and Rush, 1986). Ultrasonography, in addition to chest roentgenography, is helpful in documenting mediastinal involvement. Hemorrhage, fibrosis, and chronic inflammation can alter a cystic lymphatic anomaly of the neck and mediastinum and belie its true nature (Sumner and associates, 1981).

The characteristic history of a lymphatic malformation is enlargement commensurate with the child's growth. Determination of a lesion's growth pattern is, therefore, the critical step toward an accurate diagnosis (Fig. 66–41). This may require multiple office visits, examination of early photographs, and other means of historical documentation. Periodic variations in the size of a lymphatic anomaly are common, but proportionate growth is the rule. A lymphatic malformation may suddenly expand; this often occurs coin-

cident with an upper respiratory tract infection.

Bacterial infection (cellulitis) occurred in 16 per cent of 126 cases (Ninh and Ninh, 1974). The inflamed lymphatic lesion is tense, warm, and erythematous and enlarged lymph nodes are often found nearby. Acute infection of a lymphatic malformation within the tongue or floor of the mouth can cause upper airway obstruction and/or interference with swallowing. Alarming respiratory distress may result, secondary to extrinsic compression of the trachea and pulmonary parenchyma by an infected mediastinal lymphatic malformation (Sumner and associates, 1981; Grosfeld, Weber, and Vane, 1982). Death may result from respiratory embarrassment and recurrent infections (Csicsko and Grosfeld, 1974). Repeated bouts of inflammation cause fibrosis and may produce further expansion of the lymphatic anomaly.

A lymphatic malformation can also enlarge abruptly, secondary to intralesional hemorrhage; this happens in 8 to 12.6 per cent of lesions (Ninh and Ninh, 1974; Broomhead, 1964).

Lymphatic anomalies also occur in the orbit, eyelids, and conjunctiva, often with contiguous involvement of the frontotemporal skin and musculature (Jakobiec and Jones, 1979). A characteristic feature is exacerbation of exophthalmos concomitant with an upper respiratory tract infection. Rupture

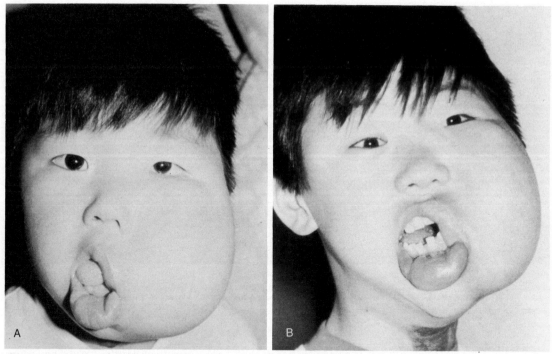

Figure 66–41. *A,* Hemifacial lymphatic anomaly in a 3 year old infant. *B,* Twelve years later, the malformation has grown commensurately with the patient. Note the associated congenital cervical nevus and malocclusion. (From Mulliken, J. B., and Young, A. E.: Vascular Birthmarks: Hemangiomas and Malformations. Philadelphia, W. B. Saunders Company, 1988.)

and hemorrhage into the lymphatic spaces produce the typical subconjunctival "chocolate cysts" or ocular proptosis.

ASSOCIATED ABNORMALITIES

Soft Tissue and Skeletal Hypertrophy

Lymphatic malformation is the most common pathologic basis for an enlarged lip (*macrocheilia*), ear (*macrotia*), or tongue (*macroglossia*) (Fig. 66–42). There may be soft tissue and skeletal hypertrophy of the malar eminence (*macromala*) and large teeth (*macrodontia*) (Mulliken, 1988b).

The enlarged tongue is often covered with clear vesicles ("salmon eggs") or hemorrhagic vesicles ("caviar spots"). Multiple brownish vesicopapules stud the buccal mucosa; these periodically exude clear or blood-stained fluid. In time the tongue may protrude through the lips with resultant desiccation, ulceration, and necrosis (Fig. 66–42C).

Bone hypertrophy and distortion accompany 80 per cent of cervicofacial lymphatic anomalies (Boyd and associates, 1984). The skeletal overgrowth may be noted soon after birth and is progressive. Typically, there is maxillary and/or mandibular enlargement resulting in prognathism, open bite, or other malocclusions (Fig. 66–42D). Lymphatic anomalies of the extremities, either pure-type or combined lymphaticovenous anomalies (the Klippel-Trenaunay syndrome), are also associated with long bone hypertrophy and distortion (Young, 1988b). Scintigraphic studies show that the osseous changes are probably not the result of increased blood flow (Boyd and associates, 1984).

Midline Posterior Cervical Lymphatic Cysts and Aneuploidy

There is a well-established association between cystic lymphatic lesions of the posterior cervical midline region and chromosomal abnormalities (Chervenak and associates, 1983; Garden and associates, 1986). This highly lethal complex of anomalies can be diagnosed by ultrasonography as early as 12 to 14 weeks of gestation. The sonographic hallmarks are a thin-walled, multiseptated, fluid-filled mass in the fetal head and the nuchal region, located asymmetrically with respect to the long axis of the spine (Phillips and McGahan,

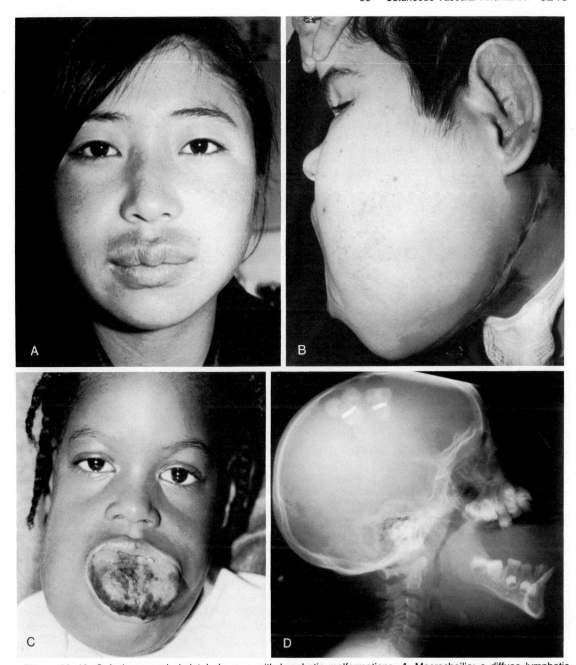

Figure 66–42. Soft tissue and skeletal changes with lymphatic malformations. *A,* Macrocheilia: a diffuse lymphatic anomaly of the upper lip with hypertrophy and periodic swelling. *B,* Macrotia: a diffuse lymphatic anomaly of the lower face with bone and auricular cartilage overgrowth. *C,* Macroglossia: hemorrhagic vesicles on the protruding tongue with mandibular prognathism and open bite. The malocclusion is, in part, secondary to the large tongue; skeletal overgrowth may be noted in infancy. (Courtesy of G. H. Gifford, Jr.) *D,* Lateral radiograph of the patient in *C* demonstrates overgrowth, particularly in the mandibular body region. (From Mulliken, J. B., and Young, A. E.: Vascular Birthmarks: Hemangiomas and Malformations. Philadelphia, W. B. Saunders Company, 1988.)

1981). There may be a midline septum, corresponding to the nuchal ligament (Fig. 66–43*A*). There is often fetal hydrops, seen on sonography as ascites and edematous skin (Fig. 66–43*B*). In this setting, amniocentesis for karyotyping is essential in order to counsel the parents. Approximately 50 per cent of such fetuses have Turner's syndrome; others have trisomy 13, 18, or 21 or Roberts syndrome (Greenberg, Carpenter, and Ledbetter,

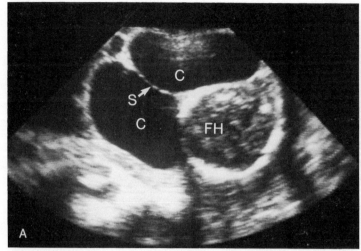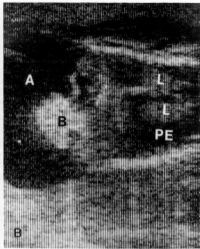

Figure 66–43. Lethal posterior cervical lymphatic malformation. *A,* Sonogram of a 22 week old fetus. The fetal head (FH) on the right is seen as a bright, echogenic structure. Adjacent is a bilobed cystic anomaly (C) with characteristic midline septum (S). The fetus has Turner's syndrome, lymphangiectasia, and skin edema. (Courtesy of B. Benacerraf.) *B,* Longitudinal sonogram of an 18 week fetus with posterior cystic lymphatic anomaly and generalized hydrops. L = lung; PE = pleural effusion; B = bowel; A = ascites. (Courtesy of F. A. Chervenak.) (From Mulliken, J. B., and Young, A. E.: Vascular Birthmarks: Hemangiomas and Malformations. Philadelphia, W. B. Saunders Company, 1988.)

1983; Graham, Stephens, and Shepard, 1983; Chervenak and associates, 1983; Garden and associates, 1986). The prognosis for a fetus with this malformation complex is poor. In the presence of hydrops, most die either in utero or in the early neonatal period.

On the basis of the studies of Singh and Carr (1966) and van der Putte (1977), Graham and associates (1983) hypothesized a "jugular lymphatic obstruction sequence" to explain the association between cystic nuchal lymphatic anomalies and hydroptic fetuses. If the jugular lymph sacs were to fail to communicate with the internal jugular veins, the posterior skin of the fetus would become distended. Later, with reestablishment of lymphaticovenous drainage, the jugular lymph sac would collapse, leaving a webbed neck and puffiness of the distal extremities, findings typical of Turner's syndrome. Another curious correlation is that patients with Turner's syndrome may have capillary-venular ectasia of the small and large bowel that can cause life-threatening gastrointestinal hemorrhage during childhood (Burge and associates, 1981; Rutlin and associates, 1981).

DIMINUTION IN SIZE

Growth proportionate to that of the child is the characteristic natural history of a lymphatic anomaly. However, there are reports of remarkable "regression" (Williams, 1979).

Broomhead noted spontaneous resolution in seven of 44 patients with cervical lymphatic anomalies; the improvement usually began early in life, continued steadily, and was complete by the age of 2 years (Broomhead, 1964). Grabb and colleagues (1980) followed 70 patients with lymphatic malformations and documented amelioration in 15 to 90 per cent. Figure 66–44*A,B* illustrates an infant with a posterior cervical lesion that literally vanished overnight. An example of a diffuse facial lesion that gradually diminished with time is seen in Figure 66–44*C,D.*

Until the mechanism is elucidated, use of the terms "resolution" or "deflation" seems more appropriate than labeling the cases as examples of "involution" or "regression" of lymphatic malformations. Lymphaticovenous shunts may be responsible or possibly drainage may occur through newly opened lymphatic channels. Other explanations proposed for deflation include rupture of cystic lesions or sclerosis secondary to infection (Figi, 1929; Gross and Goeringer, 1939).

TREATMENT OF LYMPHATIC MALFORMATIONS

The list of treatments for lymphatic anomalies includes the *injection of sclerosing agents*, e.g., boiling water (Reder, 1920), sodium morrhuate (Harrower, 1933), hyper-

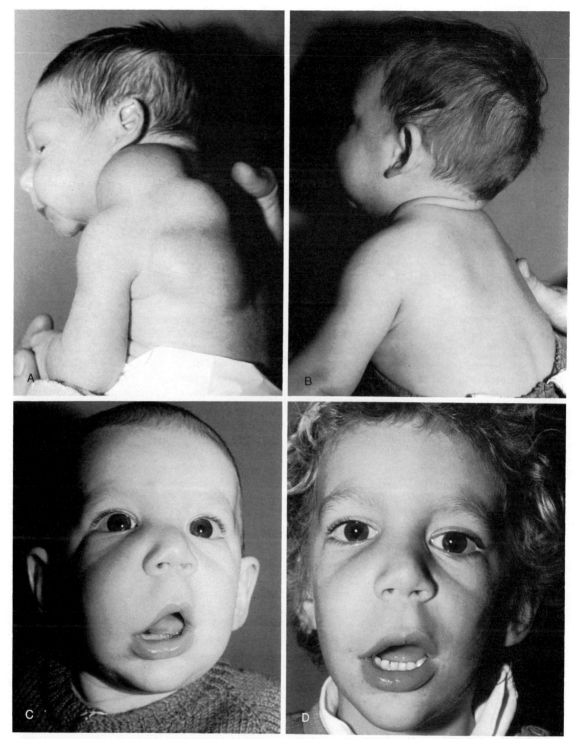

Figure 66–44. Natural shrinkage of lymphatic malformation. *A,* A 1 month old child with a multicystic lymphatic anomaly of the posterior shoulder and thorax. *B,* The same child at 3 months of age; the lesion "miraculously" disappeared (over a 48 hour period). *C,* A 6 month old boy with a diffuse lymphatic anomaly of the right face. *D,* The same boy at age 4 years. Note the improvement in contour; there is maxillary hypertrophy. (From Mulliken, J. B., and Young, A. E.: Vascular Birthmarks: Hemangiomas and Malformations. Philadelphia, W. B. Saunders Company, 1988.)

tonic salt or sugar solutions (Gross and Goeringer, 1939), iodized oil (Vaughan, 1934), and bleomycin (Ikeda and associates, 1977); *cautery* (Crawford and Vivakananthan, 1973); and *irradiation* (Figi, 1929). None of these therapies can be recommended today. Infections should be treated aggressively with antibiotics, and the mainstay of therapy, when indicated, is surgical excision.

Obstruction. A newborn infant with a cervicofacial lesion may present with rapid enlargement of the tongue or floor of the mouth, resulting in respiratory obstruction. The situation demands immediate attention to the airway. Aspiration or incision and drainage of a cystic sublingual lesion can be useful as an emergency maneuver (Fonkalsrud, 1974); however, this is rarely more than a temporizing measure (Chait and associates, 1974). A tracheostomy may be necessary, particularly when the lymphatic anomaly impinges on the oropharynx, or the obstruction occurs secondary to intralesional hemorrhage or sepsis. A large cervicofacial anomaly may also compromise function of the tongue and upper alimentary tract, necessitating the placement of a feeding tube or gastrostomy.

Sepsis. Rapid increase in the size of a lymphatic malformation usually indicates cellulitis, and is accompanied by erythema, tenseness, tenderness, and fever. This situation requires prompt initiation of penicillin therapy, on the presumption that the mouth flora are responsible (gram-positive and anaerobic microorganisms). Severe or recurrent cellulitis necessitates systemic antibiotic therapy. If the patient is unable to tolerate penicillin, either clindamycin or erythromycin should be given. The clinical response is often protracted, and recrudescent infection frequently occurs. Prophylactic antibiotics probably should not be used because of the likelihood of selection for more resistant bacterial strains. After the inflammation subsides, the involved area usually remains edematous and firm for an extended time.

Carious primary teeth may be the source of bacterial contamination of a lymphatic anomaly. Therefore, dental care is an especially important prophylactic measure in these children. If the palatine tonsils are suspected as the origin of repeated sepsis, tonsillectomy may be indicated.

Excision. Given that there may be improvement in certain lesions, watchful waiting seems justified. This is advisable for small-channel anomalies with diffuse in-

volvement throughout the face and neck, for which surgical excision is hazardous. On the other hand, a well-localized cystic lymphatic anomaly can be dissected from surrounding tissue, and this type of lesion is unlikely to deflate, no matter how long it is observed.

A lymphatic anomaly is not neoplastic. It does not slowly invade normal tissues, but involves adjacent tissues that are apparently normal. Therefore, wide and complete resection is the surgical goal. For a diffuse malformation, staged excision is recommended, limiting each procedure to a defined anatomic area. In planning, the surgeon should set restrictions, not only for the extent of dissection, but also for the duration of the operation and limit of blood loss.

The coronal incision may be useful in approaching a *fronto-orbital* lymphatic malformation; resection is often necessary during infancy in order to preserve vision (Fig. 66–45A,B). Anomalous lymphatic tissue in the upper eyelid is removed via an incision in the supratarsal fold. Conjunctival lesions can be locally excised, but recurrent cyst formation is common. Removal of a *hemifacial* anomaly is best undertaken via a preauricular incision, and requires tedious dissection of the facial nerve in continuity with resection of the superficial portion of the parotid gland. Azzolini, Salimbeni Ughi, and Riberti (1984) recommended temporary occlusion of the external carotid artery during such a dissection. *Cervical* lymphatic malformation requires a radical neck type of dissection. As in cervical lymphadenectomy, the marginal mandibular branch of the facial nerve must be isolated early in the procedure. The internal jugular vein usually must be taken; the sternocleidomastoid muscle can be spared if it is not riddled with lymphatic cysts. All important nerves in the neck must be identified, including the cervical sympathetic chain. The specimen can be divided during the dissection in order to preserve these nerves (Fig. 66–45C, D). A cervical lymphatic anomaly may involve the *axilla* and dissection of the brachial plexus should be undertaken as a separate procedure. *Thoracic* wall lymphatic anomalies can usually be easily encompassed by wide resection beneath skin flaps.

A superficial lymphatic anomaly ("lymphangioma circumscriptum") usually presents in the posterior cervical area, shoulder, or axilla as multiple warty cutaneous excrescences, with repeated bleeding, purulent drainage, or irritation. The abnormal super-

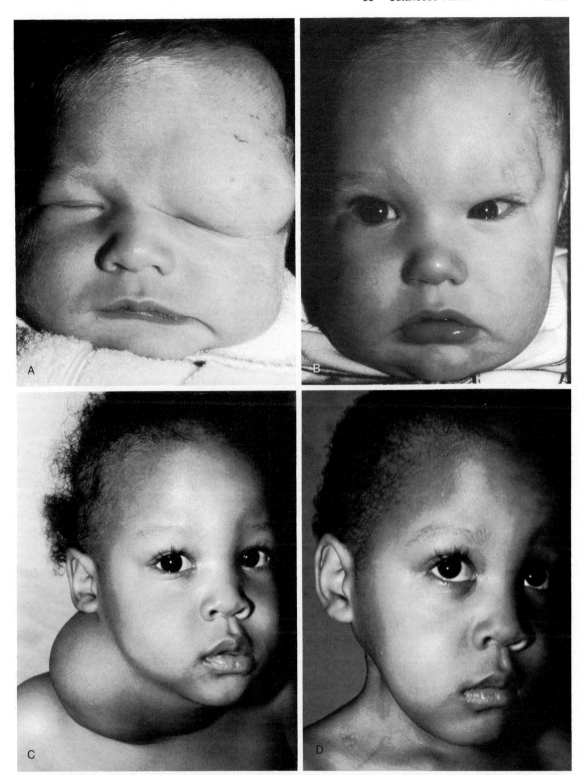

Figure 66–45. Operative treatment of lymphatic malformation. *A,* Fronto-orbital lymphatic anomaly, involving the adnexa oculi and obstructing the visual axis. *B,* Coronal and conjunctival incisions were used to resect this lesion. There is a residual intraorbital lymphatic anomaly. *C,* Cervical anomaly: a common variant that has a cystic quality and is easily transilluminated. *D,* Postoperative appearance; the sternocleidomastoid muscle could not be preserved. (*C* and *D* from Mulliken, J. B., and Young, A. E.: Vascular Birthmarks: Hemangiomas and Malformations. Philadelphia, W. B. Saunders Company, 1988.)

ficial dermal vesicles communicate with muscle-coated lymphatic cisterns, lying deep in the subcutaneous plane, that do not communicate with the deep lymphatic system (Whimster, 1976). Definitive treatment necessitates excision of both skin and subcutaneous tissue down to fascia. Frozen section monitoring of the excision margin may help to ensure removal of abnormal tissue extending beyond the territory of the skin vesicles (Bauer, Kernahan, and Hugo, 1981). The resultant defect usually requires closure with either a split-thickness skin graft or a flap. If the abnormal lymphatic tissue is not completely removed, vesicles will reappear in the scar or at the juncture of graft and skin.

Operative reduction for macroglossia may be necessary to restore the tongue into the oral cavity. A vertical or transverse wedge resection of the tongue may also mitigate the development of an anterior open bite deformity (Dingman and Grabb, 1961). However, there is no evidence that resection of a lymphatic anomaly of the tongue or cervical facial tissue will minimize mandibular overgrowth. Argon laser therapy can be used to coagulate troublesome, oozing mucosal blebs (Apfelberg and associates, 1985).

Osseous hypertrophy and distortion can interfere with dental occlusion and cause facial asymmetry. Bone contour reduction and/or osteotomies of the facial skeleton are helpful, and orthognathic procedures may be used to correct a malocclusion secondary to orofacial lymphatic malformation (see Chap. 29).

Management of lymphatic anomalies of the extremities ("lymphedema") is discussed in Chapter 83.

POSTOPERATIVE COMPLICATIONS

Wound complications after excision of a lymphatic malformation include: serosanguineous fluid collection, prolonged serous drainage, and delayed healing. Early postoperative infection or a delayed cellulitis within retained lymphatic tissue may occur. Even in the antibiotic era, the overall postoperative mortality rate is reported as 3.1 per cent (Ninh and Ninh, 1974).

Postoperative facial nerve paresis or paralysis is an obvious concern. Devastating bilateral hypoglossal nerve loss may result from repeated attempts to excise an anterior cervical lymphatic anomaly.

The appearance of vesicular blebs in the excision scar is an annoying late complication. Lymphatic cysts may reexpand within the resected area months to years after surgical removal. Two possible mechanisms could account for such "recurrences." First, there may be dilatation of persistent or preexisting channels, the result of scarring and obstruction of lymphatic drainage. Second, it is well known that lymphatics have a remarkable ability to regenerate. Incomplete excision may stimulate the proliferation of lymphatic channels within the injured tissues. It remains to be proved that anomalous lymphatics, whether damaged or not, can penetrate adjacent normal tissues.

Postoperative enlargement of a lymphatic malformation may also result if venous blood enters the anomalous vascular spaces. This phenomenon may be a consequence of rupture of vessels in the lymphatic walls or undetected lymphaticovenous connections (i.e., a combined low flow anomaly). This complication challenges the concept of a rigid distinction between venous and lymphatic vascular malformations.

Venous Malformations (VM)

TERMINOLOGY

Venous anomalies are often erroneously included under the generic mantle of "hemangioma" and labeled "cavernous hemangioma," "varicose hemangioma," or "lymphohemangioma." They are not true hemangiomas, but rather are developmental abnormalities of veins, dysmorphic in configuration and structure. Venous malformations usually occur in pure form, or they may be combined capillary-venous (CVM) or lymphaticovenous (LVM) malformations.

HISTOLOGY

Microscopic examination of a venous malformation demonstrates dilated vascular channels, varying from capillary to cavernous dimensions and lined by normal flattened endothelium. Ultrastructural examination shows a single continuous basal lamina. There is evidence of sparse smooth muscle and adventitial fibrosis in the larger anomalous channels. Organizing thrombi are frequently seen along with dystrophic calcification (phleboliths). Sections of a recent thrombus may demonstrate hypercellularity and mitoses. This finding should not be interpreted as neoangiogenesis within the malformation, nor should it be confused with angiosarcoma; it is often called "pseudosarcomatous endothelial proliferation" (Jakobiec and Jones, 1979).

CLINICAL FINDINGS

Venous anomalies present in a wide spectrum ranging from isolated skin varicosities, ectasias, or localized spongy masses to complex lesions permeating through tissue planes and presenting in diverse anatomic locations (Fig. 66–46). The skin overlying a venous malformation may be normal, although more often there is a bluish hue or dark blue color if the dermis is involved. Combined cutaneous capillary-venous malformations have a dark red to purple color. The combined lymphaticovenous lesions exhibit superficial lymphatic vesicles (often hyperkeratotic) overlying the deep venous anomaly.

Venous malformations are soft, compressible, and nonpulsatile. Cervicofacial lesions characteristically expand with a Valsalva maneuver, with the head placed in a dependent position, or with jugular vein compression (Fig. 66–47A,B). Venous anomalies of the extremities enlarge with exercise, prolonged dependency, or application of a tourniquet. They usually grow in proportion to the child, and they have little tendency to

expand unless interfered with. Rapid enlargement may follow injury or partial resection or may occur coincident with puberty, pregnancy, or antiovulant medication. Following trauma, a quiescent venous abnormality occasionally may evidence arteriovenous shunting; the lesion must be reclassified as a high flow malformation. Phlebothrombosis is a common occurrence in venous anomalies, and recurrent localized pain and tenderness are frequent presenting complaints. Phleboliths can be palpated or seen on radiographic examination (see Fig. 66–46B).

Venous anomalies may occur in skeletal muscle without involvement of the overlying skin (Scott, 1957); intramasseteric lesions are most common (Welsh and Hengerer, 1980). If a vascular lesion within the cheek becomes more prominent by tensing of the masseter, the anomaly may be either within the muscle or within the parotid gland (Faber and associates, 1978). Venous anomalies within the temporal muscle are rare (Joehl and associates, 1979). The diagnosis of intramuscular venous malformation is confirmed if phleboliths are present.

Venous anomalies are also seen in the craniofacial bones. Lesions of the frontal and parietal calvaria are supplied by the middle meningeal artery and often the superficial temporal artery (Gupta, Tiwari, and Pasupathy, 1975; Kirchhoff, Eggert, and Agnoli,

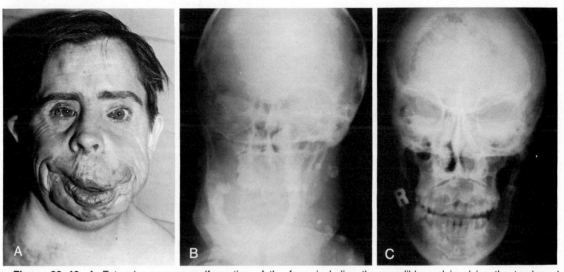

Figure 66–46. *A,* Extensive venous malformation of the face, including the mandible and involving the trunk and extremities. The patient has low grade consumptive coagulopathy and bleeds intermittently from the gingiva. *B,* Posteroanterior cephalogram of the patient demonstrates multiple bilateral phleboliths and extensive erosion of the mandible. *C,* An isolated venous anomaly of the frontal bone exhibits a characteristic "honeycomb" or "sunburst" pattern. (From Mulliken, J. B., and Young, A. E.: Vascular Birthmarks: Hemangiomas and Malformations. Philadelphia, W. B. Saunders Company, 1988.)

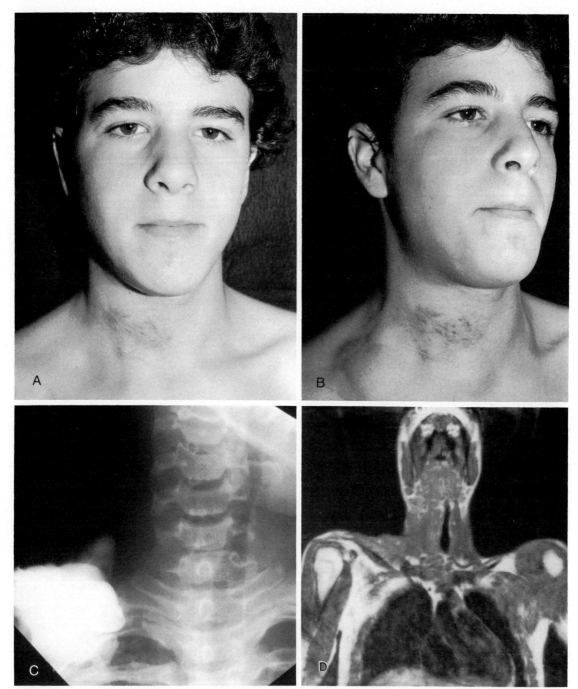

Figure 66–47. Cervical venous malformation with telangiectatic vessels in the overlying skin. *B,* The malformation is more obvious with a Valsalva maneuver. *C,* A direct intralesional dye injection, showing the large multilocular venous malformation involving the brachial plexus, fails to fill the more proximal channels in the neck. *D,* A nuclear magnetic resonance (NMR) image demonstrates that the venous anomaly (negative signal) is more extensive, involving the cervical and hypopharyngeal region and deviating the trachea. (From Mulliken, J. B., and Young, A. E.: Vascular Birthmarks: Hemangiomas and Malformations. Philadelphia, W. B. Saunders Company, 1988.)

1978). Venous anomalies also occur rarely in the nasal bones (Kanter, Brown, and Noe, 1985) and zygoma (Marshak, 1980; Schmidt, 1982). The most common craniofacial skeletal location is the mandible, and less often the maxilla. The lesions are frequently referred to as "central hemangioma" (Sadowsky and associates, 1981). Most reported anomalies are venous, although arteriovenous malformations in the mandible have also been documented (Hoey and associates, 1970; Kaban and Mulliken, 1986). Venous lesions of the mandible usually appear in the second decade as a painless, slowly growing mass. There may also be increased mobility of the teeth, expansion of the buccal cortex, or spontaneous bleeding around the gingival necks of the teeth; the lesions seldom cause paresthesia (Sadowsky and associates, 1981). Unexpected hemorrhage can follow tooth extraction or intervention for biopsy. The bleeding is either from the intraosseous vascular malformation per se or secondary to a localized coagulopathy (Kaban and Mulliken, 1986).

The radiographic appearance of craniofacial intraosseous venous anomalies is usually pathognomonic (Sherman and Wilner, 1961). Plain films demonstrate a local rarefied area with a "soap bubble" or "honeycomb" appearance, indicating the venous sinuses, which are supported by connective tissue stroma and bony trabeculae (see Fig. 66–46C). Profile or tangential films show spicules of bone radiating in a "sunburst" pattern. Computed tomography also demonstrates the intact periosteum, cortical expansion, and bony trabeculae within such an anomaly. Bone erosion is more typical of an arteriovenous malformation. Skeletal alteration, without actual intraosseous involvement, frequently occurs in association with cutaneous venous anomalies, particularly in the combined lymphaticovenous forms; bone distortion and hypertrophy are the most common changes (Boyd and associates, 1984).

TREATMENT

Venous malformations have been treated with *irradiation, electrocoagulation* (Figi, 1948), *freezing* techniques (Goldwyn and Rosoff, 1969; Huang and associates, 1972; Jarzab, 1975; Ohtsuka, Shioya, and Tanaka, 1980), *intravascular magnesium needles* (Wilflingseder, Martin, and Papp, 1981), and a long list of *sclerosants*: boiling water (Wyeth, 1903; Cole and Hunt, 1949), alcohol, sodium

morrhuate, quinine, urethan (solution of quinine and ethyl carbamate), silver nitrate, and iron or zinc chloride (Boman, 1940).

The indications for therapy are cosmetic and functional. In order to formulate a therapeutic plan, one must (1) confirm the lesion's rheologic character, (2) delineate the anatomic boundaries and channel size, and (3) evaluate the coagulation parameters. Unfortunately, given current technology, not all venous malformations can be successfully treated.

Angiography. Physical examination should be sufficient to determine whether a lesion belongs in one of the low flow malformation categories, i.e., venous (VM), capillary-venous (CVM), or lymphaticovenous (LVM). Computed tomography, with dye enhancement, is easily accomplished and may provide useful information. For a VM or CVM, direct venography under fluoroscopic control may accurately document the anatomy of the lesion (Boxt, Levin, and Fellows, 1983). The true extent of the lesion can be underestimated if there is incomplete filling of all abnormal veins or sinusoids that constitute the malformation (Fig. 66–47C). Nuclear magnetic resonance (NMR) imaging will be used more frequently as a noninvasive study of low flow vascular lesions (Fig. 66–47D) (Lea Thomas, 1988). Arteriography, either a selective or a superselective study, may be necessary to rule out an arterial component manifested by microarteriovenous shunting. In a large venous anomaly, superselective angiography may demonstrate the entire lesion, but only if sufficient contrast material is injected over a relatively long period. No abnormal "feeding" arteries are seen in a venous anomaly; delayed films reveal saccular pooling of the contrast dye, often in only a portion of the lesion.

Localized Intravascular Coagulopathy. Stasis within the low flow anomaly is probably the primary event that initiates fibrin generation. There may also be associated fibrinolysis due to plasminogen activation. The possibility of localized intravascular coagulopathy requires thorough hematologic evaluation, including a complete blood count with examination of the peripheral blood smear. PT and PTT are often within normal limits; fibrin split products and fibrinopeptide A may be elevated with concomitant decreased fibrinogen and platelet levels. Since a low grade, well-compensated consumptive coagulopathy can be exacerbated by an operation, the coagulopathy should be corrected preoperatively and the coagulation status monitored closely after a surgical procedure (Rodriguez-Erdmann and associates, 1971; Lang and Dubin, 1975). Severe systemic consumption coagulopathy may necessitate heparin therapy before a surgical procedure can be safely performed. Another approach is to begin heparin first, and follow it with antifibrinolytic therapy. Aminocaproic acid combined with cryoprecipitate is effective therapy for localized coagulopathy and may produce thrombosis and shrinkage of a venous anomaly (Warrell and Kempin, 1985).

Sclerotherapy. Although selective arterial embolization techniques have a deserved place in the management of arteriovenous malformations, embolic occlusion of the arterial inflow to a venous anomaly often causes necrosis of adjacent tissue and overlying skin (Demuth, Miller, and Keller, 1984). A more appealing stratagem is direct injection of a sclerosing solution into the epicenter of the venous anomaly during occlusion of the arterial inflow and venous outflow.

Endovascular obliteration of low flow anomalies has had a history of checkered success. Sclerosing agents, e.g., sodium morrhuate and ethyl carbamate, have not been particularly successful, except in the treatment of small local ectasias (Morgan and Schow, 1974). A liquid vegetable protein, Ethibloc (Ethicon Laboratories), has been used extensively in Europe; it is particularly effective in obliterating capillary-venous and pure venous anomalies (Fig. 66–48) (Riché

and associates, 1983; Riché and Merland, 1988). Sodium tetradecyl sulfate has been injected into venous anomalies in a small number of patients (Minkow, Laufer, and Gutman, 1979; Woods, 1987). Ethanol sclerotherapy is also at an early stage of clinical investigation (Lasjaunias and Berenstein, 1987).

Percutaneous electrodes have also been used to induce thrombosis within low flow vascular anomalies (Ogawa and Inoue, 1982). Photocoagulation with argon or yttrium-aluminum-garnet laser may be effective for tiny superficial venous or capillary-venous lesions.

Surgical Resection. Total excision is the definitive treatment for a venous malformation. All too often, anomalies extend beyond apparent boundaries, and surgical removal must be restrained by anatomic considerations with both esthetic and functional consequences. Subtotal removal can usually be safely accomplished in selected patients with capillary-venous, lymphaticovenous, or venous malformations. Resection is indicated to reduce bulk and improve contour and function (Fig. 66–49). Limited excision may also play a role in controlling chronically painful areas within a venous anomaly.

Craniectomy may be indicated for venous anomalies of the calvaria, followed by primary or secondary cranioplasty (Kirchhoff, Eggert, and Agnoli, 1978; Wojtanowski and Mandel, 1979). Venous malformations of the jaws, zygoma, or nasal bones are managed by curettage and, if necessary, packing the bone defect with hemostatic material. Bone hyper-

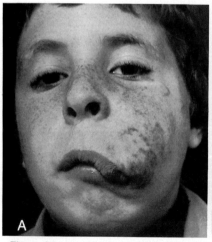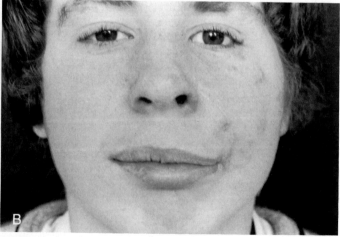

Figure 66–48. Sclerosant therapy for venous malformation. *A,* A 16 year old male with capillary-venous malformation of the upper lip and left cheek. *B,* The result after single Ethibloc injection and excision through the nasolabial fold, two years postoperatively. (From Riché, M. C., et al.: The treatment of capillary-venous malformations using a new fibrosing agent. Plast. Reconstr. Surg., *71*:607, 1983).

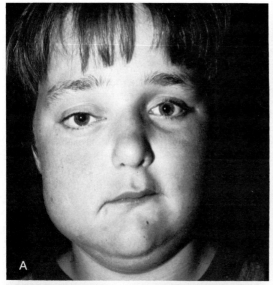

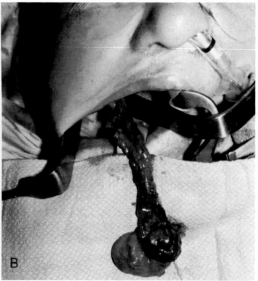

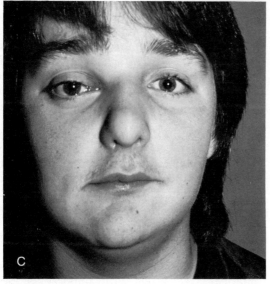

Figure 66–49. Subtotal excision of a venous malformation. *A,* Venous anomaly of the right cheek, involving the periorbital tissue. *B,* Intraoperative view of a venous anomaly within the buccal fat pad. *C,* Cheek contour improved two years postoperatively. Anomalous venous channels remain in the subconjunctival and periorbital tissues. (From Mulliken, J. B., and Young, A. E.: Vascular Birthmarks: Hemangiomas and Malformations. Philadelphia, W. B. Saunders Company, 1988.)

trophy and distortion, secondary to venous or lymphaticovenous anomalies, can be corrected by craniofacial and maxillofacial surgical procedures.

HIGH FLOW VASCULAR MALFORMATIONS

Arteriovenous Malformations (AVM)

TERMINOLOGY

The high flow vascular malformation was accurately described by Bell in his 1815 surgical text. He coined "aneurysm by anas-tomosis," an expression that later became synonymous with "pulsating angioma," "racemose aneurysm," "cirsoid aneurysm," and "pulsatile fungus hematode" (Reid, 1925a). Nineteenth century physicians were well aware of the "malignant" behavior of a pulsatile birthmark, in contrast to the benignant nevus maternus (hemangioma). "Aneurysm by anastomosis" was feared because of its propensity for hemorrhage, ulceration, and rapid enlargement, particularly after attempted extirpation.

The high flow anomalies can be subdivided: *arterial malformations* (AM)—aneurysm, ectasia, or coarctation; *arteriovenous fistulas* (AVF)—localized shunts from large (truncal) arterial branches; and *arteriovenous malfor-*

mations (AVM)—myriad small fistulas, either diffuse or localized with a "nidus" of abnormal intercalated tissue.

HISTOLOGY

Tissue from the epicenter of an arteriovenous malformation demonstrates close juxtaposition of medium-sized arteries, veins, and vessels. It is difficult, with hematoxylin and eosin stains, to determine whether any particular abnormal vascular channel is part of the original (primary) malformation or is secondarily altered because of increased flow and pressure. In time, the veins become "arterialized" and exhibit intimal thickening, increased smooth muscle within the media, and dilatation of the vasa vasorum (Reid, 1925b). There is also progressive dilatation of the proximal arteries, with fibrosis, thinning of the media, and diminished elastic tissue (Reid, 1925b). Reid (1925c) believed that the thin-walled arteries and veins could rupture into one another, forming new fistulous connections, an explanation for the rapid enlargement of arteriovenous anomalies that occurs after trauma or during pregnancy.

PHYSIOLOGY

An understanding of the natural history of congenital arteriovenous malformation is aided by the studies of post-traumatic and artificially constructed arteriovenous fistulas (Reid, 1925b; Pemberton and Saint, 1928; Holman, 1968). To some degree, congenital fistulas resemble the acquired lesions. There are differences; for example, congenital fistulas are more numerous and often microscopic in size, in comparison with acquired connections (Holman, 1968). Nevertheless, like acquired fistulas, congenital fistulas can cause cardiac enlargement over a long period as a result of the direct communication between the high resistance, high pressure arterial system and the low pressure, low resistance venous system. Arteriovenous fistulas enlarge slowly and the distal vascular bed dilates as more blood is sequestered into the circuits, causing distention of the fistulas and communicating veins. The rheologic changes also stimulate the development of collateral circulation in the region of the arteriovenous malformation. The arteries primarily involved gradually dilate further and become tortuous (presumably their walls are structurally faulty). The veins also dilate; there is

progressive fibrosis within the intima, media, and adventitia. If the fistulas between the arterial and venous circuits are quickly occluded, the heart slows—the bradycardiac phenomenon first observed by Nicoladoni (1875).

CLINICAL FINDINGS

Arteriovenous malformations occur most commonly in the head and neck region and extremities and they are rare compared with low flow vascular anomalies. The largest series of head and neck lesions was published by Malan and Azzolini (1968); other reports are based on a small number of patients (Callander, 1920; Reid, 1925a; Pemberton and Saint, 1928; Coleman and Hoopes, 1971). Arteriovenous malformations are 20 times more common in the intracerebral vasculature than in extracerebral sites (Olivecrona and Ladenheim, 1957).

Arteriovenous malformations are sometimes noted soon after birth. Symptomatic cardiac decompensation is rare in infancy, although a few neonates with large, active arteriovenous malformations develop potentially lethal cardiac failure within hours or days of birth (Flye, Jordan, and Schwartz, 1983). Years usually pass before an arteriovenous anomaly poses a threat as the ominous signs and symptoms of high flow become manifest. The lesions grow proportionately during childhood, and many go unnoticed. Some lesions lie hidden beneath an innocent-appearing cutaneous capillary stain. Rapid expansion may follow local trauma, attempted excision/ligation, or hormonal changes associated with puberty or pregnancy.

Patients with a cervicocephalic arteriovenous malformation may hear a distressing buzzing sound in the ear that prevents concentration or deprives them of sleep (Malan and Azzolini, 1968; Coleman, 1973). Pain, frequently sudden and stabbing in nature, is a common presenting complaint, especially when the vascular anomaly lies within the facial bones (Coleman, 1973).

The involved skin has an elevated temperature and usually there is a dermal stain. Palpation reveals a thrill, often transmitted along the vessels of the ipsilateral neck and head. In older lesions, pulsating veins and congestion and tortuosity of the vessels become obvious. The presence of arteriovenous shunting is confirmed by a bruit on auscultation and a constant, machinery-like murmur that is accentuated during systole.

Arteriovenous shunting (the steal phenomenon) diminishes nutritive flow to the skin so that ischemic necrosis may ensue. Repeated episodes of hemorrhage, often precipitous, follow minor trauma and may lead to a life-threatening emergency.

Destruction of adjacent osseous structures and/or actual bone involvement also occurs with craniofacial arteriovenous malformations. Within the mandible or maxilla, the anomalies may be asymptomatic or may present with pulsatile swelling in the jaw, localized throbbing pain, toothache, or sudden hemorrhage.

Disseminated intravascular coagulopathy, secondary to thrombotic consumption or destruction of clotting factors, is an insidious problem with large arteriovenous anomalies.

TREATMENT

The management of arteriovenous anomalies is potentially hazardous and the outcome is sometimes disappointing. Therapy for a purely cosmetic deformity may have to be postponed until complications arise, such as repeated hemorrhage, pain, pressure, ischemic ulceration, or congestive heart failure. The therapeutic strategy for arteriovenous anomalies consists of (1) selective embolization and (2) surgical removal, or a combination of both.

Angiography. Angiography is compulsory before one embarks on a management plan. Because the facial skeleton obscures the vascular anatomy, selective angiography and subtraction techniques are helpful for the radiologic assessment. Digital subtraction angiography allows injection of lower-strength contrast medium, instant computerized subtraction, and the potential for dynamic flow imaging. Nuclear magnetic resonance imaging is just beginning to be applied to arteriovenous anomalies and provides additional information on the extent of the lesion.

In case a major vessel needs to be sacrificed, the angiographic study must include the intracerebral circulation in order to assess the possibility of shunting between the external and internal carotid systems, the flow within the circle of Willis, and the relative contributions of the vertebral and internal carotid vessels. There is a tendency for contrast medium to shunt preferentially through the most proximal arteriovenous fistulas and fail to demonstrate the more peripheral fistulas. In addition, many of the shunts may be nonfunctional at the time of arteriography. Malan and Azzolini (1968) listed five indirect angiographic signs of arteriovenous fistulas in head and neck arteriovenous malformations:

1. Dilatation and lengthening of the afferent arteries.
2. Early and preferential flow of contrast medium toward the shunts.
3. Delayed and diminished filling of the other arteries originating from the external carotid artery.
4. Early opacification of the efferent veins, beginning at the level of the proximal fistulas.
5. Abnormal and rapid opacification of the collateral circulation.

The Fallacy of Proximal Ligation. The oldest surgical treatment of arteriovenous malformations can be traced to Hunter's successful ligation for degenerative popliteal aneurysm (Home, 1793). Examples of isolated arteriovenous fistulas, potentially curable by ligation, are exceedingly rare (Rienhoff, 1924). Halsted's patient, treated by ligation of anomalous communications between the external carotid and venous cervical plexus (Halsted, 1919), required en bloc resection 48 years later (Ravitch and Gaertner, 1960).

The hunterian concept of proximal ligation for treatment of arteriovenous malformations proved to be disastrous. Interruption of the external carotid artery or its branches results in a pressure drop in the distal tributaries, and causes collateral formation and retrograde diversion of flow from the internal carotid artery system. A "steal phenomenon" occurs, particularly in the ophthalmic artery and, to a lesser degree, from other anastomotic branches, especially the meningeal arteries. With time, the malformation becomes larger, with opening of collateral channels from the ipsilateral as well as the contralateral vessels. Carotid interruption has resulted in severe atherosclerosis in the supratentorial vessels, chronic hemispherical ischemia, and frank cerebral atrophy (Azzolini and Lechi, 1968). Horrendous examples of expansion and tissue destruction following proximal ligation for arteriovenous malformation are well documented (Coleman and Hoopes, 1971; Habal and Murray, 1972).

Embolization. Selective arteriography and embolization for intracranial anomalies were first introduced by Djindjian and associates (1977). The techniques were also applied to extracranial vascular malformations (Cunningham and Paletta, 1970; Bennett and Zook, 1972; Longacre, Benton, and Unterthiner, 1972; Haughton, 1975; Olcott and associates, 1976). On first reflection, embolization would seem to carry the same hemodynamic risk as proximal arterial ligation. Embolization, however, differs in concept because the blood delivers the embolic material into the center of the vascular malformation ("the nidus"), blocking the smallest vessels first, from the inside out (Natali and Merland, 1976; Leikensohn, Epstein, and Vasconez, 1981). Selective angiography of a facial arteriovenous malformation demonstrates that embolic occlusion of one feeding vessel causes an immediate increased flow from other facial vessels. Therefore, in theory, all micro- and macrofistulas must be obliterated in order to collapse the arteriovenous malformation permanently (Riché and Merland, 1988).

The transfemoral route is almost invariably used in order to manipulate the catheter, under fluoroscopic control, into the relevant feeding vessels. Embolic therapy for arteriovenous malformations can be either curative, palliative, or presurgical (Leikensohn, Epstein, and Vasconez, 1981). As a primary treatment modality, embolization with nonabsorbable material is used for inaccessible lesions or for extensive lesions in which surgical resection would be too mutilating. Polyvinyl alcohol foam granules are the most commonly employed nonabsorbable materials; others include lyophilized dura mater, steel coils, and detachable balloons (Debrun and associates, 1978; Riché and Merland, 1988). With obliteration of a large proportion of shunts, the arteriovenous anomaly is diminished and collateral vessels develop slowly. However, primary embolization should be regarded only as potentially curative; all too often, recanalization and reexpansion occur in time.

Intra-arterial embolization may be used to relieve symptoms of unresectable arteriovenous malformations, e.g., for hemorrhage, pain, or ischemic ulceration (Riché and Merland, 1988).

Preoperative embolization should be considered in order to diminish blood loss and facilitate surgical extirpation. Presurgical embolization should not be used in an effort to reduce the extent of resection. Temporary occlusive material is used, usually gelatin sponge (Gelfoam), and excision is arranged

for 48 to 72 hours after embolization (Azzolini, Bertani, and Riberti, 1982). Excellent results, in the short term, are possible using combined embolization and resection for extensive high flow anomalies (Schrudde and Petrovici, 1981).

The only assurance for long-term success is total resection of an arteriovenous malformation (Malan and Azzolini, 1968; Coleman, 1973; Mulliken, 1988b). Leaving behind dormant or residual anomalous channels, beyond the resection margin, invites further collateral formation, shunting, and reexpansion. Esthetic and functional considerations, particularly in the facial region, make it imperative to limit unnecessary sacrifice of tissue. Nevertheless, the goal must be radical removal of the vascular malformation. Feeding vessels may be temporarily occluded in order to diminish blood loss during the resection; however, feeding vessels should *never* be permanently ligated. Several maneuvers should be considered to minimize intraoperative hemorrhage: hypotensive anesthesia (Munro and Martin, 1980), cardiopulmonary bypass with deep hypothermic circulatory arrest (Mulliken and associates, 1978), or percutaneous transcatheter balloon occlusion of feeding vessels (Haller and associates, 1980). Placement of temporary mattress sutures around the periphery of the excision margin is a rediscovered technique (Fig. 66–50).

An arteriovenous malformation of the scalp should be widely excised (to the pericranium) and the defect closed primarily, usually with a skin graft. What appears to be a simple capillary stain of the auricle, more often than not, proves to be an underlying arteriovenous malformation. After signs and symptoms develop, treatment usually necessitates total amputation of the external ear and, if necessary, dissection of the seventh cranial nerve (Dingman and Grabb, 1965). If the arteriovenous malformation does not extend beyond the auricle, it may be possible to excise the involved skin and immediately cover the exposed cartilage framework with a temporoparietal fascial flap and split-thickness skin graft (provided the superficial temporal artery has not been sacrificed).

Following resection of an arteriovenous malformation, delayed primary closure with a skin graft is useful, particularly if bleeding is excessive, as long as vital structures are not exposed. Primary or delayed coverage with local cutaneous or musculocutaneous flaps must not involve anomalous vessels. Microvascular flap transfer should be consid-

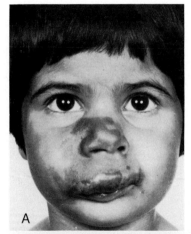

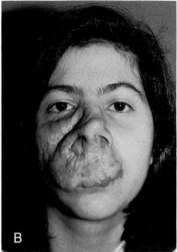

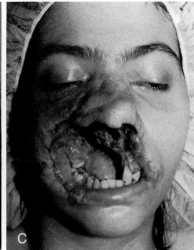

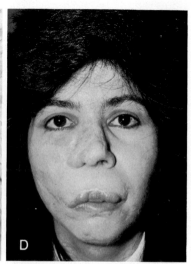

Figure 66–50. Resection and reconstruction of a facial arteriovenous malformation using tube flaps. *A,* A 3 year old girl with a port-wine stain of the nose and lip and an underlying arteriovenous malformation. *B,* At age 22 after irradiation, sclerotherapy, and several resections. She has frequent epistaxis; the right maxillary teeth are loose, indicating intraosseous vascular involvement. *C,* Forty-eight hours after embolization of the right internal maxillary artery (using Gelfoam), hemimaxillectomy, and resection of the upper lip and lower cheek accomplished under hypotensive anesthesia. *D,* Five years after staged reconstruction with a tube inner-upper arm flap and tube buccal mucosal flaps. The capillary-venous component in the nasal skin remains quiescent. (From Mulliken, J. B., and Young, A. E.: Vascular Birthmarks: Hemangiomas and Malformations. Philadelphia, W. B. Saunders Company, 1988.)

ered for coverage of large wounds with exposed nerves, vessels, or bone. Potential donor vessels for microanastomoses must be anticipated in planning preoperative embolization, and they must be preserved, if possible, during the resection (Fig. 66–51). If excision of an arteriovenous malformation is incomplete, in time it reexpands and may entangle the skin graft or flap tissue used for coverage (Puglionisi and Azzolini, 1963). Arterialized flaps may minimize reexpansion of an incompletely resected arteriovenous anomaly (Hurwitz and Kerber, 1981), although this concept has yet to be validated.

Arteriovenous anomalies of the jaws can present with frightening hemorrhage, often after tooth extraction. The most effective measure is immediate packing and pressure. There is no place for proximal arterial ligation, except perhaps as a life-saving maneuver. For elective therapy of vascular anomalies of the jaw, Azzolini, Bertani, and Riberti (1982) recommended temporary occlusion of both external carotid vessels, dental extraction, curettage, and packing with absorbable hemostatic material. Preoperative embolization is useful for mandibular arteriovenous malformations (Hoey and associates, 1970; Bryant and Maull, 1975). If these attempts fail, hemimandibulectomy is clearly indicated. Exposure to high flow anomalies of the temporal, masseter, and pterygoid muscles is via a transtemporal subfascial approach (Malan and Azzolini, 1968; Azzolini, Bertani, and Riberti, 1982).

COMBINED VASCULAR MALFORMATIONS AND HYPERTROPHY SYNDROMES

The development of the embryonic vascular system is closely integrated with morphogenesis of other mesenchymal tissues. It is, therefore, not surprising that close study of vas-

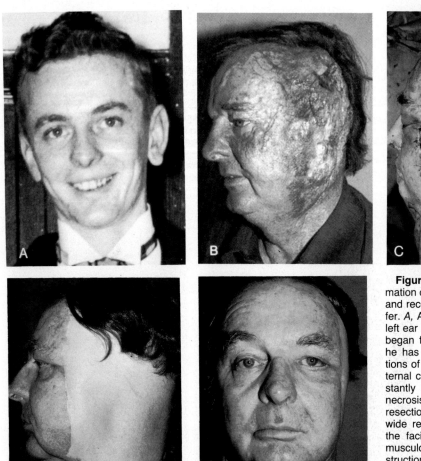

Figure 66–51. Arteriovenous malformation of the face, treated by resection and reconstruction with free flap transfer. *A,* A 21 year old male with a warm left ear and a port-wine stain; bleeding began five years later. *B,* At age 50, he has had ill-conceived staged ligations of both vertebral arteries and external carotid vessels. He bleeds constantly from an area of ischemic necrosis that failed to heal after ear resection. *C,* Intraoperative view after wide resection of the AVM, including the facial nerve. *D,* Latissimus dorsi musculocutaneous free flap reconstruction. Resected (ligated) left facial vessels necessitated spanning the neck with vein grafts to the contralateral common carotid artery and jugular vein. (Courtesy of J. Upton, III.) *E,* Appearance after fascial sling suspension of the mouth, lower eyelid, and brow to ameliorate the facial palsy (five years postoperatively). (From Mulliken, J. B., and Young, A. E.: Vascular Birthmarks: Hemangiomas and Malformations. Philadelphia, W. B. Saunders Company, 1988.)

cular malformations reveals involvement of more than one vascular component (capillaries, arteries, lymphatics, and veins), and in addition there is often anomalous overgrowth of soft tissue and bone. Disorders in which vascular malformations are associated with gigantism are best known by eponymous syndromic designations.

An example discussed earlier is the Sturge-Weber complex, which includes combined vascular malformations and facial overgrowth. In addition to the vascular abnormalities in the craniofacial region, capillary staining may also occur on the neck, trunk, and extremities, with clinical features of the Klippel-Trenaunay syndrome.

Klippel-Trenaunay Syndrome

The association of a vascular anomaly with limb hypertrophy was first delineated as a syndrome by Klippel and Trenaunay (1900a,b). This condition should be considered a combined capillary-lymphatic-venous malformation (CLVM). In 95 per cent of patients the lower limb is involved, usually unilaterally; in 5 per cent of patients the upper limb alone is implicated; and in a few individuals the whole trunk is affected. The cutaneous (port-wine) stain ranges from pink to deep purple in color; it may be macular, minimally raised, or studded with vascular nodules (localized venous or lymphatic vesicles). The

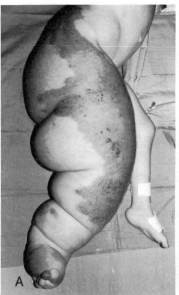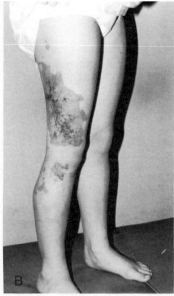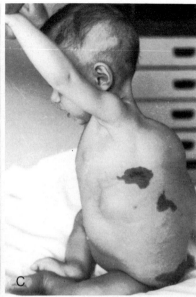

Figure 66–52. The spectrum of Klippel-Trenaunay syndrome. *A,* Infant with combined capillary-lymphatic-venous malformation of the pelvis and lower limb. *B,* Deep port-wine stain with punctate dermal ectasias, minimal soft tissue hypertrophy, and gradual limb overgrowth. *C,* Combined (capillary-lymphatic-venous) anomaly of the trunk and abdominal viscera.

distribution of the stain is often widespread and does not correspond to any cutaneous sensory nerve or other known metameric distribution (Fig. 66–52) (Young, 1978).

Varicosities of the greater and lesser saphenous system occur commonly, the most frequent pattern being the lateral venous anomaly of the calf (Young, 1988b). Incompetent perforating veins are seen, and in 25 to 50 per cent of patients deep vein abnormalities can also be documented (Lindenauer, 1965; Servelle, 1985; Young, 1988b). Although calf blood flow is within normal limits, flow in the abnormal limb is greater than in the normal limb (Ackroyd and associates, 1984). In the absence of arteriovenous fistulas, the increase in flow is ascribed to the presence of the capillary dermal malformation (Baskerville, Ackroyd, and Browse, 1985). Whether or not there is clinically apparent lymphatic involvement, most patients with the Klippel-Trenaunay syndrome have lymphatic hypoplasia by demonstrable lymphography (Young, 1988b); obvious lymphedema is observed in 25 per cent of patients (Kinmonth, 1982). If the trunk is involved, there may be vascular anomalies of the solid viscera, and intestinal lymphangiectasia may occur with associated protein-losing enteropathy (Fig. 66–52C).

Limb hypertrophy is in length (72 per cent)

or girth (58 per cent) (Young, 1988b). Gigantism is obvious at birth (Fig. 66–52A); more commonly, mild degrees of hypertrophy and elongation may not be noted until late infancy or adolescence (Fig. 66–52B). The limb enlargement is often disproportionate in parts of the limb, especially in the toes and feet. Increased girth of the limb is due to muscle hypertrophy, thickened skin, and excessive fat, in association with ectatic lymphaticovenous channels. A few patients, with otherwise classic Klippel-Trenaunay syndrome, may have a short and/or hypotrophic limb. The management of this syndrome is well presented by Young (1988c).

Parkes Weber Syndrome

The Parkes Weber syndrome is substantially less common than the Klippel-Trenaunay syndrome. Both are combined capillary-lymphatic-venous anomalies. The distinction is that in the Klippel-Trenaunay syndrome the primary vascular lesion is venous, whereas in the Parkes Weber syndrome (Weber, 1907a,b) the primary vascular anomaly is arteriovenous (Vollmar, 1974). The Parkes Weber syndrome more commonly affects the upper than the lower limb (Fig. 66–53) (Robertson, 1956). Infants with clinically obvious

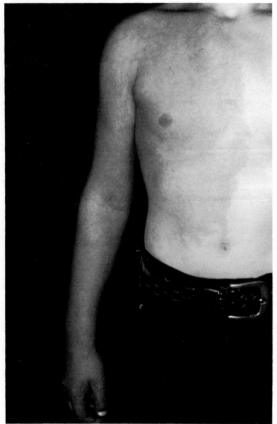

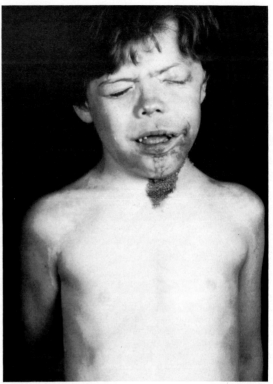

Figure 66–55. Epidermal nevus syndrome: 5 year old boy with cervicofacial verrucous nevus, capillary staining, and hemifacial skeletal and soft tissue overgrowth. Following a transient ischemic attack, an arteriogram demonstrated narrowing of the distal internal carotid artery with collaterals in the anterior cerebral territories ("moyamoya" syndrome). The patient presented with a giant cell tumor of the left maxilla at age 7 years.

Figure 66–53. Parkes Weber syndrome: dense port-wine stain of the upper extremity with overgrowth in length and girth. The limb is warm, indicating diffuse microarteriovenous shunting.

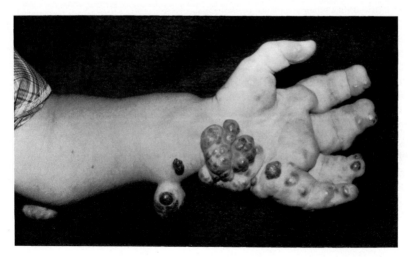

Figure 66–54. Maffucci's syndrome: exophytic venous anomalies with bone exostoses and enchondromatoses.

arteriovenous fistulas are likely to develop clinically important limb length disparity.

Maffucci's Syndrome

This syndrome is defined by the coexistence of vascular malformations and dyschondroplasia (Ollier's disease; multiple enchondromatosis). The first case was described by Maffucci in 1881; he also noted the increased risk of sarcomatous degeneration shared by Ollier's disease. In Maffucci's syndrome the long bones are foreshortened and deformed, with exostoses appearing on the fingers and toes, as well as on the proximal extremities. There are complex vascular anomalies in the subcutaneous tissues, usually venous but sometimes lymphatic in type (Fig. 66–54) (Loewinger and associates, 1977). Venous anomalies may also present in bone, leptomeninges, and the gastrointestinal tract (Cremer, Gullotta, and Wolf, 1981). Malignant tumors develop in 20 per cent of the patients (Lewis and Ketcham, 1973). These are usually chondrosarcoma; others include vascular sarcoma, glioma, fibroadenoma, and ovarian teratoma (Loewinger and associates, 1977; Cremer, Gullotta, and Wolf, 1981; Cheng and associates, 1981).

Multiple Dysplasia Syndromes

There are other rare entities, characterized by dysplasia of multiple tissues, that fall within the continuum of the Klippel-Trenaunay, Sturge-Weber, and Maffucci syndromes.

The *epidermal nevus syndrome* denotes patchy, linear, or sebaceous pigmented nevi in association with vascular anomalies of the skin and central nervous system and skeletal abnormalities, e.g., digital gigantism, craniofacial bone overgrowth, hemifacial hypertrophy, and vertebral defects (Fig. 66–55) (Solomon, Fretzin, and Dewald, 1968). Benign tumors as well as malignant degeneration are reported in this neurocutaneous syndrome (Solomon and Esterly, 1975). The fa-

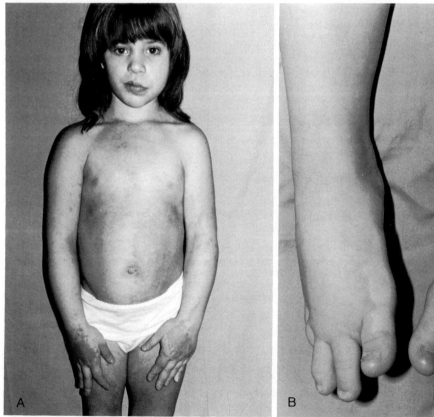
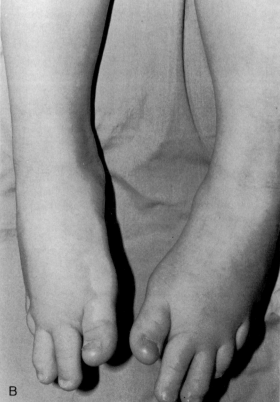

Figure 66–56. Proteus syndrome. *A, B,* A 5 year old girl with left hemicraniofacial hypertrophy (including premature dental eruption), widespread cutaneous capillary staining, and asymmetric gigantism of the fingers and toes.

milial *Riley-Smith syndrome* combines macrocephaly with pseudopapilledema and multiple subcutaneous vascular malformations (Riley and Smith, 1960).

Bannayan's syndrome also includes macrocephaly in conjunction with multiple subcutaneous lipomas, vascular malformations, and lymphedema (Bannayan, 1971). Similar cases have been reported noting the increased risk of intracranial neoplasms (Higginbottom and Schultz, 1982).

The *Proteus syndrome*, named after the polymorphic Greek god, is characterized by partial gigantism of the hands and/or feet, hemifacial hypertrophy, macrocephaly with localized exostoses, pigmented nevi, and thickening of the palms and soles, in association with subcutaneous lipomas and vascular malformations (Fig. 66–56) (Wiedemann and associates, 1983). The overgrowth of cellular elements of all three germ layers has a random distribution with a wide phenotypic range. Asymmetric growth is perhaps the only constant feature of this syndrome. Additional cases have expanded the already broad spectrum of the Proteus phenotype and revealed overlapping of stigmatic features with other vascular syndromes. For example, cutaneous capillary-lymphatic-venous lesions typical of the Klippel-Trenaunay syndrome (Clark and associates, 1987) and visceral vascular malformations (Viljoen and associates, 1987) are seen in the Proteus syndrome. "Benign lipomatosis," a rare type of facial hemihypertrophy (Slavin and associates, 1983), may present with similar capillary staining and maxillary overgrowth. "Encephalocraniocutaneous lipomatosis" (Haberland and Perou, 1970; Fishman, Chang, and Miller, 1978) is probably a circumscribed form of the Proteus syndrome (Wiedemann and Burgio, 1986). There are also reports of the Proteus syndrome exhibiting lipomatosis of the trunk (Mücke and associates, 1985) and pelvis (Costa, Fitch, and Azouz, 1985).

REFERENCES

Abernethy, J.: The Surgical Works of. Vol. 2. Part 1. London, Longman, Hurst, Rees, Orme and Brown, 1811, pp. 224–230.

Ackroyd, J. S., Baskerville, P. A., Young, A. E., and Browse, N. L.: The pathophysiology of the Klippel-Trenaunay syndrome. 5th International Workshop for Vascular Anomalies, Milan, 1984.

Albert, L. I., and Benisch, B.: Hemangioendothelioma of the liver associated with microangiopathic hemolytic anemia. Report of four cases. Am. J. Med., *48*:624, 1970.

Albrecht, E.: Die Grundprobleme der Geschwülstlehre. Part I. Frankf. Z. Pathol., *1*:221, 1907.

Alderson, M. R.: Spider naevi—their incidence in healthy school children. Arch. Dis. Child., *38*:286, 1963.

Allen, P. W., and Enzinger, F. M.: Hemangioma of skeletal muscle. Cancer, *29*:8, 1972.

Aminoff, M. J.: Vascular malformations of the central nervous system. *In* Mulliken, J. B., and Young, A. E. (Eds.): Vascular Birthmarks: Hemangiomas and Malformations. Philadelphia, W. B. Saunders Company, 1988, pp. 277–300.

Amir, J., Metzker, A., Krikler, R., and Reisner, S. H.: Strawberry hemangioma in preterm infants. Pediatr. Dermatol., *3*:131, 1986.

Ammann, A. J., Cain, W. A., Ishizaka, K., Hong, R., and Good, R. A.: Immunoglobulin E deficiency in ataxia-telangiectasia. N. Engl. J. Med., *281*:469, 1969.

Anderson, C. R.: Treatment of vascular naevi. J. Pediatr., *25*:148, 1944.

Andreev, V. C., and Pramatarov, K.: Cutis marmorata telangiectatica congenita in two sisters. Br. J. Dermatol., *101*:345, 1979.

Andrews, G. C., Domonkos, A. N., Torres-Rodriguez, V. M., and Bembenista, J. K.: Hemangiomas—treated and untreated. J.A.M.A., *165*:1114, 1957.

Andrews, G. C., and Kelly, R. J.: Treatment of vascular nevi by injection of sclerosing solutions. Arch. Dermat. Syphil., *26*:92, 1932.

Apfelberg, D. B., Greene, R. A., Maser, R., Lash, H., Rivers, J. L., and Laub, D. R.: Results of argon laser exposure of capillary hemangiomas of infancy—preliminary report. Plast. Reconstr. Surg., *67*:188, 1981.

Apfelberg, D. B., Maser, M. R., Lash, H., and White, D. N.: Benefits of CO_2 laser in oral hemangioma excision. Plast. Reconstr. Surg., *75*:46, 1985.

Ardissone, P., Pecco, P., and Italiano, F.: Attuali aspetti patogenetici e terapeutici della sindrome di Kasabach-Merritt. Minerva. Pediatr. *32*:1047, 1980.

Argenta, L. C., Bishop, E., Cho, K. J., Andrews, A. F., and Coran, A. G.: Complete resolution of life-threatening hemangioma by embolization and corticosteroids. Plast. Reconstr. Surg., *70*:739, 1982.

Argenta, L. C., Watanabe, M. J., and Grabb, W. C.: The use of tissue expansion in head and neck reconstruction. Ann. Plast. Surg., *11*:31, 1983.

Azizkhan, R. G., Azizkhan, J. C., Zetter, B. R., and Folkman, J.: Mast cell heparin stimulates migration of capillary endothelial cells in vitro. J. Exp. Med., *152*:931, 1980.

Azzolini, A., Bertani, A., and Riberti, C.: Superselective embolization and immediate surgical treatment: our present approach to treatment of large vascular hemangiomas of the face. Ann. Plast. Surg., *9*:42, 1982.

Azzolini, A., and Lechi, A.: Circoli anastomotici dall'arteria carotide interna all'esterna nelle malformazioni artero-venose della faccia. Considerazioni clinico-arteriografiche. Minerva. Cardioangiol., *16*:182, 1968.

Azzolini, A., and Nouvenne, R.: Nuove prospettive nella terapia degli angiomi immaturi dell'infanzia. 115 lesioni trattate con infiltrazioni intralesionali di triamcinolone acetonide. Ateneo Parmense, Sezione 1, Acta Bio-Medica, *41*:51, 1970.

Azzolini, A., Riberti, C., Orsoni, G. J., and Porta, R.: Protocollo terapeutico combinato chirurgico-oculistico nel trattamento degli angiomi palpebrali dell'infanzia. Minerva. Chir., *38*:925, 1983.

Azzolini, A., Salimbeni Ughi, G., and Riberti, C.: Present approach to large lymphangiomatous malformations of parotid and submandibular regions in infancy and childhood. Chir. Plast., 7:233, 1984.

Bannayan, G. A.: Lipomatosis, angiomatosis, and macrencephalia. A previously undescribed congenital syndrome. Arch. Pathol., 92:1, 1971.

Barsky, S. H., Rosen, S., Geer, D. E., and Noe, J. M.: The nature and evolution of port wine stains: a computer-assisted study. J. Invest. Dermatol., 74:154, 1980.

Barter, R. H., Letterman, G. S., and Schurter, M.: Hemangiomas in pregnancy. Am. J. Obstet. Gynecol., 87:625, 1963.

Bartoshesky, L. E., Bull, M., and Feingold, M.: Corticosteroid treatment of cutaneous hemangiomas: how effective? A report on 24 children. Clin. Pediatr., 17:625, 1978.

Baskerville, P. A., Ackroyd, J. S., and Browse, N. L.: The etiology of Klippel-Trenaunay syndrome. Ann. Surg., 202:624, 1985.

Bauer, B. S., Kernahan, D. A., and Hugo, N. E.: Lymphangioma circumscriptum—a clinicopathological review. Ann. Plast. Surg., 7:318, 1981.

Bauer, S.: Pediatric neuro-urology. In Krane, R. J., and Siroky, M. B. (Eds.): Clinical Neuro-Urology. 2nd Ed. Boston, Little, Brown, & Company, 1988.

Bean, W. B.: Vascular Spiders and Related Lesions of the Skin. Springfield IL, Charles C Thomas, 1958.

Beard, G. M.: Cases of naevi treated by electrolysis. N.Y. Med. J., 26:616, 1877.

Bek, V., and Zahn, K.: Cataract as a late sequel of contact roentgen therapy of angiomas in children. Acta Radiol., 54:443, 1960.

Bell, J.: The Principles of Surgery. London, Longman, Hurst, & Rees, 1815, pp. 456–489.

Benjamin, B., and Carter, P.: Congenital laryngeal hemangiomas. Ann. Otol. Rhinol. Laryngol., 92:448, 1983.

Bennett, J. E., and Zook, E. G.: Treatment of arteriovenous fistulas in cavernous hemangiomas of face by muscle embolization. Case report. Plast. Reconstr. Surg., 50:84, 1972.

Bennett, R. G., Keller, J. W., and Ditty, J. F., Jr.: Hemangiosarcoma subsequent to radiotherapy for a hemangioma in infancy. J. Dermatol. Surg. Oncol., 4:881, 1978.

Berman, B., and Lim, H. W. P.: Concurrent cutaneous and hepatic hemangiomata in infancy: report of a case and a review of the literature. J. Dermatol. Surg. Oncol., 4:869, 1978.

Bhattacharyya, N. C., Yadav, K., Mitra, S. K., and Pathak, I. C.: Lymphangiomas in children. Aust. N.Z. J. Surg., 51:296, 1981.

Bill, A. H., and Sumner, D. S.: A unified concept of lymphangioma and cystic hygroma. Surg. Gynecol. Obstet., 120:79, 1965.

Blackfield, H. M., Torrey, F. A., Morris, W. J., and Low Beer, B. V. A.: The management of hemangiomata. A plea for conservatism in infancy. Plast. Reconstr. Surg., 20:38, 1957.

Blair, J.: Naevus treated successfully by local application of liquor arsenicalis. Br. Med. J., 1:761, 1884.

Bobbs, J. S.: Two cases of naevi in infants, treated by ligature and excision; and excision alone. Indiana J. M., 1:33, 1870–1871.

Boman, K.: A clinico-histologic investigation on hemangioma. Acta Chir. Scand., 83:185, 1940.

Bona, G., Mussa, G. C., Mora, P., and Silvestro, L.: Studio della sequentrazione piastrinica con piastrine marcate con 99m-Tc in un caso di sindrome di Kasabach-Merritt. Minerva. Pediatr., 32:215, 1980.

Bonnet, P., Dechaume, J., and Blanc, E.: L'anévrysme cirsoïde de la retiné (anévrysme racemeux), ses relations avec l'anévrysme cirsoïde de la face et avec l'anévrysme cirsoïde du cerveau. J. Med. Lyon, 18:165, 1937.

Bowers, R. E.: Treatment of haemangiomatous naevi with thorium X. Br. Med. J., 1:121, 1951.

Bowers, R. E., Graham, E. A., and Tomlinson, K. M.: The natural history of the strawberry nevus. Arch. Dermatol., 82:667, 1960.

Bowles, L. J., Kostopoulos-Farri, E., and Papageorgiou, A. N.: Perinatal hemorrhage associated with Kasabach-Merritt syndrome. Clin. Pediatr., 20:428, 1981.

Boxt, L. M., Levin, D. C., and Fellows, K. E.: Direct puncture angiography in congenital venous malformations. AJR, 140:135, 1983.

Boyd, J. B., Mulliken, J. B., Kaban, L. B., Upton, J., III, and Murray, J. E.: Skeletal changes associated with vascular malformations. Plast. Reconstr. Surg., 74:789, 1984.

Boyer, A.: A Treatise on Surgical Diseases and the Operations Suited to Them. Vol. I. Translated by A. H. Stevens. New York, T. & J. Swords, 1815, pp. 322–326.

Bradley, S. M.: Large veno-cutaneous naevus treated successfully by repeated injections with carbolic acid. Br. Med. J., 1:443, 1876.

Brain, R. T., and Calnan, C. D.: Vascular naevi and their treatment. Br. J. Dermatol., 64:147, 1952.

Braverman, I. M., and Ken-Yen, A.: Ultrastructure and three-dimensional reconstruction of several macular and papular telangiectases. J. Invest. Dermatol., 81:489, 1983.

Broomhead, I. W.: Cystic hygroma of the neck. Br. J. Plast. Surg., 17:225, 1964.

Brown, B. Z., and Huffaker, G.: Local injection of steroids for juvenile hemangiomas which disturb the visual axis. Ophthalmic Surg., 13:630, 1982.

Brown, J. B., and Byars, L. T.: Interstitial radiation treatment of hemangiomata. Am. J. Surg., 39:452, 1938.

Brown, J. B., Cannon, B., and McDowell, A.: Permanent pigment injection of capillary hemangiomata. Plast. Reconstr. Surg., 1:106, 1946.

Brown, S. H., Jr., Neerhout, R. C., and Fonkalsrud, E. W.: Prednisone therapy in the management of large hemangiomas in infants and children. Surgery, 71:168, 1972.

Bryant, W. M., and Maull, K. I.: Arteriovenous malformations of the mandible. Graduated surgical management. Plast. Reconstr. Surg., 55:690, 1975.

Bunch, J. L.: The treatment of 300 naevi by freezing. Br. Med. J., 1:247, 1911.

Burge, D. M., Middleton, A. W., Kamath, R., and Fasher, B. J.: Intestinal haemorrhage in Turner's syndrome. Arch. Dis. Child., 56:557, 1981.

Burke, E. C., Winkelmann, R. K., and Strickland, M. K.: Disseminated hemangiomatosis. The newborn with central nervous system involvement. Am. J. Dis. Child, 108:418, 1964.

Burman, D., Mansell, P. W. A., and Warin, R. P.: Miliary hemangiomata in the newborn. Arch. Dis. Child., 42:193, 1967.

Burrows, P. E., Lasjaunias, P. L., Ter Brugge, K. G., and Flodmark, O.: Urgent and emergent embolization of lesions of the head and neck in children: indications and results. Pediatrics, *80*:386, 1987.

Burrows, P. E., Mulliken, J. B., Fellows, K. E., and Strand, R. D.: Childhood hemangiomas and vascular malformations: angiographic differentiation. AJR, *141*:483, 1983.

Callander, C. L.: Study of arteriovenous fistula with analysis of 447 cases. Ann. Surg., *71*:428, 1920.

Caplan, A. I., and Koutroupas, S.: The control of muscle and cartilage development in the chick limb: the role of differential vascularization. J. Embryol. Exp. Morphol., *29*:571, 1973.

Cartwright, J. D., and Van Coller, J. D.: Conservative management of the Kasabach-Merritt syndrome (cavernous haemangioma and thrombocytopenia). S. Afr. Med. J., *60*:670, 1981.

Chait, D., Yonkers, A. J., Beddoe, G. M., and Yarington, C. T., Jr.: Management of cystic hygromas. Surg. Gynecol. Obstet., *139*:55, 1974.

Chandler, D.: Pulmonary and cerebral arteriovenous fistula with Osler's disease. Arch. Intern. Med., *116*:277, 1965.

Cheng, F. C., Tsang, P. H., Shum, J. D., and Ong, G. B.: Maffucci's syndrome with fibroadenomas of the breasts. J. R. Coll. Surg. Edinb., *26*:181, 1981.

Chervenak, F. A., Isaacson, G., Blakemore, K. J., Breg, W. R., Hobbins, J. C., et al.: Fetal cystic hygroma. Cause and natural history. N. Engl. J. Med., *309*:822, 1983.

Clark, R. D., Donnai, D., Rogers, J., Cooper, J., and Baraitser, M.: Proteus syndrome: an expanded phenotype. Am. J. Med. Genet., *27*:99, 1987.

Clemmensen, O.: A case of multiple neonatal hemangiomatosis successfully treated by systemic corticosteroids. Dermatologica, *159*:495, 1979.

Clodius, L.: Excision and grafting of extensive facial haemangiomas. Br. J. Plast. Surg., *30*:185, 1977.

Clodius, L.: Surgery for the facial port-wine stain: technique and results. Ann. Plast. Surg., *16*:457, 1986.

Clodius, L., and Smahel, J.: Resurfacing denuded areas of the beard with full-thickness scalp grafts. Br. J. Plast. Surg., *32*:295, 1979.

Cobb, S.: Haemangioma of the spinal cord, associated with skin naevi of the same metamere. Ann. Surg., *62*:641, 1915.

Coget, J. M., and Merlen, J. F.: Klippel-Trenaunay, syndrome ou maladie? Phlebologie, *33*:37, 1980.

Cohen, S. R., and Wang, C. I.: Steroid treatment of hemangioma of the head and neck in children. Ann. Otol. Rhinol. Laryngol., *81*:584, 1972.

Cole, P. P., and Hunt, A. H.: The treatment of cavernous haemangiomas and cirsoid aneurysms by the injection of boiling water. Br. J. Surg., *36*:346, 1949.

Coleman, C. C., Jr.: Diagnosis and treatment of congenital arteriovenous fistulas of the head and neck. Am. J. Surg., *126*:557, 1973.

Coleman, C. C., Jr., and Hoopes, J. E.: Congenital arteriovenous anomalies of the head and neck. Plast. Reconstr. Surg., *47*:354, 1971.

Conway, H.: Evolution of treatment of capillary hemangiomas of the face with further observation on the value of camouflage by permanent pigment injection (tattooing). Surgery, *23*:389, 1948.

Conway, H., McKinney, P., and Climo, M.: Permanent camouflage of vascular nevi of the face by intradermal injection of insoluble pigments (tattooing): experience through twenty years with 1022 cases. Plast. Reconstr. Surg., *40*:457, 1967.

Cooke, D. A.: Renal arteriovenous malformation demonstrated angiographically in hereditary haemorrhagic telangiectasia (Rendu-Osler-Weber disease). J. R. Soc. Med., *79*:744, 1986.

Coombs, C.: A new method of treating subcutaneous naevi. Lancet, *2*:374, 1881.

Cooper, A. G., and Bolande, R. P.: Multiple hemangiomas in an infant with cardiac hypertrophy. Pediatrics, *35*:27, 1965.

Cosman, B.: Clinical experience in the laser therapy of port-wine stains. Lasers Surg. Med., *1*:133, 1980.

Costa, T., Fitch, N., and Azouz, E. M.: Proteus syndrome: report of two cases with pelvic lipomatosis. Pediatrics, *76*:984, 1985.

Costello, M. J.: Management of vascular nevi. Pediatrics, *4*:825, 1949.

Crawford, B. S., and Vivakananthan, C.: The treatment of giant cystic hygroma of the neck. Br. J. Plast. Surg., *26*:69, 1973.

Cremer, H., Gullotta, F., and Wolf, L.: The Maffucci-Kast syndrome. Dyschondroplasia with hemangiomas and frontal lobe astrocytoma. J. Cancer Res. Clin. Oncol., *101*:231, 1981.

Crum, R., Szabo, S., and Folkman, J.: A new class of steroids inhibits angiogenesis in the presence of heparin or a heparin fragment. Science, *230*:1375, 1985.

Csicsko, J. F., and Grosfeld, J. L.: Cervicomediastinal hygroma with pulmonary hypoplasia in the newly born. Am. J. Dis. Child., *128*:557, 1974.

Cunningham, D. D., and Paletta, F. X.: Control of arteriovenous fistulae in massive facial hemangioma by muscle emboli. Plast. Reconstr. Surg., *46*:305, 1970.

Curling, T. B.: Observations on the treatment of naevi materni—with cases of removal of these growths from different parts of the face without deformity. London Med. Gazette, *45*:133, 1850.

Dana, M., and Beyer, J.: Résultats lointains de traitement par le radium de 820 angiomes cutanés tubereix. J. Radiol. Electr., *47*:325, 1966.

Darcel, C. le Q., and Franks, L. M.: Angiomatoid lesions of the skin in young chicks. J. Path. Bact., *66*:499, 1953.

David, T. J., Evans, D. I., and Stevens, R. F.: Haemangioma with thrombocytopenia (Kasabach-Merritt syndrome). Arch. Dis. Child., *58*:1022, 1983.

Davies, M. G., and Marks, R.: Dermo-epidermal relationships in pyogenic granuloma. Br. J. Dermatol., *99*:503, 1978.

Davis, J. S., and Wilgis, H. E.: The treatment of hemangiomata by excision. South. Med. J., *27*:283, 1934.

Debrun, G., Lacour, P., Caron, J. P., Hurth, M., Comoy, J., and Keravel, Y.: Detachable balloon and calibrated-leak balloon techniques in the treatment of cerebral vascular lesions. J. Neurosurg., *49*:635, 1978.

Dehner, L. P., and Ishak, K. G.: Vascular tumors of the liver in infants and children. Arch. Pathol., *92*:101, 1971.

deLorimier, A. A.: Hepatic tumors of infancy and childhood. Surg. Clin. North Am., *57*:443, 1977.

deLorimier, A. A., Simpson, E. B., Baum, R. S., and Carlsson, E.: Hepatic-artery ligation for hepatic hemangiomatosis. N. Engl. J. Med., *277*:333, 1967.

Demuth, R. J., Miller, S. H., and Keller, F.: Complications of embolization treatment for problem cavernous hemangiomas. Ann. Plast. Surg., *13*:135, 1984.

Denekamp, J.: Vasculature as a target for tumour therapy. Angiogenesis. *In* Hammersen, F., and Hudlicka, O. (Eds.): Progress in Applied Microcirculation Vol. 4. Basel, Karger, 1984, pp. 28–38.

Desnick, R. J., and Sweeley, C. C.: Fabry's disease: alpha-galactosidase—a deficiency (angiokeratoma corporis diffusum universale). *In* Fitzpatrick, T. B., Eisen, A.

Z., Wolff, K., et al. (Eds.): Dermatology in General Medicine. 3rd Ed. New York, McGraw-Hill Book Company, 1987, p. 1739.

deTakats, G.: Vascular anomalies of the extremities. Surg. Gynecol. Obstet., *55*:227, 1932.

Dethlefsen, S. M., Mulliken, J. B., and Glowacki, J.: An ultrastructural study of mast cell interactions in hemangiomas. Ultrastruct. Pathol., *10*:175, 1986.

De Venecia, G., and Lobeck, C. C.: Successful treatment of eyelid hemangiomas with prednisone. Arch. Ophthalmol., *84*:98, 1970.

Dingman, R. O., and Grabb, W. C.: Lymphangioma of the tongue. Plast. Reconstr. Surg., *27*:214, 1961.

Dingman, R. O., and Grabb, W. C.: Congenital arteriovenous fistulae of the external ear. Plast. Reconstr. Surg., *35*:620, 1965.

Djindjian, M., Djindjian, R., Hurth, M., Rey, A., and Houdart, R.: Spinal cord arteriovenous malformations and the Klippel-Trenaunay-Weber syndrome. Surg. Neurol., *8*:229, 1977.

Doppman, J. L., Wirth, F. P., Jr., DiChiro, G., and Ommaya, A. K.: Value of cutaneous angiomas in the arteriographic localization of spinal-cord arteriovenous malformations. N. Engl. J. Med., *281*:1440, 1969.

Duncan, J.: On galvano-puncture of naevus. Edinburgh Med. J., *15*:777, 1870.

Durand, P., Borrone, C., and Della Cella, G.: A new mucopolysaccharide lipid-storage disease? Letter. Lancet, *2*:1313, 1966.

Edgerton, M. T.: The treatment of hemangiomas: with special reference to the role of steroid therapy. Ann. Surg., *183*:517, 1976.

Ellis, P. O.: Occlusion of the central retinal artery after retrobulbar corticosteroid injection. Am. J. Ophthalmol., *85*:352, 1978.

Enjolras, O., Riché, M. C., and Merland, J. J.: Facial port-wine stains and Sturge-Weber syndrome. Pediatrics, *76*:48, 1985.

Enzinger, F. M., and Weiss, S. W.: Benign tumors and tumor-like lesions of blood vessels. *In* Enzinger, F. M., and Weiss, S. W. (Eds.): Soft Tissue Tumors. St. Louis, C. V. Mosby Company, 1983, pp. 379–421.

Esterly, N. B.: Kasabach-Merritt syndrome in infants. J. Am. Acad. Dermatol., *8*:504, 1983.

Evans, H. W.: Angioma of the scrotum (Fordyce lesion). Arch. Intern. Med., *110*:520, 1962.

Evans, J., Batchelor, A. D. R., Stark, G., and Uttley, W. S.: Haemangioma with coagulopathy: sustained response to prednisone. Arch. Dis. Child., *50*:809, 1975.

Faber, R. G., Ibrahim, S. Z., Drew, D. S., and Hobsley, M.: Vascular malformations of the parotid region. Br. J. Surg., *65*:171, 1978.

Fabry, J.: Über einen Fall von Angiokeratoma circumscriptum am linken Oberschenkel. Derm. Ztschr., *22*:1, 1915.

Figi, F. A.: Radium in the treatment of multilocular lymph cysts of the neck in children. Am. J. Roentgenol., *21*:473, 1929.

Figi, F. A.: Treatment of hemangiomas of the hand and neck. Plast. Reconstr. Surg., *3*:1, 1948.

Finn, M. C., Glowacki, J., and Mulliken, J. B.: Congenital vascular lesions: clinical application of a new classification. J. Pediatr. Surg., *18*:894, 1983.

Fishman, M. A., Chang, C. S., and Miller, J. E.: Encephalocraniocutaneous lipomatosis. Pediatrics, *61*:580, 1978.

Fitzsimmons, J. S., and Starks, M.: Cutis marmorata telangiectatica congenita or congenital generalized phlebectasia. Arch. Dis. Child., *45*:724, 1970.

Flores, J. T., Apfelberg, D. B., Maser, M. R., Lash, W.,

and White, D.: Angiokeratoma of Fordyce: successful treatment with the argon laser. Plast. Reconstr. Surg., *74*:835, 1984.

Flye, M. W., Jordan, B. P., and Schwartz, M. Z.: Management of congenital arteriovenous malformations. Surgery, *94*:740, 1983.

Folkman, J.: Tumor angiogenesis factor. Cancer Res., *34*:2109, 1974.

Folkman, J.: The vascularization of tumors. Sci. Am., *234*:58, 1976.

Folkman, J., and Cotran, R.: Relation of vascular proliferation to tumor growth. Int. Rev. Exp. Pathol., *16*:207, 1976.

Folkman, J., and Haudenschild, C.: Angiogenesis in vitro. Nature, *288*:551, 1980.

Folkman, J., and Klagsbrun, M.: Angiogenic factors. Science, *235*:442, 1987.

Folkman, J., Langer R., Linhardt, R. J., Haudenschild, C., and Taylor, S.: Angiogenesis inhibition and tumor regression caused by heparin or a heparin fragment in the presence of cortisone. Science, *221*:719, 1983.

Fonkalsrud, E. W.: Surgical management of congenital malformations of the lymphatic system. Am. J. Surg., *128*:152, 1974.

Fordyce, J. A.: Angiokeratoma of the scrotum. J. Cutan. Genito-urin. Dis., *14*:81, 1896.

Forster, J. C.: The Surgical Diseases of Children. London, John W. Parker & Son, 1860, pp. 206–249.

Fost, N. C., and Esterly, N. B.: Successful treatment of juvenile hemangiomas with prednisone. J. Pediatr., *72*:351, 1968.

Garden, A. S., Benzie, R. J., Miskin, M., and Gardner, H. A.: Fetal cystic hygroma colli: antenatal diagnosis, significance, and management. Am. J. Obstet. Gynecol., *154*:221, 1986.

Glowacki, J., and Mulliken, J. B.: Mast cells in hemangiomas and vascular malformations. Pediatrics, *70*:48, 1982.

Goetsch, E.: Hygroma colli cysticum and hygroma axillae: pathologic and clinical study and report of twelve cases. Arch. Surg., *36*:394, 1938.

Goldwyn, R. M., and Rosoff, C. B.: Cryosurgery for large hemangiomas in adults. Plast. Reconstr. Surg., *43*:605, 1969.

Good, T. A., Carnazzo, S. F., and Good, R. A.: Thrombocytopenia and giant hemangiomas in infants. Am. J. Dis. Child., *90*:260, 1955.

Grabb, W. C., Dingman, R. O., Oneal, R. M., and Dempsey, P. D.: Facial hamartomas in children: neurofibroma, lymphangioma, and hemangioma. Plast. Reconstr. Surg., *66*:509, 1980.

Grabb, W. C., MacCollum, M. S., and Tan, N. G.: Results from tattooing port-wine hemangiomas. A long-term follow-up. Plast. Reconstr. Surg., *59*:667, 1977.

Graham, J. M., Jr., Stephens, T. D., and Shepard, T. H.: Nuchal cystic hygroma in a fetus with presumed Roberts syndrome. Am. J. Med. Genet., *15*:163, 1983.

Greenberg, F., Carpenter, R. J., and Ledbetter, D. H.: Cystic hygroma and hydrops fetalis in a fetus with trisomy 13. Clin. Genet., *24*:389, 1983.

Greenhouse, J. M.: In discussion of a paper by B. Yaffe. A.M.A. Arch. Dermatol., *72*:89, 1955.

Grosfeld, J. L., Weber, T. R., and Vane, D. W.: One-stage resection for massive cervicomediastinal hygroma. Surgery, *92*:693, 1982.

Gross, R. E.: Cystic hygroma. *In* The Surgery of Infancy and Childhood. Philadelphia, W. B. Saunders Company, 1953, pp. 960–970.

Gross, R. E., and Goeringer, C. F.: Cystic hygroma of the

neck. Report of twenty-seven cases. Surg. Gynecol. Obstet., *59*:48, 1939.

Gross, S. D.: System of Surgery: Pathological, Diagnostic, Therapeutic, and Operative. Vol. I. Philadelphia, Blanchard & Lea. 1859, pp. 968–975.

Gunn, T., Reece, E. R., Metrakos, K., and Colle, E.: Depressed T cells following neonatal steroid treatment. Pediatrics, *67*:61, 1981.

Gupta, S. D., Tiwari, I. N., and Pasupathy, N. K.: Cavernous haemangioma of the frontal bone: case report. Br. J. Surg., *62*:330, 1975.

Habal, M. B., and Murray, J. E.: The natural history of a benign locally-invasive hemangioma of the orbital region. Plast. Reconstr. Surg., *49*:209, 1972.

Haberland, C., and Perou, M.: Encephalocraniocutaneous lipomatosis. Arch. Neurol., *22*:144, 1970.

Haik, B. G., Jakobiec, F. A., Ellsworth, R. M., and Jones, I. S.: Capillary hemangioma of the lids and orbit: an analysis of the clinical features and therapeutic results in 101 cases. Ophthalmology, *86*:760, 1979.

Hales, M. R.: Multiple small arteriovenous fistulae of the lungs. Am. J. Pathol., *32*:927, 1956.

Haller, J. A., Jr., Pickard, L. R., Kumar, A. J., and White, R. I., Jr.: A new percutaneous technique for occluding arterial flow to massive congenital A-V malformation to prevent major hemorrhage during resection. J. Pediatr. Surg., *15*:523, 1980.

Halsted, W. S.: Congenital arteriovenous and lymphaticovenous fistulae: unique clinical and experimental observations. Trans. Am. Surg. Assoc., *37*:262, 1919.

Hammond, W. A.: Three cases of the successful treatment of vascular tumors by injection with the fluid extract of argot. Arch. Clin. Surg., *1*:123, 1876.

Hanes, F. M.: Multiple hereditary telangiectases causing hemorrhage (hereditary hemorrhagic telangiectasia). Am. J. Derm. Genito-Urinary Dis., *13*:249, 1909.

Harkins, G. A., and Sabiston, D. C., Jr.: Lymphangioma in infancy and childhood. Surgery, *47*:811, 1960.

Harrower, G.: Treatment of cystic hygroma of the neck by sodium morrhuate. Br. Med. J., *2*:148, 1933.

Haughton, V. M.: Hemoclip-Gelfoam emboli in the treatment of facial arteriovenous malformations. Neuroradiology, *10*:69, 1975.

Healy, G. B., Fearon, B., French, R., and McGill, T.: Treatment of subglottic hemangioma with the carbon dioxide laser. Laryngoscope, *90*:809, 1980.

Healy, G. B., McGill, T., and Friedman, E. M.: Carbon dioxide laser in subglottic hemangioma. An update. Ann. Otol. Rhinol. Laryngol., *93*:370, 1984.

Hidano, A., and Nakajima, S.: Earliest features of the strawberry mark in the newborn. Br. J. Dermatol., *87*:138, 1972.

Higginbottom, M. C., and Schultz, P.: The Bannayan syndrome: an autosomal dominant disorder consisting of macrocephaly, lipomas, hemangiomas, and risk for intracranial tumors. Pediatrics, *69*:632, 1982.

Hill, G. J., 2nd, and Longino, L. A.: Giant hemangioma with thrombocytopenia. Surg. Gynecol. Obstet., *114*:304, 1962.

Hobby, L. W.: Further evaluation of the potential of the argon laser in the treatment of strawberry hemangiomas. Plast. Reconstr. Surg., *71*:481, 1983.

Hodges: Injection of a naevus with perchloride of iron. Boston Med. Surg. J., *70*:60, 1864.

Hoey, M. F., Courage, G. R., Newton, T. H., and Hoyt, W. F.: Management of vascular malformations of the mandible and maxillae. Review and report of two cases treated by embolization and surgical obliteration. J. Oral. Surg., *28*:696, 1970.

Holden, K. R., and Alexander, F.: Diffuse neonatal hemangiomatosis. Pediatrics, *46*:411, 1970.

Holgate, T. H.: The treatment of naevus by the intrainjection of alcohol. Arch. Pediatr., *6*:379, 1889.

Holman, E.: Abnormal Arteriovenous Communications. 2nd Ed. Springfield, IL, Charles C Thomas, 1968.

Holmdahl, K.: Cutaneous hemangiomas in premature and mature infants. Acta Paediatr., *44*:370, 1955.

Home, E.: An account of Mr. Hunter's method of performing the operation for the cure of the popliteal aneurism. Trans. Soc. Impr. Med. Chir. Know., *1*:138, 1793.

Hooper, R.: Lexicon Medicum (Medical Dictionary). Vol. 1. New York, Harper & Brothers, 1838.

Höpfel-Kreiner, H.: Histogenesis of hemangiomas—an ultrastructural study on capillary and cavernous hemangiomas of the skin. Pathol. Res. Pract., *170*:70, 1980.

Howell, J. S.: The experimental production of vascular tumours in the rat. Br. J. Cancer, *17*:663, 1963.

Huang, T., Kim, K. A., Lynch, J. B., Doyle, J. E., and Lewis, S. R.: The use of cryotherapy in the management of intra-oral hemangiomas. South. Med. J., *65*:1123, 1972.

Hurvitz, C. H., Alkalay, A. L., Sloninsky, L., Kallus, G., and Pomerance, J. J.: Cyclophosphamide therapy in life-threatening vascular tumors. J. Pediatr., *109*:360, 1986.

Hurwitz, D. J., and Kerber, C. W.: Hemodynamic considerations in the treatment of arteriovenous malformations of the face and scalp. Plast. Reconstr. Surg., *67*:421, 1981.

Hutchinson, J.: A peculiar form of serpiginous and infective naevoid disease. Arch. Surg. (Lond.), *1*:Plate IX, 1889–1890.

Ikeda, K., Suita, S., Hayashida, Y., and Yakabe, S.: Massive infiltrating cystic hygroma of the neck in infancy with special reference to bleomycin therapy. Z. Kinderchir., *20*:227, 1977.

Imperial, R., and Helwig, E. B.: Angiokeratoma. A clinicopathological study. Arch. Dermatol., *95*:166, 1967a.

Imperial, R., and Helwig, E. B.: Verrucous hemangioma. A clinicopathologic study of 21 cases. Arch. Dermatol., *96*:247, 1967b.

Imperial, R., and Helwig, E. B.: Angiokeratoma of the scrotum (Fordyce type). J. Urol., *98*:379, 1967c.

Iwamoto, T., and Jakobiec, F. A.: Ultrastructural comparison of capillary and cavernous hemangiomas of the orbit. Arch. Ophthalmol., *97*:1144, 1979.

Jacobs, A. H.: Strawberry hemangiomas: the natural history of the untreated lesion. Calif. Med., *86*:8, 1957.

Jacobs, A. H., and Walton, R. G.: The incidence of birthmarks in the neonate. Pediatrics, *58*:218, 1976.

Jahnke, V.: Ultrastructure of hereditary telangiectasia. Arch. Otolaryngol., *91*:262, 1970.

Jakobiec, F. A., and Jones, I. S.: Vascular tumors, malformations, and degenerations. *In* Jones, I. S., and Jakobiec, F. A. (Eds.): Diseases of the Orbit. Philadelphia, J. B. Lippincott Company, 1979, pp. 276–283, 286.

Jargiello, D. M., and Caplan, A. I.: The fluid flow dynamics in the developing chick wing. *In* Fallon, J. F., and Caplan, A. I. (Eds.): Limb Development and Regeneration. Part A. New York, Alan R. Liss, 1983, pp. 143–154.

Jarzab, G.: Clinical experience in the cryosurgery of haemangioma. J. Maxillofac. Surg., *3*:146, 1975.

Jessen, R. T., Thompson, S., and Smith, E. B.: Cobb syndrome. Arch. Dermatol., *113*:1587, 1977.

Joehl, R. J., Miller, S. H., Davis, T. S., and Graham, W. P., III: Hemangioma of the temporalis muscle: a case report and review of the literature. Ann. Plast. Surg., 3:372, 1979.

Johnston, M. C. A.: Radioautographic study of the migration and fate of cranial neural crests in the chick embryo. Anat. Rec., 156:143, 1966.

Jönsson, G.: New method of treating capillary haemangiomas. Acta Chir. Scand., 95:275, 1947.

Kaban, L. B., and Mulliken, J. B.: Vascular anomalies of the maxillofacial region. J. Oral Maxillofac. Surg., 44:203, 1986.

Kagan, A. R., Jaffe, H. D., and Kennamer, R.: Hemangioma of the liver treated by irradiation. J. Nucl. Med., 12:835, 1971.

Kalischer, S.: Demonstration des Gehirns eines Kindes mit Teleangiectasie der linksseitigen Gesichts-Kopfhaut und Hirnoberfläche. Berl. Klin. Wchnschr., 34:1059, 1897.

Kampmeier, O. F.: Evolution and Comparative Morphology of the Lymphatic System. Springfield, IL, Charles C Thomas, 1969.

Kanter, W. R., Brown, W. C., and Noe, J. M.: Nasal bone hemangiomas: a review of clinical, radiologic, and operative experience. Plast. Reconstr. Surg., 76:774, 1985.

Kaplan, E. N.: Vascular malformation of the extremities. In Williams, H. B. (Ed.): Symposium on Vascular Malformations and Melanotic Lesions. St. Louis, C. V. Mosby Company, 1983, p. 144.

Kasabach, H. H., and Merritt, K. K.: Capillary hemangioma with extensive purpura: report of a case. Am. J. Dis. Child., 59:1063, 1940.

Keller, L., and Bluhm, J. F., III: Diffuse neonatal hemangiomatosis: a case with heart failure and thrombocytopenia. Cutis, 23:295, 1979.

Kessler, D. A., Langer, R. S., Pless, N. A., and Folkman, J.: Mast cells and tumor angiogenesis. Int. J. Cancer, 18:703, 1976.

Kingston, S.: Treatment of naevus by adhesive or suppurative inflammation. Lancet, 1:420, 1862.

Kinmonth, J. B.: The Lymphatics. 2nd Ed. London, Edward Arnold, 1982.

Kinmonth, J. B., and Eustace, P. W.: Lymph nodes and vessels in primary lymphedema. Their relative importance in aetiology. Ann. R. Coll. Surg. Engl., 58:278, 1976.

Kinmonth, J. B., and Wolfe, J. H.: Fibrosis in the lymph nodes in primary lymphoedema. Histological and clinical studies in 74 patients with lower-limb oedema. Ann. R. Coll. Surg. Engl., 62:344, 1980.

Kirchhoff, D., Eggert, H. R., and Agnoli, A. L.: Cavernous angiomas of the skull. Neurochirurgia, 21:53, 1978.

Klippel, M., and Trenaunay, P.: Du naevus variqueux ostéo-hypertrophique. Rev. Gen. Med., Paris, 14:65, 1900a.

Klippel, M., and Trenaunay, P.: Du naevus variqueux ostéo-hypertrophique. Arch. Gen. Med., Paris, 3:641, 1900b.

Knott, S. J.: Forty cases of naevi successfully treated with electrolysis. Lancet, 1:402, 1875.

Koerper, M. A., Addiego, J. E., Jr., deLorimier, A. A., Lipow, H., Price, D., and Lubin, B. H.: Use of aspirin and dipyridamole in children with platelet trapping syndromes. J. Pediatr., 102:311, 1983.

Kontras, S. B., Green, O. C., King, L., and Duran, R. J.: Giant hemangioma with thrombocytopenia. Am. J. Dis. Child., 105:188, 1963.

Krabbe, K. H.: Facial and meningeal angiomatosis associated calcifications of brain cortex: a clinical and anatomicopathologic contribution. Arch. Neurol. Psychiat., 32:737, 1934.

Kraemer, K. H.: Ataxia-telangiectasia. In Fitzpatrick, T. B., Eisen, A. Z., Wolff, K., et al. (Eds.): Dermatology in General Medicine. 3rd Ed. New York, McGraw-Hill Book Company, 1987, p. 1796.

Kromayer: Die Behandlung der roten Muttermale mit Licht und Radium nach Erfahrungen und 40 Fällen. Dtsch. Med. Wochenschr., 36:299, 1910.

Kurczynski, T. W.: Hereditary cutis marmorata telangiectatica congenita. Pediatrics, 70:52, 1982.

Kushner, B. J.: Local steroid therapy and adnexal hemangioma. Ann. Ophthalmol., 11:1005, 1979.

Kushner, B. J.: The treatment of periorbital infantile hemangioma with intralesional corticosteroid. Plast. Reconstr. Surg., 76:517, 1985.

Kwaan, H. C., and Silverman, S.: Fibrinolytic activity in lesions of hereditary hemorrhagic telangiectasia. Arch. Dermatol., 107:571, 1973.

Laidlaw, G. F., and Murray, M. R.: Melanoma studies. III. A theory of pigmented moles. Their relation to the evolution of hair follicles. Am. J. Pathol., 9:827, 1933.

Laird, W. P., Friedman, S., Koop, C. E., and Schwartz, G. J.: Hepatic hemangiomatosis. Successful management by hepatic artery ligation. Am. J. Dis. Child., 130:657, 1976.

Lampe, I., and Latourette, H. B.: The management of cavernous hemangiomas in infants. Postgrad. Med., 19:262, 1956.

Lang, P. G., and Dubin, H. V.: Hemangioma-thrombocytopenia syndrome: a disseminated intravascular coagulopathy. Arch. Dermatol., 111:105, 1975.

Larcher, V. F., Howard, E. R., and Mowat, A. P.: Hepatic hemangiomata: diagnosis and management. Arch. Dis. Child., 56:7, 1981.

Lasjaunias, P., and Berenstein, A. (Eds.): Surgical Neuroangiography. Vol. II. Heidelberg, Springer-Verlag, 1987, p. 394.

Lea Thomas, M.: Radiological assessment of vascular malformations. In Mulliken, J. B., and Young, A. E. (Eds.): Vascular Birthmarks: Hemangiomas and Malformations. Philadelphia, W. B. Saunders Company, 1988, pp. 141–169.

Leikensohn, J. R., Epstein, L. I., and Vasconez, L. O.: Superselective embolization and surgery of noninvoluting hemangiomas and A-V malformations. Plast. Reconstr. Surg., 68:143, 1981.

Lewis, F. T.: The development of the lymphatic system in rabbits. Am. J. Anat., 5:95, 1905–1906.

Lewis, R. J., and Ketcham, A. S.: Maffucci's syndrome: functional and neoplastic significance. J. Bone Joint Surg., 55A:1465, 1973.

Li, F. P., Cassady, J. R., and Barnett, E.: Cancer mortality following irradiation in infancy for hemangioma. Radiology, 113:177, 1974.

Lindenauer, S. M.: The Klippel-Trenaunay syndrome: Varicosity, hypertrophy and hemangioma with no arteriovenous fistula. Ann. Surg., 162:303, 1965.

Lister, W. A.: The natural history of strawberry naevi. Lancet, 1:1429, 1938.

Loewinger, R. J., Lichtenstein, J. R., Dodson, W. E., and Eisen, A. Z.: Maffucci's syndrome: a mesenchymal dysplasia and multiple tumour syndrome. Br. J. Dermatol., 96:317, 1977.

Longacre, J. J., Benton, C., and Unterthiner, R. A.: Treatment of facial hemangioma by intravascular embolization with silicone spheres. Case report. Plast. Reconstr. Surg., 50:618, 1972.

MacCollum, D. W.: Treatment of hemangiomas. Am. J. Surg., 29:32, 1935.

MacCollum, D. W., and Martin, L. W.: Hemangiomas in

infancy and childhood. A report based on 6479 cases. Surg. Clin. North Am., *36*:1647, 1956.

Maffucci, A.: Di un caso di encondroma ed angioma multiplo contribuzione al a genesi embrionale dei tumor. Movimento Med. Chir. (Naples), *3*:399, 1881.

Malan, E.: Vascular Malformations (Angiodysplasias). Milan, Carlo Erba Foundation, 1974.

Malan, E., and Azzolini, A.: Congenital arteriovenous malformations of the face and scalp. J. Cardiovasc. Surg., *9*:109, 1968.

Mangus, D. J.: Continuous compression treatment of hemangiomata. Evaluation in two cases. Plast. Reconstr. Surg., *49*:490, 1972.

Margileth, A. M., and Museles, M.: Cutaneous hemangiomas in children: diagnosis and conservative management. J.A.M.A., *194*:523, 1965.

Marks, R. M., Roche, W. R., Czerniecki, M., Penny, R., and Nelson, D. S.: Mast cell granules cause proliferation of human microvascular endothelial cells. Lab. Invest., *55*:289, 1986.

Marriott, P. J., Munro, D. D., and Ryan, T.: Angioma serpiginosum—familial incidence. Br. J. Dermatol., *93*:701, 1975.

Marshak, G.: Hemangioma of the zygomatic bone. Arch. Otolaryngol., *106*:581, 1980.

Marshall, J.: The naevus maternus (or mark of the mother) cured by vaccination. London Med. Surg. J., *5*:52, 1830.

Martini, G. A.: The liver in hereditary haemorrhagic telangiectasia: an inborn error of vascular structure with multiple manifestations: a reappraisal. Gut, *19*:531, 1978.

Matolo, N. M., and Johnson, D. G.: Surgical treatment of hepatic hemangioma in the newborn. Arch. Surg., *106*:725, 1973.

Matthews, D. N.: Treatment of haemangiomata. Br. J. Plast. Surg., *6*:83, 1954.

Matthews, D. N.: Hemangiomata. Plast. Reconstr. Surg., *41*:528, 1968.

McCabe, W. P., and Kelly, A. P., Jr.: Management of epistaxis in Osler-Weber-Rendu disease: recurrence of telangiectases within a nasal skin graft. Plast. Reconstr. Surg., *50*:114, 1972.

McGrae, J. D., Jr., and Winkelmann, R. K.: Generalized essential telangiectasia: report of a clinical and histochemical study of 13 patients with acquired cutaneous lesions. J.A.M.A., *185*:909, 1963.

McLean, R. H., Moller, J. H., Warwick, W. J., Satran, L., and Lucas, R. V., Jr.: Multinodular hemangiomatosis of the liver in infancy. Pediatrics, *49*:563, 1972.

Merlob, P., and Reisner, S. H.: Familial nevus flammeus of the forehead and Unna's nevus. Clin. Genet., *27*:165, 1985.

Mibelli, V.: Di una nuova forma de cheratosi "Angiocheratoma." Gior. Ital. d. Mal. Ven., *30*:285, 1889.

Miller, S. H., Smith, R. L., and Shochat, S. J.: Compression treatment of hemangiomas. Plast. Reconstr. Surg., *58*:573, 1976.

Mills, S. E., Cooper, P. H., and Fechner, R. E.: Lobular capillary hemangioma: the underlying lesion of pyogenic granuloma. A study of 73 cases from the oral and nasal mucous membranes. Am. J. Surg. Pathol., *4*:470, 1980.

Minkow, B., Laufer, D., and Gutman, D.: Treatment of oral hemangiomas with local sclerosing agents. Int. J. Oral Surg., *8*:18, 1979.

Modlin, J. J.: Capillary hemangiomas of the skin. Surgery, *38*:169, 1955.

Monlux, W. S., and Delaplane, J. P.: Hemangiomas in the skin of the chicken. Cornell Vet., *42*:193, 1952.

Moore, A. M.: Pressure in the treatment of giant hemangioma with purpura. Case report and observations. Plast. Reconstr. Surg., *34*:606, 1964.

Morel-Fatio, D.: Essai de traitement des angiomes plans par ponçage coloré de la peau congelée. Ann. Chir. Plast., *9*:326, 1964.

Morgan, J. F., and Schow, C. E., Jr.: Use of sodium morrhuate in the management of hemangiomas. J. Oral Surg., *32*:363, 1974.

Morris, M.: Lymphangioma circumscriptum. *In* Unna, P. G., Morris, M., Duhring, L. A., et al. (Eds.): International Atlas of Rare Skin Diseases. London, H. K. Lewis, 1889, p. 2.

Morton, E. R.: The treatment of naevi and other cutaneous lesions by electrolysis, cautery, and refrigeration. Lancet, *2*:1658, 1909.

Mücke, J., Willgerodt, H., Kunzel, R., and Brock, D.: Variability in the Proteus syndrome: report of an affected child with progressive lipomatosis. Eur. J. Pediatr., *143*:320, 1985.

Mulliken, J. B.: Pathogenesis of vascular birthmarks. *In* Williams, H. B. (Ed.): Symposium on Vascular Malformations and Melanotic Lesions. St. Louis, C. V. Mosby Company, 1982, pp. 27–35.

Mulliken, J. B.: Cutaneous vascular lesions of children. *In* Serafin, D., and Georgiade, N. G. (Eds.): Pediatric Plastic Surgery. St. Louis, C. V. Mosby Company, 1984, pp. 137–154.

Mulliken, J. B.: Diagnosis and natural history of hemangiomas. *In* Mulliken, J. B., and Young, A. E. (Eds.): Vascular Birthmarks: Hemangiomas and Malformations. Philadelphia, W. B. Saunders Company, 1988a, pp. 41–62.

Mulliken, J. B.: Vascular malformations of the head and neck. *In* Mulliken, J. B., and Young, A. E. (Eds.): Vascular Birthmarks: Hemangiomas and Malformations. Philadelphia, W. B. Saunders Company, 1988b, pp. 301–342.

Mulliken, J. B., and Glowacki, J.: Hemangiomas and vascular malformations in infants and children: a classification based on endothelial characteristics. Plast. Reconstr. Surg., *69*:412, 1982.

Mulliken, J. B., Murray, J. E., Castaneda, A. R., and Kaban, L. B.: Management of a vascular malformation of the face using total circulatory arrest. Surg. Gynecol. Obstet., *146*:168, 1978.

Mulliken, J. B., and Young, A. E.: Vascular birthmarks in folklore, history, art, and literature. *In* Mulliken, J. B., and Young, A. E. (Eds.): Vascular Birthmarks: Hemangiomas and Malformations. Philadelphia, W. B. Saunders Company, 1988, pp. 3–23.

Mulliken, J. B., Zetter, B. R., and Folkman, J.: In vitro characteristics of endothelium from hemangiomas and vascular malformations. Surgery, *92*:348, 1982.

Munro, I. R., and Martin, R. D.: The management of gigantic benign craniofacial tumors: the reverse facial osteotomy. Plast. Reconstr. Surg., *65*:776, 1980.

Munro, R., and Munro, H. M.: Scrotal haemangiomas in boars. J. Comp. Pathol., *92*:109, 1982.

Murray, J. J.: Removal by ligature of large subcutaneous naevi without loss of skin. Lancet, *1*:321, 1864.

Natali, J., and Merland, J. J.: Superselective arteriography and therapeutic embolisation for vascular malformations (angiodysplasias). J. Cardiovasc. Surg., *17*:465, 1976.

Nicoladoni, C.: Phlebarteriectasie der rechten oberen Extremität. Arch. Klin. Chir., *18*:252, 1875.

Ninh, T. N., and Ninh, T. X.: Cystic hygroma in children: report of 126 cases. J. Pediatr. Surg., *9*:191, 1974.

Novick, N. L.: Angiokeratoma vulvae. J. Am. Acad. Dermatol., *12*:561, 1985.

Nozue, T., and Tsuzaki, M.: Further studies on distribution of neural crest cells in prenatal or postnatal development in mice. Okajimas Folia Anat. Jpn., *51*:131, 1974.

Nussbaum, M., and Buchwald, R. P.: Adult cystic hygroma. Am. J. Otolaryngol., 2:159, 1981.

Ogawa, Y., and Inoue, K.: Electrothrombosis as a treatment of cirsoid angioma in the face and scalp and varicosis of the leg. Plast. Reconstr. Surg., *70*:310, 1982.

Ohtsuka, H., Shioya, N., and Tanaka, S.: Cryosurgery for hemangiomas of the body surface and oral cavity. Ann. Plast. Surg., *4*:462, 1980.

Olcott, C., Newton, T. H., Stoney, R. J., and Ehrenfeld, W. K.: Intra-arterial embolization in the management of arteriovenous malformations. Surgery, *79*:3, 1976.

Olivecrona, H., and Ladenheim, J.: Congenital Arterio-Venous Aneurysms of the Carotid and Vertebral Arterial Systems. Berlin, Springer-Verlag, 1957, p. 14.

Order, S. E.: Hemangioma and the risk/benefit ratio. Int. J. Radiat. Oncol. Biol. Phys., *5*:143, 1979.

Osler, W.: On a family form of recurring epistaxis, associated with multiple telangiectases of the skin and mucous membranes. Johns Hopkins Hosp. Bull., *12*:333, 1901.

Øster, J., and Nielsen, A.: Nuchal naevi and interscapular telangiectases. Acta Paediatr. Scand., *59*:416, 1970.

Overcash, K. E., and Putney, F. J.: Subglottic hemangioma of the larynx treated with steroid therapy. Laryngoscope, *83*:679, 1973.

Padilla, R. S., Orkin, M., and Rosai, J.: Acquired "tufted" angioma (progressive capillary hemangioma). Am. J. Dermatopathol., *9*:292, 1987.

Park, W. C., and Phillips, R.: The role of radiation therapy in the management of hemangiomas of the liver. J.A.M.A., *212*:1496, 1970.

Pasyk, K. A., Argenta, L. C., and Schelbert, E. B.: Angiokeratoma circumscriptum: successful treatment with argon laser. Ann. Plast. Surg., *20*:183, 1988.

Pasyk, K. A., Cherry, G. W., Grabb, W. C., and Sasaki, G. H.: Quantitative evaluation of mast cells in cellularly dynamic and adynamic vascular malformations. Plast. Reconstr. Surg., *73*:69, 1984.

Paterson, R., and Tod, M. C.: The radium treatment of angiomas in children. Am. J. Roentgenol., *42*:726, 1939.

Patten, B. M.: Human Embryology. 3rd Ed. New York, McGraw-Hill Book Company, 1968, pp. 532–537.

Patterson, A. B.: Spontaneous cure of a naevus maternus—large vascular tumor occupying side of neck. South. Med. Rec., *24*:477, 1894.

Pauli: Ueber das Fuermal und die einzig sichere Methode, diese Entstellung zu heilen. Siebold Archiv. f. Geburtshilfe, Frauenzimmer und Kinderkrank, *15*:66, 1835.

Payne, M. M., Moyer, F., Marcks, K. M., and Trevaskis, A. E.: The precursor to the hemangioma. Plast. Reconstr. Surg., *38*:64, 1966.

Pemberton, J., and Saint, J. H.: Congenital arteriovenous communications. Surg. Gynecol. Obstet., *46*:470, 1928.

Pereyra, R., Andrassy, R. J., and Mahour, G. H.: Management of massive hepatic hemangiomas in infants and children: a review of 13 cases. Pediatrics, *70*:254, 1982.

Petrozzi, J. W., Rahn, E. K., Mofenson, H., and Greensher, J.: Cutis marmorata telangiectatica congenita. Arch. Dermatol., *101*:74, 1970.

Phillips, H. E., and McGahan, J. P.: Intrauterine fetal cystic hygromas: sonographic detection. A.J.R., *136*:799, 1981.

Poser, C. M., and Taveras, J. M.: Cerebral angiography in encephalotrigeminal angiomatosis. Radiology, *68*:327, 1957.

Pratt, A. G.: Birthmarks in infants. Arch. Dermatol., *67*:302, 1967.

Price, A. C., Coran, A. G., Mattern, A. L., and Cochran, R. L.: Hemangioendothelioma of the pelvis. A cause of cardiac failure in the newborn. N. Engl. J. Med., *286*:647, 1972.

Puglionisi, A., and Azzolini, A.: Caratteri dei nevi vascolari e transformazione angiomatosa de innesti e trapianti cutanei in soggetti portatori di fistole arterovenose congenite. Minerva Cardioangiol., *11*:493, 1963.

Pusey, W. A.: The use of carbon dioxide snow in the treatment of nevi and other lesions of the skin. J.A.M.A., *49*:1354, 1907.

Radcliffe-Crocker, H.: Diseases of the Skin. Philadelphia, Blakiston Press, 1893, p. 646.

Ravitch, M. M., and Gaertner, R. A.: Congenital arteriovenous fistula in the neck—48 year follow-up of a patient operated upon by Dr. Halsted in 1911. Bull. Johns Hopkins Hosp., *107*:31, 1960.

Ravitch, M. M., and Rush, B. F., Jr.: Cystic hygroma. *In* Welch, K. J., Randolph, J. G., Ravitch, M. M., et al. (Eds.): Pediatric Surgery. 4th Ed. Chicago, Year Book Medical Publishers, 1986, pp. 533–539.

Reder, F.: Hemangioma and lymphangioma, their response to the injection of boiling water. Med. Rec. N.Y., *98*:519, 1920.

Reid, M. R.: Studies on abnormal arteriovenous communications, acquired and congenital. I. Report of a series of cases. Arch. Surg., *10*:601, 1925a.

Reid, M. R.: Abnormal arteriovenous communications, acquired and congenital. II. The origin and nature of arteriovenous aneurysms, cirsoid aneurysms and simple angiomas. Arch. Surg., *10*:996, 1925b.

Reid, M. R.: Abnormal arteriovenous communications, acquired and congenital. III. The effects of abnormal arteriovenous communications on the heart, blood vessels and other structures. Arch. Surg., *11*:25, 1925c.

Rendu, M.: Epistaxis répetées chez un sujet porteur de petits angiomes cutanés et muqueux. Bull. Soc. Méd. Hôp. Paris, *13*:731, 1896.

Riché, M. C., Hadjean, E., Tran-Ba-Huy, P., and Merland, J. J.: The treatment of capillary-venous malformations using a new fibrosing agent. Plast. Reconstr. Surg., *71*:607, 1983.

Riché, M. C., and Merland, J. J.: Embolization of vascular malformations. *In* Mulliken, J. B., and Young, A. E. (Eds.): Vascular Birthmarks: Hemangiomas and Malformations. Philadelphia, W. B. Saunders Company, 1988, pp. 436–453.

Rienhoff, W. F., Jr.: Congenital arteriovenous fistula, an embryologic study, with the report of a case. Bull. Johns Hopkins Hosp., *35*:271, 1924.

Rigdon, R. H.: Spontaneous regression of neoplasms: an experimental study in the duck. South. Med. J., *47*:303, 1954.

Rigdon, R. H.: Spontaneous regression of hemangiomas, an experimental study in the duck and chicken. Cancer Res., *15*:77, 1955.

Rigdon, R. H., Walker, J., and Teddlie, A. H.: Hemangiomas. An experimental study in the duck. Cancer, *9*:1107, 1956.

Riley, H. D., Jr., and Smith, W. R.: Macrocephaly, pseudopapilledema and multiple hemangiomata. Pediatrics, *26*:293, 1960.

Robb, R. M.: Refractive errors associated with hemangiomas of the eyelids and orbit in infancy. Am. J. Ophthalmol., *83*:52, 1977.

Robertson, D. J.: Congenital arteriovenous fistulae of the extremities. Ann. R. Coll. Surg. Engl., *18*:73, 1956.

Rocchini, A. P., Rosenthal, A., Issenberg, H. J., and Nadas, A. S.: Hepatic hemangioendothelioma: hemodynamic observations and treatment. Pediatrics, *57*:131, 1976.

Rodriguez-Erdmann, F., Button, L., Murray, J. E., and Moloney, W. C.: Kasabach-Merritt syndrome: coagulo-analytical observations. Am. J. Med. Sci., *261*:9, 1971.

Ronchese, F.: The spontaneous involution of cutaneous vascular tumors. Am. J. Surg., *86*:376, 1953.

Rook, A. J., Wilkinson, D. S., and Ebling, F. J. G. (Eds.): Textbook of Dermatology. 3rd Ed. Oxford, Blackwell Scientific Publications, 1979, p. 969.

Rosai, J., Gold, J., and Landy, R.: The histiocytoid hemangiomas: a unifying concept embracing several previously described entities of skin, soft tissue, large vessels, bone and heart. Hum. Pathol., *10*:707, 1979.

Rush, B. F., Jr.: Treatment of giant cutaneous hemangioma by intra-arterial injection of nitrogen mustard. Ann. Surg., *164*:921, 1966.

Rutlin, E., Wisloff, F., Myren, J., and Serck-Hanssen, A.: Intestinal telangiectasis in Turner's syndrome. Endoscopy, *13*:86, 1981.

Ryan, T. J., and Barnhill, R. L.: Physical factors and angiogenesis. In Development of the Vascular System. London, Pitman, 1983, pp. 80–94.

Sabin, F. R.: On the origin of the lymphatic system from the veins and the development of the lymph hearts and thoracic duct in the pig. Am. J. Anat., *1*:367, 1902.

Sabin, F. R.: On the development of the superficial lymphatics in the skin of the pig. Am. J. Anat., *3*:183, 1904.

Sabin, F. R.: The development of the lymphatic nodes in the pig and their relation to the lymph hearts. Am. J. Anat., *4*:355, 1905.

Sabin, F. R.: The lymphatic system in human embryos, with a consideration of the morphology of the system as a whole. Am. J. Anat., *9*:43, 1909.

Sabin, F. R.: Studies on the origin of blood vessels and of red blood-corpuscles as seen in the living blastoderm of chicks during the second day of incubation. Contrib. Embryol., Carnegie Inst., *9*:213, 1920.

Sadowsky, D., Rosenberg, R. D., Kaufman, J., Levine, B. C., and Friedman, J. M.: Central hemangioma of the mandible. Oral Surg. Oral Med. Oral Pathol., *52*:471, 1981.

Sasaki, G. H., Pang, C. Y., and Wittliff, J. L.: Pathogenesis and treatment of infant skin strawberry hemangiomas: clinical and in vitro studies of hormonal effects. Plast. Reconstr. Surg., *73*:359, 1984.

Saunders, W. H.: Septal dermoplasty for control of nosebleeds caused by hereditary hemorrhagic telangiectasia or septal perforations. Trans. Am. Acad. Ophthalmol. Otolaryngol., *64*:500, 1960.

Schmidt, G. H.: Hemangioma in the zygoma. Ann. Plast. Surg., *3*:330, 1982.

Schnyder, U. W.: Zur Klinik und Histologie der Angiome. Arch. Derm. Syph., *200*:483, 1955.

Schrudde, J., and Petrovici, V.: Surgical treatment of giant hemangioma of the facial region after arterial embolization. Plast. Reconstr. Surg., *68*:878, 1981.

Scott, J. E. S.: Haemangiomata in skeletal muscle. Br. J. Surg., *44*:496, 1957.

Sehgal, V. N., Ghorpade, A., and Koranne, R. V.: Angiokeratoma corporis naeviforme. Dermatologica, *168*:144, 1984.

Semon, H. C.: Treatment of angiomas with the carbon dioxide snow pencil. Lancet, *1*:1167, 1934.

Servelle, M.: Klippel and Trenaunay's syndrome. 768 operated cases. Ann. Surg., *102*:365, 1985.

Shannon, K., Buchanan, G. R., and Votteler, T. P.: Multiple hepatic hemangiomas: failure of corticosteroid therapy and successful hepatic artery ligation. Am. J. Dis. Child., *136*:275, 1982.

Shapshay, S. M., and Oliver, P.: Treatment of hereditary hemorrhagic telangiectasia by Nd-YAG laser photocoagulation. Laryngoscope, *94*:1554, 1984.

Sherman, R. S., and Wilner, D.: The roentgen diagnosis of hemangioma of bone. Am. J. Roentgenol., *86*:1146, 1961.

Simpson, J. R.: Natural history of cavernous haemangiomata. Lancet, *2*:1057, 1959.

Singh, R. P., and Carr, D. H.: The anatomy and histology of XO human embryos and fetuses. Anat. Rec., *155*:369, 1966.

Skalkeas, G., Gogas, J., and Pavlatos, F.: Mammary hypoplasia following radiation to an infant breast. Case report. Acta Chir. Plast., *14*:240, 1972.

Slavin, S. A., Baker, D. C., McCarthy, J. G., and Mufarrij, A.: Congenital infiltrating lipomatosis of the face: clinicopathologic evaluation and treatment. Plast. Reconstr. Surg., *72*:158, 1983.

Smith, D. W.: Recognizable Patterns of Human Malformation: Genetic, Embryologic and Clinical Aspects. 3rd Ed. Philadelphia, W. B. Saunders Company, 1982, p. 472.

Smith, E. B., Graham, J. L., Ledman, J. A., and Snyder, R. D.: Fucosidosis. Cutis, *19*:195, 1977.

Smith, M. A., and Manfield, P. A.: The natural history of salmon patches in the first year of life. Br. J. Dermatol., *74*:31, 1962.

Smith, R. B., Prior, I. A., and Park, R. G.: Angiokeratoma of Mibelli: a family with nodular lesions of the leg. Aust. J. Dermatol., *9*:329, 1968.

Smoller, B. R., and Rosen, S.: Port-wine stains: a disease of altered neural modulation of blood vessels? Arch. Dermatol., *122*:177, 1986.

Solomon, L. M., and Esterly, N. B.: Epidermal and other congenital organoid nevi. Curr. Probl. Pediatr., *6*:1, 1975.

Solomon, L. M., Fretzin, D. F., and Dewald, R. L.: The epidermal nevus syndrome. Arch. Dermatol., *97*:273, 1968.

Sondel, P. M., Ritter, M. W., Wilson, D. G., and Lieberman, L. M.: Use of 111In platelet scans in the detection of treatment of Kasabach-Merritt syndrome. J. Pediatr., *104*:87, 1984.

South, D. A., and Jacobs, A. H.: Cutis marmorata telangiectatica congenita (congenital generalized phlebectasia). J. Pediatr., *93*:944, 1978.

Squire, B.: An improvement in the treatment of port-wine mark by linear scarification. Br. Med. J., *2*:732, 1879.

Stern, J. K., Wolf, J. E., Jr., and Jarratt, M.: Benign neonatal hemangiomatosis. J. Am. Acad. Dermatol., *4*:442, 1981.

Stevenson, R. F., Thomson, H. G., and Morin, J. D.: Unrecognized ocular problems associated with port wine stain of the face in children. Can. Med. Assoc. J., *111*:953, 1974.

Stigmar, G., Crawford, J. S., Ward, C. M., and Thomson, H. G.: Ophthalmic sequelae of infantile hemangiomas of the eyelids and orbit. Am. J. Ophthalmol., *85*:806, 1978.

Stone, H. H., and Nielson, I. C.: Hemangioma of the liver in the newborn. Report of a successful outcome following hepatic lobectomy. Arch. Surg., *90*:319, 1965.

Stout, A. P., and Lattes, R. S.: Tumors of the Soft Tissues. Washington, D. C., Armed Forces Institute of Pathology, fascicle 1, second series, 1967.

Sturge, W. A.: A case of partial epilepsy, apparently due to a lesion of one of the vaso-motor centres of the brain. Trans. Clin. Soc. Lond., *12*:162, 1879.

Sumner, T. E., Volberg, F. M., Kiser, P. E., and Shaffner, L. D.: Mediastinal cystic hygroma in children. Pediatr. Radiol., *11*:160, 1981.

Swerlick, R. A., and Cooper, P. H.: Pyogenic granuloma (lobular capillary hemangioma) within port-wine stains. J. Am. Acad. Dermatol., *8*:627, 1983.

Szilagyi, D. E., Smith, R. F., Elliott, J. P., and Hageman, J. H.: Congenital arteriovenous anomalies of the limbs. Arch. Surg., *111*:423, 1976.

Tan, K. L.: Nevus flammeus of the nape, glabella and eyelids. A clinical study of frequency, racial distribution, and association with congenital anomalies. Clin. Pediatr., *11*:112, 1972.

Taylor, S., and Folkman, J.: Protamine is an inhibitor of angiogenesis. Nature, *297*:307, 1982.

Tefft, M.: The radiotherapeutic management of subglottic hemangiomas in children. Radiology, *86*:207, 1966.

Tegtmeyer, C. J., Smith, T. H., Shaw, A., Barwick, K. W., and Kattwinkel, J.: Renal infarction: a complication of Gelfoam embolization of hemangioendothelioma of the liver. Am. J. Roentgenol., *128*:305, 1977.

Théron, J., Newton, T. H., and Hoyt, W. F.: Unilateral retinocephalic vascular malformations. Neuroradiology, 7:185, 1974.

Thoma, R.: Untersuchungen über die Histogenese und Histomechanik des Gefässystems. Stuttgart, F. Enke Publ., 1893. Cited by Malan, E.: In Vascular Malformations. Milan, Carlo Erba Foundation, 1974, pp. 21–22.

Thomson, H. G., Ward, C. M., Crawford, J. S., and Stigmar, G.: Hemangiomas of the eyelid: visual complications and prophylactic concepts. Plast. Reconstr. Surg., *63*:641, 1979.

Thomson, H. G., and Wright, A. M.: Surgical tattooing of the port wine stain. Operative technique, results, and critique. Plast. Reconstr. Surg., *48*:113, 1971.

Thornton, S. C., Mueller, S. N., and Levine, E. M.: Human endothelial cells: use of heparin in cloning and long-term serial cultivation. Science, *222*:623, 1983.

Toth, B., Magee, P. N., and Shubik, P.: Carcinogenesis study with dimethylnitrosamine administered orally to adult and subcutaneously to newborn BALB/C mice. Cancer Res., *24*:1712, 1964.

Toth, B., and Wilson, R. B.: Blood vessel tumorigenesis by 1,2-dimethylhydrazine dihydrochloride (symmetrical). Gross, light and electron microscopic descriptions. Am. J. Pathol., *64*:585, 1971.

Touloukian, R. J.: Hepatic hemangioendothelioma during infancy: pathology, diagnosis, and treatment with prednisone. Pediatrics, *45*:71, 1970.

Trélat, U., and Monod, A.: De l'hypertrophie unilatérale partielle ou totale du corps. Arch. Gen. Med., *13*:636, 1869.

Trell, E., Johansson, B. W., Linell, F., and Ripa, J.: Familial pulmonary hypertension and multiple abnormalities of large systemic arteries in Osler's disease. Am. J. Med., *53*:50, 1972.

Turner, D.: De Morbis Cutaneis. A Treatise of Diseases Incident to the Skin. London, R. Bonwicke, W. Freeman, T. Goodwin, et al., 1714, pp. 120–128.

Ulsø, C., Vase, P., and Stoksted, P.: Long-term results of dermatoplasty in the treatment of hereditary haemorrhagic telangiectasis. J. Laryngol. Otol., *97*:223, 1983.

van der Putte, S. C.: The development of the lymphatic system in man. Adv. Anat. Embryol. Cell Biol., *51*:3, 1975.

van der Putte, S. C.: Lymphatic malformation in human fetuses. A study of fetuses with Turner's syndrome or status Bonnevie-Ullrich. Virchows Arch. [Pathol. Anat.], *376*:233, 1977.

van Lohuizen, C. H. J.: Über eine seltene angeborene Hautanomalie (Cutis marmorata telangiectatica congenita). Acta Dermatovener., *3*:202, 1922.

Vaughan, A. M.: Cystic hygroma of the neck. Am. J. Dis. Child., *48*:149, 1934.

Viljoen, D. L., Nelson, M., de Jong, G., and Beighton, P.: Proteus syndrome in southern Africa: natural history and clinical manifestations in six individuals. Am. J. Med. Genet., *27*:87, 1987.

Virchow, R.: Angiome. In Die krankhaften Geschwülste. Vol. 3. Berlin, August Hirschwald, 1863, pp. 306–425.

Vollmar, J.: Zur Geschichte and Terminologie der Syndrome nach F. P. Weber und Klippel-Trenaunay. VASA, *3*:231, 1974.

Vracko, R., and Benditt, E. P.: Capillary basal lamina thickening. Its relationship to endothelial cell death and replacement. J. Cell Biol., *47*:281, 1970.

Wagget, J., Inkster, J. S., and Ashcroft, T.: Hemangioendothelioma of the liver of an infant—hypotensive crisis during resection. Surgery, *65*:352, 1969.

Wallace, H. J.: The conservative treatment of haemangiomatous naevi. Br. J. Plast. Surg., *6*:78, 1953.

Wallace, H. J.: Anderson-Fabry disease. Br. J. Dermatol., *88*:1, 1973.

Waller, T., and Rubarth, S.: Haemangioendothelioma in domestic animals. Acta Vet. Scand., *8*:234, 1967.

Wallerstein, R. O.: Spontaneous involution of giant hemangioma. Am. J. Dis. Child., *102*:233, 1961.

Walsh, T. S., Jr., and Tompkins, V. N.: Some observations on the strawberry nevus of infancy. Cancer, *9*:869, 1956.

Walter, J.: On the treatment of cavernous hemangioma with special reference to spontaneous regression. J. Fac. Radiol., *5*:134, 1953.

Ward, C. M., and Buchanan, R.: Haemangiosarcoma following irradiation of a haemangioma of the face. J. Maxillofac. Surg., *5*:164, 1977.

Wardrop, J.: Some observations on one species of naevus maternus with the case of an infant where the carotid artery was tied. Med.-Chirurg. Trans, *9*:199, 1818.

Warrell, R. P., Jr., and Kempin, S. J.: Treatment of severe coagulopathy in the Kasabach-Merritt syndrome with aminocaproic acid and cryoprecipitate. N. Engl. J. Med., *313*:309, 1985.

Warren, J. C.: Surgical Observations on Tumours with Cases and Operations. Boston, Crocker & Brewster, 1837, pp. 413–427.

Watson, W. L., and McCarthy, W. D.: Blood and lymph vessel tumors: a report of 1,056 cases. Surg. Gynecol. Obstet., *71*:569, 1940.

Way, B. H., Herrmann, J., Gilbert, E. F., Johnson, S. A., and Opitz, J. M.: Cutis marmorata telangiectatica congenita. J. Cutan. Pathol., *1*:10, 1974.

Weber, F. P.: Multiple hereditary developmental angiomata (telangiectases) of the skin and mucous membranes associated with recurring haemorrhages. Lancet, *2*:160, 1907a.

Weber, F. P.: Angioma formation in connection with hypertrophy of limbs and hemi-hypertrophy. Br. J. Dermatol., *19*:231, 1907b.

Weber, F. P.: Right-sided hemihypertrophy resulting

from right-sided congenital spastic hemiplegia, with a morbid condition of the left side of the brain, revealed by radiograms. J. Neurol. Psychopathol., *3*:134, 1922.

Wegner, G.: Ueber Lymphangiome. Arch. klin. Chir., Berl., *20*:641, 1876–1877.

Wells, G. A., and Morgan, G.: Multifocal haemangioma in a pig. J. Comp. Pathol., *90*:483, 1980.

Welsh, D., and Hengerer, A. S.: The diagnosis and treatment of intramuscular hemangiomas of the masseter muscle. Am. J. Otolaryngol., *1*:186, 1980.

Wenzl, J. E., and Burgert, E. O., Jr.: The spider nevus in infancy and childhood. Pediatrics, *33*:227, 1964.

Wernher, A.: Die angebornen Kysten-Hygrome und die ihnen verwandten Geschwülste in anatomischer, diagnosticher und therapeutischer Beziehung. Giessen, G. F. Heyer, Vater, 1843.

Whimster, I. W.: The pathology of lymphangioma circumscriptum. Br. J. Dermatol., *94*:473, 1976.

Wiedemann, H. R., and Burgio, G. R.: Encephalocraniocutaneous lipomatosis and Proteus syndrome. Am. J. Med. Genet., *25*:403, 1986.

Wiedemann, H. R., Burgio, G. R., Aldenhoff, P., Kunze, J., Kaufmann, H. J., and Schirg, E.: The Proteus syndrome: partial gigantism of the hand and/or feet, nevi, hemihypertrophy, subcutaneous tumors, macrocephaly, or other skull anomalies and possible accelerated growth and visceral affections. Eur. J. Pediatr., *140*:5, 1983.

Wilflingseder, P., Martin, R., and Papp, Ch.: Magnesium seeds in the treatment of lymph- and haemangiomata. Chir. Plast., *6*:105, 1981.

Williams, H. B.: Hemangiomas of the parotid gland in children. Plast. Reconstr. Surg., *56*:29, 1975.

Williams, H. B.: Facial bone changes with vascular tumors in children. Plast. Reconstr. Surg., *63*:309, 1979.

Willis, R. A.: Pathology of Tumors. 3rd Ed. London, Butterworth & Co., 1960, p. 716.

Wishnick, M. M.: Multinodular hemangiomatosis with partial biliary obstruction. J. Pediatr., *92*:960, 1978.

Wojtanowski, M. H., and Mandel, M. A.: Seizures abolished by excision of a cavernous hemangioma of the scalp and skull. Case report. Plast. Reconstr. Surg., *64*:831, 1979.

Woods, J. E.: Extended use of sodium tetradecyl sulfate in treatment of hemangiomas and other related conditions. Plast. Reconstr. Surg., *79*:542, 1987.

Woollard, H. H.: The development of the principal arterial system in the forelimb of the pig. Contrib. Embryol., Carnegie Inst., *14*:139, 1922.

Woollard, H. H., and Harpman, J. A.: The relationship between the size of an artery and the capillary bed in the embryo. J. Anat., *72*:18, 1937.

Wright, T. L., and Bresnan, M. J.: Radiation-induced cerebrovascular disease in children. Neurology, *26*:540, 1976.

Wyburn-Mason, R.: Arteriovenous aneurysm of midbrain and retina, facial naevi and mental changes. Brain, *66*:163, 1943.

Wyeth, J. A.: The treatment of vascular tumours by the injection of water at a high temperature. J.A.M.A., *40*:1778, 1903.

Wyman, L. C., Fulton, G. P., and Shulman, M. H.: Direct observations on the circulation in the hamster cheek pouch in adrenal insufficiency and experimental hypercorticolism. Ann. N.Y. Acad. Sci., *56*:643, 1953.

Young, A. E.: Congenital mixed vascular deformities of the limbs and their associated lesions. Birth Defects; Original Article Series, *14*:289, 1978.

Young, A. E.: Pathogenesis of vascular malformations. *In* Mulliken, J. B., and Young, A. E. (Eds.): Vascular Birthmarks: Hemangiomas and Malformations. Philadelphia, W. B. Saunders Company, 1988a, pp. 107–113.

Young, A. E.: Combined vascular malformations. *In* Mulliken, J. B., and Young, A. E. (Eds.): Vascular Birthmarks: Hemangiomas and Malformations. Philadelphia, W. B. Saunders Company, 1988b, pp. 246–274.

Young, A. E.: Vascular malformations of the lower limb. *In* Mulliken, J. B., and Young, A. E. (Eds.): Vascular Birthmarks: Hemangiomas and Malformations. Philadelphia, W. B. Saunders Company, 1988c, pp. 400–423.

Zak, T. A., and Morin, D. J.: Early local steroid therapy of infantile eyelid hemangiomas. J. Pediatr. Ophthalmol. Strabismus, *18*:25, 1981.

Zarem, H. A., and Edgerton, M. T.: Induced resolution of cavernous hemangiomas following prednisolone therapy. Plast. Reconstr. Surg., *39*:76, 1967.

Zetter, B. R.: Migration of capillary endothelial cells is stimulated by tumour-derived factors. Nature, *285*:41, 1980.

Zinn, K. M.: Iatrogenic intraocular injection of depot corticosteroid and its surgical removal using the pars plana approach. Ophthalmology, *88*:13, 1981.

Zweifach, B. W., Shor, E., and Black, M. M.: The influence of the adrenal cortex on the behavior of the terminal vascular bed. Ann. N.Y. Acad. Sci., *56*:626, 1953.

Irving M. Polayes

Surgical Treatment of Diseases of the Salivary Glands

HISTORICAL BACKGROUND

Hippocrates was the first to describe the clinical signs accompanying the inflammation of epidemic parotitis in the fifth century B.C. and was also the first to describe ranula as a "stone in the mouth." However, he failed to relate his clinical findings to the anatomic structures of the parotid, sublingual, or submandibular glands. It is not known who first described the anatomic structure of the parotid and other major salivary glands. From the early theories of the Greeks until the seventeenth century A.D., the salivary glands were referred to as "emunctories" (excretory organs) of the brain for circulation of "humors" similar to what was thought to be the origin of urine, gastric juice and bile (Ambroise Paré, 1594).

The first to recognize the glandular substance of the parotid was Riolan in 1648. Niels Stensen has been recorded as being the first to have dissected a sheep's head and to discover the duct of the parotid gland in 1660. In 1656 Thomas Wharton was the first to identify the submandibular gland and duct. Bartholinus (1669) discovered the major sublingual gland and its duct, while Ravinus described the multiple ductules emanating from the sublingual gland into the floor of the mouth in 1677. It was not until 1910–1913 that Weber, Figri, Carmalt, Churchill, and Florence first described the microscopic and topographic anatomy of the salivary glands.

In 1802 Bertrandi outlined the first surgical plan of parotidectomy for the treatment of parotid masses. Morestin proposed ligation of Stensen's duct in 1818 to produce glandular atrophy and eliminate salivary fistulas. In

1830 von Langenbeck suggested that the injured salivary duct be repaired by dissecting the duct to its source of fistula formation, excising the fistulous tract, and repairing the severed ends of the duct.

The surgeons of the late eighteenth and early nineteenth centuries also proposed total resection of the submandibular and sublingual glands to remove tumor masses involving the floor of the mouth. The technique of submandibular gland resection was best described by Velpeau and served as the model for modern-day techniques. Submandibular and sublingual gland resection did not pose the technical problems involved with the more difficult parotid resection, and until the early twentieth century the correlation of clinical and anatomic findings with the pathologic condition encountered was not fully appreciated.

Through the early nineteenth century, most parotid surgery was confined to either small local excisions or superficial segmental resections. In 1825 Heyfelder was able to avoid facial paralysis while carrying out a parotidectomy. Velpeau (1830) was the first to demonstrate a method of locating and identifying the trunk of the facial nerve. Along with Bell, he emphasized that the facial nerve was the prime force of facial muscle activity and coursed through the parotid gland. At the same time, Velpeau and Bell noted that sensory supply to the face was through the fifth nerve. In 1869 the need for preservation of the facial nerve in parotidectomy for benign tumors was emphasized by Erichsen, and the first total parotidectomy with preservation of the facial nerve was reported by Codreanu (1892). With the advent of the electric nerve stimulator proposed by Clausen and Henley in 1948 and demonstrated as effective by Buxton and associates in 1949, surgical technique improved markedly in both segmental and total resection of all major salivary glands with preservation of the facial nerve.

Billroth (1856) was the first to describe cylindroma or adenoid cystic carcinoma of the salivary glands; Warthin's tumor of the salivary glands was first noted in the United States in 1929 by Warthin, although it had been clearly described by Albrecht and Arzt in Germany in 1910. Virchow described a mixed tumor of the salivary glands in 1863, and Nasse (1901) first reported that the acinic cell adenoma originated from the cells of the ducts and acini of the salivary glands.

SURGICAL ANATOMY

The salivary glands arise from the ingrowth of oral ectoderm into an underlying dense mesenchyme. The major glands are generally ectodermal derivatives while the minor glands may be either ectodermal or entodermal, depending on their respective oral or pharyngeal locations. The oral primordium develops as an epithelial bud from which branching ducts and terminal secretory acini develop. The mesenchymal elements encapsulate and divide the glandular units into segments and provide their vascular support. The parotid and submandibular glands appear in the sixth fetal week and extend from their respective main excretory ducts in the mouth to form glandular structures in front of the ear or below the mandible. The sublingual glands arise independently about the eighth week as a group of buds that develop into 10 or 12 minor ducts and one major duct, the duct of Bartholin, emptying alongside the tongue in the floor of the mouth and/or into the submandibular duct. The diffuse minor salivary glands are found in the oral pharynx, within the lips, the palate, the cheeks, the base of the tongue, the tonsillar fossa, and the accessory paranasal sinuses. They arise at approximately the third month from multiple epithelial ectodermal buds.

Parotid Gland. The parotid gland is the largest of the salivary glands and occupies a roughly triangular bony space between the external auditory canal, the ramus of the mandible, and the mastoid process. The gland rests upon the styloid process and the transverse process of the second cervical vertebra. It overflows these bony confinements into a space between the medial and lateral pterygoid, digastric, and stylohyoid muscles and superficially onto the sternocleidomastoid and masseter muscles (Fig. 67–1). Single or multiple accessory parotid glands may be present and lie along the path of the main parotid duct on the masseter muscle and the anterior border of the parotid gland (Fig. 67–2). The main parotid duct runs forward to the anterior border of the masseter muscle and passes medially through the buccinator muscle to open into the buccal mucosa alongside the maxillary second molar tooth. An imaginary line drawn from beneath the external nares to the tragus indicates the position of the main parotid or Stensen's duct, which is palpable against the examining finger when

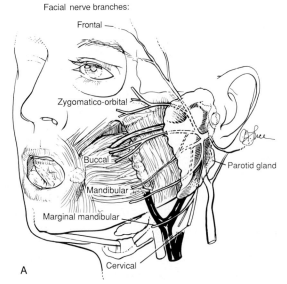

Facial nerve branches:

Frontal

Zygomatico-orbital

Buccal

Mandibular

Marginal mandibular

Cervical

Parotid gland

Figure 67–1. Anatomic relationships of the major salivary glands. *A*, Facial nerve. *B*, Portion of mandible removed. Note the minor salivary glands in the palate.

A

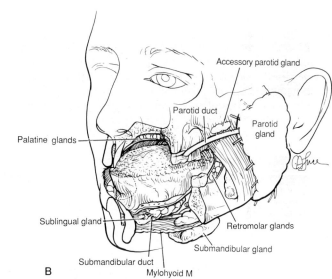

Accessory parotid gland

Parotid duct

Parotid gland

Palatine glands

Sublingual gland

Retromolar glands

Submandibular gland

Submandibular duct

Mylohyoid M

B

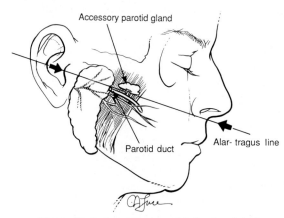

Accessory parotid gland

Parotid duct

Alar-tragus line

Figure 67–2. Accessory parotid gland and duct.

the skin overlying the masseter muscle bulk is gently rolled (see Fig. 67–2).

A firm sheath encases the parotid gland beneath the subcutaneous fat and is derived from the anterior or superficial layer of the deep cervical fascia. This sheath is attached above to the zygomatic arch and is thickened below into a stylomandibular ligament that extends from the styloid process downward and forward to the posterior border of the mandible, separating the parotid from the submandibular gland.

The facial nerve is a structure of primary consideration by the surgeon when operating on the parotid gland. Fear of surgical injury to the nerve has long been a deterrent to adequate drainage of infections as well as the adequate removal of tumors. The general concept that the gland is divided into a superficial and deep "lobe" by the facial nerve has been shown to be anatomically inaccurate and is an artificial division. The parotid gland in its entirety is a single mass. Gasser (1970) demonstrated the encirclement of the facial nerve that appears in the fourth to fifth fetal week by an ingrowth of the developing parotid primordium. Accordingly, the anatomic terms superficial (lateral) and deep (medial) *portions* of the gland suggested by McKenzie in 1948 have *replaced* the terms superficial and deep *lobes* in the 1966 edition of the Nomina Anatomica. The parotid gland, then, is referred to as having a superficial or lateral *segment* and deep or medial *segment,* indicating that it is a single (unitary) structure, indented by the ascending ramus of the mandible, and containing the facial nerve between the superficial and deep segments (Fig. 67–3).

The *facial nerve* exits from the skull at the stylomastoid foramen posterior to the base of the styloid process to enter the deep surface of the parotid gland inferior to the auditory meatus (see Chap. 42). From this point, the nerve gradually becomes more superficial as it passes across the masseter muscle to innervate the muscles of facial expression and the buccinator muscle. Immediately after emerging from the stylomastoid foramen, the main trunk of the facial nerve gives branches to the posterior digastric and stylohyoid muscles. The main trunk of the nerve measures approximately 4 mm in diameter and, after penetrating the deep segment, divides into the two main branches, the temporofacial and cervicofacial branches. Beyond this point, branching of the nerve is accompanied by intercommunicating arborization to form five groups of nerves or branches: (1) the *temporal* or *frontal,* passing to the lateral brow; (2) the *zygomatico-orbital,* to the orbit and palpebral sphincter; (3) the *buccal,* parallel to the parotid duct and innervating the cheek and upper lip; (4) the *mandibular,* passing along the inferior mandible to the oral commissure; and (5) the *cervical,* which passes to the platysma muscle (see Fig. 67–1).

Temporary or permanent paralysis may follow invasion by tumor or severe trauma to the face or gland along the course of the facial nerve. Incisions behind the angle of the mandible in the upper neck below the earlobe must not pass beneath the subcutaneous fat

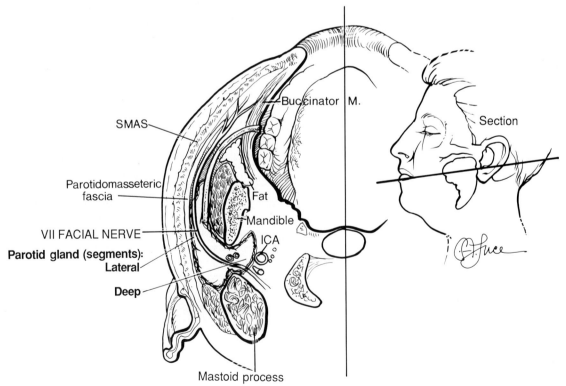

Figure 67–3. The segments of the parotid gland and their relationship to the facial nerve, ascending mandibular ramus, pharynx, and jugulodigastric structures. ICA = internal carotid artery.

in *children,* otherwise the unprotected main trunk of the facial nerve may be divided. The later development of the mastoid process in children over age 10 years displaces the facial nerve trunk into a deeper, protected plane, making it more difficult to injure this nerve trunk at the subcutaneous level. Similarly, the incisions through the parotid fascia should be parallel to the peripheral branches of the facial nerve. When incising the parotid gland for drainage, it is best to elevate the skin through a preauricular incision and to make the appropriate incision into the abscess bluntly through the parotid fascia in a direction *parallel* to the *nerve branches.*

Lymphatics and Lymph Nodes. Just as the facial nerve is surrounded and enveloped by the developing parotid parenchyma, so too are the lymphatics and lymph nodes. The parotid lymph nodes are divided into the *extraglandular* or *superficial paraglandular* and *deep intraglandular groups.* The *extraglandular* nodes are *preauricular* on the parotid fascial sheath, and drain the temporal and frontal scalp, the eyelids, and the anterior auricle. These lymphatics empty posteriorly into a superficial cervical chain of nodes along the external jugular vein. The *deep intraglandular* lymphatics drain the glandular substance, the eustachian tube, the external auditory canal, and the deeper portions of the face anteriorly via the subparotid nodes or posteriorly along the retromandibular vein into a deep cervical chain, which follows the

spinal accessory or 11th cranial nerve. The subparotid nodes drain into the deep upper cervical nodal chain or jugulodigastric group of nodes, closely attached to the internal jugular vein (Fig. 67–4).

Submandibular Gland. The submandibular gland (Fig. 67–5) is approximately one-half the size of the parotid gland and is a paired structure. The submandibular gland presents as a cervical portion and as an intraoral portion by wrapping itself around the posterior border of the mylohyoid muscle. The gland is indented by that muscle so that from the posterior superior cervical portion the major, or Wharton's, duct passes forward toward the midline anteriorly on the mylohyoid muscle, beneath the mucosa of the floor of the mouth; the major inferior cervical portion lies below the mylohyoid muscle and within the digastric triangle between the anterior and posterior bellies of the digastric muscle. The gland is enclosed in the anterior (superficial) layer of the deep cervical fascia, which runs from the hyoid bone to the lower border of the mandible. In some cases, a projection of the gland may extend along the main duct beyond the free posterior border of the mylohyoid muscle and may terminate proximal to the more anteriorly and laterally placed sublingual gland. Associated with any dissection of the submandibular gland is the mandibular branch of the facial nerve, passing between the platysma muscle and facial vessels along the inferior border of the body of the

Lymph nodes draining salivary glands

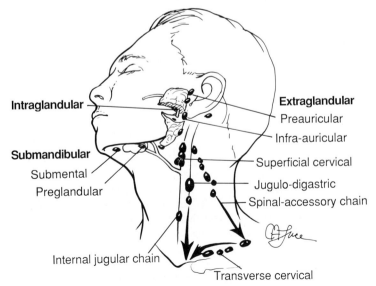

Figure 67–4. Lymphatic drainage of the salivary glands, including the drainage of the submandibular and sublingual glands.

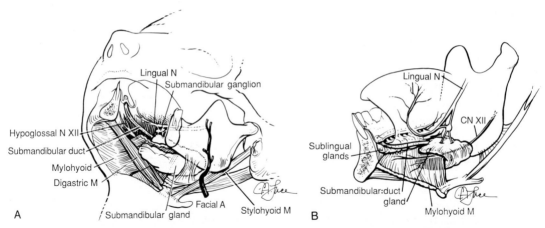

Figure 67–5. *A,* Relationships of the submandibular and sublingual glands to the floor of the mouth. *B,* Submandibular and sublingual glands and relationships with the floor of the mouth and the lingual and hypoglossal nerves.

mandible and the laterosuperior surface of the submandibular salivary gland. The medial surface of the submandibular gland rests upon the hyoglossus muscle and the hypoglossal nerve, the submandibular ganglion, the lingual nerve, and the main duct of the gland itself.

The *hypoglossal nerve* is the motor nerve of the tongue and passes beneath the posterior belly of the digastric muscle onto the hyoglossus muscle (see Fig. 67–5). It runs adjacent to the lingual veins and may be injured during submandibular gland surgery. Ipsilateral paralysis of the tongue follows injury or compression of this nerve.

The *lingual nerve* (Fig. 67–5) is at the uppermost surface of the submandibular gland and is also subject to surgical injury, as well as to compression by tumor from either the floor of the mouth, the tongue, or the submandibular gland itself. Injury to the lingual nerve results in anesthesia of the ipsilateral anterior two-thirds of the tongue.

The submandibular duct proceeds forward and upward behind the posterior free border of the mylohyoid muscle to open through the mucous membrane in the ipsilateral sublingual papilla adjacent to the anterior midline of the floor of the mouth. The submandibular gland is innervated by the lingual nerve, the sympathetic plexus from the facial artery, and the submandibular ganglion, which contains the parasympathetic secretory fibers from the chorda tympani. The external facial (or maxillary) artery provides the arterial supply to the submandibular gland, while the facial veins drain the gland.

The lymphatic drainage of the submandibular gland is to a group of submandibular lymph nodes adjacent to the gland and to a second group at the facial notch along the inferior border of the mandible. These lymph nodes receive the lymphatic drainage from the lips, cheeks, gingiva, teeth, lower face, tongue, and submandibular gland. The efferent vessels of these nodes pass to the deep cervical chain, notably the jugulodigastric and occasionally the jugulo-omohyoid nodes along the internal jugular vein (see Fig. 67–4). The fibrous fascial sheath, forming a capsule-like covering of the submandibular gland, lacks the strong septa that permeate the parotid gland and therefore allows for a more simple enucleation of the submandibular gland from its bed.

In completing a submandibular gland resection, the relationship of the submandibular gland is noteworthy in that the fascia on the floor of the submandibular fossa is the hyoglossal myofascial covering inferior to which pass the hypoglossal nerve, the venae comitantes, and the hyoglossus muscle. Superior to the resected glandular site is the mylohyoid muscle on which the duct passes forward into the floor of the mouth and which paired muscle also forms the floor of the mouth and roof over the submandibular fossa. In this fossa one notes superiorly the lingual nerve as it crosses the submandibular duct from a posterior to an anterior direction in its course to the tongue. This path of the lingual nerve should also be carefully studied in its relationship to the submandibular duct as well as the submandibular (or submaxillary) ganglion, which is attached to the lingual nerve and submaxillary gland by its pre- and postganglionic fibers. Care must be taken in separating an intact lingual nerve from the submaxillary gland by severing the post-ganglionic fibers extending from the submaxillary ganglion into the gland itself. In this way, the ganglion is left attached to the lingual nerve without injuring the nerve structure (see Fig. 67–5).

Sublingual Gland. The sublingual gland is one-half the size of the submandibular gland and is the smallest of the paired six major salivary glands. The sublingual gland lies along the anterolateral portion of the floor of the mouth beneath the mucosa and rests against the lingual surface of the mandible. It is separated from the cervical portion of the submandibular gland by the mylohyoid muscle, and its medial surface lies against the anteriormost portion of the submandibular duct and the lingual nerve. The genioglossus muscle lies medial to the sublingual gland, and approximately 20 small ducts pass from the gland to open into the mouth in the oral mucosa of the sublingual fold or plica sublingualis. Occasionally, several of these small ducts become confluent and may empty as a single Bartholin duct into the major submandibular, or Wharton's, duct. Obstruction of any of the ducts of the sublingual gland can produce a cystic swelling in the floor of the mouth, known for many years as a ranula. In performing surgery for removal of a ranula, it is best to remove both the cystic mass and the entire sublingual gland.

The sublingual artery is a branch of the lingual artery and is the chief arterial supply to the sublingual gland. This artery, along with the lingual nerve, is particularly vulnerable to surgical trauma. The sublingual gland is supplied with sympathetic fibers from the sublingual artery as well as parasympathetic fibers from the submandibular ganglion.

The lymphatic vessels of the sublingual salivary gland drain into the preglandular submandibular nodes as they penetrate the mylohyoid muscle. The preglandular nodes and the efferent lymphatics of the posterior portion of the sublingual gland empty into the subdigastric nodes along the internal jugular vein in a fashion similar to that of the submandibular nodes. It is because of these drainage pathways that the rare, but more often malignant, solid tumors of the sublingual gland metastasize readily into the deep jugular chain.

Minor Salivary Glands. The minor salivary glands are numerous submucosal aggregates of salivary tissue that are mucous or seromucous in nature. They are present in the lips, the palate, the buccal mucosa, the floor of the mouth, the tongue, the retromolar or glossopharyngeal area, the nasopharynx, the paranasal sinuses, and the tracheobronchial tree. In contrast to the parotid gland, which is mainly serous in the type of secretion produced, these glandular elements are mucous or seromucous. The minor salivary glands are subject to the same types of salivary gland disorders as the major salivary glands. However, when the minor salivary glands are involved with a malignant lesion, the latter tend to be "more malignant" than those occurring in the parotid and submandibular glands; they are, however, equal in malignancy to the solid tumors appearing in the sublingual gland.

DIAGNOSIS

A reliable history and careful physical examination are basic to the clinical evaluation of all disease entities of the salivary glands.

The salivary glands should be evaluated by leading questions. Is there pain associated with glandular swelling or with meals? Does swelling occur after ingestion of certain foods? Are there allergies that produce pain or swelling in the salivary glands? Is there weakness of the facial nerve, lingual nerve, or hypoglossal nerve? Does the patient perceive some drooping or weakness in moving one side of the face? Is it difficult to talk because the tongue does not move in a normal fashion? Is there numbness or loss of taste on one side of the tongue? These leading questions may provide hints as to the diagnosis of the salivary gland nodule or mass.

The physical examination is commenced with a careful inspection of the patient's head and neck area, facial expression, and tongue motion during speech. The examination should include the nodes in the head and neck area and the axillary region, as well as palpation of the liver, spleen, and thyroid and a comprehensive neurologic examination. In general, involvement of multiple glands points toward a systemic problem, in contrast to involvement of a single salivary gland, which more often suggests the presence of inflammatory duct obstruction or a possible neoplasm. Diffuse enlargement of a single salivary gland suggests a chronic inflammatory disease, whereas multiple gland enlargement suggests a lymphoepithelial disorder such as Sjögren's syndrome.

Palpation of the major salivary glands and their ducts for evidence of tenderness and intraductal masses can be performed using bimanual techniques. In the submandibular gland, bimanual palpation of the floor of the mouth may elicit a calculus in the submandibular duct. All branches of the facial nerve should be carefully examined for active function. Any compression or limitation of function by invasion of the hypoglossal and lingual nerves can also be evaluated through examination of the tongue for sensation as well as deviation in protrusion.

A mass in the salivary gland should be evaluated for its degree of fixation, the mobility of the overlying skin, and the consistency relative to surrounding soft tissues. Bimanual external and intraoral palpation can help identify masses involving the deep parotid segment in that they may appear as a glossopalatal, glossopharyngeal, or pharyngotonsillar enlargement. The lymph nodes in the submandibular area as well as the parotid nodes should be carefully palpated and examined for consistency and size. One must be suspicious of tumor involvement when lymph nodes measure more than 1.5 cm in diameter.

Masses involving the parotid gland are usually located in the tail of that gland, and appear to elevate the overlying ear lobule or to extend over the angle of the mandible into the retromandibular area (Fig. 67–6). Masses in the anterior midcheek area or at the anterior limits of the parotid gland may represent tumor involvement of an accessory parotid gland (Fig. 67–7). Masses appearing anterior to the tragus may represent a metastatic carcinoma in a preauricular lymph node and signal the need for careful head and neck examination to identify a primary lesion elsewhere (Fig. 67–8). The nature of the mass relative to its surrounding tissue in the parotid gland can provide a clue as to its benign or malignant potential. Warthin's tumor, for example, may be soft or firm and is well defined, while the pleomorphic adenoma may be quite firm and also well circumscribed.

A mass of salivary gland origin can be evaluated further by CT scan, or computed tomography, which, coordinated with sialography, offers an excellent means of evaluating a mass in any of the salivary glands. Sialography alone may define the ductal system and demonstrate evidence of obstruction;

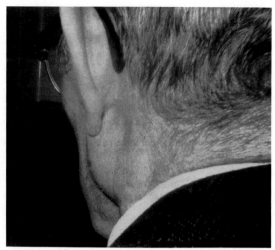

Figure 67–6. Appearance of a parotid mass elevating the ear lobule and filling the retromandibular space.

its main value as a diagnostic tool alone is in detecting calcareous ductal obstruction and defining a Sjögren's type of syndrome. However, to delineate the location of a salivary gland mass, the best radiographic study is through the CT scan with simultaneous sialography. This method clearly identifies small lesions that are not easily palpable and relates the lesions to surrounding tissues, both in the longitudinal and the coronal projections. It is most useful in detecting lesions involving the deep parotid segment and the parapharyngeal areas. However, in combination with sialography, it may also define the actual location, size, and configuration of a benign pleomorphic adenoma or a malignant invading neoplasm. One may eliminate sialography and use perfusion techniques in combination with the CT scan by taking the same scanning views with intravenous contrast enhancement. However, if one wishes to outline the ductal system, CT scanning with simultaneous sialography provides a useful study of the major salivary gland system.

The appearance of cystic masses in the area of the salivary glands may or may not be indicative of a benign or malignant lesion. A branchial cleft cyst arising from the first branchial arch (Fig. 67–9) may present in the preauricular area, in the postauricular sulcus, in the upper neck adjacent to the angle of the mandible and overlying or underlying the tail (posterior aspect) of the parotid gland, or in the stylomastoid recess. Another mass presenting as a posterior parotid lesion is the

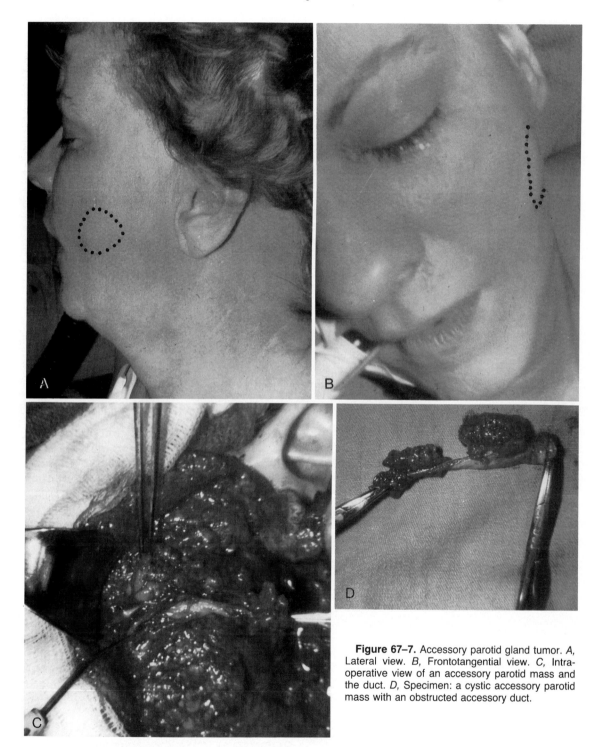

Figure 67–7. Accessory parotid gland tumor. *A,* Lateral view. *B,* Frontotangential view. *C,* Intraoperative view of an accessory parotid mass and the duct. *D,* Specimen: a cystic accessory parotid mass with an obstructed accessory duct.

neurilemoma (Fig. 67–10) (Polayes and Robson, 1978). In addition, Warthin's tumor may present in the tail of the parotid gland or it can be palpated as a firm cystic mass involving the lower portion of the superficial parotid segment. Warthin's tumor can be diagnosed

from a technetium scan in many (78 per cent) but not all cases (Grove and DiChiro, 1968; Gates, 1972; Garcia, 1974).

Hemangiomas, lymphangiomas, lipomas, and masseteric hypertrophy may present as solid or cystic parotid masses, arousing sus-

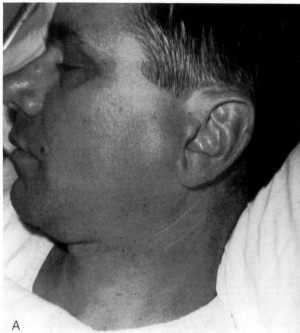
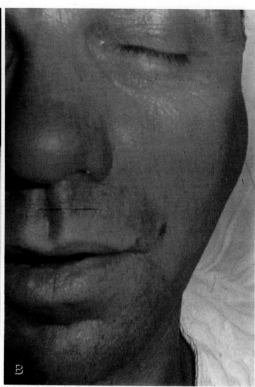

Figure 67–8. Metastatic small cell carcinoma from the lung to the left parotid lymphatics. *A,* Lateral view. *B,* Frontal view.

picion that they are tumors of either benign or malignant potential. CT scanning with intravenous contrast enhancement can differentiate and delineate the hemangioma, and often outlines the presence of a lymphangioma in a diagnostic pattern.

Metastatic lesions can also appear in the lymph nodes involving the intraglandular as well as the paraglandular portions of the parotid, and thus appear as parotid tumors. Metastatic melanoma and squamous cell cancer, especially from the external ear, the scalp, or the eyelids, may involve the paraglandular or "extracapsular" nodes of the parotid, and thus appear as nodular masses. One can often detect the primary lesions as well as evidence of simultaneous metastatic node involvement in the upper neck. In the absence of such nodal involvement, open biopsy of the node or total parotidectomy including the nodes may be indicated. However, one must search the head and neck area integument, the lungs, and the genitourinary and gastrointestinal systems carefully for any primary lesion before progressing to a parotidectomy.

The one fact that should be obvious at this point is that it is difficult to determine whether a lesion is benign or malignant, and the longer one deals with lesions involving the salivary glands, the more obvious it becomes that benign and malignant solid or cystic lesions do not present any differentiating warning symptoms in their early stages of formation. Indeed, in most cases the symptomatology is usually lacking until late in the disease. One symptom complex that can occur and should alert one to the possibility of a malignant lesion is the appearance of weakness in a single branch of the facial nerve. Paresis or paralysis of the 12th nerve should also arouse the suspicion of a malignant lesion involving the hypoglossal nerve at the tongue level or within the submandibular triangle. Therefore, lesions of the sublingual gland or submandibular gland, if accompanied by ipsilateral hypoglossal nerve weakness or paralysis, should be highly suspect of being malignant.

SURGICAL TREATMENT OF SALIVARY GLAND TUMORS

The overall incidence of tumors of the salivary glands is one to three per 100,000 of the population (Eneroth, 1971) in all regions of the world. Tumors of the salivary glands

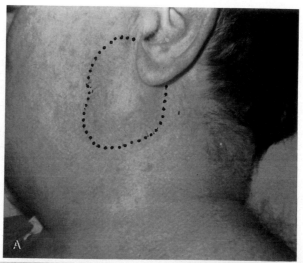

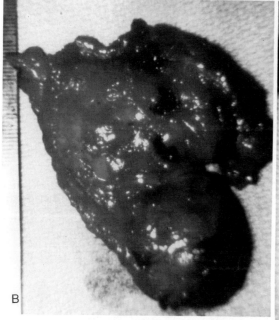

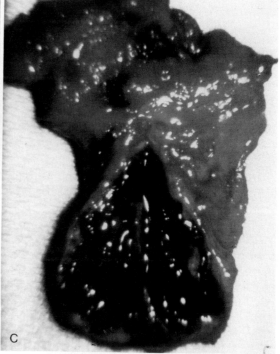

Figure 67–9. Branchial cleft cyst. *A,* Cystic mass overlying the tail and retromandibular parotid. *B,* Branchial cleft cyst specimen. *C,* Open cyst with contents.

account for only 3 per cent of all malignant and benign tumors involving the total body. Tumors of the parotid gland are found more often in nonwhites, with a slightly higher incidence in the female than in the male nonwhite patient; otherwise, the sex distribution of parotid tumors shows no significant difference between male and female. Approximately 85 per cent of parotid tumors are benign, 45 per cent of submandibular gland tumors are benign, and between 10 and 15 per cent of sublingual gland tumors are be-

nign (Thackray, 1968). The incidence of salivary gland tumors is recorded as 85 per cent in the parotid gland, 10 per cent in the submandibular gland, and 1 per cent in the sublingual gland. However, the incidence of malignancy is stated to be 10 to 15 per cent of all parotid tumors, 55 per cent of submandibular gland tumors, and approximately 80 to 85 per cent of sublingual gland tumors. The incidence of malignancy is approximately 60 per cent of all tumors arising from the minor salivary glands of the cheek, lips, and

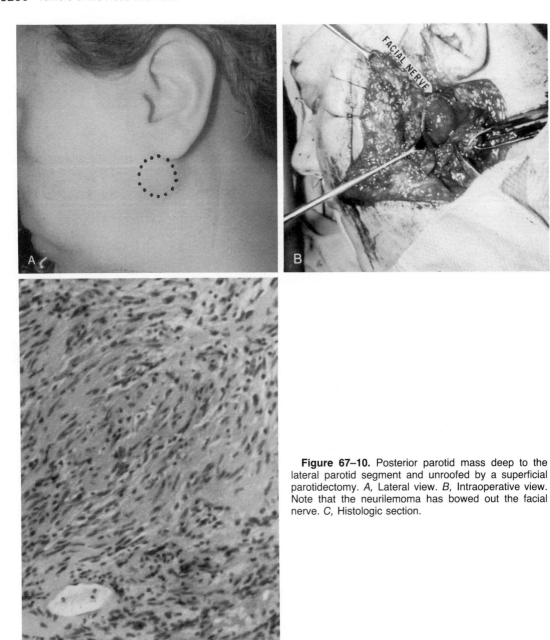

Figure 67–10. Posterior parotid mass deep to the lateral parotid segment and unroofed by a superficial parotidectomy. *A,* Lateral view. *B,* Intraoperative view. Note that the neurilemoma has bowed out the facial nerve. *C,* Histologic section.

buccal surfaces. From the above information, it is apparent that as one progresses from the parotid to the submandibular, sublingual, and minor salivary gland elements, there is an increasing incidence of malignancy. Most tumors in the parotid gland are benign, although the incidence of tumors in the parotid gland is ten times higher than in the sub-mandibular gland and 100 times higher than in the sublingual gland (Thackray, 1968).

For many years the presence of the facial nerve between the superficial and deep segments of the parotid gland and within the parenchymal parotid portions served as a deterrent to adequate parotid gland surgery for extirpation of tumors. McFarland (1943) noted the high incidence of local surgical recurrence due to *multicentric tumor origin* and, since surgical treatment would not improve the prognosis for malignant tumors in the parotid gland, advocated radiation therapy. After McFarland's declaration, work by Bailey (1941), Brown, McDowell, and Fryer (1950), and Martin (1952) provided technical improvements for adequately extirpating lesions of the parotid gland and at the same time preserving the facial nerve. The results of such surgery demonstrated that the higher rate of recurrences in the past was due mainly to inadequate wedge excisions and enucleations that left tumor behind or implanted tumor cells within the remaining tissues. The concept of total resection of the gland or gland segment containing the tumor mass without violating the pathologic entity of the mass enabled the surgeon to base the surgical or follow-up plan directly on the pathologic diagnosis of the lesion and its adequacy of removal.

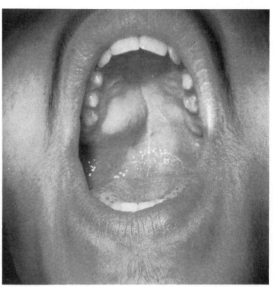

Figure 67–11. Low grade mucoepidermoid cancer of the minor salivary glands of the palate.

In the smaller salivary glands such as the submandibular and sublingual, adequate excision was recognized early as being a total gland removal rather than a segmental removal of the tumor itself. Mixed tumors of the submandibular gland were best removed by total resection of the gland without violating the tumor capsule.

Biopsy Specimen. Most *parotid tumors* (80 per cent) occur in the more abundant superficial portion of the parotid gland lying lateral to the facial nerve. A biopsy specimen should be obtained by removing the *entire superficial parotid segment,* which allows for preservation of the facial nerve (Rankow and Polayes, 1976a,b).

Tumors involving the *submandibular* and *sublingual glands* should be removed as a specimen composed of the *entire gland containing the area of pathology* that is not violated. A higher percentage of solid tumors are malignant in the submandibular gland (55 per cent) and in the sublingual gland (85 per cent), most of these tumors are either mucoepidermoid or adenoid cystic carcinomas.

The *minor salivary glands* may be involved by tumors, approximately 55 to 60 per cent of these being malignant. The lesions involving the minor salivary glands appear as firm masses beneath the mucous membrane, producing a raised mass covered by the oral or pharyngeal mucosa. They are found in the hard and soft palate (Fig. 67–11), lips, buccal

mucosa, base of the tongue, supraglottic glands, and paranasal sinuses. Often it is impossible because of their distribution and (at times) hidden location to obtain an adequate excisional biopsy unless the lesion is small and the mass is accessible. It is therefore advisable to obtain an incisional biopsy and wait for the definitive pathologic diagnosis on permanent section. After this has been obtained, the histopathology will dictate the appropriate surgical therapy. As a general rule, wide radical local resection of the submucosal gland involvement including underlying bone is essential to avoid a high incidence of local recurrence. Most of these malignancies appear to be adenoid cystic carcinomas, and postoperative radiation is an acceptable part of the treatment plan, especially if one is dealing with a recurrent tumor. The primary excision of minor salivary gland lesions, especially an adenoid cystic carcinoma, may often include a radical neck dissection if regional lymph nodes are clinically involved. However, it is noteworthy that metastases of adenocystic carcinoma are as likely to be found in distant sites as in the regional lymph nodes.

Needle Aspiration Biopsy. The use of fine needle biopsy technique for lesions involving the salivary glands is a controversial subject. The main objection to this technique is that one has to withdraw enough material precisely from the lesion to provide the pathologist with sufficient material from which to make a diagnosis. Additionally, the diagnostic accuracy is directly related to the experience of the pathologist. The tumor may be missed and peripheral tissue obtained for biopsy that could provide a misleading diagnosis. It is also thought by many that penetration of tumor and withdrawal of the needle may provide a tract of tumor cells that can seed and provide recurrence or spread of the lesion. It is the author's opinion that biopsy techniques should all be through an open approach and should be incisional or excisional in order to provide an adequate specimen for diagnosis. The goal in surgery of the salivary gland mass is to remove the entire tumor with an adequate margin of normal tissue. Therefore, a biopsy specimen should be performed as an open biopsy and should represent the entire mass within the superficial segment of the parotid gland, or indeed even the entire parotid, submandibular, or sublingual gland, if so indicated.

Inflammatory Masses

The term "salivary gland mass" conveys the impression of a possible malignant lesion. However, there are masses of inflammatory origin that must be differentiated from masses resulting from benign or malignant neoplasia. Any obstructive phenomenon that prevents the normal passage of salivary gland secretions can induce formation of a mass, which often is cystic or fibrotic and usually results from obstruction of the main duct by a calculus or by a mucous plug (Fig. 67–12). Palpation often defines the cystic nature of an obstructed gland, but the chronicity of such obstruction may be misleading in that a cyst within the gland parenchyma can become quite firm owing to persistent surrounding chronic inflammatory reaction. This finding can provide a confusing differential diagnosis between a mixed tumor, Warthin's tumor, and an obstructed salivary gland cyst. However, the obstructed salivary gland cyst is most often accompanied by pain as the degree of obstruction increases. Increasing size of the salivary gland in itself can produce pain; however, tenderness and pain and their recurrent nature relating to food ingestion should lead one to suspect an inflammatory basis.

A history of recurrent pain, swelling, and infection may or may not be associated with calculi in the main salivary gland duct of either the submandibular, sublingual, or parotid glands. Chronically recurrent parotitis usually indicates some form of obstruction, which might be associated with an enlarging tumor mass but is more often associated with obstructing calculi. Sialography is of some aid toward the diagnosis, although most calculi are visible on plain radiographs.

In the case of sialadenitis, conservative treatment with antibiotics, maintaining the patient on a bland diet, and improving oral hygiene with attentive mouth care and saline rinses, often provide relief and resolution of the inflammatory process.

When obstruction is due to an enlarging or infiltrating tumor mass, symptoms will recur or may not respond to conservative measures in any case. In these patients, superficial parotidectomy to remove the entire mass as the biopsy specimen would be diagnostic. If the lesion is a chronic inflammatory mass or benign tumor, the patient will be cured. If it is a low grade malignant mass, cure is possible. However, a wider resection by total parotidectomy and, if nodes are palpable in the neck, a combined radical neck procedure would be the indicated treatment of choice.

Chronic recurrent inflammatory processes producing indurated masses in the submandibular and sublingual glands are best cured by total resection of the sublingual or the submandibular gland, or both glands, as the case may be.

Ascending Duct Infection. In debilitated and dehydrated patients, especially the elderly, who are often in electrolyte imbalance and have poor oral hygiene, there is an increased incidence of acute suppurative parotitis or submaxillary gland infection. Careful examination of the oral cavity and palpation of the salivary glands may reveal other masses, which may be metastatic or represent a primary infiltrating and expanding malignant lesion. The need for culture diagnosis of secretions from the salivary gland duct is important in determining appropriate antibiotic therapy. Progression of the disease with increasing pain and swelling over a period of 48 hours is an indication for prompt incision and drainage to release the pressure from the fascial envelope surrounding the salivary gland and relieve the pain. At the same time, correction of the electrolyte and fluid balance is important.

The parotid gland is frequently involved with *acute purulent processes*. When it is necessary to drain a parotid abscess, the

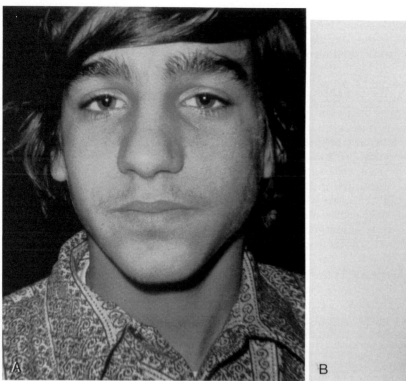

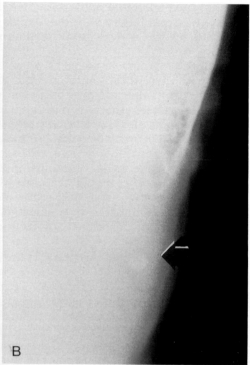

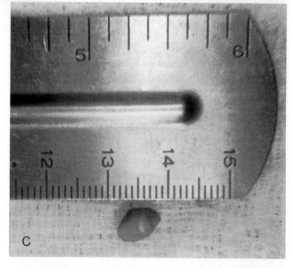

Figure 67–12. Obstructive left parotitis with cyst formation due to a calculus in the proximal portion of Stensen's duct. *A,* Frontal view. *B,* Calculus visible *(arrow)* in a posteroanterior radiograph. *C,* Specimen: calculus from Stensen's duct.

gland is approached through an anterior preauricular skin flap, as one would for a superficial parotidectomy, by elevating the skin flap and incising through the overlying fascial or capsular layer *parallel to the branches of the facial nerve.* By spreading the underlying parenchymal substance parallel to the facial nerve branches, the abscess can be adequately drained. A biopsy of any suspected mass can be performed at the same time.

Usually the acute suppurative parotitis occurs bilaterally, but it may occur in a single gland, thereby adding confusion to the diagnosis of an enlarging firm mass within the gland. However, the presence of purulent material in the duct confirms the diagnosis, although one must not ignore the possibility that a coexisting tumor mass may also be present. Close follow-up is, of course, indicated over a period of several months to make certain that there are no other masses present within the gland. Final cure of the "tumor mass" is often accomplished by superficial parotidectomy to remove the entire chronically involved portion of the parotid gland, or by total submandibular and sublingual gland resection when either of those glands are involved by the same chronic suppurative process.

Epidemic parotitis (mumps) is often associated with involvement of the parotid gland bilaterally, but may involve other salivary glands as well as the pancreas and liver. Mumps, however, may involve only one gland in unilateral epidemic parotitis. Adults can present with unilateral mumps without involvement of other salivary glands or other organs (Fig. 67–13). In the evaluation of a mass in the parotid gland, part of the differential diagnosis must include questions of exposure to the infectious diseases in children as well as in adults.

Solitary or clustered *calculi* within the duct of the parenchymal portions of the salivary glands can produce a localized purulent inflammatory process (Fig. 67–14). This lesion can present as a solitary mass in the parotid gland and be interpreted as a *cystic tumor mass* or possible malignancy. The surrounding fascial layers are involved with chronic inflammatory fibrosis and may cause fibrotic adherence of the mass to the skin as well as to the underlying structures (Fig. 67–15).

Approximately 80 per cent of salivary calculi occur in the submandibular gland (Blatt, 1964) and a smaller percentage in the parotid and sublingual glands. One may also find small dense calculi that appear as particles in minor salivary glands and are palpable directly beneath the mucosa.

Calculi are best palpated bimanually when they occur in the submandibular gland or duct as well as in the sublingual gland. In the parotid gland, Stensen's duct may be totally obstructed by a calcareous mass at the opening of the duct into the oral cavity. The calculus, of course, is easily palpated bimanually and can often be detected by a plain radiograph.

If the duct is accessible, as in the floor of the mouth, the calculi can be located by a cannula placed within the duct, and a simple incision through the mucosa and partially through the duct facilitates removal in most cases. This maneuver can also be employed for stones appearing in the distal aspect of Stensen's duct. By placing a cannula or probe in the parotid duct, the obstructing mass is located, and by temporarily ligating the duct proximal to the mass one can make an incision through mucosa and into the duct to remove the stone. The duct can then be either marsupialized through the mucosa or repaired over a stent. This type of repair is also possible in the submandibular duct. The stent (usually a No. 6 or small diameter Silastic tube) remains in situ for eight to ten days.

Recurrent calculi in the submandibular gland are an indication for total removal of that gland. The same principle applies to calculi found in the sublingual gland, in which case total excision of that gland is curative, since recurrent calcareous obstruction is usually the case (Polayes and Rankow, 1976).

Benign and Malignant Neoplasms—Surgical Considerations

In planning a surgical approach to the treatment of salivary gland masses, it is important to relate the clinical pathologic findings and histologic characteristics of the tumor at the time of surgery. To do so demands a frozen section of the tumor specimen, in which case the segmental parotid resection, including its tumor mass, is submitted to the pathologist for a frozen section diagnosis and for evaluation of the adequacy of the surgical margins. By India inking the margins of the specimen, one can then determine the adequacy of the margins at selected sites. It

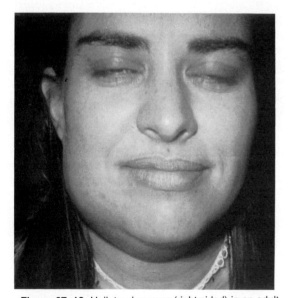

Figure 67–13. Unilateral mumps (right-sided) in an adult (epidemic parotitis).

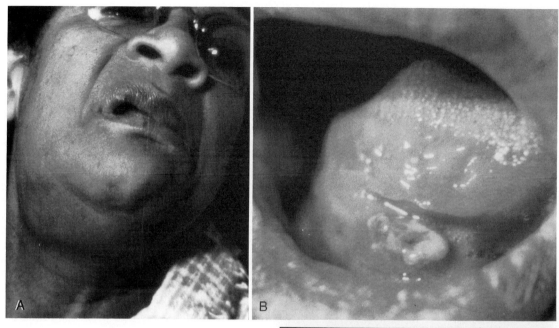

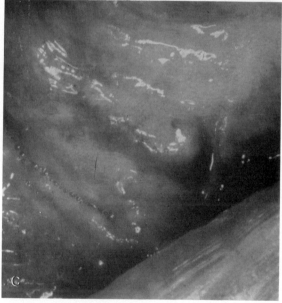

Figure 67–14. *A,* Obstruction of the right submandibular gland and duct. *B,* Purulence from the duct (intraoral view). *C,* Calculus at the opening to the submandibular duct after the cellulitis was controlled.

remains for the multiple permanent sections to determine the adequacy of resection several days later. However, the initial frozen section report is important to the surgeon for determining the extent of surgical treatment. If diagnosis by frozen section is difficult, it is best to defer extensive radical surgery until there is histologic support for that decision through study of the permanent sections. From the foregoing, it is a fundamental maxim that an adequate excisional biopsy involves the *total* removal of the tumor in its

glandular segment with adequate safe margins.

In summary, when treating tumors of the parotid gland, the lateral segment that harbors most of the tumors occurring in that gland must first be totally resected as the biopsy specimen, i.e., a lateral segment parotidectomy must be performed. Second, if the lesion lies in the retromandibular portion of the parotid gland, one must be certain that the deep segment is not involved. Therefore, the specimen should be the entire parotid

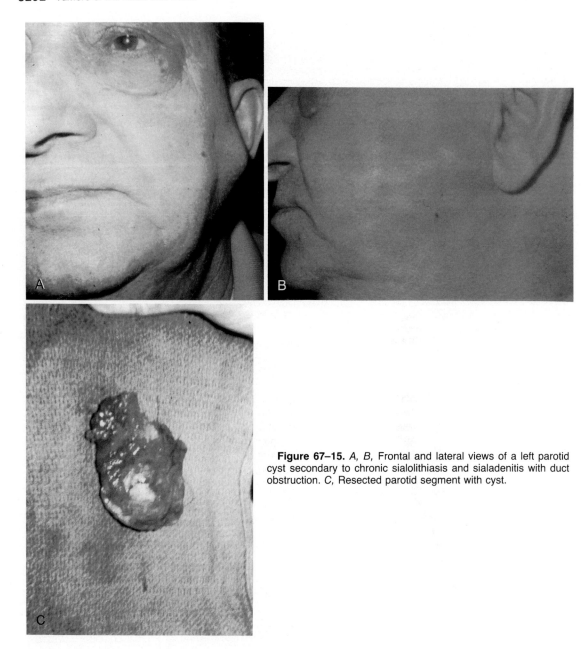

Figure 67–15. *A, B,* Frontal and lateral views of a left parotid cyst secondary to chronic sialolithiasis and sialadenitis with duct obstruction. *C,* Resected parotid segment with cyst.

gland, including the lateral, retromandibular, and deep parotid segment medial to the facial nerve with *preservation* of the facial nerve, unless tumor has directly invaded into the nerve.

The position of the facial nerve and the distribution of its main trunk into its two major divisions and the five peripheral (superficial) branches serves as a plane separating the lateral from the deep segment of the parotid gland. The preservation of the facial nerve is best accomplished by direct identification of the main facial nerve trunk as it

exits through the stylomastoid foramen. Although there are techniques in which the nerve is traced from a retrograde approach, i.e., identification of the terminal branches of the facial nerve first anteriorly and then posteriorly toward the trunk, this method of dissection is fraught with danger. It is therefore safer to identify forthwith the facial nerve trunk as it exits through the stylomastoid foramen, and then separate the gland from each of the nerve branches as one dissects from the larger proximal to the distal smaller peripheral nerve branches, always keeping the facial nerve in direct view and maintaining a plane of dissection in the often thin fibrofatty layer between nerve and glandular tissue.

If it is not possible to identify or to dissect the trunk of the facial nerve (and this is rarely if ever the case), one may identify the posterior facial vein located inferior to the posterior surface of the gland and follow it superiorly until the cervicofacial division of the nerve trunk crosses above the vein. Another alternative method is to trace the position of the parotid duct and dissect the buccal branch of the facial nerve distally. Dissection of the buccal facial nerve branch proximally toward the retromandibular portion of the gland leads to the junction of the buccal branch and the trunk of the facial nerve at or near the division of the trunk into its cervicomandibular and temporofrontal-zygomatic branches. As stated previously, these alternative methods are not as safe or precise as identifying the trunk first and dissecting from a proximal to a distal direction.

The anatomic landmarks used to identify the trunk of the facial nerve and its point of exit from the stylomastoid foramen include (1) the second cervical vertebra lying beneath the posterior belly of the digastric muscle, (2) the tip of the mastoid process, (3) the tympanomastoid fissure, and (4) the styloid process, all of which encircle the stylomastoid foramen. Within this circle lies the (5) "tragal pointer" to the nerve itself in the form of a triangular cartilaginous process at the deepest edge of the cartilaginous external auditory canal, with its point directed medially and downward exactly at the facial nerve as

it exits the stylomastoid foramen (Fig. 67–16). By following this pointer, one comes upon the main trunk by noting a surrounding area of fat, approximately 1 cm deep to the "tragal pointer." By careful dissection with a moist cotton pledget, the surgeon will encounter the neurovenous plane superficial to the facial nerve trunk, and this can easily be separated from the nerve itself. After the trunk is identified, it remains the task of the surgeon to remove the overlying parenchymal tissue from the nerve, branch by nerve branch from the proximal position proceeding distally. In this manner, the entire lateral segment of the parotid gland can be removed.

If a tumor is encountered in the deep segment or involves the retromandibular segment, one must first perform a superficial parotidectomy before removing the deep segment. If the tumor is in continuity with the deep segment and after the superficial parotidectomy is completed, the parenchymal tissue must not be separated until the nerve trunk is carefully dissected free of and elevated from the deep segment. By moving the mandible into a protrusive position while at the same time applying intraoral pressure with a finger against the lateral pharyngeal wall, the surgeon can elevate the deep segment from behind the ramus of the mandible and out of its deep fossa. Only occasionally is it necessary to dislocate the mandible from the temporomandibular joint, or in some instances to incise the stylomandibular ligament to aid in gaining access to the deep segment. The skin incisions are illustrated in Figure 67–17.

The surgical approach to the submandibu-

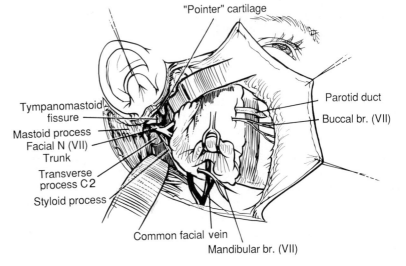

Figure 67–16. Anatomic landmarks for identification of the facial nerve trunk at the stylomastoid foramen.

"Pointer" cartilage

Tympanomastoid fissure
Mastoid process
Facial N (VII) Trunk
Transverse process C2
Styloid process

Parotid duct
Buccal br. (VII)

Common facial vein
Mandibular br. (VII)

lar gland is through a "digastric" incision following the upper cervical skin crease (Fig. 67–17). The depth or concavity of this incision is at the hyoid bone and it curves posteriorly, following the posterior belly of the digastric muscle and anteriorly following the anterior belly of the digastric muscle. The excised total gland is the *specimen* for any tumor mass lying within the submandibular gland parenchyma or involving the parenchymal duct area above the mylohyoid muscle. Incisional biopsies are dangerous in that a much higher percentage of solid submandibular gland masses are malignant, i.e., approximately 60 per cent.

The *sublingual gland* presents with the highest incidence of malignant solid tumor masses. The lesions are mostly mucoepidermoid and adenoid cystic carcinomas and account for an 85 per cent incidence of malignancy in the solid tumors occurring in that gland. The recommended biopsy specimen for a solid mass of the sublingual gland is complete removal of the entire gland. Sublingual glands may be removed through an intraoral approach. At times this is difficult when the mandibular dental arch is narrow and often is met with injury to the sublingual branch of the lingual artery. When one considers that the sublingual gland lies directly beneath the mucosa and against the lingual plate of the mandible (see Fig. 67–5*B*), the difficulty of achieving an adequate resection of a malignant lesion requiring an incontinuity wide resection along with a radical neck dissection poses an obvious problem of surgical access. To rely on an intraoral approach alone would provide a basis for limiting the adequacy of surgery. It is best to utilize the intraoral approach for obtaining the biopsy specimen (total sublingual gland including tumor mass) and, after permanent sections have been studied, return the patient to the operating room for a definitive surgical resection, if indicated.

Before pathologic sections of a tumor in the *sublingual gland* are obtained, a malignant lesion is a presumptive diagnosis. It is advisable to approach the gland through a submandibular or upper neck digastric incision (Fig. 67–17). The tumor in the sublingual gland probably involves the terminal end of the submandibular duct, or Wharton's duct; therefore, resection of the submandibular gland would be indicated. For this reason, an upper neck incision along the cervical crease should be the surgical approach for excision

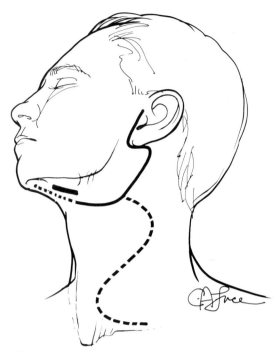

Figure 67–17. Various skin incisions for parotidectomy and resection of the submandibular gland.

of the submandibular gland, the duct, the involved portion of the mylohyoid muscle, and the mucosa overlying the sublingual gland as well as the nodes in the upper cervical area, including the upper jugular nodes (en bloc specimen). If the nodes show no evidence of microscopic metastasis, the procedure is terminated. If, however, there is evidence of microscopic metastasis, a full neck dissection should be completed.

The adenoid cystic and mucoepidermoid carcinomas represent highly likely diagnoses of the infrequent solid tumor within the sublingual gland. Thus, the cautious approach of including an upper neck dissection with removal of both sublingual and submandibular glands in continuity with any tissue that appears attached to the tumor is the preferred treatment for these malignant lesions. In any case, the cervicomandibular branches of the facial nerve should be preserved, as should the lingual and hypoglossal nerves unless they are directly invaded by the tumor. Nerve grafts obtained from the great auricular nerve may be used to replace segments of facial nerve that must be sacrificed.

Solid tumors of the sublingual gland are infrequent, even though their incidence of malignancy is the *highest of all the salivary glands*. In contrast with the parotid and submandibular glands, the highest percentage of adenoid cystic and mucoepidermoid cancers are found in the solid tumors of the sublingual glands, and there is a high incidence of local recurrence after nonsurgical therapy (Rankow and Mignogna, 1969). However, after sublingual gland excision was advocated not only to remove en bloc the gland and its surrounding suspected tissues but also to clear the entire upper neck of the adjacent submandibular gland, as well as the glandular nodes in the surgical field, the subparotid or common facial vein lymph nodes, and the submental and the upper jugular nodes, a better chance for cure is provided. Certainly, if the nodes are positive for metastatic disease, i.e., mucoepidermoid cancer, a complete neck dissection is indicated. In the low grade mucoepidermoid carcinomas, metastasis more often is *not* the case, and only the nodes adjacent to the submandibular gland and in the digastric triangle should be included with the resection.

BENIGN NEOPLASMS

The benign neoplasms occurring in the parotid, submandibular, and sublingual major salivary glands, as well as in the minor salivary glands, require adequate but not radical resection. In all these cases, the lesion requires either a segmental parotidectomy, a total submandibular gland resection, or a total sublingual gland resection. If the minor salivary glands are involved, a local resection of the minor salivary glands in the involved area is indicated. All the specimens must have adequate margins, and all resections should be performed with preservation of the facial nerve branches and/or the hypoglossal and lingual nerves.

Benign neoplasms of the salivary gland include:
1. Pleomorphic adenoma (benign mixed tumor).
2. Warthin's tumor (papillary adenocystoma lymphomatosum).
3. Oncocytoma.
4. Monomorphic adenomas (variant of mixed tumor):
   a. Basal cell adenoma.
   b. Sebaceous cell lesions.
   c. Sialadenoma papilliferum (papillary ductal adenoma).
5. Hemangioma.
6. Lymphangioma.
7. Lipoma.

8. Myxoma.
9. Neurilemoma.
10. Neurofibroma.

Since most benign salivary gland tumors occur in the parotid gland and 80 per cent of such tumors arise in the lateral parotid segment, particularly the tail of the parotid, it is prudent to suspect that any mass arising at the angle of the mandible and below the ear lobule is a benign parotid tumor (see Fig. 67–6).

The treatment of benign lesions in any of the major salivary glands is an adequate excision for cure. In the *parotid,* a lateral segmental parotidectomy is curative for most of the benign lesions, and for those lesions involving the retromandibular or deep segment of the parotid, total parotidectomy would be curative, with *preservation* of the facial nerve. In the *submandibular gland,* the treatment for any of the benign lesions would be total excision of the submandibular gland with its tumor mass, and preservation of the lingual and hypoglossal nerves and the ramus mandibularis of the facial nerve. For benign salivary gland tumors occurring in the *sublingual gland,* resection of the entire gland is curative, but in some cases inclusion of the submandibular duct and submandibular gland is also indicated. Since the sublingual gland often empties into the submandibular duct, and since the benign lesion is most commonly a mixed tumor or pleomorphic adenoma, recurrence is a possibility, unless an adequate resection of all contiguous tissue is completed by sacrifice of both sublingual and submandibular glands, including the submandibular duct. When small benign tumors involve the sublingual gland and are well contained within that gland, the submandibular gland may be spared as well as its major Wharton's duct.

It is important to be well acquainted with the pertinent statistics involving the location and incidence of salivary gland tumors. Eighty to 85 per cent of all masses in the parotid gland are *benign.* Fifty to 55 per cent of submandibular gland masses, in the author's experience, have been *benign* and only 15 to 20 per cent of sublingual gland solid tumors have been *benign.* As for the minor salivary glands, 45 per cent of the lesions are *benign.* The incidence and occurrence rates in the various glands indicate that 85 per cent of salivary gland tumors occur in the parotid gland, 10 per cent in the submandibular gland, 1 per cent in the sublingual gland,

and approximately 4 to 5 per cent in the minor salivary glands. Eighty-five per cent of all solid tumors occurring in the sublingual gland are *malignant;* 50 per cent of the solid tumors in the submandibular gland are *malignant;* 15 per cent of solid tumors in the parotid gland are *malignant;* and 50 per cent of all solid tumors in the minor salivary glands are *malignant* (Eneroth, 1971).

Studies on the derivation of these tumors indicate that, in benign as well as malignant epithelial tumors, the cells forming the tumor mass arise from the intercalated duct reserve cells and are not differentiated from their mature epithelial counterparts (Eversole, 1971). These findings were corroborated by electron microscopic studies indicating that all salivary gland epithelial neoplasms arise from one of two cells: the reserve cell of the intercalated duct or the reserve cell of the excretory duct in the major salivary glands (Regezi and Batsakis, 1977). It is therefore assumed that neoplasia is a result of changes in the reserve cells that are responsible for salivary duct and glandular tissue renewal, and not a result of changes in the fully differentiated epithelial cell. The development of the reserve cells into either benign or malignant lesions is considered to be predetermined and not due to changes in the normally developed adult cell.

Pleomorphic Adenoma. The *pleomorphic adenoma (benign mixed tumor)* has its origin in two cell types: the myoepithelial cell and the epidermoid cell. Ultrastructural studies indicate that both cells originate from one basic cell, the intercalated duct reserve cell. Other immunohistochemical studies suggest that the cell in a pleomorphic adenoma has two different origins. Therefore, the controversy regarding whether this is a tumor arising from one cell of origin and differentiating into a myoepithelial and an epithelial cell is still unsettled.

This neoplasm is the most common of all salivary gland tumors and accounts for 65 per cent of benign tumors in the parotid gland. Of the benign tumors of the submandibular gland, the pleomorphic adenoma accounts for approximately 50 per cent. In the sublingual gland, very few solid tumors are benign, but 20 per cent of those that are benign are pleomorphic adenomas. In the minor salivary glands, pleomorphic adenoma accounts for 56 per cent of all tumors. The tumors of the minor salivary glands occur in the submucosal glands of the oral cavity,

mostly in the palate, upper lip, and buccal mucosa. On the palate, these lesions are located mainly in the posterior third of the hard palate and on the soft palate. The *basal cell adenoma* is defined as a monomorphic type of tumor, but it nonetheless is a variant of the pleomorphic adenoma.

Treatment of the mixed tumor consists of wide resection, since the lesions are encapsulated by a pseudocapsule. "Lumpectomy" is to be avoided in that the pseudocapsule contains cells of the tumor that, if left behind, recur in a high percentage of cases. Most of the lesions are located in the lateral parotid segment (Fig. 67–18), a finding that indicates that a lateral parotidectomy should be performed to ensure cure. In the less common location involving the deep retromandibular portion of the parotid gland, a total parotidectomy is the preferred treatment.

For mixed tumors in the sublingual and submandibular glands, total gland removal is indicated. If the mass involves only the submandibular gland, the entire submandibular gland and duct should be removed, and the sublingual gland can be spared. The reverse, however, is not true in that tumors in the sublingual gland often involve the duct and may involve portions of the submandibular gland in its intraoral segment above the mylohyoid muscle.

Recurrence of mixed tumors with adequate resection is low and perhaps should be nil. If there is recurrence, it often means that inadequate resection was performed or violation of tumor occurred at the time at which

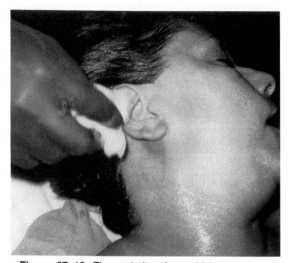

Figure 67–18. The majority of parotid lesions as they appear in the lateral parotid segment with displacement of the ear lobule.

the specimen and its tumor mass were removed. The treatment of all pleomorphic adenomas or mixed tumors is surgical, and wide resection is necessary to provide the greatest chance of cure. If there *is* recurrence, secondary surgical resection is required, but in this situation the surgical procedure is hampered by the scarring resulting from the original resection. Again, the branches of the seventh cranial nerve and the lingual and hypoglossal nerves must be preserved. The recurrent pleomorphic adenoma or mixed tumor is also noted to be less benign and can behave more as a malignant lesion. This is clinically demonstrated when recurrence is noted more than once in the same patient. Each recurrence tends to grow at a more rapid rate and appears to spread with a more desmoplastic and infiltrating quality than the original lesion. Neither radiation nor chemotherapy is an effective method of treatment. The first chance for resection is the best chance.

Warthin's Tumor. The second most common benign tumor involving the parotid gland is *Warthin's tumor,* described as an adenolymphoma by the World Health Organization and the Armed Forces Institute of Pathology. It is thought to originate from salivary gland tissue and ductal tissue entrapped within the lymph node during embryologic formation of the parotid gland. The lesion is more common in the male, occurring in a 5:1 male:female ratio, and it is noted more commonly between the fourth and sixth decades. Cases have been reported in young children as well as in the aged. It occurs bilaterally in 10 per cent of cases and accounts for 8 to 10 per cent of all parotid tumors. There are cases of multifocal occurrence within the same gland, and of Warthin's tumor occurring simultaneously with a mixed tumor as well as with a mucoepidermoid carcinoma in the same parotid gland. The adenolymphomas are well encapsulated and benign; adequate resection is curative. There are few associated findings, except for the increasing size of the mass, which patients variably noted as present for one to five years.

The lesion should be considered an exclusive pathologic entity for the parotid gland or accessory parotid glandular tissue. The tumor is most often found in the lateral parotid segment, and a lateral parotidectomy is the treatment of choice to remove the glandular tissue containing the tumor mass (Fig. 67–19). There are very few reported Warthin's tumors extending from the retromandibular area to the deep segment. Therefore, resection of the retromandibular parotid with the lateral segment including the tumor mass is acceptable treatment. This lesion may occasionally be multicentric or multifocal in the same gland (Chaudhry and Gorlin, 1958).

Resection of an adenolymphoma by segmental parotidectomy is indicated in that there have been documented lymphoma and malignant epithelial changes within a Warthin's tumor mass. The tumor mass, on gross examination, presents as a round or oval encapsulated tumor that on sectioning contains a "pea soup" brown mucoid material (Fig. 67–19*B*). The histopathologic sections demonstrate numerous cystic papillary forms in which a vascular core is covered by a double layer of granular eosinophilic epithelium. The inner epithelial layer consists of small round cells, and the outer epithelial layer is composed of tall columnar cells. The papillary epithelium usually occurs in projections separated by what appears to be lymphoid tissue with germinal centers. On histologic examination it is sometimes difficult to make a definitive pathologic diagnosis between Warthin's tumor and an oncocytoma, although often the differentiation can be made by technetium uptake, which is positive for Warthin's tumor and not specific for the oncocytoma. Although the great majority of the lesions are located in the parotid tissue or in accessory parotid glands, they rarely may be found in extra parotid sites such as the submandibular gland, the submucosal glands of the lips, the larynx, the pharyngeal wall, and the maxillary sinus (Johns, Batsakis, and Short, 1973). Recurrence has been reported to be as high as 12 per cent, although most surgeons report a recurrence rate in the neighborhood of 4 to 6 per cent.

Recurrence of Warthin's tumor, when there has been an adequate resection of the involved parotid gland, suggests that the lesion was multicentric in origin and that adequate resection of the existing tumor was performed, leaving behind a possible multicentric site of origin. One then is faced with the choice of a total parotidectomy or a segmental gland resection. Since the lesion is benign, it is best to perform lateral segment resection including the tumor mass unless the mass is located in the retromandibular portion, in which case a total parotidectomy would not be a wrong decision. The author's preference is to perform an adequate lateral parotidec-

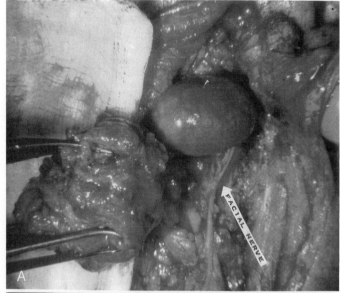

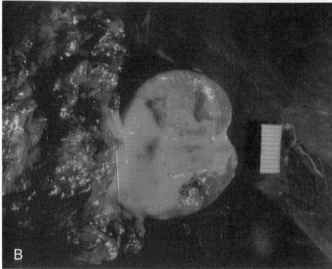

Figure 67–19. *A,* Lateral parotidectomy disclosing an oval-shaped and encapsulated Warthin's tumor. Note the underlying facial nerve. *B,* Gross specimen, sliced to show the "pea soup" contents.

tomy to include normal gland with the tumor. It is again emphasized that 90 per cent of these lesions are cured by segmental resection, and the remaining 10 per cent are either multicentric in origin or represent recurrence due to inadequate surgical resection.

Oncocytoma. The *oncocytoma* is a benign lesion confined principally to the parotid gland. The lesion appears as an encapsulated lobular mass, usually occurring after the fifth decade of life and often at the age of 70. It appears to be a normal finding in aging salivary tissue, particularly in the parotid salivary gland.

The gross lesion is usually a solid mass, but may appear as cystic forms defined as an oncocystic cystadenoma, which mimics the histologic appearance of Warthin's tumor. The origin of this lesion has been defined by electron microscopy, and its particular cellular structure is acquired by a disturbance of mitochondrial enzyme organization. Regardless of the theory of origin, the lesions are probably due to hyperplasia with aging and not to neoplasia. The oncocytoma accounts for less than 1 per cent of all salivary gland tumors. It is usually found in the parotid gland between the sixth and seventh decades of life, and resection of the involved segment is curative in almost all cases. A rare malignant variant of the solid oncocytoma has been described but is difficult to differentiate from the benign lesion on microscopic examination (Johns, Batsakis, and Short, 1973). However, in the malignant oncocytoma the lesion is *solid* and not *cystic*.

Basal Cell Adenoma. *Basal cell adenomas* are usually found in a superficial location of the parotid, usually in the lateral segment (Bernacki, Batsakis, and Johns, 1974). The probable origin of these cells is the intercalated duct reserve cell. The lesions may occur in the minor salivary glands, but one common finding is that all are benign. Most of the lesions are 3 cm or less in diameter, and they are located mainly in the parotid gland and in the submucosal glands of the lip, especially the upper lip. The basal cell adenoma is a solid, round, encapsulated tumor, occurring most often in the sixth decade of life with equal sex distribution. It should be carefully differentiated from the adenoid cystic carcinoma or the nonpleomorphic form of the pleomorphic adenoma.

Surgical treatment involves adequate resection of the involved area. In the case of the parotid, a lateral parotidectomy is indicated, and when the minor salivary glands are involved, a generous resection with an adequate amount of surrounding normal glandular tissue is the treatment of choice. The experienced pathologist differentiates this lesion as benign by its characteristic strands and islands of small round or spindle cells with a radially oriented peripheral cell row, findings similar to those seen in the basal cell epithelioma of the skin. A variant of the basal cell adenoma is seen in the tubular and trabecular varieties, both of which are also benign. The basal cell adenoma is *well encapsulated,* does *not* show any signs of invasion, has *no microcyst* formation, and is benign. Total excision is curative.

Sebaceous Cell Lesions. The *sebaceous cell lesions* described as sebaceous adenoma, sebaceous lymphadenoma, and the very rare sebaceous carcinoma are unusual (Batsakis, Littler, and Leahy, 1972). Ectopic sebaceous glands are commonly seen in the parotid gland in one-third of all adults and at times may be found as a small entity or intermixed with the cellular structures of pleomorphic adenomas, mucoepidermoid carcinomas, and Warthin's tumors. True neoplasms arising from sebaceous cells are very rare. The sebaceous lymphadenoma resembles Warthin's tumor in that sebaceous glands are found in a lymphoid stroma identical in appearance to that of Warthin's tumor. The ductal tissue is surrounded by lymphoid tissue and the ducts may be branching. The latter are partially lined by both squamous and sebaceous types of epithelium. The existence of a pure sebaceous carcinoma in the salivary gland is open to question and is so rare that this entity has not been seriously included. A suspected sebaceous tumor in salivary glands or suspected carcinoma of sebaceous origin stained with *lipid stains* should be *positive* and *PAS stain after diastase* should be *negative,* in order to qualify the lesions as being a carcinoma of sebaceous origin. Total resection of the lesion is curative whether it is located in the minor salivary glands or in the parotid.

Clear Cell Adenoma. Another type of monomorphic adenoma is the rare, glycogen-rich *clear cell adenoma* (Goldman and Klein, 1942). This lesion is characterized by histologic demonstration of ductal spaces lined with cuboidal cells and surrounded by larger polygonal clear cells resting on a basement membrane, which delineates small groups of such cells. Mucin and lipid stains are negative and the clear cells contain a diastase labile glycogen. The clear cells are accompanied by ductal structures, and this tumor must be differentiated from other clear cell–containing tumors such as the mucoepidermoid carcinoma, the acinic cell tumor, and the metastatic clear cell carcinoma of renal origin. The differentiation lies in the fact that mucus production and epidermoid features are not part of the clear cell adenoma, while the acinic cell tumor lacks ducts.

Sialadenoma Papilliferum. The *sialadenoma papilliferum* (McCoy and Eckert, 1980) is another rare tumor showing a predilection for the parotid gland and the palate. The parotid lesion appears as a pale circumscribed mass, while the lesion on the palate appears to be exophytic and occasionally is accompanied by painful symptoms. The lesion on section reveals papillary folds of epithelium with dilated tortuous ducts. The epithelial cells are often mucous but also may be of the squamous variety. Excision with an adequate margin is usually curative.

Hemangioma. Fifty per cent of all parotid tumors in children are hemangiomas (Fig. 67–20) (Williams, 1975; Touloukian, 1976). They are often present at birth or appear within the first two months of life. The lesion is described as a capillary, cavernous, or mixed hemangioma; the capillary is a neoplastic type of vascular malformation while the cavernous is either a reaction to trauma

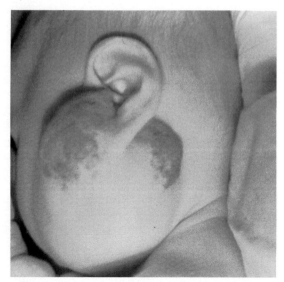

Figure 67–20. Mixed capillary and cavernous hemangioma involving the left parotid gland with compression-obstruction of the external auditory canal.

or due to vascular malformation (see also Chap. 66). The capillary type of hemangioma is more common and a large percentage of these undergo spontaneous resolution. The capillary hemangioma and mixed hemangioma undergo rapid growth during the first six months of life to become quite firm, and can obstruct the external auditory canal. The hemangioma infiltrates the involved salivary gland and most often appears in the parotid, although it may less frequently involve the submandibular gland and minor salivary glands. The lesion is unencapsulated, and there is evidence of endothelial proliferation along the dilated vessels and sinusoids lined by endothelium. Because a large number of capillary hemangiomas involute within the first five years of life, it behooves one to wait until the hemangioma has reached its maximal growth, i.e., until the patient is 5 years of age, before proceeding with surgical treatment.

When treating hemangiomas involving salivary glands, one is dealing mainly with lesions involving the parotid glands of children. Conservative treatment is therefore recommended: the growth potential of the lesion should be observed before any surgery is contemplated. When there is hemorrhage within the lesion due to trauma or spontaneous onset, there may be pain as well as occlusion of the adjacent external auditory canal requiring surgical intervention. Historically the facial nerve trunk has been the

main deterrent to parotid surgery in the adult. Because of the subcutaneous location of this nerve in a child there is even greater risk of facial nerve injury in parotid surgery. If it is possible to wait until the mastoid process is pneumatized and developed at 6 years of age, parotid surgery is safer, but still dangerous, since growth has not allowed for the facial nerve to be fully protected in depth as in the adult. Therefore, surgery before age 5 years is contraindicated unless it is made absolutely necessary by uncontrollable bleeding, trauma, or excessive tumor growth producing compression of vital structures such as the external auditory canal. Radiation is of no value in the treatment of salivary gland hemangiomas, but involution of the hemangioma may be helped in early childhood by steroid therapy (Fost and Esterly, 1968).

Lymphangioma. Lymphangiomas (Harkins and Sabiston, 1960; Touloukian, 1976) are malformations and not true neoplasms that appear as endothelium-lined spaces having a connective tissue stroma and forming multiloculated lesions containing fluid. Fifty per cent of all lymphangiomas occur in the neck, but they only rarely involve or are confined to the salivary gland. A low percentage of lymphangiomas involute compared with capillary hemangiomas. Lymphangiomas may appear at birth but more often are noted within the first to second year of life. They may be unilocular or multilocular and encapsulated. Those that are localized and encapsulated offer the best chance for a cure, whereas the multiloculated and diffuse varieties often require multiple surgical procedures. As for hemangiomas, one should not interfere surgically until it is absolutely necessary, as when there are symptoms indicating compression of vital structures, or severe cosmetic distortion. One should again wait until the facial nerve is well protected by the mastoid process.

Lipoma. Lipomas (Walts and Perzik, 1976) are uncommon tumors involving salivary glands. They account for 4 per cent of parotid tumors (Fig. 67–21) and less than 1 per cent of submandibular gland tumors (Fig. 67–22). They are more often found in the male and usually are recognized in the fourth and fifth decades of life as an expanding mass. They present with few, if any, symptoms until they expand, causing compression and obstruction of the involved gland.

Treatment consists of resection of the lipoma, often including the entire submandib-

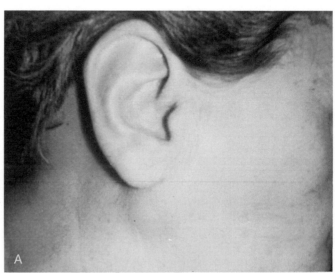

Figure 67–21. *A,* Lipoma in the tail and lateral parotid segment. *B,* Specimen.

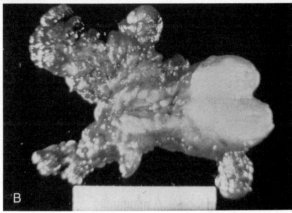

ular or sublingual gland as the case may be. Excision of a parotid lipoma should include the surrounding involved parotid segment, most often the lateral segment of the parotid gland. The lipoma usually involves the lateral parotid segment extending into the parotid tail. Preservation of a portion of the lateral segment is possible if the lipoma can be removed with an adequate cuff of normal parotid tissue. The tumor should not be excised as a "lumpectomy" since the "capsule" of a lipoma in the parotid area is not safely distinct from the parotid tissue, and portions of the lipomatous mass may be left behind.

Myxoma. The benign true myxoma (Stout, 1948) is a rare tumor occurring in the parotid gland; it is slow growing but infiltrative. The lesion is usually asymptomatic until it reaches large size or infiltrates a large portion of the parotid parenchyma. Its presence within the salivary gland produces areas of fibrosis or desmoplastic reaction to the growth and infiltration of its cells. Since the lesion is slow growing and is infiltrative, wide excision is indicated. Most of these rare lesions occur in the lateral segment of the parotid gland, and a lateral or superficial parotidectomy, including the tumor mass with a generous surrounding margin of normal parotid tissue, is curative.

Neurilemoma. Neurilemomas (Polayes and Robson, 1978) are slow-growing solitary tumors that produce few if any symptoms until they compress adjacent structures. The term neurilemoma was introduced by Stout (1935) to describe tumors originating from Schwann cells or schwannomas. The origin of these tumors was confirmed by tissue culture (Murray and Stout, 1940), demonstrating that indeed a neurilemoma derived its origin from the neural sheath of Schwann's cell rather than from the connective tissue fibroblast. The neurilemoma is a round or fusiform encapsulated tumor that may be firm, but

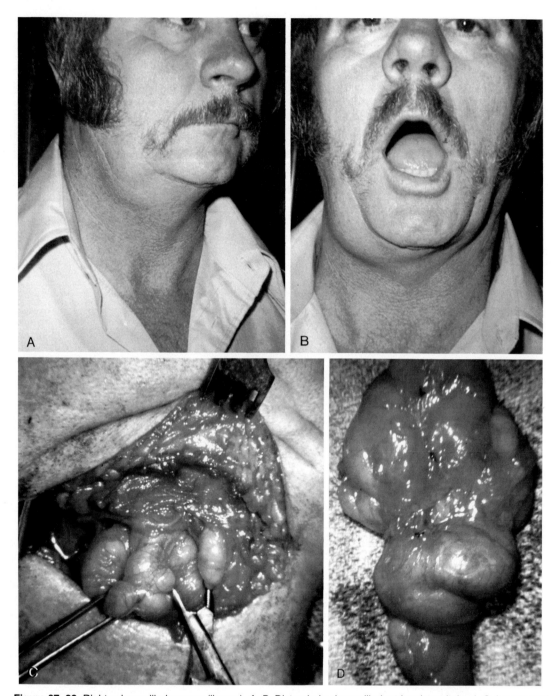

Figure 67–22. Right submandibular mass (lipoma). *A, B,* Distended submandibular triangle and gland. *C,* Intraoperative view of a lipoma compressing the submandibular gland. *D,* The specimen consisting of a lipoma and an obstructed submandibular salivary gland.

may at times indicate cystic formation (see Fig. 67–10). It is usually attached to the involved peripheral or cranial nerve sheath at or near its site of presentation. The tumor mass enlarges at its point of origin and may cause a splaying out of the nerve.

The tumor is benign, and approximately 37 per cent of all neurilemomas occur in the head and neck region. Symptoms, if any, occur late and usually manifest as pain due to compression of the surrounding sensory nerves. When adjacent to major vessels, the mass may produce a bruit in the compressed vessel, namely, in the jugulodigastric area, or displace the pharyngeal wall.

Treatment of these lesions consists of careful total resection of the neurilemoma, using loupe or microscopic magnification to dissect the mass free of the involved peripheral nerve. Neurilemomas have involved cranial nerves in the jugulodigastric area including the ninth, tenth, eleventh, and twelfth nerves and have also involved the intraparotid peripheral branches of the facial nerve (see Fig. 67–10). Careful dissection of this benign lesion is curative unless portions of the neurilemoma are left behind. It is often possible to preserve the involved peripheral nerve, and only rarely is sacrifice of the nerve necessary in order to resect the entire mass. In that case, immediate nerve graft repair is indicated, especially when it involves the facial nerve. Increasing size of the tumor mass, when the facial nerve is involved, is responsible for the appearance of facial nerve weakness; however, with careful dissection, removal of the mass is often followed by return of function. Alternative means of treatment are not effective and radiation is of no value.

The *accessory parotid glands* (Polayes and Rankow, 1979) may be involved with any of the benign masses already described. The one point to remember is that these masses are usually located along the alar-tragus line in the midcheek, directly parallel to the buccal branch of the facial nerve and the parotid duct (see Fig. 67–7). They lie within or on the parotid fascia anterior to the anterior border of the parotid gland, and usually have connections to the parotid duct. Benign lesions involving the accessory parotid gland require that the entire lateral parotid segment along with the involved accessory glands be removed. In the case in which the nonepithelial benign lesions are confined solely to the accessory parotid gland, resection of the accessory parotid gland and its accessory duct alone are adequate for control and cure of the lesion. When dealing with mixed tumors involving the accessory parotid glands, one must perform a total lateral parotid segment resection to ensure that the tumor mass within the accessory parotid gland demonstrates a sufficient cuff of normal parotid tissue without violation of the pseudocapsule of the tumor. In general, it is safer to remove the entire accessory parotid gland along with the lateral parotid segment and ensure preservation of the facial nerve.

The *submandibular* and *sublingual glands* may be involved with the same benign tumors that have already been noted. The pleomorphic adenoma is the most common tumor of the submandibular gland. Ten per cent of all salivary gland neoplasms occur in the submandibular gland, 40 per cent of these being a pleomorphic adenoma. The tumors are usually slow growing, and complete excision demands total removal of the submandibular gland along with its duct.

Benign tumors account for only 20 per cent of the tumors occurring in the sublingual gland. Eighty to 85 per cent of tumors in the sublingual gland are malignant. The benign tumors in the sublingual gland are mainly pleomorphic adenomas requiring complete excision of that gland along with its duct, often including the submandibular gland and duct as part of the specimen. A small pleomorphic adenoma within the sublingual gland can be approached intraorally and totally removed as a curative procedure. However, if there is any question of adequacy of margins, the adjacent submandibular duct and gland should be removed through an external submandibular neck incision.

The minor salivary glands are also involved with many of the same benign lesions already described. The most common location of these benign lesions is in the oral cavity, including the palate, lips, and buccal mucosa. The posterior third of the hard palate and the soft palate account for most of the minor salivary gland benign neoplasms. Fifty-six per cent of all minor salivary gland tumors are pleomorphic adenomas. The treatment of choice is wide local resection and coverage by a skin graft or flap.

The *benign tumors* occurring in the *salivary glands of children* (Touloukian, 1976; Polayes, 1982) include mainly the hemangioma, the lymphangioma, the pleomorphic adenoma, and Warthin's tumor. The most common tumor of the salivary glands in children is the hemangioma (50 per cent of all parotid tumors in children). The most frequent epithelial neoplasm involving the parotid gland in children is the pleomorphic adenoma. Although lymphangiomas as well as lipomas may occur, they are uncommon and treatment is not indicated unless the tumor mass is symptomatic.

After a mass has appeared, suggesting that the parotid or even the more uncommon submandibular glands are involved with a pleomorphic adenoma, resection is indicated. If tumor growth is slow and the patient is carefully monitored, surgery can be delayed until the child has passed age 4 or 5 years. The majority of benign neoplasms may appear between 8 and 10 years of age, although there are reports of lesions occurring in children as young as 3 to 4 years of age. The same surgical requirements that apply in the adult apply to the child. If the pleomorphic adenoma involves the parotid gland, a segmental resection with preservation of the facial nerve is indicated. Since the lesion most often involves the lateral parotid segment, a lateral parotidectomy or superficial segment parotidectomy is performed. If it involves the submandibular gland (rare in children), the lesion demands total excision of the submandibular gland and duct. If the sublingual gland is involved, both sublingual and submandibular glands are removed to ensure cure.

MALIGNANT NEOPLASMS

The malignant lesions involving the salivary glands include mucoepidermoid carcinoma, adenoid cystic carcinoma, malignant pleomorphic adenoma, acinous cell carcinoma, squamous cell carcinoma, adenocarcinoma, undifferentiated carcinoma, malignant oncocytoma, clear cell carcinoma, nonsalivary malignant neoplasms, and metastatic lesions to the salivary glands.

Malignant neoplasms of the salivary glands are less frequently encountered than are the benign lesions (Thackray, 1968; Eneroth, 1971; Richardson and associates, 1975). Approximately 15 per cent of the parotid tumors are malignant, 45 to 50 per cent of submandibular gland tumors, 80 per cent of sublingual gland neoplasms, and 55 per cent of the minor salivary gland tumors. The prognosis is most favorable in malignant lesions of the palate, less favorable for lesions in the parotid, and least favorable for lesions in the submandibular and sublingual glands. In many cases, the lesions are slow growing and present with few, if any, symptoms until late in their development. They most often occur in the fifth to sixth decades of life, although 2 per cent occur in children from 1 to 10 years of age, and approximately 16 per cent in people under 30 years of age. Fifty per cent of intraoral salivary neoplasms occur on the palate, and approximately 86 per cent of salivary gland tumors appear without associated signs or symptoms for many years.

Pain is not a distinguishing characteristic in malignant lesions of the salivary glands, but if a lesion is known to be malignant and is associated with pain, the prognosis is less favorable. Facial nerve paralysis associated with a malignant tumor carries a most grave prognosis. The rate of tumor growth does not truly reflect the degree of malignancy. A low grade mucoepidermoid carcinoma as well as an adenoid cystic carcinoma may show slow growth at the primary site but nonetheless is accompanied by distant metastases, even though the local lesion has been brought under control. The metastatic lesions may often appear several years after the primary lesion has been resected and controlled.

The site of distant metastases from salivary gland tumors is primarily to the lungs and secondarily to bones. It has been reported that women with a documented salivary gland cancer have a significantly increased risk of developing breast cancer; conversely, those with breast cancer have an increased risk of also having a salivary gland cancer. It has also been noted that exposure to low and medium doses of radiation increases the incidence of salivary neoplasia in the parotid gland. The difficulty in relying on a five-year cure rate when dealing with salivary gland cancer is thus obvious in that the growth and spread of the lesion is slow in many cases. The patient can survive in the presence of multiple metastases from salivary gland lesions in the lung as well as the bone for up to 15 to 20 years. This observation has been especially true in the adenoid cystic carcinomas involving the parotid and submandibular glands, and also in low grade mucoepidermoid cancer.

Mucoepidermoid Carcinoma. Mucoepidermoid carcinoma consists of two predominant cell types: mucous cells and epidermoid cells, which apparently arise from the excretory duct reserve cell. This type of carcinoma accounts for approximately 6 per cent of *all* salivary gland tumors and 18 per cent of *all* malignant salivary gland tumors. It is the most common malignant neoplasm of the parotid gland, accounting for 21 per cent of all parotid malignant cancers. Sixty-five per cent of all mucoepidermoid cancers are found in the parotid gland.

All mucoepidermoid carcinomas are currently classified as malignant lesions although they are divided into *low, intermediate,* and *high grade* malignant lesions on the basis of their microscopic appearance. Low grade lesions have predominantly mucous cells and cysts, while high grade lesions demonstrate few mucous cells and cystic spaces but many more squamous cells. The intermediate grade contains a mixture of mucous and squamous cells. Although low grade lesions are considered less malignant, they can behave as aggressive lesions, while high grade lesions may occasionally be slow growing.

The low grade mucoepidermoid carcinomas usually present as firm to hard, gray-white or grayish-red masses circumscribed by a desmoplastic or firm connective tissue accumulation that is not a true capsule. The more malignant high grade carcinomas, in contrast, have ill-defined margins. The intermediate grade of mucoepidermoid cancer shows areas with a fibrous peripheral envelope of pseudocapsule, as well as areas of tumor having an extension of neoplastic tissue strands directly into the parenchyma of the salivary gland without a circumscribed type of fibrous tissue. The intermediate classification should be dropped in favor of a high grade lesion if there is any area of mucoepidermoid carcinoma demonstrating extension in an ill-defined manner into the parenchymal tissue.

The *low grade* lesion may demonstrate (and on palpation may suggest) cystic areas, which are not unusual, whereas in the high grade lesion such cystic areas are few, and solid strands or areas of cells make up the firm consistency of the lesion. Mucoepidermoid carcinoma appears in the fourth to sixth decade of life, and the low grade variety usually has been present as a mass of changing size over months to years before a definitive diagnosis is made, often with little associated symptomatology. The lesion, on clinical examination, is often suggestive of a pleomorphic adenoma or mixed tumor. However, in the low grade mucoepidermoid carcinoma, up to 8 per cent of patients have facial nerve involvement with variable degrees of paresis. Less than 10 per cent of low grade mucoepidermoid carcinomas have been found to have microscopic metastasis in the local or first echelon lymph nodes, especially the parotid and submandibular nodes.

Since the low grade mucoepidermoid carcinoma behaves in a manner similar to that of the mixed tumor, early detection of this lesion allows one to achieve a high rate of cure by parotidectomy with preservation of the facial nerve (Thorvaldsson and associates,

1970; Healey, Perzin, and Smith, 1970). Resection of a low grade mucoepidermoid carcinoma in the lateral parotid segment by means of a lateral parotidectomy may offer a cure if sections of the total block reveal no evidence of tumor at the margins. However, if there is tumor at the margins, there is a significant degree of recurrence, which should be treated aggressively. It is therefore the author's preference when treating mucoepidermoid carcinoma to perform a total parotidectomy (Fig. 67–23). If the lesion is detected early and if the local area lymph nodes are negative, a lateral parotidectomy with all margins free of tumor and with preservation of the facial nerve could also be a curative procedure. Radiation to the ipsilateral neck, as well as to the surgical site postoperatively, is a preferred method of adjunctive treatment, especially if any of the compartmental nodes associated with the specimen are suspicious clinically, although not proved histologically to be affected.

When dealing with the intermediate grades of mucoepidermoid cancer, a total parotidectomy is recommended, including a sample of the compartmental nodes. If the latter are negative, there is no need for an ipsilateral radical neck dissection. In any case, preser-

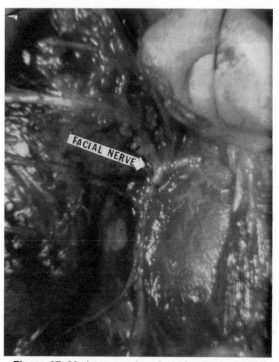

Figure 67–23. Intraoperative view after total parotidectomy for mucoepidermoid carcinoma with preservation of the facial nerve.

vation of the facial nerve, if not involved by the tumor, should be the rule in the treatment of this lesion. The recurrence rate of mucoepidermoid cancer in the parotid gland is reported as 15 per cent, a rate reflecting an inadequate primary surgical resection. The cure rate is reasonably high, although one must be careful in alluding to a five year survival rate since this grade of lesion is often slow growing.

High grade mucoepidermoid cancer is usually detected earlier. Its growth is generally more rapid and the margins are less distinct on palpation. In the high grade lesion, approximately 25 per cent of patients demonstrate facial paralysis and half of those studied demonstrated cervical metastases on initial presentation. Treatment demands total resection of the parotid gland along with the associated compartmental nodes and the preservation of the facial nerve, unless there is evidence of paralysis and direct invasion of the facial nerve branches or trunk. If the compartmental or primary drainage sites demonstrate no evidence of metastasis, a radical neck resection is not indicated. Radiation to the site of surgery as well as to the neck should be considered in every case of a high grade mucoepidermoid carcinoma involving the parotid gland. Long-term follow-up care in these patients (i.e., in patients having either low grade or high grade mucoepidermoid carcinoma) is advisable, since 25 per cent of the recurrences and 20 per cent of the deaths were noted after the first five years of follow-up.

The *submandibular gland* demonstrates the same histologic type of mucoepidermoid carcinoma as that described in the parotid gland. However, a mucoepidermoid carcinoma within the submandibular gland is more aggressive, and metastases, direct extension, and involvement of local nodes occur more frequently. Therefore, it behooves the surgeon to perform a complete local resection of both the submandibular and adjacent sublingual glands in continuity with an upper neck dissection. If the nodes in the area are negative for metastasis, the chance of cure is more realistic. Consideration should be given to supervoltage radiation therapy to the ipsilateral neck and site of surgery postoperatively. The five year survival rate in mucoepidermoid carcinoma involving the submandibular gland has been reported as only 17 per cent.

The *sublingual gland* rarely is involved with solid tumors. However, such tumors in the sublingual gland demonstrate malignancy in 80 per cent of cases; 40 per cent of the malignant lesions are mucoepidermoid carcinomas. Treatment requires resection of the sublingual gland, submandibular duct, submandibular gland, and upper neck nodes in continuity as a block, with preservation of branches of the facial nerve as well as the lingual and hypoglossal nerves.

Adenoid Cystic Carcinoma. The adenoid cystic carcinoma, originally termed "cylindroma," accounts for 4 per cent of all neoplasms involving the major salivary glands. Approximately 4 to 5 per cent of all parotid tumors are adenoid cystic carcinomas, 35 per cent of all malignant minor salivary gland tumors, and between 50 and 60 per cent of all sublingual gland tumors. The most common malignant tumor of the submandibular gland is the adenoid cystic carcinoma. The lesion appears as an asymptomatic mass, which has been reported to have been present for any period from one month to several years. Approximately 25 to 30 per cent are associated with the early appearance of either paresthesia or paralysis involving branches of the facial nerve. The adenoid cystic carcinoma has a special affinity for perineural invasion, which is the most common finding in this insidious lesion (Fig. 67–24). The tu-

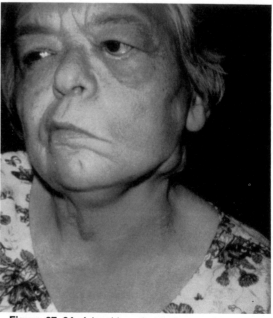

Figure 67–24. Adenoid cystic carcinoma of the left parotid gland with perineural invasion and spread to the neck. There is advanced disease with facial nerve paresis.

mor is slow growing in most cases and appears as a unilobular lesion that is not encapsulated. It is composed of basaloid type of cells classically arranged in a cribriform pattern and with pseudocystic type of spaces, which are extracellular spaces lined by several basement membranes. The cut surface of this lesion is usually moist and grayish pink, and the cribriform pattern on histologic section is diagnostic (Leafstedt and associates, 1971; Spiro, Huvos, and Strong, 1974).

The adenoid cystic carcinoma behaves in an unpredictable fashion, some cases proving rapidly fatal while others follow a protracted course with metastatic lesions appearing in the lungs. Involvement of a surprisingly large area of lung tissue is tolerated by the patient for up to 20 years or more. The long-term prognosis is grave. In many reported series, the five to ten year survival period is meaningless, whereas the 15 to 20 year survival rate demonstrates the poor prognostic implication of this diagnosis. For example, at five years, 3 per cent of survivors had metastases and local recurrence, 3 per cent had local recurrence only, and 18 per cent had metastases only. At ten years, 25 per cent of survivors demonstrated metastases and local recurrence, 25 per cent had local recurrence only, and 18 per cent had metastases only. At 20 years, 28 per cent of the survivors had metastases and local recurrence. These figures indicate that the morbid course of this disease is continuous and relentless, metastases most commonly being to the lung followed by metastases to bone (Spiro, Huvos, and Strong, 1974).

Many cases studied demonstrate that despite the widespread metastases to lung, the ominous outcome of adenoid cystic carcinoma is delayed for several years. This lesion produced a fatal outcome in approximately one-third of cases within one year. However, between 20 and 25 per cent of patients with a diagnosis of adenoid cystic carcinoma live more than five years even though metastatic disease is evident despite proven control of the primary lesion. Lymph node involvement is not commonly seen except for the first echelon nodes adjacent to the site of the original tumor (Allen and Marsh, 1976). Such nodal involvement occurred in 15 per cent of cases and was thought to be more a result of direct extension than of embolic metastases.

Surgical treatment requires complete excision of the tumor, recognizing that it appears to travel significant distances along the perineural lymphatic root of the nerves. It is difficult to recognize the complete extent of nerve involvement. Therefore, it has been advocated that all nerves in the path of this lesion should be sacrificed even if this involves partial temporal bone resection where a main branch or trunk of the facial nerve is involved. When there is local recurrence, this too is resected, following the same premise that resection of the involved nerve and tumor offers the best chance of cure. When recurrence is unresectable, radiation therapy is suggested as a means of controlling the ultimate outcome (Smith, Lane, and Rankow, 1965). In another type of approach, the surgical resection is much more radical; the widest resection is made in the case of the parotid gland, including a total parotidectomy; sacrifice of the facial nerve; resection of the masseter muscle, the ascending ramus of the mandible, and part of the temporal bone; and an incontinuity radical neck dissection. Recurrent lesions are resected in the same radical fashion if possible, and if not, radiation is also adminstered. The above therapeutic approach has been associated with a five year survival rate of 82 per cent and a 20 year survival rate of 13 per cent; the second more radical approach produced a five year survival rate of 89 per cent and 20 year survivals of 20 per cent (Chang, 1976).

Radiation therapy has long been considered of limited use in the treatment of salivary gland malignant lesions, but it has been found that the adenoid cystic carcinoma appears to be radiosensitive although not radiocurable. Responses noted in the treatment of recurrent disease appear to be good for a span of 3.8 to 14 years following radiation after surgical failure to control recurrent adenoid cystic carcinoma. It has been recommended that a combined surgical and supervoltage radiation approach should be planned when this lesion is diagnosed. The findings in many large series show that the lesion can be tolerated by the patient for many years, widespread metastases to lung and bone and ultimate death occurring 20 or more years after the original surgical procedure has been performed (Chang, 1976).

The adenoid cystic carcinoma, as noted, is the most common malignant lesion of the submandibular gland. However, it accounts for up to 60 per cent of all sublingual gland tumors, as well as 35 per cent of all malignant minor salivary gland tumors. Complete removal of the salivary gland is necessary to ensure the best possible control of the local lesions. Careful follow-up observation to detect any evidence of local recurrence, as well as distant metastases to lung and bone, is necessary if one is to attempt cure or prolong the survival of these patients.

Malignant Pleomorphic Adenoma (Malignant Mixed Tumor). *Carcinoma ex pleomorphic adenoma* is a malignant mixed tumor that is a transformation of the epithelial component of a benign pleomorphic adenoma into a carcinoma with metastasis by the epithelial component only (Beahrs and associates, 1957). Another variety of malignant pleomorphic adenoma is the histologically benign mixed tumor or pleomorphic adenoma, which is accompanied by metastases of mixed tumor cells to the liver as well as to the lung even though the primary lesion has been totally removed (Youngs and Scheuer, 1973). Another rare variant is the malignant mixed tumor demonstrating malignant epithelial as well as myoepithelial components, which might better be classified as carcinosarcoma. Both epithelial and myoepithelial components metastasize to systemic areas as well as to bone and lung.

The malignant rare carcinoma ex pleomorphic adenoma makes up 3 to 5 per cent of the pleomorphic adenomas and most often appears in the parotid. It may also appear in the submandibular gland and less often on the palate, lip, paranasal sinuses, and nasopharyngeal and tonsillar areas. It is difficult to diagnose this tumor on frozen section as it is often interpreted as a benign mixed tumor. The lesion is more commonly found in the 50 to 60 year age group, the average duration of the lesion before resection being ten years. The lesion thus may well develop from a benign mixed tumor that has not been resected. In other words, the transformation of epithelial components within a preexisting mixed tumor becomes a possibility *if the mixed tumor has been present for ten or more years* (Eneroth, Blanck, and Jakobsson, 1968).

The carcinoma ex pleomorphic adenoma is more malignant than the more common salivary gland carcinomas and there is local recurrence after initial resection in 30 per cent of patients treated. There is a tendency toward perineural invasion, and distant metastases are noted in 45 per cent of patients. The tumor appears with a pseudocapsule, similar to that in the mixed tumor, which is often found to contain tumor cells. Total par-

otidectomy with sacrifice of invaded nerve segments, followed by immediate repair of the facial nerve with nerve grafts and a radical neck dissection, is advisable for the treatment of this lesion. Whether postoperative radiation is also administered depends on the findings of nodal involvement in the neck and the extent of local disease. The five year survival rate has been reported as 55 to 58 per cent. However, the 20 year survival rate is close to zero, being less than 1 per cent (LiVolsi and Perzin, 1977).

Acinous (Acinic) Cell Carcinoma. The acinous cell carcinoma is divided into *low, intermediate,* and *high grade varieties.*

The *high grade* lesion demonstrates intravascular extension and a tubular type of growth pattern with finger-like extensions, and primarily involves the parotid gland, the salivary glands of the oral cavity being involved to a lesser extent. These lesions make up 2 to 5 per cent of all salivary gland neoplasms, 3 per cent appearing bilaterally. The acinous cell carcinoma appears between the ages of 30 and 60 years and is more common in the female, although many studies show an equal sex distribution (Fox, ReMine, and Woolner, 1963).

The lesion appears as a painless, slow growing, solid or cystic mass that is histologically unencapsulated and may present with calcifications within the tumor. Thirty per cent of these lesions have an accompanying lymphoid component, and metastases by hematogenous routes to lungs and bones, especially the vertebra, are common. The incidence of metastases to the cervical lymph nodes is approximately 10 per cent. Recurrence of the lesion has been reported as early as one year and as late as 50 years after the initial resection.

Treatment of an acinous cell carcinoma of the parotid gland consists of total parotidectomy with resection of involved facial nerve segments, immediate repair of the nerve, and a radical neck dissection, if there is palpable cervical adenopathy. Radiation is not effective treatment of an acinous cell carcinoma. Recurrence must be treated vigorously since widespread and rapid involvement of surrounding tissues is the rule (Chong, Beahrs and Woolner, 1974; Levin, Robinson, and Lin, 1975).

Squamous Cell Carcinoma. Squamous cell carcinoma is an unusual primary tumor of the salivary glands. When present, its origin must be ruled out as arising either from a high grade mucoepidermoid carcinoma or from a metastatic squamous cell lesion stemming from a primary tumor elsewhere in the head and neck. The lesion appears as a firm, indurated mass fixed to the surrounding structures in 50 per cent of cases, often extending beyond the confines of the gland with metastasis to the cervical nodes of the neck. One-third of the patients demonstrate evidence of facial nerve paresis or paralysis at the time of presentation. Patients are usually over 60 years of age, and males are more frequently involved than females. Radical total parotidectomy with sacrifice of the facial nerve, if necessary, should be accompanied by a radical neck dissection and postoperative radiation to improve the chances of five year survival. The reported ten year survival rate has been approximately 45 per cent with the radical approach, as noted above (Woods, Chong, and Beahrs, 1975).

Adenocarcinoma. Adenocarcinomas occurring primarily in salivary glands can be classified as those that are not found to be an adenoid cystic carcinoma, an acinous cell carcinoma, or a mucoepidermoid carcinoma. The adenocarcinomas make up approximately 2.8 per cent of all parotid neoplasms and may be papillary, mucus secreting, or a ductal type of carcinoma demonstrating frequent invasion of the lymphatics and blood vessels (Blanck, Eneroth, and Jakobsson, 1971). The adenoid cystic carcinoma, acinous cell carcinoma, and mucoepidermoid carcinoma are distinct entities and are given a separate classification from that of the broad classification of adenocarcinomas.

These lesions present as firm masses, are slow growing, are present for many years, and are usually fixed to surrounding structures. They involve the 30 to 60 year age group, with males predominating over females. Facial nerve paresis is seen in 22 per cent of patients on first examination, 25 per cent already demonstrating regional metastasis and 20 per cent showing systemic metastasis. The lesion spreads outside the parotid gland or into the deep parotid segment in a large number of patients, metastasis to bone and lung being fairly common.

The treatment of an adenocarcinoma consists of wide resection with sacrifice of any involved facial nerve structures followed by immediate nerve graft. A radical neck dissection is indicated, and postoperative radiation is advisable since recurrence is often widespread and rapid. Fifty to 75 per cent of

treated patients demonstrate a five year survival following parotid gland resection with radical neck dissection and postoperative radiation.

Undifferentiated Carcinoma. The undifferentiated cancers (Koss, Spiro, and Hajdu, 1972; Cornog and Gray, 1976) are those tumors that cannot be classified as either adenocarcinomas or of squamous cell cancer origin. They are uncommon lesions and occur mostly in the 70 to 80 year age group, males being more involved than females. One-third of these lesions arise from a pleomorphic adenoma that has been present for many years. They consist of small round or spindle cells ("oat cells") and are highly malignant, 33 per cent of patients demonstrating partial or total facial paralysis and spread beyond the parotid gland into adjacent tissue at the time of presentation. Regional metastases are noted in 13 per cent of patients.

Radical resection including total parotidectomy, radical neck dissection, sacrifice of invaded nerves, and postoperative radiation is indicated. The five year survival rate is only 25 to 30 per cent.

Malignant Oncocytoma. The oncocytomas (Johns, Batsakis, and Short, 1973; Cornog and Gray, 1976) for the most part are benign lesions and make up less than 1 per cent of salivary gland neoplasms. The malignant oncocytoma is a rare tumor. It is often solid rather than cystic, and its growth is aggressive and infiltrative. Multiple recurrences and regional metastases are reported in patients treated by radical methods. The best chance for survival, however, is to control these lesions through wide resection, including a radical neck dissection, and removal of all contiguous tissue where evidence of involvement can be demonstrated histologically.

Clear Cell Carcinoma. The true clear cell carcinoma (Goldman and Klein, 1942) is undifferentiated but may originate from the myoepithelial cell of the intercalated duct cellular lining. It is a rare, low grade cancer that acts like a low grade mucoepidermoid carcinoma, but it must be differentiated from a renal cell carcinoma that has metastasized to the parotid gland. Resection is best accomplished by total parotidectomy.

NONSALIVARY MALIGNANCIES

The primary *fibrosarcomas* are rare and can be treated by wide excision of the total gland followed by radiation. The *malignant neurogenous* tumors include the *neuroblastoma* and the *neurogenous sarcomas*. Treatment by radical surgery is indicated. However, the mortality rate is high and there are very few surgical cures.

The primary *melanoma* is another rare entity that can occur within the parotid, but one must first rule out the more common metastasis from elsewhere, mainly in the parotid nodes. The primary melanoma occurs within the node-bearing tissue of the parotid parenchyma. Radical neck dissection in continuity with the parotid gland is the treatment recommended. Primary lymphomas may occur although they are rare, and these are all Stage 1 lesions of lymphoma with a fair prognosis.

When dealing with metastatic disease to the parotid gland, one must recall that there are paraglandular nodes as well as intraglandular lymphoid accumulations that communicate freely with each other within the parotid gland. The paraglandular nodes are located in the subcutaneous layer above the parotid fascia and are usually pretragal or supratragal in location. These drain the lateral surface of the auricle and the adjacent scalp and cheek areas. The intraglandular nodes, which are located within the parenchymal substance of the parotid gland lateral to the facial vein, drain the afferent channels from the nose, eyelid, conjunctiva, frontotemporal scalp, external auditory meatus and middle ear, lacrimal gland, and sinuses, as well as the nasopharyngeal and oropharyngeal cavities. When a lesion appears to be in the paraglandular node, the possibility of metastasis from elsewhere must be entertained in the differential diagnosis of the lesion. Since the intraglandular nodes are lateral to the facial vein and closely approximate the facial nerve, resection for metastatic disease may necessitate excision of the branches of the facial nerve or the trunk itself. One must, however, be prepared to repair the nerve either by nerve graft or by anastomosis with adjacent nerve segments.

Patients with invasive melanoma and poor to moderately differentiated squamous cell carcinoma of the eyelid, conjuctiva, frontotemporal scalp, posterior cheek, or anterior ear are at high risk for metastatic spread to the parotid nodes. Most often, melanoma metastasizes to the paraglandular nodes, while squamous cell carcinoma appears to spread to the intraglandular nodes. In these cases, dissemination or spread to the cervical nodes is common, and resection of the total gland in continuity with a radical neck dissection should therefore be considered (Conley and Arena, 1963; Storm and associates, 1977).

MALIGNANT LESIONS INVOLVING THE DEEP PAROTID SEGMENT

When one is dealing with tumors involving the deep parotid segment of the parotid gland (Thorvaldsson and associates, 1970; Richardson and associates, 1975), total parotidectomy is indicated. Deep segment tumors of the parotid usually present as a mass below the ear or as an intraoral parapharyngeal mass, although a combination of both can produce the so-called dumbbell-type tumor (see Fig. 67–10). Most of the lesions in the deep parotid segment are benign, as is true of the lateral segment. However, 15 to 20 per cent of parotid masses are malignant, and the most common of these lesions are the mucoepidermoid and the acinous cell carcinomas. When the deep segment is involved with either of these lesions, a total parotidectomy with as much of a cuff of normal tissue as possible around the deep segment is indicated. Usually, the facial nerve can be spared if the lesion is confined to the deep segment; however, a total parotidectomy is necessary. Whether an in continuity radical neck dissection is indicated depends on the presence of cervical node involvement. Since the deep segment is so close to the pharyngeal wall, short of resecting the lateral pharyngeal wall in continuity with the deep segment, one should plan postoperative radiation to control the possibility of leaving tumor behind in such a narrow margin of mucosal wall.

MALIGNANT LESIONS INVOLVING THE SUBMANDIBULAR, SUBLINGUAL, AND MINOR SALIVARY GLANDS

As described earlier in this chapter, 50 per cent of submandibular gland tumors are malignant (Rankow, 1973; Richardson and associates, 1975; Rankow and Polayes, 1976a,b). These lesions are of the same histologic type as occur in the parotid, but when found in the submandibular gland they appear to be more aggressive in behavior. The adenoid cystic carcinoma is more often found in the submandibular gland, as is the mucoepidermoid carcinoma and the adenocarcinoma. The treatment of carcinomas primarily occurring in the submandibular gland is a composite resection that involves removing the submandibular gland, the adjacent mylohyoid muscle segment, the overlying mucosa of the floor of the mouth, a portion of the tongue, the submandibular duct, and the sublingual gland, all in continuity with the radical neck dissection. Postoperative radiation is strongly recommended as a means of controlling possible areas of microscopic metastasis to nodal neck tissue.

In the sublingual gland, 80 per cent of tumors are malignant, and most of these are adenoid cystic or mucoepidermoid carcinomas. The treatment of cancer in the sublingual gland consists of radical removal of the gland in continuity with the submandibular duct, the submandibular gland, the involved mylohyoid muscle, and a portion of the adjacent mandible, if involved, in continuity with an ipsilateral radical neck dissection.

The minor salivary glands are involved by primary malignant lesions more often than are the submandibular glands. Fifty-five to 60 per cent of these lesions are malignant, most tumors occurring in the minor salivary glands of the oral cavity, predominantly those of the palate. These lesions appear as a mass covered by smooth overlying mucosa that may be painful, although in most cases they are annoying only because of their size. In all locations of the minor salivary glands, the predominant carcinoma is the adenoid cystic carcinoma, followed in frequency by the mucoepidermoid carcinoma. In general, lesions in the minor salivary glands are identical to those in the parotid or submandibular glands, although they appear to be more aggressive when located in the minor salivary glands. Wide local resection with as wide a margin as possible is the treatment of choice.

EXCESSIVE SALIVATION AND TRANSPOSITION OF PAROTID DUCT

Although originally described as a method of managing uncontrolled drooling in spastic children (Wilkie, 1967), surgical transposition of Stensen's duct into the tonsillar fossa has been recommended for treating drooling or excessive salivation from a variety of causes. Loss of the oral sphincter and mandibular symphysis from either trauma or surgical extirpation predisposes to virtually un-controlled drooling, and can be relatively controlled by redirecting the salivary flow into the tonsillar fossa where it can be more easily swallowed.

The surgical technique consists of the creation of a mucosal flap based on the opening of Stensen's duct (Fig. 67–25A). The flap is then tubed with a simple continuous suture of fine catgut (Fig. 67–25B). The tubed flap containing the opening of Stensen's duct in its base is tunneled into the tonsillar fossa just beneath the anterior tonsillar pillar. It is important that the tube be directed slightly downward as well as posteriorly to facilitate drainage into the tonsillar fossa (Fig. 67–25C). The use of a polyethylene stent may be of some help in the formation and tubing of the mucosal flap, but it is not essential. Furthermore, the stent should not be left in place after completion of the procedure.

COMPLICATIONS OF SALIVARY GLAND SURGERY

The possible complications arising from surgery of the salivary glands can be divided into those resulting from diagnostic procedures, those following operative exposure, and those appearing early or later in the postoperative period.

The diagnosis of lesions involving the salivary glands relies on a tissue diagnosis. When lesions appear to be accompanied by obstruction of the salivary gland duct, the use of a sialogram is helpful in outlining the parenchymal segments and duct system of the gland to locate the site of obstruction. The use of radiopaque contrast material for this study may evoke sensitivity reactions or severe allergic reactions to the iodine compounds. Aside from the allergic reaction to the radiopaque material, the patient often experiences pain as the contrast material is introduced into the duct. Water-soluble contrast materials are preferred to oil-based contrast solutions in that they are more easily drained and absorbed and do not remain as a source of irritation in the gland.

Perforations of the duct as well as oral fistulization can be detected and outlined by introducing such contrast material into the major duct of the gland, thereby defining an oral mucosal or oral cutaneous salivary fistula. The fistulous tract can be traced to its origin and to its points of communication with either the oral cavity or the skin surface. The

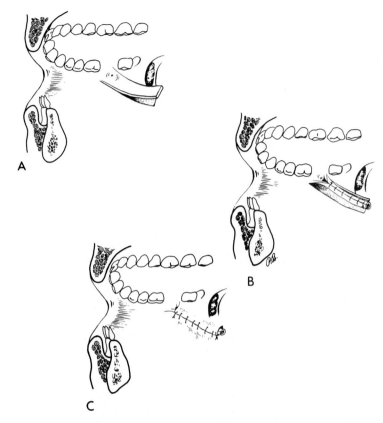

Figure 67–25. Transposition of the parotid duct. *A,* Transposition of the salivary duct to the tonsillar fossa is accomplished by the construction of an oral mucosa–lined flap with its base including the opening of Stensen's duct. *B,* The flap is tubed, establishing a mucosa–lined tube from the duct opening to the tonsillar fossa. *C,* Mobilization and closure of the adjacent oral soft tissue over the mucosa–lined tube allow salivary secretion to drain into the base of the tonsillar fossa.

instillation of contaminated contrast solutions into the salivary duct should be avoided, since this can lead to severe sialadenitis. It is therefore advisable to use sterile technique.

The drainage of postoperative salivary gland abscesses, in which acute bacterial infections may involve the parenchymal elements of the gland, poses the surgical problem of avoiding injury to the facial nerve branches. Drainage of a parotid parenchymal abscess is accomplished through a routine parotidectomy type of incision and care is exercised to avoid injury to the facial nerve branches. In the case of the submandibular gland, care should be taken to perform an incision and drainage through a submandibular cervical crease incision and to approach the gland as one would for a submandibular gland resection, incising through the capsule and dissecting carefully into the gland to promote drainage. The mandibular and cervical branches of the facial nerve are subject to injury and must be carefully protected.

If probing of a duct has been too vigorous, it is possible to lacerate the duct and produce a fistula into the oral mucosa or even through the skin, especially if the remaining portions of the duct are obstructed. Fistulization into

the oral mucosal surface is acceptable and usually provides adequate drainage of the gland by emptying the salivary contents into the oral and pharyngeal cavity. However, if the fistula occurs through the skin surface, one must identify the points of injury to the duct. Through a routine cutaneous parotid approach, or if possible through a buccal mucosal incision, the distal parotid duct can be exposed and a Silastic tube (stent) placed across the area of injury so that the duct can be repaired. The fistulous tract can be excised and closed when the duct is patent and functional. This type of complication can also be corrected by opening the severed duct into the oral cavity if it has adequate length to pass through the buccal mucosa. However, if there are a sufficient distal segment of parotid duct and a normal meatus at the opening to Stensen's duct, it is better to achieve a repair of the duct over a stent and allow for drainage through its normal path.

Calculi or cysts appearing in the submandibular duct from either the sublingual or the submandibular gland have often been treated intraorally by marsupialization of the duct into the floor of the mouth. However, repeated bouts of submandibular duct obstruction by calculi, tumor, or repeated cyst formation dictate total excision of the involved gland with its duct, be it the submandibular or sublingual gland, or both (Fig. 67–26). Multiple episodes of obstructive sialadenitis are a surgical indication for resection of the involved salivary gland and duct.

When the obstructed parotid gland is being dealt with, calculi may be found in the parotid duct. The approach to the duct can be either through the mouth or through a routine parotidectomy incision, isolating the duct and tracing it distally. Those stones that can be palpated under the mucosa of the distal duct can be approached directly through the buccal

oral mucosa. In this case, a probe is passed into the duct up to the point of the stone and a traction suture is placed around the more proximal portion of the duct, proximal to the stone itself, to prevent the stone from being pushed back into the gland or into the duct. After the calculus has been removed, the duct can be repaired over a Silastic stent, which is left in place for ten days. However, if the stone is pushed back into the glandular substance, a routine parotidectomy approach to isolate the calculus is indicated and occasionally it may be necessary to perform a lateral parotidectomy.

The major, most common intraoperative

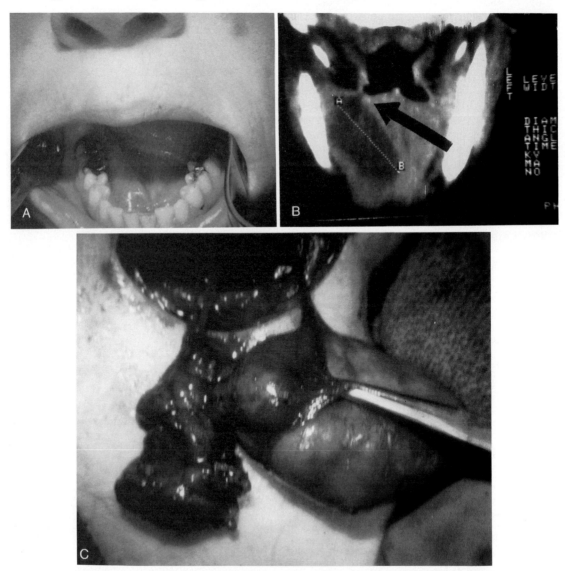

Figure 67–26. *A,* Cyst or ranula involving the right floor of the mouth, sublingual gland, and submandibular gland and duct. *B,* CT scan showing the full extent of the ranula into the cervical-submandibular triangle. *C,* Intraoperative view of the specimen, including the sublingual and submandibular glands and duct.

complication is that of injury to the branches of the facial nerve. Earlier in the chapter, it was pointed out that direct identification of the trunk of the facial nerve, and distal dissection to expose its branches and remove the glandular tissue from around the branches, is the safest way to perform a parotidectomy. There are situations, however, in which the tumor mass is large or has infiltrated the area, producing a fibrous reaction around the branches of the nerve and making it difficult to identify or approach the trunk. With careful technique one can usually identify the facial nerve trunk and dissect the nerve branches distally. However, it is safer to resort to identification of the most distal portions of the facial nerve branches (either the buccal or ramus mandibularis) and trace them proximally to the trunk, rather than blindly resect parotid tissue. It should be borne in mind that with this alternative method of identifying the facial nerve there is more likely to be paresis. Another cause of facial nerve weakness is repeated galvanic stimulation of the facial nerve by a nerve stimulator. The stimulator should be applied at the lowest current that is sufficient to demonstrate nerve function. When one has to resort to repeated high levels of current transmitted through the nerve to demonstrate function, there is often an accompanying paresis, which may last for several months.

Hypoesthesia of the ear lobule after a parotidectomy usually is associated with injury to the greater auricular nerve. This hypoesthesia appears to resolve, but at times there may be neuroma formation that is tender to touch or palpation.

Gustatory sweating, or Frey's syndrome (Fig. 26–27), usually follows parotidectomy when there has been disturbance of reflex pathways from both the greater auricular and the auriculotemporal nerves to the skin. If Frey's syndrome is severe and persistent over many months or years, reelevation of the original skin flap interrupts the spurious connections between the parasympathetic and sympathetic nerve endings to the skin, and gustatory sweating ceases. Gustatory sweating may recur, but reelevation of the parotidectomy skin flap is usually beneficial.

Injury to the hypoglossal nerve or the lingual nerve may also occur in submandibular and sublingual gland surgery. With injury of the hypoglossal nerve, the atrophic tongue may deviate to the side of injury, producing

abnormal speech. If the lingual nerve is involved, there is both loss of sensation in the tongue and partial loss and differentiation of taste.

Injury to the sublingual branch of the lingual artery can also produce hematoma formation and postoperative hemorrhage. Usually the bleeding arises from multiple points over a generalized area in which ligation can be dangerous and possibly produce injury to the facial nerve. *Only if the vessel can be clearly identified and separated from the facial nerve branches is ligation possible.* Bleeding can often be controlled by simply evacuating the clots and maintaining a pressure dressing over a drain.

Violation of the tumor mass, especially if a

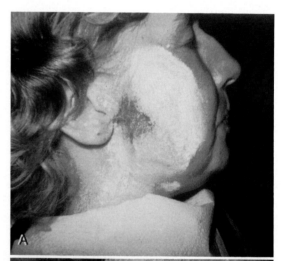
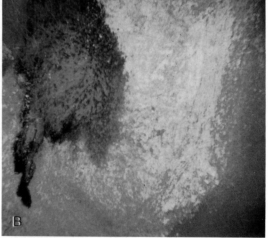

Figure 67–27. *A, B,* Frey's syndrome (gustatory sweating). Postparotidectomy patient with beads of sweat appearing as she ate an apple. Note the starch iodine reaction beginning in the preauricular area as the moistened starch reacts with the dry tincture of iodine applied before the patient ate the apple.

mixed tumor is involved, usually results in spillage of its contents and seeding of tumor cells throughout the area of dissection. A recurrent mixed tumor arising in this manner appears as multiple small nodules attached to the underlying areolar tissue and to the facial nerve branches. With each recurrence of a mixed tumor, the tumor cell becomes more malignant and cure is less likely unless surgery is more radical.

Lesions such as a mucoepidermoid cancer involving the lateral parotid segment with continuity in the retromandibular portion is often removed by a lateral parotidectomy. In this case, one must be suspicious of possible involvement of the deep segment, which, if left behind, often presents with a recurrent tumor mass that demands a more radical surgical approach, with possible sacrifice of the involved facial nerve. The attempt to remove a deep parotid segment tumor mass involves removal of the lateral parotid segment and careful dissection deep to the facial nerve in order to remove the entire deep segment. If the nerve is involved, it is often necessary to sacrifice that portion of the nerve. In this case, immediate repair by nerve graft is advocated, unless one is dealing with a tumor mass that has been incompletely removed and may require further surgical treatment.

Soft tissue losses resulting from vascular compromise following elevation of a parotidectomy skin flap can be reconstructed by the use of local cervical flaps. The postoperative soft tissue "hollow" resulting from parotidectomy or submandibular gland resection can often be treated by rotation of deepithelized cervical composite flaps or sternomastoid muscle flaps into the defect as a satisfactory means of restoring contour.

REFERENCES

Allen, M. S., Jr., and Marsh, W. L., Jr.: Lymph node involvement by direct extension in adenoid cystic carcinoma. Absence of classic embolic lymph node metastasis. Cancer, *38*:2017, 1976.

Bailey, H.: The treatment of tumors of the parotid gland with special reference to total parotidectomy. Br. J. Surg., *28*:337, 1941.

Batsakis, J. G., Littler, E. R., and Leahy, M. S.: Sebaceous cell lesions of the head and neck. Arch. Otolaryngol., *95*:151, 1972.

Beahrs, O. H., Woolner, L. B., Kirklin, J. W., and Devine, K. D.: Carcinomatous transformation of mixed tumor of the parotid gland. Arch. Surg., *75*:605, 1957.

Bernacki, E. G., Batsakis, J. G., and Johns, M. E.: Basal cell adenoma. Distinctive tumor of salivary glands. Arch. Otolaryngol., *99*:84, 1974.

Blanck, C., Eneroth, C. M., and Jakobsson, P. A.: Mucus-producing adenopapillary (nonepidermoid) carcinoma of the parotid gland. Cancer, *28*:676, 1971.

Blatt, I. M.: Studies of sialolithiasis. Part 3. Pathogenesis, diagnosis and treatment. South. Med. J., *57*:723, 1964.

Brown, J. B., McDowell, F., and Fryer, M. P.: Direct operative removal of benign mixed tumors of anlage origin in the parotid region. Surg. Gynecol. Obstet., *90*:257, 1950.

Brunetti, F., Fiori, Ratti, L., et al.: La Ghiondole Salivari: Patologia e Clinica. Atti del 57th Cong. 25–27 September 1969, Assisi, Porziuncola, 1969.

Chang, Chu H.: Radiation therapy. *In* Rankow, R. M., and Polayes, I. M. (Eds.): Diseases of the Salivary Glands. Philadelphia, W. B. Saunders Company, 1976, pp. 343–355.

Chaudhry, A. P., and Gorlin, R. J.: Papillary cystadenoma lymphomatosum (adenolymphoma). Am. J. Surg., *95*:923, 1958.

Chong, G. C., Beahrs, O. H., and Woolner, L. B.: Surgical management of acinic cell carcinoma of the parotid gland. Surg. Gynecol. Obstet., *138*:65, 1974.

Conley, J., and Arena, S.: Parotid gland as a process of metastasis. Arch. Surg., *87*:757, 1963.

Cornog, J. L., and Gray, S. R.: Surgical and clinical pathology of salivary gland tumors. *In* Rankow, R. M., and Polayes, I. M. (Eds.): Diseases of the Salivary Gland. Philadelphia, W. B. Saunders Company, 1976, pp. 99–142.

Eneroth, C. M.: Salivary gland tumors in the parotid gland, submandibular gland, and the palate region. Cancer, *27*:1415, 1971.

Eneroth, C. M., Blanck, C., and Jakobsson, P. A.: Carcinoma in pleomorphic adenoma of the parotid gland. Acta Otolaryngol., *66*:477, 1968.

Eversole, L. R.: Histogenic classification of salivary tumors. Arch. Pathol., *92*:433, 1971.

Fost, N. C., and Esterly, N. B.: Successful treatment of juvenile hemangiomas with prednisone. J. Pediatr., *72*:351, 1968.

Fox, N. M., Jr., ReMine, W. H., and Woolner, L. B.: Acinic cell carcinoma of the major salivary glands. Am. J. Surg., *106*:860, 1963.

Garcia, R. R.: Differential diagnosis of tumor of the salivary glands with radioactive isotopes. Int. J. Oral Surg., *3*:330, 1974.

Gasser, R. F.: The early development of the parotid gland around the facial nerve and its branches in man. Anat. Rec., *167*:63, 1970.

Gates, G. A.: Radiosialographic aspects of salivary gland disorders. Laryngoscope, *82*:115, 1972.

Goldman, R. L., and Klein, H. Z.: Glycogen-rich adenoma of the parotid gland. An uncommon benign clear-cell tumor resembling certain clear-cell carcinomas of salivary origin. Cancer, *30*:749, 1942.

Grove, A. S., Jr., and DiChiro, G.: Salivary gland scanning with technetium 99m pertechnetate. Am. J. Roentgen., *102*:109, 1968.

Hanna, D. C., Gaisford, J. C., Richardson, G. S., and Bindra, R. N.: Tumors of the deep lobe of the parotid gland. Am. J. Surg., *116*:524, 1968.

Harkins, G. A., and Sabiston, D. C., Jr.: Lymphangioma in infancy and childhood. Surgery, *47*:811, 1960.

Healey, W. V., Perzin, K. H., and Smith, L.: Mucoepidermoid carcinoma of salivary gland origin: classification, clinicopathologic correlation, and results of treatment. Cancer, *26*:368, 1970.

Jaques, D. A., Krolls, S. O., and Chambers, R. G.: Parotid tumors in children. Am. J. Surg., *132*:469, 1976.

Johns, M. E., Batsakis, J. G., and Short, C. D.: Oncocytic and oncocytoid tumors of the salivary glands. Laryngoscope, *83*:1940, 1973.

Koss, L. G., Spiro, R. H., and Hajdu, S.: Small cell (oat cell) carcinoma of minor salivary gland origin. Cancer, *30*:737, 1972.

Leafstedt, S. W., Gaeta, J. F., Sako, K., Marchetta, F. C., and Shedd, D. P.: Adenoid cystic carcinoma of major and minor salivary glands. Am. J. Surg., *122*:756, 1971.

Levin, J. M., Robinson, D. W., and Lin, F.: Acinic cell carcinoma. Collective review including bilateral cases. Arch. Surg., *110*:64, 1975.

LiVolsi, V. A., and Perzin, K. H.: Malignant mixed tumors arising in salivary glands. I. Carcinomas arising in benign mixed tumors: a clinicopathologic study. Cancer, *39*:2209, 1977.

Major, R. H.: The seventeenth century. *In* A History of Medicine. Springfield, IL, Charles C Thomas, 1954a, p. 543.

Major, R. H.: The nineteenth century—first half. *In* A History of Medicine. Springfield, IL, Charles C Thomas, 1954b, pp. 706–707.

Martin, H.: The operative removal of tumors of the parotid salivary gland. Surgery, *31*:670, 1952.

McCoy, J. M., and Eckert, E. F., Jr.: Sialadenoma papilliferum. J. Oral Surg., *38*:691, 1980.

McFarland, J.: Treatment of mixed tumors of the salivary gland by roentgen rays and radium. Am. J. Roentgen., *46*:507, 1941.

McFarland, J.: The mysterious mixed tumors of the salivary glands. Surg. Gynecol. Obstet., *76*:23, 1943.

McKenzie, J.: The parotid gland in relation to the facial nerve. J. Anat., *82*:183, 1948.

Micheli-Pellegrini, V., and Polayes, I. M.: Historical background. *In* Rankow, R. M., and Polayes, I. M. (Eds.): Diseases of the Salivary Glands. Philadelphia, W. B. Saunders Company, 1976, pp. 1–16.

Morestin, H.: Contribution à l'étude du traitement des fistules salivaires consecutives aux blessures de guerre. Bull. Mem. Soc. Chir. Paris, *43*:845, 1917.

Murray, M. R., and Stout, A. P.: Schwann cell versus fibroblast as origin of specific nerve sheath tumor—observations upon normal nerve sheaths and neurilemmoma in vitro. Am. J. Pathol., *71*:60, 1940.

Paré, A.: Opera Chirurgica. Francofurti, 1594.

Polayes, I. M.: Salivary gland tumors in children. *In* Gellis, S. S., and Kagan, B. M. (Eds.): Current Pediatric Therapy. Philadelphia, W. B. Saunders Company, 1982, pp. 161–162.

Polayes, I. M., and Rankow, R. M.: Inflammatory disorders. Part 2. Surgical management. *In* Rankow, R. M., and Polayes, I. M. (Eds.): Diseases of the Salivary Glands. Philadelphia, W. B. Saunders Company, 1976, pp. 229–238.

Polayes, I. M., and Rankow, R. M.: Cysts, masses and tumors of the accessory parotid gland. Plast. Reconstr. Surg., *64*:17, 1979.

Polayes, I. M., and Robson, M. C.: Neurilemmoma presenting as a tumor in the tail of the parotid. Plast. Reconstr. Surg., *61*:225, 1978.

Rankow, R. M.: Surgical decisions in the treatment of major salivary gland tumors. Plast. Reconstr. Surg., *51*:514, 1973.

Rankow, R. M., and Mignogna, F.: Cancer of the sublingual salivary gland. Am. J. Surg., *118*:790, 1969.

Rankow, R. M., and Polayes, I. M.: Surgical anatomy and diagnosis. *In* Rankow, R. M., and Polayes, I. M. (Eds.): Diseases of the Salivary Glands. Philadelphia, W. B. Saunders Company, 1976a, pp. 156–184.

Rankow, R. M., and Polayes, I. M.: Surgical treatment of salivary gland tumors. *In* Rankow, R. M., and Polayes, I. M. (Eds.): Diseases of the Salivary Glands. Philadelphia, W. B. Saunders Company, 1976b, pp. 239–283.

Regezi, J. A., and Batsakis, J. G.: Histogenesis of salivary gland neoplasms. Otolaryngol. Clin. North Am., *10*:297, 1977.

Richardson, G. S., Dickason, W. L., Gaisford, J. C., and Hanna, D. C.: Tumors of salivary glands. Plast. Reconstr. Surg., *55*:131, 1975.

Smith, L. C., Lane, N., and Rankow, R. M.: Cylindroma (adenoid cystic carcinoma), a report of 58 cases. Am. J. Surg., *110*:519, 1965.

Spiro, R. H., Huvos, A. G., and Strong, E. W.: Adenoid cystic carcinoma of salivary origin: a clinicopathologic study of 242 cases. Am. J. Surg., *128*:512, 1974.

Stensen (Stenonis), N.: De Glandulis Oris & Novis Earundem Vasis. Observationes Anatomicae 1661. *In* Garrett, J. R.: Changing attitudes on salivary secretion—a short history on spit. Proc. R. Soc. Med., *68*:553, 1975.

Storm, F. K., Eilber, F. R., Sparks, F. C., and Morton, D. L.: A prospective study of parotid metastases from head and neck cancer. Am. J. Surg., *134*:115, 1977.

Stout, A. P.: Peripheral manifestations of specific nerve sheath tumors (neurilemmoma). Am. J. Cancer, *24*:751, 1935.

Stout, A. P.: Myxoma: the tumor of primitive mesenchyme. Ann. Surg., *127*:706, 1948.

Thackray, A. C.: Salivary gland tumors. Proc. R. Soc. Med., *61*:1089, 1968.

Thorvaldsson, S. E., Beahrs, O. H., Woolner, L. B., and Simons, J. N.: Mucoepidermoid tumors of the major salivary glands. Am. J. Surg., *120*:432, 1970.

Touloukian, R. J.: Salivary gland diseases in infancy and childhood. *In* Rankow, R. M., and Polayes, I. M. (Eds.): Diseases of the Salivary Glands. Philadelphia, W. B. Saunders Company, 1976, pp. 284–303.

Velpeau, A. L. M.: Traite d'anatomie chirurgicale Paris 1823. *In* Major, R. H. (Ed.): The nineteenth century—second half. *In* A History of Medicine. Vol. II. Springfield, IL, Charles C Thomas, 1954, pp. 773–774.

Walts, A. E., and Perzik, S. L.: Lipomatous lesions of the parotid area. Arch. Otolaryngol., *102*:230, 1976.

Wharton, T.: Adenographia, 1656, and quoted in Garrett, J. R.: Changing attitudes on salivary secretion—a short history on spit. Proc. R. Soc. Med., *68*:553, 1975.

Wilkie, T. F.: The problem of drooling in cerebral palsy: a surgical approach. Can. J. Surg., *10*:60, 1967.

Williams, H. B.: Hemangiomas of the parotid gland in children. Plast. Reconstr. Surg., *56*:29, 1975.

Woods, J. E., Chong, G. C., and Beahrs, O. H.: Experience with 1360 primary parotid tumors. Am. J. Surg., *130*:460, 1975.

Youngs, G. R., and Scheuer, P. J.: Histologically benign mixed parotid tumor with hepatic metastasis. J. Pathol., *109*:171, 1973.

68

Phillip R. Casson
Philip Bonanno
Joseph Fischer

Tumors of the Maxilla

The first total maxillectomy, which included an orbital exenteration, was performed by Syme in 1828. In 1842 Fergusson described the classic anterior surgical approach to the maxilla, a technique with which his name is still associated. The first large series of patients treated by maxillectomy for tumors of the maxilla was reported by Öhngren in 1933 and consisted of a group of 187 individuals initially treated with surgery and then with radiation therapy. The reported five year survival rate was 39 per cent. In the succeeding 50 years the treatment of neoplastic disease of the maxilla has not improved the five year survival rate and remains discouraging in spite of increasingly aggressive therapy. The current management of this disease consists of a trimodal approach of surgical ablation, postoperative radiation therapy, and chemotherapy; this has improved the survival rate. The surgical approach has been extended beyond that originally described by Fergusson to allow the surgeon access to the pterygomaxillary fossa via a temporal approach (Attenborough, 1980).

INCIDENCE

Malignant tumors of the paranasal sinuses (see also Chap. 70) are relatively uncommon and make up approximately 0.2 per cent of all malignancies and 3 per cent of cancers of the upper respiratory and alimentary tract. At least 80 per cent of the tumors in the paranasal sinuses arise in the maxillary sinus, the remainder developing in the nasal cavity and the ethmoid sinuses.

The average annual rate of incidence of paranasal sinus cancer in the United States is 0.8 per 100,000 in males and 0.5 per 100,000 in females. The incidence of the disease is similar in Caucasians and blacks. There are approximately 1300 new cases of paranasal sinus cancer each year in the United States. It is encountered most frequently in the age group between 60 and 70 years, with a median age of 64 years. The rate increases as the age of the population increases, with a peak of four to five per 100,000 in individuals over the age of 75 (Schottenfeld and Fraumeni, 1982).

The incidence of the disease varies in different geographic areas. It is much more common in Japan and parts of Africa, especially Uganda and Zimbabwe, where rates of between two and three per 100,000 in males have been reported. Hawaiian males and female American Indians also appear to have an increased incidence but the series are small and may not be statistically significant (Schottenfeld and Fraumeni, 1982). Long-term trends do indicate, however, a slight increase in the incidence of this disease over the years.

ETIOLOGY

The etiology of most tumors of the maxilla is not known. The rarity of the disease in the general population makes identification of an increased risk factor difficult and it has usually been based on the recognition of a few cases in an exposed group. Workers in the nickel refining industry have a risk of developing carcinoma of the maxilla up to 800 times greater than that of the general population. Other occupations in which there is an increased risk include chromic pigment manufacturing, mustard gas manufacturing, and isopropyl alcohol production. Workers in the furniture, woodworking, and boot manufacturing industries also seem to be in a higher risk group (Schottenfeld and Fraumeni, 1982).

Various lesions such as polyps, chronic sinusitis, and hypertrophic changes in the mucosa of the sinus itself have been suggested as leading to the development of carcinoma. The only lesion that has been proved to be associated with the development of paranasal sinus carcinoma is the inverted papilloma of the mucosa, which may become malignant after multiple recurrences over several years (Lawson and associates, 1983) or may contain carcinoma on histologic examination (Weissler and associates, 1986). Previous radiation for other tumors in the area such as retinoblastoma in childhood (Rowe, Lane, and Snow, 1980) and fibrous dysplasia of the maxilla may also have as a sequela an increased incidence of osteogenic sarcoma of the maxilla. Burkitt's (1958) lymphoma, which may involve the maxilla or mandible and present as a malignant tumor, is associated with infection by the Epstein-Barr virus.

CLASSIFICATION

Neoplasms of the maxilla may be divided into three main groups: carcinomas, sarcomas, and odontogenic tumors (Table 68–1).

PATHOLOGY

In a review of the histologic diagnosis of malignant tumors of the nose and paranasal sinuses in 840 cases, 792 (92 per cent) involved the maxilla (Sakai, Fuchihata, and Hamasaki, 1976). Of their cases 70 per cent were squamous cell carcinoma, 3 per cent were adenocarcinoma, 1.2 per cent were adenocystic carcinoma, and 4 per cent were anaplastic carcinomas. Mucoepidermoid carcinoma (0.6 per cent) and transitional cell carcinoma (0.7 per cent) made up the remainder of the carcinomas in the series. In the sarcoma group, which constituted 4.5 per cent of the entire series, the most common was reticulum cell sarcoma (1.4 per cent). Twenty-one per cent of the tumors in the series were not histologically classified.

The predominant morphologic type, squamous cell carcinoma (Fig. 68–1), arises from the pseudostratified columnar epithelium lining the sinus. The next most common tumor, the adenocarcinoma, has its origin in the mucus-secreting glands of this same mucous membrane lining. The maxilla may also be invaded by secondary extensions of tumors, which may be benign or malignant, such as osteomas, ossifying fibromas, osteogenic sarcoma, and chondrosarcoma (Fig. 68–2). Tu-

Table 68–1. Classification of Maxillary Neoplasms

Carcinomas	Squamous cell carcinoma
	Adenocarcinoma
	Adenoid cystic carcinoma (formerly basal cell epithelioma)
	Mucoepidermoid carcinoma
	Anaplastic carcinoma
	Transitional cell carcinoma
Sarcomas	Reticulum cell sarcoma
	Osteogenic sarcoma
	Chondrosarcoma
	Fibrosarcoma
	Liposarcoma
	Rhabdomyosarcoma
Odontogenic tumors	Odontoma
	Ameloblastoma
Others	Melanoma
	Lymphoma
	Burkitt's lymphoma
	Metastatic

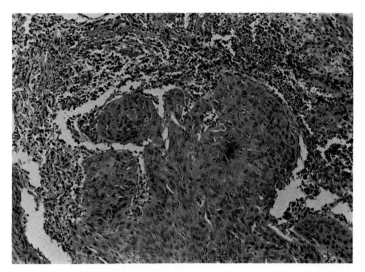

Figure 68–1. Photomicrograph of squamous cell carcinoma of the maxillary sinus.

mors of similar pathology may arise in adjacent sinus cavities or the palate and invade the maxilla by direct extension.

The paper-thin, bony walls and the confined anatomy of the region allow early involvement of these structures with invasion of surrounding soft tissues, and the exact site of origin may be difficult to determine.

Metastases

The anatomic factors mentioned above account for the high incidence of death by local invasion of vital structures rather than by metastases. Autopsy findings demonstrate that only 25 per cent of patients with maxillary carcinoma show evidence of spread beyond the local area. The silent invasion of adjacent structures is additionally complicated by the lymphatic drainage of the maxillary sinus to clinically inaccessible lymph nodes in the retropharyngeal space, and only later to the superior cervical nodes. Tumors that involve the superior and medial walls of the antrum tend to metastasize to the retropharyngeal group, while cancers involving the floor and lateral wall of the antrum may metastasize to cervical lymph nodes, which are more readily palpable (Robin and Powell, 1980). In the Memorial Hospital series (Lewis and Castro, 1972), 15 per cent of patients presenting with this disease complex had palpable cervical lymph nodes, and another 14 per cent developed lymph node metastases during the follow-up period.

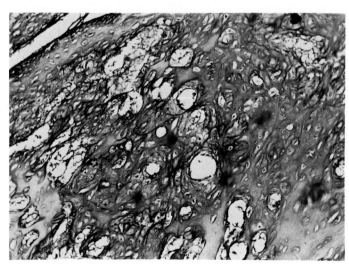

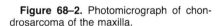

Figure 68–2. Photomicrograph of chondrosarcoma of the maxilla.

EXAMINATION AND DIAGNOSIS

Early symptoms and signs of paranasal tumors may be confused with those of acute and chronic inflammation or allergic conditions of the upper respiratory tract, and thus many neoplasms are far advanced before they produce definitive symptoms. As a result, cancer of the maxilla is rarely diagnosed early in its course, a factor leading to its poor prognosis.

The most common symptoms and signs are as follows but they do not necessarily occur in this sequence.

Pain. Pain is not a prominent early symptom, although there may be a complaint of discomfort over the maxillary sinus aggravated at night by the recumbent position. Pain in the upper molar teeth, especially if it is not relieved by tooth extraction, may be significant, and as the destructive lesion advances to the pterygopalatine and infratemporal fossae, severe pain may be experienced over the eye and cheek as the trigeminal nerve branches become involved.

External Swelling. This occurs as the tumor increases in size, involving the cheek and the periorbital tissues with upward displacement of the globe, and interfering with eye muscle function. The palate may be expanded and the buccogingival sulcus obliterated by direct extension of tumor. Such swelling is a late manifestation of the disease and indicates the erosion of bony walls and the spread of tumor into surrounding soft tissues. This may be accompanied by local signs of cellulitis and osteomyelitis.

Unilateral Nasal Obstruction. This may be partial or complete, accompanied by a sense of fullness in the nose. It is a common presenting symptom, indicating expansion of the medial wall of the maxilla into the nasal cavity. There may be accompanying symptoms such as mucopurulent or serosanguineous nasal discharge and hemorrhage.

Other less frequent symptoms and signs include excessive lacrimation, a fetid odor, disturbances in olfaction, paresthesia or anesthesia in the distribution of the infraorbital nerve, increasing nasality, and trismus.

A high index of suspicion toward the following relatively insignificant symptoms is essential to improve the low cure rate of this disease:

1. Pain in the maxillary sinus or upper teeth out of proportion to clinical findings, with or without tenderness of the teeth on biting or occlusal percussion.

2. Complaints of poor-fitting dentures, caused by expansion of the underlying bone or obliteration of the buccal sulcus.

3. Dull pain in the maxilla that increases in the recumbent position.

4. Chronic nasal polyps, particularly when accompanied by excessive hemorrhage. All polypoid and presumably benign tissue removed from the nose should be submitted for histopathologic examination.

5. Nasal obstruction of recent onset, usually unilateral but occasionally bilateral.

6. Recurrent mucopurulent, serosanguineous discharge or epistaxis.

7. Chronic sinus infection that fails to respond to adequate local and systemic therapy within a reasonable time.

8. Unilateral swelling of the cheek, with or without tenderness.

Patients who present with these symptoms or signs, particularly those in an older age group, should not be dismissed until the presence of paranasal sinus cancer has been excluded.

Radiographic Examination

In the asymptomatic patient, early tumors of the maxilla are occasionally identified by the alert dentist interpreting routine dental radiographs. If available, preexisting dental radiographs should be obtained and evaluated, as they may provide an indication of the site of origin.

Before the development of the computed tomographic (CT) scan, neoplasms of the maxilla were diagnosed by conventional radiography and tomography, which were of value only when there were bony changes produced by the tumor.

Computed tomography (Fig. 68–3) without the addition of contrast material provides significant information to the clinician even in early cases and makes it possible to pinpoint the location of the tumor when no physical signs are evident. The technique also allows the treating physician to correlate tumor extension into the orbit, ethmoid sinuses, pterygopalatine fossa, and nasal cavity, as demonstrated by CT changes, with clinical findings; treatment planning is thus more precise and surprises in the operating room are kept to a minimum. Retropharyngeal lymph node disease may also be visual-

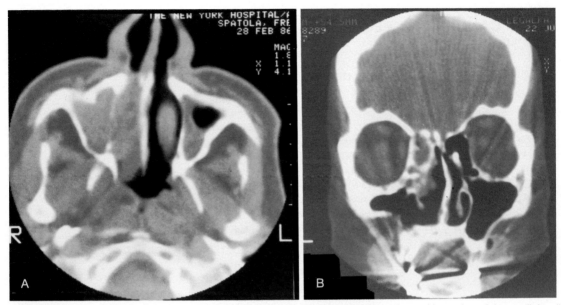

Figure 68–3. CT scans. *A,* Axial cut demonstrating a tumor of the right maxillary sinus with erosion of the medial wall and extension into the nose. *B,* Coronal cut with evidence of a tumor of the maxillary and ethmoid sinuses and nasal cavity.

ized at an early stage, permitting the radiation therapist to plan treatment fields accordingly.

CT examination is also useful in the monitoring of the postmaxillectomy patient, and recurrent disease may be detected much earlier than by physical examination. A baseline examination should be obtained after complete healing has occurred. Any alteration in the appearance of the CT scan should be followed by biopsy (Som, Shugar, and Biller, 1982). This type of examination is not a substitute for meticulous follow-up at frequent intervals, in view of the high local recurrence rate in malignant disease of the paranasal sinuses.

Follow-up examination consists of visual examination of the operative defect with careful digital palpation. It should be ascertained from the patient at each visit whether there is any change in the fit and comfort of the prosthesis.

The detection of recurrent disease on both clinical and radiologic grounds is rendered more difficult by the postradiation sequelae, which are an accompaniment of a full cancericidal course of radiation therapy in this location.

The continuing development of magnetic resonance imaging (MRI) will, in the future, provide valuable information about the soft tissue component of these tumors, their origin, and their spread. The evaluation of bone changes, in terms of both destruction and deformity, still necessitates the use of the CT scan.

Biopsy

A definitive diagnosis of a neoplasm is established only by biopsy of suspected tumor and examination of the pathologic material obtained. The physical examination and CT findings provide information indicating where the biopsy should be made and the optimal surgical approach to be used. In some individuals the procedure is made simple because of the breakthrough of tumor into the nasal cavity, the overlying skin, or the palate, these areas being readily accessible by punch biopsy, aspiration biopsy, or maxillary sinus irrigation. In the maxillary sinus itself adequate material may be obtained by a Caldwell-Luc approach through the anterior wall of the maxilla. Fine needle aspiration biopsy may also provide sufficient tissue to enable the pathologist to make a diagnosis without the necessity for a preliminary surgical procedure. Definitive surgery should be performed only in the presence of a positive biopsy of malignant disease, and the resection, performed soon thereafter, should include the previous biopsy site.

STAGING OF PARANASAL SINUS CANCER BY SPECIFIC ANATOMIC SITE

American Joint Committee on Cancer Classification, 1983

Using the anatomic plane originally described by Öhngren (1933), as illustrated in Figure 68–4, the maxillary sinus may be divided into an anteroinferior portion or infrastructure and a superoposterior portion or suprastructure. Staging of the disease is determined by the evaluation of a physical examination of the head and neck, including indirect laryngoscopy and nasal pharyngoscopy. A complete radiographic study of the paranasal sinuses, a biopsy of the primary tumor, and a chest radiograph are also necessary. The primary tumor classification is as follows:

T-X. Minimal requirements to assess the primary tumor cannot be met.

T-0. No evidence of tumor.

T-1. Tumor confined to the antral mucosa of the infrastructure with no bone erosion or destruction.

T-2. Tumor confined to the suprastructure mucosa without bone destruction, or to the infrastructure with destruction of the medial or inferior bony walls only.

T-3. More extensive tumor invading the

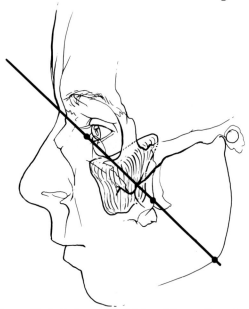

Figure 68–4. Radiographic division of the maxillary sinus into an anteroinferior (infrastructure) and superoposterior (suprastructure) portion (Öhngren, 1933). The line extends from the medial canthus to the angle of the mandible.

skin of the cheek, the orbit, the anterior ethmoid sinuses, or the pterygoid muscles.

T-4. Massive tumor with invasion of the cribriform plate, the posterior ethmoids, the sphenoid, the nasopharynx, the pterygoid plate, or the base of the skull.

The classification of the cervical nodes and distant metastases is the same as that for other tumors of the head and neck (see Chap. 70).

TREATMENT

The modern treatment of this highly lethal form of cancer involves the judicious use of a trimodal therapy consisting of surgery, radiation, and chemotherapy.

After the diagnosis has been established, the site of origin of the neoplasm and the extent of invasion of adjacent structures should be determined as accurately as possible. A careful study of the CT films and the clinical findings enables the surgeon to construct a three-dimensional picture of the extent of the disease process and to plan the optimal treatment sequence.

The earliest recorded methods of treatment of maxillary cancer were surgical. The results were discouraging but with the development of radiation therapy, they became more acceptable. Results of treatment by radiation therapy alone also proved to be disappointing, with a 15 per cent five year cure rate (Frazell and Lewis, 1963). The cancericidal doses of radiation in this region using the equipment available at that time led to serious complications, such as panophthalmitis and ocular edema, with subsequent loss of the eye in many patients. Radiation necrosis of the bony structures in the radiation field was also a problem accompanied by severe pain and chronic drainage. Modern radiation therapy plays an important role in the overall management of the disease and may again become the primary treatment of choice (Catterall, Blake, and Rampling, 1984).

At the present time the treatment of malignant tumors of the paranasal sinuses consists of surgical resection followed by radiation therapy and chemotherapy. A three year survival rate of 85.2 per cent and a five year survival rate of 71.1 per cent were obtained in a series of 52 cases of squamous cell carcinoma treated with surgery, radiation therapy, and chemotherapy (Konno, Togawa, and Inoue, 1980). The chemotherapeutic agents most commonly used have been methotrexate, bleomycin, 5-fluorouracil (5-FU), and (more recently) cisplatin. The arterial infusion of 5-FU and methotrexate has been combined with radiation therapy in some advanced lesions with an acceptable long-term survival (Goepfert, Jesse, and Lindberg, 1973).

Surgery

Operative treatment of this disease is planned by careful analysis of the CT scans to resect the entire disease process without transgression of the tumor itself. The involved tissues may include the contents of the orbit, the ethmoid air cells, the lateral and medial pterygoid muscles, and the contents of the pterygopalatine and infratemporal fossae. If the overlying skin is involved, this also requires resection. When the tumor is found to approach closely or extend beyond the margins of the en bloc resection, the patient is given radiation therapy in the immediate postoperative period. In far advanced T-4 disease, consideration should be given to a combined craniofacial approach (see Chap. 69) (Wilson and Westbury, 1973).

Such radical procedures are surprisingly well tolerated by the patients. The mortality rate for these lesions is reported as 10 per cent, four out of eight patients surviving for five years (Terz, Young, and Lawrence, 1980).

Position and Anesthesia. The procedure is performed with the patient in the supine position, the head of the table being moderately elevated to reduce venous pressure and subsequent bleeding. In addition, hypotensive anesthesia with arterial line monitoring reduces total blood loss, lowering the need for blood transfusion. The respiratory tract is protected by the use of an inflatable cuff on the endotracheal tube in combination with oropharyngeal packing.

Surgical Procedures. The choice of the surgical procedure depends on the preoperative evaluation of the patient, as described above. The findings of the CT scan may enable the surgeon to modify the procedure to preserve, for example, the hard palate or the orbital floor, depending on the location and extent of the tumor. In smaller tumors a complete maxillectomy is not mandatory; without it, the postoperative morbidity is reduced and the quality of life after the sur-

gery is improved (Sessions and Humphreys, 1983).

The pathologic condition also influences surgical planning; those tumors known to be more aggressive with a higher local recurrence rate, e.g., osteogenic sarcomas, require more extensive procedures (Russ and Jesse, 1980).

The surgical techniques may be one of four types:

1. Total maxillectomy with orbital resection.
2. Total maxillectomy preserving the eye but resecting the floor of the orbit.
3. Maxillectomy with preservation of the floor of the orbit.
4. Subtotal maxillectomy in which the procedure is modified according to the location of the tumor and to a certain extent the pathologic diagnosis.

Total Maxillectomy. It is advisable to obtain the preoperative consent of the patient for the removal of the eye regardless of the type of procedure planned, although it should be explained that every effort will be made to preserve the eye.

Before surgery the eyelids should be sutured together with a lid occlusal suture to protect the cornea during the operation.

The initial incision follows the classic Weber-Fergusson-Longmire approach to expose the anterior surface of the maxilla. The procedure begins with a lip-splitting incision offset at the vermilion border and extended upward along the lateral fold of the philtrum into the alar groove. It is continued in the paranasal angle to within 2 mm of the medial canthus, then laterally below the palpebral margin to the zygoma (Fig. 68–5). The incision is extended to the bone along its entire length. When invasion of the zygoma is suspected, the incision is extended laterally to expose this area. If it becomes necessary to reflect the nose to obtain better exposure, particularly if involvement of the ethmoid sinuses is suspected, the incision is carried medially across the nasofrontal angle from its apex and the nasal bones are mobilized with an osteotome. In the intraoral location the incision begins at the superior aspect of the lip split after extraction of the incisor teeth, and is extended laterally and posteriorly in the buccogingival sulcus until the tuberosity of the maxilla is reached. If a previous Caldwell-Luc procedure has been performed for diagnostic purposes, the entire healed incision must be included in the re-

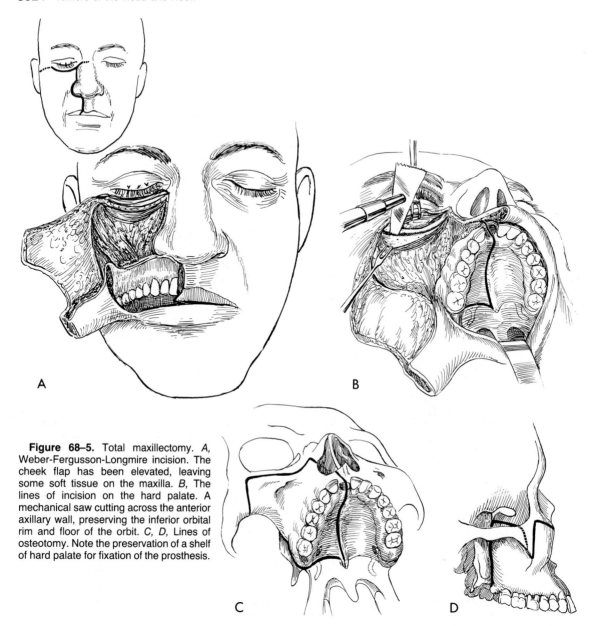

Figure 68–5. Total maxillectomy. *A,* Weber-Fergusson-Longmire incision. The cheek flap has been elevated, leaving some soft tissue on the maxilla. *B,* The lines of incision on the hard palate. A mechanical saw cutting across the anterior axillary wall, preserving the inferior orbital rim and floor of the orbit. *C, D,* Lines of osteotomy. Note the preservation of a shelf of hard palate for fixation of the prosthesis.

section. The cheek flap formed in this fashion is reflected laterally. If it is considered that the anterior wall of the maxilla is involved with tumor, an adequate margin of subcutaneous tissue should be left on the bone, and if the tumor has already invaded the overlying skin, the excision should include the involved area with an adequate margin of uninvolved tissue. The sacrifice of skin will necessitate an additional reconstructive procedure at the conclusion of the resection.

The next step in the procedure is the division of the hard palate, and depending on the location of the tumor, the palate is divided leaving a shelf of bone on the side of the tumor, if possible; this makes the future positioning of the palatal prosthesis more stable. Examination of the dry skull confirms that in most examples of this disease a portion of the hard palate on the ipsilateral side is readily preserved. The incision is extended to the bone with either a scalpel or a cautery knife (Fig. 68–5*A,B*) and carried laterally following the posterior border of the hard palate until the tuberosity of the maxilla is again reached; this joins the incision on the palate with that already made in the buccal sulcus. Bleeding may be encountered at this point owing to the division of the descending palatine artery as it exits from the greater palatine foramen. This is controlled by inserting the electrocautery point into the foramen.

The bony hard palate is next divided with either a chisel, a Gigli saw, a Stryker saw, or an air driven cutting drill. The junction of the nasal bone and the frontal process of the maxilla is divided and the osteotomy is continued laterally below the orbital rim to the zygoma when it is planned to preserve the floor of the orbit (Fig. 68–5C,D). With the same technique the maxilla is separated from the prominence of the zygoma, which should be preserved when possible to enhance the esthetic result. The pterygomaxillary disimpaction that is necessary to complete the mobilization of the maxilla is accomplished by the use of a curved osteotome placed between the maxilla and the pterygoid process. All bony connections between the maxilla and the surrounding skull should have been divided at this point, and the maxilla may be removed. The judicious use of an osteotome and a mallet assist in this maneuver. Gentle mobilization of the bone is necessary to avoid breaking into tumor. Hemorrhage is controlled with a pack, which is withdrawn slowly, exposing the terminal branches of the pterygopalatine portion of the internal maxillary artery. Vessels should be clamped and ligated where possible; however, electrocoagulation of some vessels and suture ligatures may be necessary. To complete the procedure the mucoperichondrium of the septum is removed (Fig. 68–6A) and a split-thickness skin graft is sutured to the wound edges and held in place by packing (Fig. 68–6B). A prosthesis is inserted to hold the packing in place (Fig.

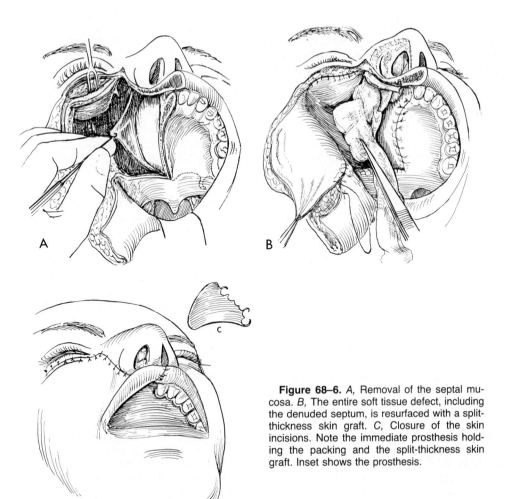

Figure 68–6. *A,* Removal of the septal mucosa. *B,* The entire soft tissue defect, including the denuded septum, is resurfaced with a split-thickness skin graft. *C,* Closure of the skin incisions. Note the immediate prosthesis holding the packing and the split-thickness skin graft. Inset shows the prosthesis.

68–6C) and closure of the external wound is completed.

The procedure as described above is indicated for tumors involving the lower maxilla or infrastructure, and should be modified to resect the floor of the orbit if the tumor is in the upper portion of the maxilla. The resection is completed through the inferior orbital fissure and is modified to resect the anterior and posterior ethmoid sinuses if the tumor approaches these structures. The entire cavity is lined by a split-thickness skin graft held in place by suitable packing and a prosthesis supplied by the prosthodontist.

Exenteration of Orbit. This procedure, indicated for tumors that originate in the upper portion of the maxillary sinus, involves removal of the orbital contents in continuity with the maxilla and the anterior and posterior ethmoid sinuses. The decision to perform orbital exenteration and maxillectomy is made after careful clinical examination, looking for signs of involvement of the orbit as evidenced by muscle dysfunction, proptosis, and displacement of the globe. CT scans provide further information regarding the necessity for the more radical procedure (location of the tumor in the superior portion of the maxilla, or bony destruction of the floor or medial wall of the orbit).

The basic incisions outlined above are employed with modifications. A double-limbed incision is made to circumscribe the palpebral margin, leaving the skin containing the lashes on the specimen. The upper lid is elevated from the tarsus to the superior orbital rim. At this point the periosteum is incised and with an elevator the periosteum is separated from the roof of the orbit until the optic nerve is reached. The subperiosteal dissection is continued until the anterior and posterior ethmoid foramina are visualized. In radical maxillectomy it is advisable to include the anterior and posterior ethmoid sinuses in the resection, and care should be taken to avoid injury to the cribriform plate, the level of which is located just below a line joining the anterior and posterior ethmoid foramina. Using an osteotome, one can separate the anterior and posterior ethmoid air cells from the frontal bone, the osteotome entering the nasal cavity. If the tumor extends through the posterior wall of the maxilla or through the inferior orbital fissure into the infratemporal fossa, as determined in advance by examination of the CT scans, resection of the pterygoid process with the lateral and medial pterygoid muscles is indicated. The zygomatic arch is severed more laterally, close to the articulation with the temporal bone (Fig. 68–7A,B). As a final step the optic stalk is divided (Fig. 68–7C). The specimen may be removed; bleeding is controlled by the insertion of a pack, which is slowly removed, and the bleeding vessels are ligated securely.

Closing of Wound. After bleeding has been controlled, a meticulous search is made for evidence of residual cancer. Any suspicious areas are excised and submitted for frozen section, and further resection is performed if indicated. The wound is then ready for closure. As mentioned above, the entire cavity should be lined with a split-thickness skin graft, preferably as a single sheet, to obtain prompt postoperative healing; this reduces the morbidity, improves the cosmetic result, and makes the early tolerance of a dental prosthesis possible. Skin grafts may be applied to exposed bone, the cheek flap, the dura, and the cerebral cortex if this is exposed, as it may be in the middle cranial fossa.

A dual set-up is used to obtain the graft, the donor site selected being non–hair-bearing wherever possible. The graft is applied to all raw areas and is held in place by sutures and appropriately placed packing. The skin flap is returned to its original position and closed with interrupted nylon sutures.

It is the opinion of the authors that the defect should not be reconstructed after the orbital contents have been removed, but allowed to remain open to facilitate observation of the area for possible local recurrence. The cavity also provides for the more stable fitting of a cosmetic prosthesis. If it is elected not to use an eye prosthesis, an eye patch provides adequate camouflage of the defect. In addition, the delivery of the planned radiation therapy is more accurate and it is not delayed by the need to complete a reconstructive procedure.

Postoperative Management. At the completion of the procedure before the patient is extubated, a nasogastric tube is inserted, the oral packing is removed, and the pharynx is inspected and aspirated. A tracheostomy is rarely necessary in a standard maxillectomy. However, if there is any possibility of obstruction to the airway from postoperative edema or if a radical neck dissection is to be performed at the same time, a tracheostomy may be indicated.

A high protein, high calorie diet is admin-

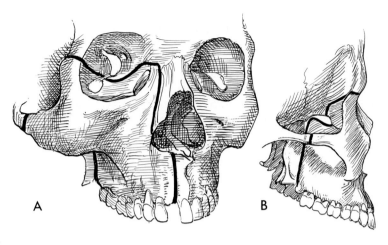

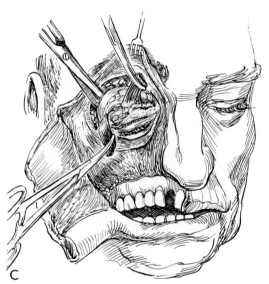

Figure 68–7. Total maxillectomy with orbital exenteration. *A, B,* Lines of osteotomy. Note that the entire floor of the orbit is resected. *C,* En bloc removal of the orbital contents and maxilla.

istered for three to four days postoperatively through the nasogastric tube, which may be removed as soon as swallowing is resumed. This function requires the provision of a palatal prosthesis, which enables the patient to swallow liquid and soft foods. Solid foods usually are not taken until the permanent dental prosthesis has been prepared and inserted, a task that may take several weeks.

The pack is removed from the operative defect in five to six days, and thereafter the operative area is scrupulously cleansed daily, being irrigated with dilute solutions of hydrogen peroxide and warm saline. The packing is replaced at each dressing to prevent shrinkage of the cavity and contraction of the cheek flap. Impressions for the insertion of a transitional appliance are obtained as soon as the patient can tolerate manipulation in the operative site; preoperative dental impressions facilitate the early construction of such an appliance. As the tissues heal, adjustments are made by the prosthodontist to aid in the closure of the defect and retention of the appliance. The presence of sound teeth on the remaining alveolus enhances the ability of the patient to maintain a stable prosthesis, as does the presence of a palatal shelf on the ipsilateral side. In the completely edentulous patient, various undercuts in the operative field can be utilized, and the sealing function of the soft palate can be employed for retention of the prosthesis. The acceptance and successful management of a prosthetic device by the patient depend to a large extent on the interest and ingenuity of the prosthodontist.

When the disease process involves the soft tissues in the skin overlying the maxilla, it may be necessary to sacrifice the skin. At times the lip may be involved and also resected in continuity with the maxilla. This type of substantial defect that interferes with function necessitates some form of immediate reconstruction. The surgeon has a choice of several readily available myocutaneous flaps and microvascular free flaps as discussed in Chapters 29 and 70.

MAXILLECTOMY VIA A MIDFACIAL DEGLOVING INCISION

The midfacial degloving technique (Casson, Bonanno, and Converse, 1974) may be employed as a surgical approach for either subtotal or total maxillectomy, including removal of the orbital floor (Fig. 68–8). The

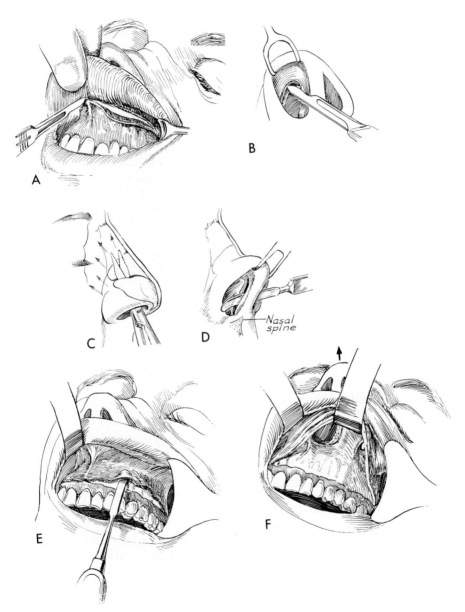

Figure 68–8. The midfacial degloving technique. *A,* Incision in the labiogingival sulcus. *B,* Intercartilaginous incision. *C,* Elevation of the soft tissue. *D,* Transfixion incision that communicates with the labiogingival incision. *E, F,* Elevation of the soft tissue over the anterior wall of the maxilla.

technique has the advantage of avoiding external incisions and, when used with an immediately fitted prosthodontic appliance, it provides rapid rehabilitation of the patient. The technique is reserved for patients who show no evidence of involvement of the infraorbital nerve or extraocular muscles, conjunctival edema, diplopia, trismus, or facial skin invasion. The surgical approach combines a buccal incision with a transfixion incision and separates the membranous from the cartilaginous septum and the lateral wall of the nose as far superiorly as the level of the nasal bones. It permits the complete exposure of the maxilla to the level of the orbital rim and the zygomatic process of the temporal

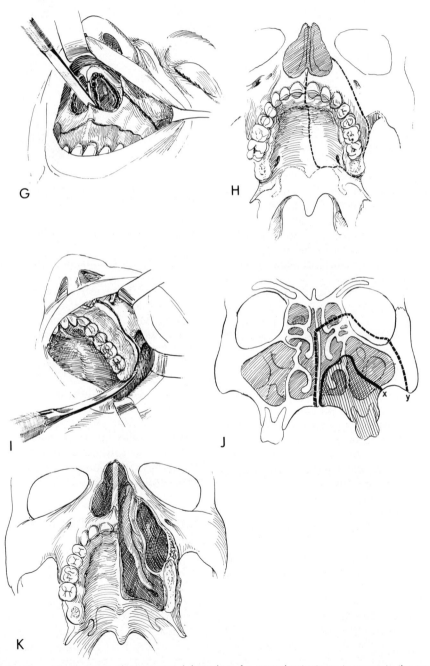

Figure 68–8 *Continued G, H,* Lines of osteotomy. *I,* Insertion of a curved osteotome to separate the posterior wall of the maxilla from the pterygoid process. *J,* Lines of resection: *x,* subtotal maxillectomy; *y,* total maxillectomy. *K,* Resulting defect.

bone (Fig. 68–8*A–F*). The appropriate osteotomies may then be performed under direct vision (Figs. 68–8*G–K*, 68–9). Feeding tubes are not used and the patient is permitted a liquid diet when recovery from anesthesia is complete (Figs. 68–10, 68–11).

Radiation Therapy

The place of radiation therapy in the management of tumors of the maxilla has varied over the years. The treatment of choice in the 1930's, it was superseded by surgery because of the disappointing comparative results (Frazell and Lewis, 1963). The techniques were primitive by present-day standards. Modern supervoltage therapy either alone (Shibuya and associates, 1984) or as a planned postoperative adjuvant (Korzeniowski, Reinfuss, and Skoyszewski, 1985) is providing cure rates in the 35 per cent range, even in patients with T-4 stage disease. Some clinicians have favored preoperative radiation therapy using dosages of 5000 to 6000 rads, five year survival rates being in the 28 per cent range. If no residual disease is found in the operative specimen by the pathologist, a 67 per cent five year survival rate has been reported (Bridger, Beale, and Bryce, 1978). In another series a 43 per cent five year survival rate was noted if it was possible to spare the eye, and only 10 per cent if an orbital resection was necessary (Som, 1974).

In preplanned postoperative radiation therapy, treatment is started as soon as healing of the surgical site has occurred; it should begin within three to four weeks of surgery.

The surgeon and the radiation therapist both participate in treatment planning. If residual disease or narrow surgical margins are known to be present after examination of the surgical specimen, these areas are marked for more concentrated therapy. If there is cervical node disease and a neck dissection has been performed, the neck should also be treated postoperatively. This approach may reduce the high recurrence rate that follows therapeutic node dissection (Shingaki and associates, 1985).

Promising results have also been reported with fast neutron therapy. A 94 per cent regression rate in 31 patients was noted with now obsolete equipment; most treatment failures were due to metastatic disease (Catterall, Blake, and Rampling, 1984).

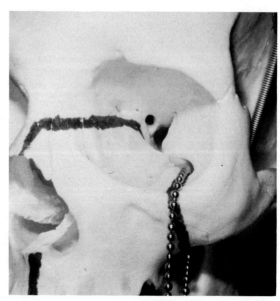

Figure 68–9. Limits of the bony resection (midfacial degloving technique). The Gigli saw is introduced at the level of the infraorbital fissure.

Adjuvant Chemotherapy

At present the best results in managing malignant tumors of the maxilla are obtained with a combination of surgical resection of the lesion followed by postoperative radiation therapy and adjuvant chemotherapy. Commonly used agents include bleomycin and methotrexate (Moseley and associates, 1981), 5-FU (Sakai and associates, 1983), and cisplatin (Carter, 1977).

Regional perfusion is the most popular method of chemotherapy administration in these patients; this route is advocated because high levels of drug concentration are achieved. Significant palliation and prolonged survival may be achieved (Goepfert, Jesse, and Lindberg, 1973).

Management of Cervical Metastases

The incidence of cervical node metastases with squamous cell carcinoma of the maxillary sinus is 10 to 20 per cent and varies according to the tumor stage at the initial presentation (Frazell and Lewis, 1963; Robin and Powell, 1980). If enlarged lymph nodes are palpable at the time of surgery, a radical neck dissection should be performed at the same time as the maxillectomy. If lymph nodes prove positive on pathologic examina-

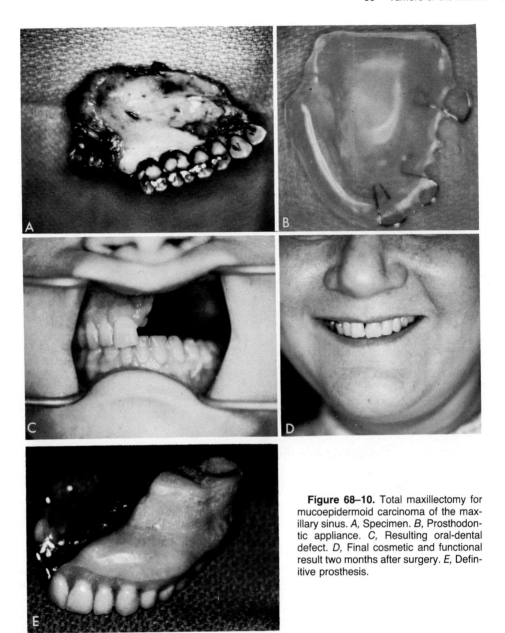

Figure 68–10. Total maxillectomy for mucoepidermoid carcinoma of the maxillary sinus. *A*, Specimen. *B*, Prosthodontic appliance. *C*, Resulting oral-dental defect. *D*, Final cosmetic and functional result two months after surgery. *E*, Definitive prosthesis.

tion of the neck dissection specimen, a full course of radiation therapy should be administered to the neck as soon as the incisions from the radical neck dissection have healed. If cervical lymph nodes become enlarged at any time after surgery, it should be assumed that they are involved with metastatic cancer. Aspiration needle biopsy (see Chap. 70) may help to establish the diagnosis, but if this technique is not available a radical neck dissection is indicated. When retropharyngeal lymph nodes are involved, the patient should be given radiation therapy and chemotherapy.

The presence of cervical node metastases at the time of surgery or during the period of follow-up is of serious import; an already unfavorable prognosis is worsened with a five year survival rate of 11.3 per cent (Lewis and Castro, 1972).

COMPLICATIONS

Surgical treatment of paranasal sinus cancer may be attended by serious complications, especially in the presence of previous radiation therapy. The extensive surgical expo-

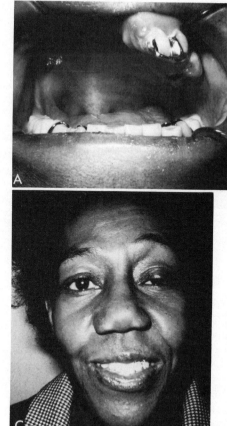
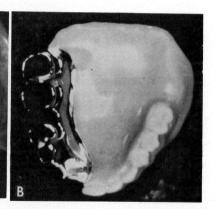

Figure 68–11. Bilateral subtotal maxillectomy for squamous cell carcinoma. *A,* Resultant defect. *B,* Large palatomaxillary prosthodontic appliance. *C,* Final appearance.

sure, the contiguity to vital structures, and contamination from the oral cavity are significant factors that contribute to the complications.

Bleeding. Hemorrhage during the procedure can be prevented by attention to anatomic details. Bleeding deep in the wound can be treated initially by packing, which is slowly removed, the bleeding being controlled by suture ligatures. Electrocoagulation may be necessary and, if all else fails, packing may be inserted and left in place for some days. Routine ligation of the external carotid artery is not recommended unless a neck dissection is being done, as it has little influence on the volume of bleeding that occurs.

Secondary hemorrhage, occurring five to seven days after the operation, is most commonly related to wound infection with the necrosis of the walls of large vessels that had been managed by electrocoagulation. This problem may be controlled by direct pressure, or a return to the operating room may be necessary.

Infection. Among the more serious post-operative complications of this type of surgery is wound sepsis. Despite the contamination that always exists, serious infection is a rare occurrence and failure of the skin graft is almost unknown. The administration of perioperative antibiotics significantly reduces the incidence of wound infection. If specific organisms are identified by culture and sensitivity studies, they should be treated with appropriate antibiotics. Frequent suction irrigation in the postoperative phase with solutions of saline and hydrogen peroxide is mandatory.

Wound Healing Problems. Every attempt is made to achieve primary wound healing by careful multilayered closure of the flaps, avoiding damage to tissues, and minimizing tension when the closure is completed.

Radiation Therapy. When radiation therapy has preceded the surgical procedure, skin damage and bone necrosis may be present and wound healing may be delayed. This is more significant if radiation treatment has failed and surgery is undertaken months or years after the original therapy. In the presence of an already precarious blood supply, it may be a wise decision by the surgeon to sacrifice the overlying skin and reconstruct the soft tissue defect at the completion of surgery. This problem should not arise in planned preoperative radiation therapy in which surgery six to eight weeks after completion of therapy is part of the overall treatment plan.

Diabetes Mellitus. Diabetes increases the problems of managing the postmaxillectomy patient. The incidence of wound infection and delayed healing is increased, and pre- and postoperative control of the disease is essential. In the severe diabetic patient, despite these measures, recovery can be associated with serious surgical and medical complications.

Nutritional Status. Some degree of preoperative nutritional insufficiency is encountered in many cancer patients. Attention should be given to improving the nutritional status of the patient before surgery with vitamin supplements and a high protein, high calorie diet. This approach helps promote wound healing and overall recovery. In the early postoperative period, tube feeding must be sufficient to maintain a positive nitrogen balance until the fitting of a dental prosthesis enables the patient to resume an adequate oral intake. Rapid oral rehabilitation promotes both physical and psychologic recovery.

Local Injuries. During the surgical procedure every precaution should be taken to avoid injury to surrounding structures.

Corneal Injury. This can be avoided by occlusive suturing of the lids before surgery or by insertion of a corneal shield. An ophthalmic ointment should be routinely instilled into the conjunctival sac before lid closure. Corneal abrasion must be treated with occlusive dressings and the appropriate instillation of ophthalmic ointment and drops.

Nerve Injury. Since the operative procedure is extensive and the dissection may not be along anatomic planes, injury to nerves may be unavoidable. The fifth and seventh nerves are at risk but remain a secondary consideration in relation to the more important goal of total excision of the tumor. Injury to the seventh cranial nerve occurs and usually involves specific peripheral branches. The frontalis and the orbital branches may be either weakened or paralyzed in the more aggressive resections when exposure is being obtained. Complete loss of muscle function is

rare and the spontaneous return of function commonly results within several months. The mandibular division of the fifth nerve is also at risk in the more extensive tumors when the contents of the infratemporal fossa are resected.

Trismus. This is an occasional distressing complication of maxillary surgery, often secondary to radiation fibrosis, although it may be the result of static spasm of the masseter, the pterygoid muscles, and the temporalis muscle. The late occurrence of trismus may also indicate recurrent disease involving the lateral and medial pterygoid muscles.

Injury to Dura Mater. If the cribriform plate is either resected or damaged during surgery, a cerebrospinal fluid leak results from injury to the dura. The leak may be controlled by a combination of suturing and the application of split-thickness skin grafts to the area. Decompression by continuous spinal drainage is indicated in the immediate postoperative period. If a leak persists despite these measures, neurosurgical intervention may become necessary.

Nasolacrimal Duct Obstruction. Transient or permanent obstruction of the lacrimal duct resulting in epiphora is a complication of both total and partial maxillectomy. It has been shown that the two areas most vulnerable to surgical injury are the lacrimal sac and duct located beneath the medial canthus tendon and the duct ostium in the inferior meatus. Dacryocystorhinostomy (see Chap. 34) is the procedure of choice in reestablishing drainage after a postoperative distal obstruction (Osguthorpe and Calcaterra, 1979).

Changes in Air-Conditioning Capacity of Nose. The ability of the nose to warm and humidify the inspiratory air may be lost after maxillectomy. This function is of importance in protecting the mucosa of the lower respiratory tract, and measurements of the air-conditioning capacity of the nose have shown that in maxillectomy patients there is a considerable reduction in the vaporization of inspired air compared with patients undergoing other head and neck surgical procedures (Drettner, Falck, and Simon, 1977).

Middle Ear Complications. Middle ear effusion is a predictable sequela of radical maxillectomy in which resection of part or all of the soft palate is necessary to eradicate the tumor. Removal of these structures causes a disturbance in palatal function, specifically the tensor veli palatini muscle. In one study,

80 per cent of individuals who underwent radical maxillectomy experienced middle ear and eustachian tube dysfunction after surgery, and 23 per cent were found to have developed a perforation of the tympanic membrane or required myringotomy and tube insertion to relieve a middle ear effusion (Myers and associates, 1984). The need to treat middle ear effusion in this population of patients is important, since sensory deficits frequently coexist in this age group.

Ophthalmic Complications. In patients who undergo total maxillectomy with preservation of the globe, the inferior and medial aspects of the orbit are deprived of normal bony support. Enophthalmos occurred in 100 per cent of patients reviewed; transient diplopia was noted in 37 per cent and a cicatricial ectropion in 32 per cent. Total visual loss occurred in 16 per cent and pseudoptosis in 15 per cent. In addition, permanent diplopia was observed in 11 per cent of the patients (Smith, Lisman, and Baker, 1984). Patients who are tumor free for 18 months after maxillectomy and in whom the symptoms are distressing should undergo bone graft reconstruction of the orbital floor.

POSTMAXILLECTOMY RECONSTRUCTION

In the uncomplicated maxillectomy without orbital resection or the sacrifice of overlying skin, the defect of the palate is readily corrected by a prosthetic appliance. This may be esthetically displeasing to the fastidious patient and a functioning reconstruction by a flap and bone grafting may be more appealing. The necessity for multistage procedures, plus debulking and adjustments to accept dental appliances, make such a reconstruction unjustifiable in the authors' opinion. A more direct reconstruction of palate defects by the use of a temporalis muscle flap and a skin graft has been reported, and may be of value in both immediate and delayed repair (Wolfe, 1987).

Major resections, in which the eye, palate, and cheek skin are absent, require immediate reconstruction to restore some semblance of function. Successful reconstruction of the palate through the facial defect has been possible for many years, using a variety of flaps from the forehead (Edgerton and DeVito, 1961) or neck (Bakamjian, 1963).

With the microvascular free flaps now available (see Chap. 29), there is adequate tissue to repair the palate, cheek, and orbital defect at the time of the resection in a single stage. The presence of such flaps may delay the detection of local recurrence; what influence this delay has on the final outcome is questionable. After every effort on the part of the surgeon, the radiotherapist, and the chemotherapist, it is unlikely that a cure will be effected by additional treatment.

REFERENCES

American Joint Committee on Cancer: Manual for Staging of Cancer. Philadelphia, J. B. Lippincott Company, 1983, p. 43.

Attenborough, N. R.: Maxillectomy via a temporal approach (a new technique). J. Laryngol. Otol., 94:149, 1980.

Bakamjian, V.: A technique for primary reconstruction of the palate after radical maxillectomy for cancer. Plast. Reconstr. Surg., 31:103, 1963.

Bridger, M. W. M., Beale, F. A., and Bryce, D. P.: Carcinoma of the paranasal sinuses—a review of 158 cases. J. Otolaryngol., 7:379, 1978.

Burkitt, D.: A sarcoma involving the jaw in African children. Br. J. Surg., 46:218, 1958.

Carter, S. K.: The chemotherapy of head and neck cancer. Semin. Oncol., 4:413, 1977.

Casson, P. R., Bonanno, P. C., and Converse, J. M.: The midface degloving procedure. Plast. Reconstr. Surg., 53:102, 1974.

Catterall, M., Blake, P. R., and Rampling, R. P.: Fast neutron treatment as an alternative to radical surgery for malignant tumours of the facial area. Br. Med. J., 289:1653, 1984.

Drettner, B., Falck, B., and Simon, H.: Measurements of the air conditioning capacity of the nose during normal and pathological conditions and pharmacological influence. Acta Otolaryngol. (Stockh.), 84:266, 1977.

Edgerton, M. T., and DeVito, R. V.: Reconstruction of palatal defects resulting from treatment of carcinoma of the palate, antrum or gingiva. Plast. Reconstr. Surg., 28:306, 1961.

Frazell, E. L., and Lewis, J. S.: Cancer of the nasal cavity and accessory sinuses. Cancer, 16:1293, 1963.

Goepfert, H., Jesse, R. H., and Lindberg, R.: Arterial infusion and radiation therapy in the treatment of advanced cancer of the nasal cavity and paranasal sinuses. Am. J. Surg., 126:464, 1973.

Konno, A., Togawa, K., and Inoue, S.: Analysis of the results of our combined therapy for maxillary cancer. Acta Otolaryngol. (Suppl.), 372:1, 1980.

Korzeniowski, S., Reinfuss, M., and Skoyszewski, J.: The evaluation of radiotherapy after incomplete surgery in patients with carcinoma of the maxillary sinus. Int. J. Radiat. Oncol. Biol. Phys., 11:505, 1985.

Lawson, W., Biller, H. F., Jacobson, A., and Som, P. M.: The role of conservative surgery in the management of inverted papilloma. Laryngoscope, 93:148, 1983.

Lewis, J. S., and Castro, E. B.: Cancer of the nasal cavity and paranasal sinuses. J. Laryngol. Otol., 86:255, 1972.

Moseley, H. S., Thomas, L. R., Everts, E. C., Stevens, K. R., and Ireland, K. M.: Advanced squamous cell carcinoma of the maxillary sinus. Results of combined regional infusion chemotherapy, radiation therapy and surgery. Am. J. Surg., *141*:522, 1981.

Myers, E. N., Beery, Q. C., Bluestone, C. D., Rood, S. R., and Sigler, B. A.: Effect of certain head and neck tumors and their management on the ventilatory function of the eustachian tube. Ann. Otol. Rhinol. Laryngol. (Suppl.), *114*:3, 1984.

Öhngren, L. G.: Malignant tumors of the maxillo-ethmoid region. Acta Otolaryngol. (Suppl.), *19*:1, 1933.

Osguthorpe, J. D., and Calcaterra, T. C.: Nasolacrimal obstruction after maxillary sinus and rhinoplastic surgery. Arch. Otolaryngol., *105*:264, 1979.

Robin, P. E., and Powell, D. J.: Regional node involvement and distant metastases in carcinoma of the nasal cavity and paranasal sinuses. J. Laryngol. Otol., *94*:301, 1980.

Rowe, L. D., Lane, R., and Snow, J. B., Jr.: Adenocarcinoma of the ethmoid following radiotherapy for bilateral retinoblastoma. Laryngoscope, *90*:61, 1980.

Russ, J. E., and Jesse, R. H.: Management of osteosarcoma of the maxilla and mandible. Am. J. Surg., *140*:572, 1980.

Sakai, S., Fuchihata, H., and Hamasaki, Y.: Treatment policy for maxillary sinus carcinoma. Acta Otolaryngol., *82*:172, 1976.

Sakai, S., Hohki, A., Fuchihata, A., and Tanaka, Y.: Multidisciplinary treatment of maxillary sinus carcinoma. Cancer, *52*:1360, 1983.

Schottenfeld, D., and Fraumeni, J. F., Jr.: Cancer Epidemiology and Prevention. Philadelphia, W. B. Saunders Company, 1982, p. 519.

Sessions, R. B., and Humphreys, D. H.: Technical modifications of the medial maxillectomy. Arch. Otolaryngol., *109*:575, 1983.

Shibuya, H., Horiuchi, J., Suzuki, S., Shioda, S., and Enomoto, S.: Maxillary sinus carcinoma: result of radiation therapy. Int. J. Radiat. Oncol. Biol. Phys., *10*:1021, 1984.

Shingaki, S., Saito, R., Kawasaki, T., and Nakajima, T.: Recurrence of carcinoma of the oral cavity, oropharynx and maxillary sinus after radical neck dissection. J. Maxillofac. Surg., *13*:231, 1985.

Smith, B., Lisman, R. D., and Baker, D.: Eyelid and orbital treatment following radical maxillectomy. Ophthalmology, *91*:218, 1984.

Som, M. L.: Surgical management of carcinoma of the maxilla. Arch. Otolaryngol., *99*:270, 1974.

Som, P. M., Shugar, J. M., and Biller, H. F.: The early detection of antral malignancy in the postmaxillectomy patient. Radiology, *143*:509, 1982.

Terz, J. J., Young, H. F., and Lawrence, W., Jr.: Combined craniofacial resection for locally advanced carcinoma of the head and neck. II. Carcinoma of the paranasal sinuses. Am. J. Surg., *140*:618, 1980.

Weissler, M. C., Montgomery, W. W., Turner, P. A., and Montgomery, S. K.: Inverted papilloma. Ann. Otol. Rhinol. Laryngol., *95*:215, 1986.

Wilson, J. S., and Westbury, G.: Combined craniofacial resection for tumour involving the orbital walls. Br. J. Plast. Surg., *26*:44, 1973.

Wolfe, A. S.: Use of temporalis muscle for closure of palatal defects. Presented at American Association of Plastic Surgery annual meeting, Nashville, TN, May, 1987.

69

Ian T. Jackson
Kevin Shaw

Tumors of the Craniofacial Skeleton, Including the Jaws

Tumors of the jaws and the craniofacial skeleton include a diverse collection of benign and malignant lesions. This chapter provides a broad overview, with emphasis on the distinguishing features and the general principles of management, followed by a more detailed description of surgical planning and individual procedures. Many of the tumors can extend to multiple other areas of the facial skeleton and thus necessitate complex and extensive resections. Application of craniofacial surgical techniques to the more extensive and aggressive neoplasms has permitted more effective resections and has improved prognosis.

CYSTS AND TUMORS OF MANDIBLE AND MAXILLA

Cysts and tumors of the mandible and maxilla, excluding those of the paranasal sinuses, may be broadly classified as *odontogenic* or *nonodontogenic*. Within these two categories, there is considerable diversification. The term odontogenic is applied to lesions composed of cells normally involved in tooth development. These can be subclassified into two groups: odontogenic cysts and odontogenic tumors. They are unique to the jaws, the majority being benign. Classification controversies have led to the development of several systems. The classification proposed by Reichart and Ries (1983) is used below; it is based on the histologic and embryologic aspects of tooth development.

Tooth Development

A brief description of tooth development allows better understanding of odontogenic lesions. In the 37 day old human embryo, U-shaped bands of thickened epithelium develop in each jaw and form a series of ingrowths into the underlying ectomesenchyme (McDaniel, 1987). The epithelial ingrowths represent the dental lamina, which divides in each tooth bud to form the enamel organ, which is composed of inner and outer enamel epithelium. The condensed ectomesenchyme beneath the enamel organ is the dental papilla, which forms the dentin and pulp. The ectomesenchyme that surrounds the dental papilloma and the enamel organ differentiates into the dental follicle. Odontoblasts develop in the dental papilla and begin to form dentin, which results in the tooth root. Cells of the inner enamel epithelium differentiate into ameloblasts and begin to secrete enamel. An epithelial structure, Hertwig's root sheath, surrounds the tooth within the periodontal ligament. This epithelial structure ultimately disintegrates, leaving islands of epithelial cells: the rests of Malassez. The ectomesenchymal cells of the dental follicle develop into cementoblasts, which secrete a layer of cementum on the root surface (Ten Cate, 1980). The dental lamina also disintegrates, leaving the epithelial rests of Serres and the dental lamina rests in the gingival tissues and dental follicles (Stout, Lunin, and Calonius, 1968). An uncommon histologic feature of the dental lamina is the presence of melanocytes (Lawson, Abaci, and Zak, 1976). These are thought to be of neural crest origin, and their presence may explain the finding of melanin in certain epithelial odontogenic lesions.

Cysts of Jaws

Cysts of the jaws may be classified into two types: those arising from odontogenic epithelium, *odontogenic cysts,* and those from oral epithelium, *fissural cysts,* the latter occurring at the sites of embryonic "fusion." In addition, a third category, *nonepithelial cysts,* includes traumatic and aneurysmal bone cysts (Shear, 1983). The stimulus causing proliferation of resting epithelial cells is unknown. Several factors have been suggested: inflammation, age (Stanley, Krogh, and Pannkuk, 1965), mechanical trauma, systemic disease, and increased local vascularity (Baden, Moskow, and Moskow, 1968). Some cysts, such as keratocysts, may be aggressive, causing destruc-

tion of large portions of the jaws, interference with dentition, and destruction of neighboring structures. Cysts do not usually cause resorption of the tooth roots; this finding suggests neoplasm. The epithelial lining of cysts may rarely undergo malignant or ameloblastic change. Thus, all cysts should be examined histologically (Browne, 1975). As a rule, cysts, unless infected, are not painful. Small cysts can be found incidentally on dental radiographs, whereas large lesions can occur as painless swellings with dental disruption, bone destruction, pathologic fracture, or facial deformity.

ODONTOGENIC CYSTS

These lesions are divided into developmental and inflammatory types.

Developmental Odontogenic Cysts

Gingival Cysts. Gingival cysts in *infants* are commonly found on the palate and the alveolar ridges (Cataldo and Berkman, 1968). In the palate, they are probably fissural, whereas alveolar lesions are derived from rests of dental lamina (Stout, Lunin, and Calonius, 1968). They may be solitary or multiple and range from 1 to 5 mm in diameter. The cysts contain keratin, which is usually discharged by 3 months of age without specific treatment (Moreillon and Schroeder, 1982).

Gingival cysts in *adults* account for less than 0.2 per cent of odontogenic cysts (Browne, 1972). These probably also originate from rests of dental lamina (Wysocki and associates, 1980). They are painless, circumscribed, slowly growing, gingival swellings, 1 to 15 mm in diameter (Buchner and Hansen, 1979). On palpation, they are soft and fluctuant; radiologically they may show superficial erosion of bone. Recurrence is rare after surgical excision.

Lateral Periodontal Cysts. These lesions account for approximately 2 per cent of odontogenic cysts (Browne, 1972) and probably arise from dental lamina rests (Wysocki and associates, 1980). They are usually asymptomatic, on radiographic study appear as ovoid radiolucencies with sharply defined margins located lateral to a tooth root, and are usually less than 1 cm in diameter. Most commonly, the canine or premolar mandibular teeth are involved (Grand and Marwah, 1964). Lateral periodontal cysts are lined by a thin, nonkeratinizing squamous epithelium, which contains glycogen-rich clear cells (Wysocki and associates, 1980). The tooth remains vital. Treatment is enucleation, and recurrence is rare.

Dentigerous Cysts. Dentigerous or follicular cysts make up approximately 18 per cent of jaw cysts and are second in frequency to radicular cysts (Shear, 1983). They are usually asymptomatic and appear as radiolucent unilocular cysts encircling the crown of an unerupted tooth (Struthers and Shear, 1976). They probably result from fluid accumulation between the reduced enamel epithelium and the enamel after the root crown has completely formed (Bhaskar, 1965). If infected, they occur as a painful swelling. They range in size from 2 to 10 cm in diameter. The largest ones may cause expansion of bone cortices and displacement of adjacent teeth with root resorption. The age range at the time of diagnosis is between 20 and 50 years (Shear, 1983). Sixty-six per cent occur in the mandible, usually in the third molar region (Dachi and Howell, 1961). In the maxilla, they are observed most commonly in the canine region. Dentigerous cysts are lined by a nonkeratinizing stratified squamous epithelium. They rarely undergo ameloblastic or malignant change (Browne, 1972).

Odontogenic Keratocyst. This lesion makes up approximately 9 per cent of odontogenic cysts (Shear, 1983). Also known as a primordial cyst, it is thought to develop from two sources: dental lamina rests and basal cell hamartomas of the overlying oral mucosa (Shear, 1983). This lesion is noteworthy for several reasons. The cyst lining is composed of keratinizing stratified squamous epithelium with a well-defined basal layer, and it may show epithelial dysplasia (Brannon, 1976). Odontogenic keratocysts range in size from 1 to 9 cm (Hodgkinson and associates, 1978). Large cysts may be destructive, resulting in expansion of the jaw cortices and perforation of the cortical plate. They are seen in association with the nevoid basal cell carcinoma syndrome described by Gorlin and Goltz (1960). Recurrence rates after excision range from 20 to 60 per cent (Shafer, Hine, and Levy, 1974).

The odontogenic keratocyst can occur at any age, but most commonly in patients between 20 and 50 years of age (Brannon, 1976). Men are affected approximately twice as often as women (Brannon, 1976). It occurs three times more frequently in the mandible than in the maxilla, and it is most commonly situated in the posterior portion; however, extensive lesions may cross the midline (Brannon, 1976). Keratocysts commonly present with swelling and drainage, but pain, paresthesias, and trismus may also occur (Brannon, 1976). The radiographic appearance is that of a radiolucent unilocular or multilocular cyst with sclerotic margins. In 7 per cent of cases, there are multiple cysts, especially in the nevoid basal cell carcinoma syndrome (Brannon, 1976). The latter syndrome is inherited as an autosomal dominant trait with marked penetrance and variable expressivity. Multiple basal cell carcinomas appear at an early age in association with multiple jaw cysts, skeletal anomalies, calcification of the falx cerebri, nasal deformity, and palmar or plantar pits (Gorlin and Goltz, 1960).

Reports of treatment modalities are scanty. Some have suggested careful enucleation with aggressive curettage and close follow-up; if the lesion recurs, bony resection with 1 cm margins is advised (Ellis and Fonseca, 1987). A constant fusion of the cystic wall with the oral mucosa along the anterior border of the ascending ramus has been reported. Recurrences may thus result from invasion of the oral epithelium into the bone (Moskow and associates, 1970). Thus, the overlying oral mucosa should be excised at the enucleation. In addition, inaccessible areas are cauterized with Carnoy's solution.

A separate variety of keratocyst bursts out of the ascending ramus into the infratemporal fossa, erodes the base of the skull, and extends into the middle cranial fossa. The patient has trismus and occasionally pain, and a typical appearance on radiography and computed tomographic (CT) scan is noted (Fig. 69–1). Treatment is by total parotidectomy with preservation of the facial nerve and, if possible, en bloc excision of the involved mandible, infratemporal fossa, base of the skull, and any of the lesion present in the middle cranial fossa. Lesser surgical excision will inevitably result in recurrence and inoperability. Death can occur from involvement of the cavernous sinus, with resulting hemorrhage.

Calcifying Odontogenic Cyst (Gorlins's Cyst). This lesion represents approximately 2 per cent of jaw cysts (Altini and Farman,

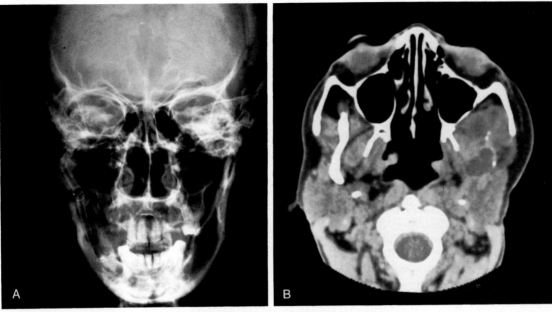

Figure 69–1. Keratocyst. *A,* Frontal plain film. *B,* CT scan.

1975) and demonstrates features of both cystic and solid neoplasms. On histologic examination it resembles the cutaneous calcifying epithelioma of Malherbe (Gorlin and associates, 1962). The epithelial lining contains masses of ghost cells undergoing keratinization and calcification. On radiographic study they appear as cysts, but they may contain calcified radiopaque material ranging from tiny flecks to large masses (Shear, 1983). One variant demonstrates extensive ameloblastic proliferations of the epithelium (Gorlin and associates, 1962). The majority are intraosseous in location. They occur at any age, but most commonly between the ages of 20 and 40 years; the mandible and maxilla are affected equally (Freedman, Lumerman, and Gee, 1975). Most are located anterior to the first molar teeth. They are painless, slowly growing swellings, ranging from 1 to 8 cm in diameter. Treatment is similar to that employed for the odontogenic keratocysts; however, these lesions do not usually recur (Shear, 1983).

Inflammatory Odontogenic Cysts

Radicular Cysts. These are the most common jaw cysts, making up 55 to 74 per cent in various series (Browne, 1972; Shear, 1983). The end result of an inflammatory process involving the dental pulp, they are preceded by the formation of a periapical granuloma. Radiographic differentiation is often difficult (LaLonde, 1970). They usually occur at the apex of a nonvital erupted tooth. Pulp vitality tests are helpful; the presence of a vital tooth rules out the diagnosis (Ellis and Fonseca, 1987). These cysts are thought to arise from the epithelial rests of Malassez in the periodontal ligament (Shear, 1983). The wall is fibrous, lined by nonkeratinizing stratified squamous epithelium with a dense chronic inflammatory infiltrate. They are found at any age, but the majority occur in the second decade (Bhaskar, 1966). Although either jaw may be involved, they occur most frequently in the anterior maxilla (LaLonde and Luebke, 1968). They are usually asymptomatic and are diagnosed on routine dental radiographs. Pain and swelling usually result from infection. On occasion, a sinus tract may develop with an oral mucosal or cutaneous opening.

On radiographic study a radicular cyst appears as an ovoid radiolucency with sclerotic margins, in continuity with a tooth root apex. Because of the difficulty in clinical differentiation from a periapical granuloma, endodontic treatment is initially advised, followed by a period of observation. If serial radiographs indicate that the lesion remains static or enlarges, a periapical surgical removal of the lesion is indicated (Ellis and Fonseca, 1987). Recurrence is rare.

Residual Cysts. If a preexisting radicular cyst is not removed at the time of extraction of its associated nonvital tooth, the cyst is termed a residual cyst (Weine and Silverglade, 1983). Further enlargement merits resection.

Lateral Periodontal Cysts. These are essentially radicular cysts that lie lateral to the tooth root (Standish and Shafer, 1958). They probably result from inflammation in the periodontal pocket; the tooth usually remains vital. Thus, if possible, the cyst should be removed surgically without injury to the adjacent tooth roots.

Paradental Cysts. These are histologically similar to radicular cysts. They arise in relation to partially erupted third mandibular molars with pericoronitis (Craig, 1976). There is a well-defined superimposed radiolucency near the buccal bifurcation of the third molar on radiographic study. They probably originate from reduced enamel epithelium or epithelial rests. Treatment is extraction and cyst removal.

FISSURAL CYSTS

Various types of fissural or inclusion cysts occur along the lines of embryologic "fusion." These epithelium-lined cysts are related to vital teeth; the teeth should be preserved when the cysts are excised (Ellis and Fonseca, 1987). Maxillary fissural cysts may be lined by respiratory or squamous epithelium.

Nasopalatine Duct Cyst. These are the most common of the fissural cysts and may grow to a large size. They must be differentiated from the normal nasopalatine canal by radiographic study. The cyst is removed via a palatal approach to avoid compromise of the blood supply to the anterior maxillary teeth.

Median Maxillary Palatal Cyst. This lesion occurs in the midline between the palatal shelves and may involve the nose and the maxillary sinus.

Globulomaxillary Cyst. This cyst occurs in the alveolus between the premaxilla and the maxilla (between the lateral incisor and the canine teeth). It frequently causes displacement of the neighboring tooth roots.

Median Mandibular Cyst. This is extremely rare and occurs at the mandibular symphysis.

MANAGEMENT OF JAW CYSTS

Except for recurrent, aggressive keratocysts, jaw cysts are enucleated when possible. The cyst is exposed by elevating a mucoperiosteal flap; on occasion, there may be factors necessitating a different surgical approach. Enucleation of large cysts may weaken the involved jaw and cause pathologic fracture, damage the inferior alveolar nerve, or establish communication with the maxillary sinus or nasal cavity. If this seems likely, the Partch procedure may be used (Hayward, 1976). In this technique a small mucoperiosteal flap is elevated for biopsy purposes. After the diagnosis of a benign lesion is established, the oral mucosa is sutured to the edge of the window made in the cyst wall. The patient is instructed to perform daily irrigations through the osseous defect to maintain patency and prevent infection. With this regimen of cyst decompression, the size of the cavity gradually decreases as followed radiographically.

When indicated, resection of the cyst is accomplished with less risk to surrounding vital structures. The inflammatory thickening of the cyst wall makes this procedure technically easy. Cysts surrounding tooth roots or occurring in inaccessible areas require aggressive curettage to remove the lining completely. Otherwise, there may be recurrence. After enucleation, the mucosa is closed directly, if possible. Serial packing is reserved for cases of breakdown of the primary closure. Enucleated cystic cavities spontaneously fill with bone over 6 to 12 months. In most cases, expanded jaws slowly remodel to a more normal contour. Primary bone grafting may be necessary when the cystic cavity is large and there is a risk of pathologic fracture. Severe destruction of bony jaw contours is also a relative indication for primary bone grafting (Ellis and Fonseca, 1987).

Odontogenic Tumors

Odontogenic tumors are benign or malignant, and they may be of epithelial or ectomesenchymal origin. Most are benign; however, some behave aggressively, with local bone destruction and invasion of related sinuses.

EPITHELIAL ODONTOGENIC TUMORS

Ameloblastic Tumors

This term refers to epithelial odontogenic tumors with minimal inductive change in the connective tissue, the stroma of these tumors consisting of mature fibrous tissue.

Ameloblastoma (Adamantinoma). Ameloblastomas account for 11 per cent of odontogenic tumors (Regezi, Kerr, and Courtney, 1978). They may originate from one of several structures, including dental lamina rests, the enamel organ, basal cells of the oral mucosa, or the epithelial lining of a dentigerous cyst (Gorlin, 1970). On histologic examination they consist of nests, strands, and cords of ameloblastic epithelium with a sparse connective tissue stroma (McDaniel, 1987). Follicular and plexiform patterns were described (Small and Waldron, 1955). Cystic degeneration may occur in the center of follicles, resulting in squamous epithelium–lined cystic cavities (Gorlin, 1970). When squamous metaplasia is extensive and keratinization occurs, the tumor is called an acanthomatous ameloblastoma (Gorlin, 1970). In the latter type a superficial biopsy specimen can be misinterpreted as a squamous cell carcinoma. Granular cells, hemangiomatous elements, or neuromatous elements may also be seen (Gorlin, 1970; Hartman, 1974).

Although cases have been reported in the newborn, affected patients are usually between 20 and 50 years (Small and Waldron, 1955). The mandible is involved four times more frequently than the maxilla. In both jaws, the tumor occurs most frequently in the posterior region (80 per cent). Tumor size ranges from 1 to 16 cm in diameter, with a mean of 4 to 5 cm. It occurs as a slowly growing, painless swelling, pain being a feature in one-third of cases. Less common findings include mobile teeth, ill-fitting dentures, malocclusion, or ulcerations. Ameloblastomas can involve the maxillary antrum and may cause nasal obstruction (Mehlisch, Dahlin, and Masson, 1972).

On radiographic examination ameloblastomas are radiolucent, unilocular, or expansile multilocular lesions, and they may or may not be associated with a tooth (Fig. 69–2). Differentiation from a dentigerous cyst is difficult (McDaniel, 1987). Ameloblastoma has the capacity for unlimited, continued local growth. It may invade cancellous bone, infiltrating between the bony trabeculae;

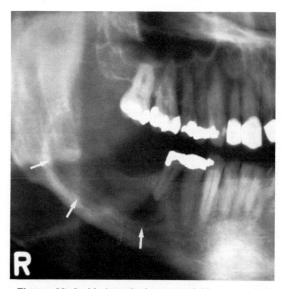

Figure 69–2. Moderately large ameloblastoma of the right angle and body of the mandible *(arrows)*. Note the relationship of the lesion to the apex of the premolar tooth.

cortical bone is not involved, although it can be eroded.

Three different clinical types of ameloblastoma exist: the conventional one and two special types, each requiring a different form of treatment (Gardner and Pecak, 1980). The first special type is *unicystic ameloblastoma,* which develops in the epithelial wall of a dentigerous cyst in the posterior mandibular region. Patients are generally less than 30 years of age. If the fibrous connective tissue wall of the lesion is uninvolved, enucleation and curettage with close follow-up is initially recommended (Ellis and Fonseca, 1987). Compared with conventional ameloblastoma, these lesions have a relatively lower rate of recurrence following this type of treatment. The second is the *peripheral* or *extraosseous ameloblastoma.* It arises from the basal cell layer of the surface epithelium overlying a tooth-bearing portion of the jaws. It is usually of the acanthomatous type and may be difficult to differentiate microscopically from basal cell or squamous cell carcinoma. The extraosseous ameloblastoma has approximately a 20 per cent postexcisional recurrence rate.

The treatment of choice for the *conventional intraosseous ameloblastoma* remains segmental or radical resection. A marginal mandibular resection is sufficient if a tumor-free inferior mandibular margin can be preserved. The teeth in relation to the tumor should be removed in continuity; the soft tissues are closed primarily. If the tumor is large, is recurrent, or involves the angle and ramus of the mandible, a partial hemimandibulectomy is indicated. The mandibular condyle should be preserved, in addition to the posterior cortex of the ramus, if possible. If perforation of the cortical plates exists, a full-thickness en bloc resection is performed with at least a 1 cm margin of uninvolved bone. Reconstruction can be performed immediately or delayed. In the latter case, a space-maintaining device is necessary. Mandibular reconstruction is discussed below (see also Chap. 29).

Ameloblastoma of Maxilla. The maxilla is less frequently involved; however, ameloblastoma in this region can be a significant problem. There is often a reluctance to resect radically because of resulting deformity and difficulty in reconstruction. This approach predisposes to a recurrence, which may involve the sinuses or the orbit, causing eye proptosis. When this occurs, a radical, occasionally intracranial, en bloc resection is necessary. In the authors' experience, it has not been necessary to remove the orbital contents, although areas of the orbit and skull base have been resected (Fig. 69–3).

Adenomatoid Odontogenic Tumor

The precise odontogenic origin of this tumor is unknown. It constitutes only 3 per cent of odontogenic tumors (Regezi, Kerr, and Courtney, 1978). Histologic examination reveals a thick-walled, cystic structure with intraluminal proliferation of odontogenic epithelium (McDaniel, 1987). The majority occur in the second decade of life, women being affected twice as often as men (Giansanti, Someren, and Waldron, 1970). The maxilla (usually the anterior region) is involved more often than the mandible. Extraosseous lesions have been reported; these occur as central labiogingival swellings without pain. There is a unilocular radiolucency around the crown of an impacted tooth. This radiographic finding makes differentiation from a dentigerous cyst difficult. Most of the tumors are between 1 and 3 cm in diameter. Treatment is by enucleation and curettage. Recurrences are rare (Courtney and Kerr, 1975).

Calcifying Epithelial Odontogenic Tumor (Pindborg's Tumor). This tumor, described by Pindborg in 1955, accounts for less than 1 per cent of odontogenic tumors (Regezi, Kerr, and Courtney, 1978). It is thought to arise from the enamel organ. The patients range in age from the first to the ninth decade (Franklin and Pindborg, 1976). It occurs mainly in the molar area in either jaw, more commonly in the mandible, often associated with an unerupted or impacted tooth (Regezi, Kerr, and Courtney, 1978). There is also an extraosseous form, which occurs as a gingival swelling in the anterior mandible (Wertheimer, Zielinski, and Wesley, 1977).

On histologic study there are clusters or sheets of polyhedral epithelial cells with occasional ringlike calcifications in a fibrous stroma (McDaniel, 1987). Infrequently, the epithelial cells are vacuolated and appear as clear cells (Anderson, Kim, and Minkowitz, 1969).

The usual presentation is that of a painless, slowly growing mass. Larger lesions may cause nasal obstruction or eye proptosis and pain (Franklin and Pindborg, 1976). The radiographic appearance is that of a unilocular radiolucency associated with an impacted tooth. Occasionally, there is calcification and radiopacity. This tumor behaves essentially like an ameloblastoma and is treated similarly. The recurrence rate is approximately 14 per cent (Franklin and Pindborg, 1976).

Squamous Odontogenic Tumor. This extremely rare lesion arises from the rests of Malassez in the periodontal ligament (Swan and McDaniel, 1983). It consists of a mature fibrous stroma, containing islands of squamous epithelium (McDaniel, 1987). There is a well-defined radiolucency involving the alveolus and surrounding the tooth roots on radiography (Pullon and associates, 1975). In the maxilla, it often perforates the cortical bone and extends into adjacent soft tissue. Conservative excision is advised (Goldblatt, Brannon, and Ellis, 1982). No recurrences have been reported.

Ameloblastic and Ectomesenchymal Tumors

These are lesions with marked inductive changes in their connective tissue stroma.

Ameloblastic Fibroma. This tumor resembles ameloblastoma on histologic study; there are scattered strands, cords, and islands of odontogenic epithelial cells in an immature cellular stroma. However, it occurs at a younger age and is less aggressive. It is

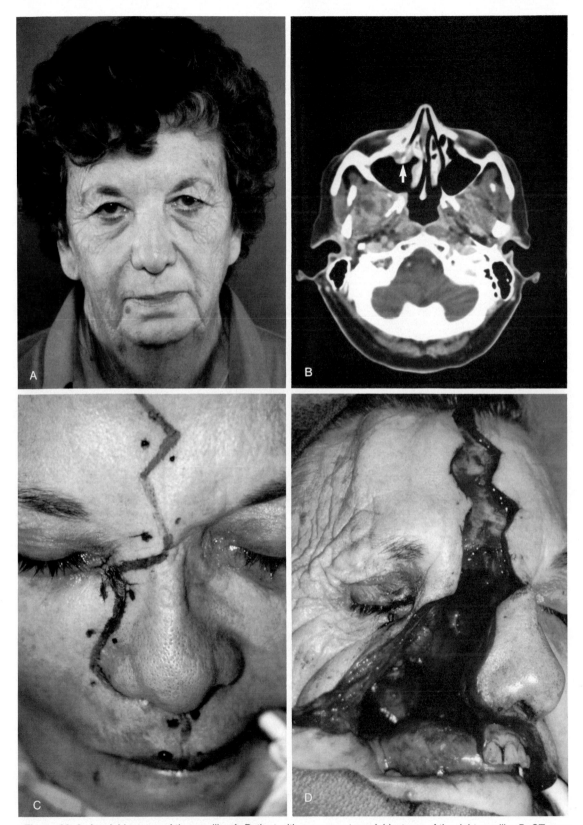

Figure 69–3. Ameloblastoma of the maxilla. *A,* Patient with a recurrent ameloblastoma of the right maxilla. *B,* CT scan shows extension of the ameloblastoma to the base of the skull *(arrow). C,* Planned surgical approach. *D,* Maxillectomy with removal of the ethmoid sinuses. The frontal W-plasty incision was designed to allow cranial base resection.

Illustration continued on following page

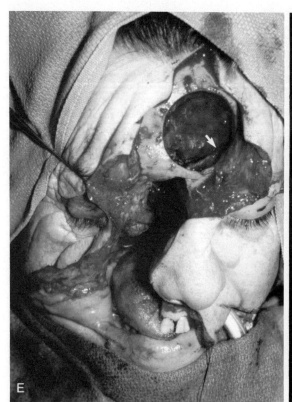

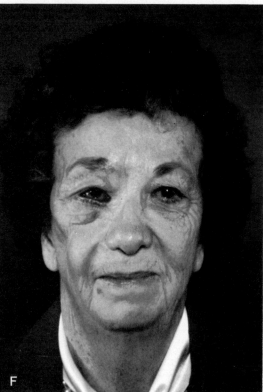

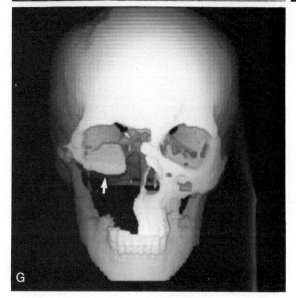

Figure 69–3 *Continued E,* Cranial base resection completed through a frontal trephine opening. The arrow indicates a galeal frontalis flap, which separates the cranial base from the nasopharynx. *F,* Postoperative result two years later prior to corrective surgery on the right lower eyelid. *G,* Three-dimensional CT scan showing the extent of the resection and reconstruction of the orbital floor with vascularized cranial bone *(arrow).* Note the cranial donor site filled with bone dust removed from the bur holes.

thought to result from a proliferation of ameloblasts that subsequently induce the formation of an ectomesenchymal stroma, which resembles that of the embryonic dental papilla (McDaniel, 1987). The patients' ages range from six months to 42 years, with an average age of 14 years (Slootweg, 1981). The sex distribution is equal. Ameloblastic fibromas make up 2 per cent of odontogenic tumors (Regezi, Kerr, and Courtney, 1978). They may affect either jaw, but most commonly involve the mandible in the posterior region (Slootweg, 1981). They occur as painless swellings; disturbances of tooth eruption occur in up to one-third of the patients (Nilsen and Magnusson, 1979); and 75 per cent are associated with unerupted teeth (Trodahl, 1972). Most appear radiographically as multilocular radiolucencies with sclerotic borders, ranging in size from 1 to 8 cm in diameter (Trodahl, 1972). The cortex is often expanded, but perforation is rare. The recurrence rate after excision is 18.3 per cent (Zallen, Preskar, and McClary, 1982). Treatment consists of enucleation and curettage. Sacrifice of teeth or tooth buds within the lesion is frequently necessary. On occasion, the tumor may recur rapidly, behaving more like an ameloblastic sarcoma. When this occurs, wide en bloc resection should be performed, with segmental resection in the mandible and partial maxillectomy in the maxilla (Ellis and Fonseca, 1987).

Ameloblastic Fibro-odontoma. This rare tumor contains elements of ameloblastic fibroma combined with features of an odontoma (McDaniel, 1987). The median age of patients is 13 years. There have been no reported recurrences after excision.

Odontoameloblastoma. This tumor contains enamel and dentin in a mature fibrous stroma with an ameloblastic epithelial component (McDaniel, 1987). There are well-defined radiolucencies with variable radiopacities on radiographic examination. It is similar to intraosseous ameloblastoma and should be treated in a similar manner (LaBriola and associates, 1980).

Odontoma. This hamartoma is classified as complex or compound (Pindborg, Kramer, and Torloni, 1971). In the complex form, all dental tissues are present, but in a disorderly pattern. In the compound variety, they are more organized; thus the lesion consists of many rudimentary dental structures. These tumors are detected most often during the

second, third, and fourth decades of life (Budnick, 1976). Complex odontomas are more common in the posterior mandible, whereas compound odontomas favor the anterior maxilla (Slootweg, 1981). They may occur in unusual locations, such as the retrotympanic area (McClatchey, Hakimi, and Batsakis, 1981) or maxillary antrum (Mendelsohn and associates, 1983). There is usually pain, expansion of the buccal plate, and frequently absence of the corresponding tooth (Stasinopoulos, 1970). The complex form is radiopaque, whereas the compound type contains multiple rudimentary dental structures. Treatment is by simple enucleation. Displacement of tooth buds and resorption of unerupted teeth may occur (McDaniel, 1987).

Odontogenic Fibroma. This rare tumor contains numerous cords of odontogenic epithelium in a stroma resembling dysplastic dentin, which may contain calcifications. There are multiloculated radiolucencies that can be associated with unerupted or displaced teeth (Dahl, Wolfson, and Haugen, 1981). Recurrence is rare after enucleation (Heimdal, Isacsson, and Nilsson, 1980).

ECTOMESENCHYMAL ODONTOGENIC TUMORS

Odontogenic Myxoma. This lesion accounts for 3 per cent of odontogenic tumors (Regezi, Kerr, and Courtney, 1978). It is composed of stellate myxoblasts in a stroma composed of basophilic mucoid ground substance (McDaniel, 1987). The tumor is locally aggressive and has a tendency to recur after conservative treatment (Killey and Kay, 1965). When this occurs, soft tissue involvement may necessitate extensive resection. Myxoma most frequently involves the posterior region of the mandible (Gorlin, Chaudhry, and Pindborg, 1961) and has a gelatinous consistency owing to its abundant mucoid matrix; this makes complete removal difficult. Small lesions may be treated by vigorous curettage; larger lesions may require partial jaw resection with immediate reconstruction (Ellis and Fonseca, 1987).

Cementoblastoma. This is the only true tumor of cemental origin. It makes up less than 1 per cent of odontogenic tumors (Regezi, Kerr, and Courtney, 1978). The tumor consists of cementoblasts, mineralized and unmineralized cementin, and a cellular fibrous stroma (McDaniel, 1987). Patients range in age from 10 to 70 years (Farman and associates, 1979). The majority of lesions are located in the mandible in the first molar region. On radiographic study there is a round, radiopaque mass, which is fused to partially resorbed tooth roots. The lesion may continue to slowly enlarge, expanding the cortex of the affected jaw to cause facial asymmetry. Pain is reported in approximately half of the cases (Corio, Crawford, and Schaberg, 1976). Endodontic treatment of the involved tooth, which is vital, is followed by periapical surgical removal of the lesion and a portion of the involved root (Ellis and Fonseca, 1987). The lesions do not tend to recur after treatment.

Periapical Cemental Dysplasia. This tumor, which accounts for 8 per cent of odontogenic tumors (Regezi, Kerr, and Courtney, 1978), has several interesting features. It may be radiolucent, radiopaque, or mixed, depending on its stage, an osteolytic stage, a calcifying stage, or a mature stage, respectively (Hamner, Scofield, and Cornyn, 1968). Seventy per cent of these lesions occur in blacks (Zegarelli and associates, 1964); 20 per cent involve the incisor or canine teeth of the mandible. The lesions are small, asymptomatic, and tend to be diagnosed incidentally on dental radiographs. They are self-limiting and require no treatment (McDaniel, 1987).

Cementifying Fibroma. This lesion consists of a cellular fibrous stroma containing islands of cementum. This accounts for its mixed radiolucent-radiopaque appearance. It accounts for approximately 2 per cent of odontogenic tumors (Regezi, Kerr, and Courtney, 1978). The patients are largely female in the third to fifth decades of life. Most lesions are located in the mandible (Waldron and Giansanti, 1973). They may grow to as large as 7 cm in diameter. Treatment consists of enucleation, and recurrence is rare.

MALIGNANT ODONTOGENIC TUMORS

Odontogenic Carcinomas. These neoplasms are extremely rare and have a poor prognosis. Five year survival rates are in the 30 to 40 per cent range (Shear, 1969). *Malignant ameloblastomas* result from malignant transformation in an intraosseous ameloblastoma, retaining the histologic features of benign ameloblastoma. They metastasize via blood vessels, by lymphatics, and occasionally by aspiration of tumor cells (Slootweg and

Muller, 1984; Ellis and Fonseca, 1987). *Ameloblastoma carcinoma* also appears to arise from conventional ameloblastoma; however, the histologic appearance is poorly differentiated when compared with that of the lesion from which it arose (Slootweg and Muller, 1984). The third type of odontogenic carcinoma is termed *primary intraosseous carcinoma* (Elzay, 1982). It occurs in a keratinizing or nonkeratinizing form and has the same histologic features as any intraoral squamous cell carcinoma. Treatment is similar to that for squamous cell carcinoma of the oral cavity that has invaded bone (Elzay, 1982). Wide resection is necessary, with ipsilateral neck dissection if metastasis to the regional lymph nodes is found. Radiation and chemotherapy may be used adjunctively.

Ameloblastic Fibrosarcoma. This rare tumor behaves as a low grade fibrosarcoma; metastases are rare (Howell and Burkes, 1977), but uncontrollable local infiltration can occur. There is a benign-appearing odontogenic epithelial component contained within a sarcomatous fibrous stroma. This lesion can arise from a preexisting benign ameloblastoma, fibroma, or ameloblastic fibro-odontoma. It may appear from the second to the eighth decade of life, but typically it occurs in the fourth decade as a painful swelling with occasional ulceration (Leider, Nelson, and Trodahl, 1972). It is a multilocular radiolucent lesion with indistinct irregular borders and root resorption. The posterior mandibular region is the most frequent site (Adekeye, Edwards, and Goubran, 1978). Treatment is radical resection; however, multiple recurrences are common (Howell and Burkes, 1977). The tumor is radioresistant, and chemotherapy is reserved for intractable cases (Goldstein, Parker, and Hugh, 1976).

Nonodontogenic Tumors

This group of skeletal tumors arise from tissue not intended for tooth formation. Their occurrence in the jaws is rare, relative to that in the remainder of the skeleton.

BENIGN NONODONTOGENIC OSSEOUS TUMORS

Osteomas. Osteomas should not be confused with exostoses, which are common in the jaws and occur in over 30 per cent of the population (Greer, Rohrer, and Young, 1987). In contrast, jaw osteomas are relatively uncommon. They are described as having three distinct histologic patterns: trabecular, compact, and osteoma durum (Batsakis, 1979). The latter shows features of both the compact and the trabecular form. A few may become sufficiently large to produce facial asymmetry, but the majority are diagnosed on dental radiographs. They occur as slowly growing central, peripheral, or subperiosteal bone-forming tumors. They occur most frequently in the mandibles of young adults, with a 2:1 male preponderance (Hallberg and Bagley, 1950). On radiographic study, they appear as well-circumscribed endosteal sclerotic masses or dense radiopaque subperiosteal lesions. Multiple osteomas are associated with a rare inherited disease, Gardner's syndrome. In this condition, there are multiple osteomas, multiple epidermoid and sebaceous cysts in the skin, supernumerary teeth, and intestinal polyposis. The significant aspect of this syndrome is malignant transformation of the intestinal polyps (Shiffman, 1962). Surgery is reserved for osteomas causing symptoms. Slowly growing central endosteal lesions discovered incidentally may be observed and followed by radiographs (Scott and Ellis, 1987). Larger osteomas, particularly the periosteal variety, may cause pain, cortical expansion, ulceration of the mucosa, interference with a dental appliance, and facial asymmetry. Treatment is enucleation; recurrence is rare.

Osteoblastoma. Osteoblastoma is a rare benign tumor of bone, which accounts for approximately 1 per cent of all primary bone tumors (McLeod, Dahlin, and Beabout, 1976). Sixty per cent occur in the long bones; the jaws are less frequently involved. The male-to-female ratio is 2:1 (Greer, Mierau, and Favara, 1983), and the lesion is detected usually in the second decade of life. The tooth-bearing areas of the mandible are most commonly affected (Smith and associates, 1982). Painful, tender swelling with expansion of the jaw may be seen. The tumors range from 2 to 10 cm in diameter and radiologically appear as spheric calcified areas surrounded by a well-defined radiolucent zone (Dahlin, 1978). Occasionally, a sun ray pattern may be noted. On histologic study, a cellular osteoblastic type of tissue is surrounded by an ample intracellular osteoid material containing abundant blood vessels. Because of its

vascularity, osteoblastoma is well defined by bone scan (Scott and Ellis, 1987). Treatment is conservative surgical excision (Lichtenstein, 1956; Shafer, Hine, and Levy, 1974).

Osteoid Osteoma. This lesion has a tendency to produce pain that is out of proportion to its size. It is slowly growing and is seldom larger than 1 cm in diameter. There is a central nidus of bone destruction surrounded by a peripheral zone of cortical bone. Jaffe (1935) postulated three stages: an initial stage showing proliferation of osteoblasts, an intermediate phase, and a mature stage in which the osteoid becomes well mineralized. The lesion occurs in either jaw (Farman, Nortje, and Grotepass, 1976); it most often involves the cortical or cancellous bone and, infrequently, the subperiosteal area. The majority occur in young adults. The radiographic appearance is usually that of a radiolucent central area of bone destruction surrounded by a dense sclerotic border. Technetium bone scans outline the lesion well (Marsh and associates, 1975). Treatment is by conservative excision; however, during surgery it may be difficult to distinguish the lesion from surrounding bone. Thus a surrounding rim of normal bone is excised. The lesions do not generally recur.

BENIGN FIBROUS AND FIBROOSSEOUS LESIONS

Fibrous Dysplasia

Although fibrous dysplasia is not strictly a neoplasm, it behaves like one. It can be described as a developmental derangement of bone resulting from an abnormal proliferation of undifferentiated mesenchymal bone-forming cells (Lichtenstein, 1975). Trauma and complex endocrine disturbances have also been postulated as causative factors (Marlow and Waite, 1965). There is proliferation of mainly fibroblasts, producing a dense collagen matrix containing trabeculae of osteoid and bone in a disorganized pattern (Greer, Rohrer, and Young, 1987). An increase in the mass of the involved bone occurs as a result of proliferation of this abnormal tissue. It may be monostotic or polyostotic; the latter may be part of the Albright syndrome (Albright and associates, 1937). Other features of the syndrome include endocrine abnormalities (e.g., precocious puberty), café au lait spots, and other extraskeletal abnormalities.

In the head and neck region, its behavior depends on the location. In the cranio-orbital area, it can be aggressive and this dictates the type of treatment (see Chap. 33); this is discussed below under Tumors of Orbits. The more common maxillary and mandibular form is usually monostotic, involving the maxilla more frequently than the mandible (Eversole, Sabes, and Rovin, 1972), and it usually becomes quiescent after puberty. Women are affected more commonly than men.

Fibrous dysplasia occurs as a unilateral slowly progressive asymmetry of the jaw. The teeth remain firmly attached to the alveolus, although they may be displaced or impacted. The lesion may cross the midline and grow into the maxillary sinus, producing nasal symptoms. Radiographic examination demonstrates a ground glass appearance with diffuse, poorly circumscribed borders. It is not restricted to any anatomic landmarks. Approximately one-fifth of lesions appear cystlike (Eversole, Sabes, and Rovin, 1972). No periosteal reaction occurs.

Treatment of fibrous dysplasia in the jaws usually consists of shaving the soft avascular bone. This is usually done for esthetic purposes, although some patients require excision to relieve the symptoms of nasal obstruction. A nasal airway can be carved through a mass of fibrous dysplasia and will remain patent and become lined with mucosa. On occasion, resection and bone graft reconstruction have been necessary (Fig. 69–4). Malignant transformation is a rare occurrence (less than 1 per cent) and appears to be related to prior radiation therapy (Gross and Montgomery, 1967). Malignant change should be suspected in any lesion that grows rapidly or becomes painful.

Cherubism

Cherubism was first described by Jones in 1933 and is a hereditary form of fibrous dysplasia, usually affecting the mandible and maxilla. Dahlin (1978) preferred to classify this lesion with the more general fibro-osseous lesions, rather than as a specific subtype of fibrous dysplasia. It is inherited as an autosomal dominant trait. Symptoms begin in early childhood and progress through adolescence. Dental disruption occurs, along with alveolar bone loss, resulting from replacement by the lesion. There is bilateral painless enlargement of the mandible and the maxilla (Fig. 69–5). With superior maxilla involvement, there is a characteristic upward rotation of the globe with inferior scleral show. Treatment is controversial. Some suggest observation only, since it may show spontaneous regression in childhood; others have recommended contouring procedures. Dubin and Jackson (1988) described the case of a 7 year old boy treated satisfactorily with curettage and suction-assisted lipectomy in combination with malar osteotomies to reduce facial width.

Central Giant Cell Granuloma

Controversy exists about whether this tumor is analogous to the true giant cell tumor of peripheral bones (Waldron and Shafer, 1966) or whether it represents a separate entity as described by Jaffe (1953). The etiology is controversial; most investigators agree that it is reactive in nature. Whether this is attributable to trauma or inflammation is not clear (Hirschl and Katz, 1974). These tumors make up only 3.5 per cent of benign tumors of the jaws (Austin, Dahlin, and Royer, 1959). They occur preponderantly in children and young adults and are more common in females (Austin, Dahlin, and Royer, 1959). The mandible is involved more often than the maxilla, and both jaws are more frequently affected in the anterior portion. Approximately one-fifth cross the midline (Waldron and Shafer, 1966). They usually occur as local painful swellings but may be asymptomatic and only be discovered on routine dental examination (Austin, Dahlin, and Royer, 1959). Radiographs show well-defined unilocular or multilocular radiolucencies. Expansion of the cortical plates is often observed with displacement of teeth and, on occasion, root resorption (Waldron and Shafer, 1966).

On histologic study there are proliferative fibroblastic connective tissue, abundant vascular tissue, collagen formation, and multinucleated giant cells in a diffuse organization with multiple foci of hemorrhage. Spicules of newly formed bone or osteoid are often seen. Mitoses in the stromal cells are common (Waldron and Shafer, 1966).

The lesions may occur with hyperparathyroidism, and it is suggested that all patients

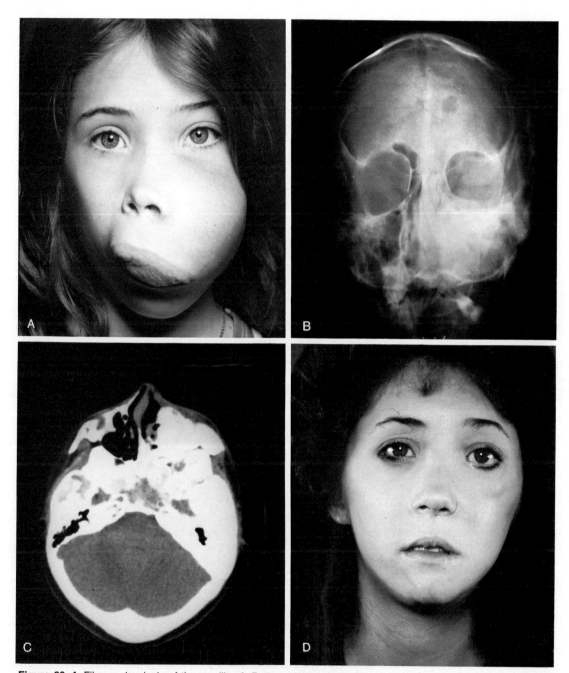

Figure 69–4. Fibrous dysplasia of the maxilla. *A,* Patient with extensive fibrous dysplasia of the left maxilla. *B,* Facial bone plain film. *C,* CT scan. *D,* Result five years after resection and reconstruction with split rib grafts in association with contouring of the mandible and the palate.

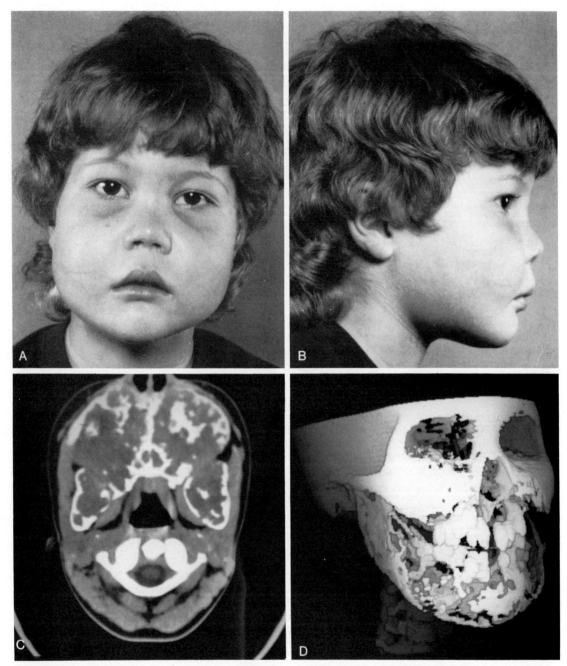

Figure 69–5. Cherubism. *A, B,* Frontal and profile views. *C,* CT scan demonstrating involvement of the maxilla. *D,* Three-dimensional CT scan showing extensive involvement of the maxilla and the mandible.

with this diagnosis should have preoperative serum calcium and phosphate screening (Scott and Ellis, 1987). In this situation, excision of parathyroid adenomas rather than the jaw cysts is indicated. From the majority of the lesions, the treatment of choice is local excision and curettage. Dental splinting for mobile teeth may be necessary. Because of the vascularity of these granulomas, considerable bleeding may be encountered during resection. Recurrence after removal is rare.

Aneurysmal Bone Cysts

Aneurysmal bone cysts are rapidly growing, expansile, solitary lesions; they are often observed in patients less than 20 years of age (Biesecker and associates, 1970). They are much more common in the vertebral column and long bones. The etiology is unknown. Trauma has been implicated; others have refuted this cause, since aneurysmal cysts occur with other benign bone lesions. They account for 1.5 per cent of nonodontogenic jaw cysts (El Deeb, Sedano, and Waite, 1980), and they occur as localized painless swellings with occasional malocclusion. The most common location is the body of the mandible. On radiographic study there is a unilocular cystic mass; it can also be multilocular, with a honeycombed appearance (Lichtenstein, 1950). The lesion characteristically erodes through the cortex, but it is limited by a thin shell of new subperiosteal bone not visible on standard radiographs (Tillman and associates, 1968).

Histologic examination shows cavernous, blood-filled spaces lined by compressed fibrous tissue (Dahlin, 1978). Frequently, multinucleated giant cells occur within the wall of the cyst, but the most common cell type is the fibroblast (Steiner and Kantor, 1977).

Treatment is surgical removal. When size and access permit, the tumor bed should be curetted and cauterized (Lovely, 1983). When the lesion is large or less accessible, such as in the ramus, en bloc excision may be necessary. Preoperative fine needle aspiration biopsy should be performed. Considerable bleeding may be encountered on removal. Radiotherapy is contraindicated and may cause sarcomatous change (Tillman and associates, 1968; Daugherty and Eversole, 1971).

Desmoplastic Fibroma

Desmoplastic fibroma is a benign, but locally aggressive intraosseous tumor of connective tissue. There are bundles of abundant collagen fibers separated by spindle-shaped fibroblasts on histologic examination. Cellularity is sparse. Occasional mitoses can be seen. It can be difficult to distinguish from a well-differentiated fibrosarcoma (Stout, 1962). The usual presentation is that of a slowly expanding tumor, with swelling often being the only finding (Hinds, Kent, and Fechner, 1969). Seventy per cent of the lesions occur in the ramus and posterior body of the mandible (Freedman and associates, 1978). Although it may occur in any age group, it is found principally in young adults, with a female-to-male ratio of 3:1. Radiographic study shows that it is radiolucent and usually large; and the cortical plates may be thinned and have a honeycombed appearance. There is penetration into the soft tissues and muscles with resulting trismus (Hinds, Kent, and Fechner, 1969). Because of the growth pattern and radiographic features, the tumors are often mistaken for malignancies. Treatment for most lesions is en bloc surgical resection, including removal of adjacent surrounding normal tissue. If the cortical plates have not been destroyed and there is no invasion of soft tissues, enucleation and curettage with appropriate follow-up may be considered. The tumors often recur. The possibility of a missed fibrosarcoma must always be considered (Masson and Soule, 1966).

Histiocytosis X

This group of lesions consists of three different clinical complexes that are grouped together because of their similar histologic appearance. There is a proliferation of histiocytes, usually in sheets, with a variable number of eosinophils, plasma cells, lymphocytes, multinucleated giant cells, and foam cells. Necrosis is often present (Oberman, 1961). The etiology of histiocytosis X is obscure; however, a popular theory implicates a defect in the immunoregulatory mechanisms. The proliferating cell in histiocytosis X is the Langerhans cell, a dendritic histiocyte. Electron microscopy can confirm the diagnosis by detecting the presence of Langerhans' or Birbeck's granules within the cytoplasm of

Langerhans' cells (Newton and Hamoudi, 1973). The inclusion bodies are not present in normal histiocytes.

Histiocytosis X disorders can be subdivided into (1) eosinophilic granuloma, monostotic or polyostotic; (2) Hand-Schüller-Christian disease, and (3) Letterer-Siwe syndrome (Lichtenstein, 1953).

Eosinophilic granuloma is a localized form of histiocytosis X. It usually occurs within the first two decades of life and affects males twice as often as females (Huvos, 1979). In the polyostotic form multiple bones are involved. The most common symptoms are swelling and pain. Gingival lesions are often associated wtih adjacent bone involvement and are characterized by a nonspecific, erythematous swelling with ulceration. The radiograph shows unilocular well-defined radiolucencies. Skull lesions are characterized by a punched-out appearance and are often multiple. In the monostotic form, treatment consists of vigorous curettage with long-term follow-up (Scott and Ellis, 1987). The adjacent teeth are often sacrificed because of the loss of alveolar support. A radiographic skeletal survey is recommended to rule out the presence of other lesions. The prognosis is usually good.

Hand-Schüller-Christian disease is a chronic disseminated form of histiocytosis X. The classic triad of skull lesions, exophthalmos, and diabetes insipidus occurs in less than 10 per cent of cases (Nolph and Luikin, 1982). The initial findings occur later than with eosinophilic granuloma, sometimes being observed in adults. A number of extraosseous organs may be involved, including liver, spleen, lymph nodes, and bone. Radiation therapy and local curettage have been employed for treatment of the bone lesions. Chemotherapy has been used for extraosseous organ involvement. The median survival is 10 to 15 years (Scott and Ellis, 1987).

Letterer-Siwe syndrome is an acute disseminated form of histiocytosis X. It generally occurs in infants less than 3 years of age. There is multiple organ involvement, with extraskeletal lesions predominating. The clinical course is rapid and usually fatal. Chemotherapy with cytotoxic drugs has been employed with limited success (Scott and Ellis, 1987).

Hemangiomas

Jaw hemangiomas are extremely rare lesions, which are probably hamartomas or developmental malformations rather than true neoplasms. Most frequently, they occur during the second decade of life. The female-to-male ratio is 2:1 (Lund and Dahlin, 1964). The molar region of the mandible is most frequently affected. The lesions may be discovered as an incidental finding, such as a radiolucency on dental radiographs. The most common clinical presentation is expansion of the buccal cortex, gingival bleeding from around the necks of mobile teeth, or severe hemorrhage after dental extraction, gingival biopsy, or eruption of a tooth. Severe epistaxis may be the initial symptom of a maxillary lesion. The majority grow slowly and are painless. Hemangiomas of the jaw most commonly appear radiographically as multilocular radiolucencies with a honeycombed appearance (Worth and Stoneman, 1979). On occasion, a sunburst appearance, represented by a radiolucent cystic lesion with bony trabeculae radiating from the center, may be observed. Since the multilocular radiolucent appearance is not diagnostic of hemangiomas, this finding underlines the importance of needle aspiration of radiolucent lesions before biopsy. After the diagnosis of an hemangiomatous lesion of the jaws is made, carotid angiography is essential to demonstrate the extent of the lesion, to identify the supplying vessels, and to determine the rate of blood flow and shunt. This information allows correct treatment planning.

Hemangiomas have been classically described as capillary, cavernous, or mixed in type or as arteriovenous malformations (see Chap. 66). Cavernous hemangiomas are composed of large, thin-walled vascular spaces filled with red blood cells and lined by a single layer of endothelial cells in a connective tissue stroma. Capillary hemangiomas, in contrast, are composed of numerous capillary channels. In practice, this classification is of academic interest only, since the histologic type bears no relation to clinical behavior, response to treatment, or prognosis. A more useful classification is that related to the hemodynamics observed on angiography. Examination of the arterial and venous phases allows grouping according to the rate of flow through the lesion and the degree of arteriovenous (AV) shunting. The flow is the amount of blood coming into the lesion, and the shunt is the rapidity of transfer from the arterial to the venous system. When the shunt is high, the arterial and venous phases of the angiogram can be seen on the same x-ray plate.

Hemangiomas are largely in one of two categories: low flow, low shunt lesions and high flow, high shunt arteriovenous malformations. Low flow, low shunt lesions elsewhere in the body usually lend themselves to treatment with sclerosing agents (sodium tetradecyl sulfate [Sotradecol]) injected directly into the lesion. However, within bone they are best treated in the same way as the high flow, high shunt lesions because of the dangers of severe hemorrhage. The optimal treatment is preoperative, superselective embolization, using an absorbable gelatin sponge (Gelfoam) or occasionally ivalon, and followed, usually within 48 hours, by segmental resection. Immediate reconstruction is the rule in this setting. It may be possible to remove the hemangioma from the resected segment of jaw and use this as an autogenous bone tray filled with iliac cancellous bone in the reconstruction. Alternatively, a microvascular bone transfer may be used. Finally, the mandible may be stabilized to the maxilla by intermaxillary fixation; a spacer may be placed in the mandible and a delayed reconstruction performed. In the past, ligation of the external carotid supply was recommended; this causes a siphon effect resulting in the development of a new supply from the internal carotid system. This makes resection virtually impossible without severe neurologic sequelae. It is now believed that these lesions should be resected after embolization with minimal disturbance of the local vasculature to prevent this consequence (Fig. 69–6). Embolization may also be necessary as an emergency procedure to control acute hemorrhage, which can occur with tooth extraction when a previously undiagnosed lesion is present (Forbes and associates, 1986; Jackson, French, and Tolman, 1988).

PRIMARY MALIGNANCIES

Malignant odontogenic tumors are discussed above. Excluding tumors of the paranasal sinuses, the remainder of the primary malignancies of the jaws are made up mainly of sarcomas and lymphomas. Soft tissue sarcomas, squamous cell carcinoma, basal cell carcinoma, malignant melanoma, and metastatic lesions may also involve the jaws and craniofacial regions.

Osteosarcoma

Osteosarcoma accounts for 20 per cent of all primary bone malignancies (Coley, 1960); however, it represents only 6 per cent of jaw malignancies (Garrington and associates, 1967). The peak incidence is during the third and fourth decades of life, it is rare in children. There is a 2:1 male-to-female preponderance (Finkelstein, 1970). Radiation, preexisting bone disorders, and trauma have been implicated as causative factors (Greer, Rohrer, and Young, 1987). Paget's disease and fibrous dysplasia (Slow and Friedman, 1971) are the most common preexisting benign lesions associated with this tumor, although the role of the latter is extremely doubtful. Multicentric jaw lesions have also been reported (Stroncek and associates, 1981). Juxtacortical and periosteal forms are exceedingly rare (Banerjee, 1981).

The most common presentation is a painful swelling with associated paresthesias, occurring more often in the body of the mandible than in the maxilla (Curtis, Elmore, and Sotereanos, 1974). Maxillary lesions usually occur along the alveolar ridge, and there may be ulceration of the gingiva. With large lesions, there may be facial swelling, nasal obstruction and discharge, and, in maxillary lesions, epistaxis has been noted. Approximately 20 per cent of patients have elevated alkaline phosphatase levels (Caron, Hajdu, and Strong, 1971).

The radiographic appearance is variable. Some appear radiolucent and poorly delineated, whereas others show a dense radiopaque mass, with or without a prominent sunburst appearance. The latter is not a specific finding in malignancy and may also be seen in such conditions as fibrous dysplasia and osteomyelitis. Evidence of a symmetrically widened periodontal membrane space may be a significant early finding in osteosarcoma of the jaws (Garrington and associates, 1967). Although it is not diagnostic, it increases the index of suspicion. These findings, along with rapid growth over a period of six to eight weeks with associated pain and often paresthesias, are usually present. Computed tomography is the most useful investigation for determining the anatomic limits of this tumor. Three-dimensional reformatting of the CT scan may be helpful, as this can accurately show tumor size and shape (Fig. 69–7). Histologic examination demonstrates a sarcomatous connective tissue stroma, producing tumor osteoid and bone. Four histologic subtypes (fibroblastic, chondroblastic, osteoblastic, and telangiectatic) have been described (Greer, Rohrer, and Young, 1987).

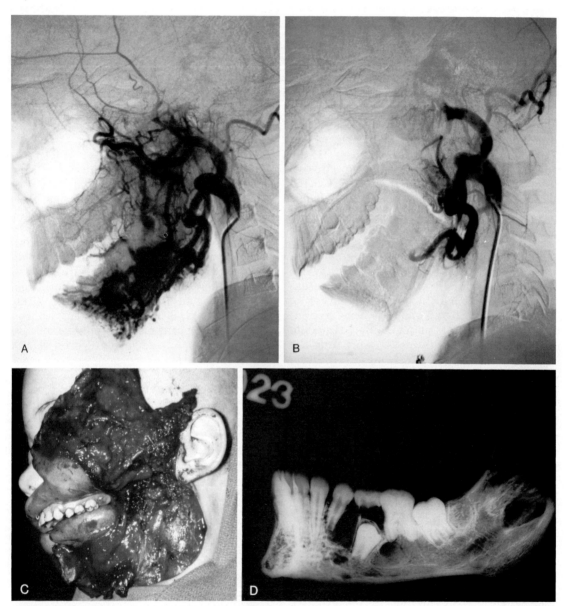

Figure 69–6. High flow AV malformation involving the left mandible and the pterygoid fossa. *A,* Left carotid angiogram of a patient with life-threatening bleeding associated with molar tooth eruption. There is extensive involvement of the left ascending ramus, the body of the mandible, and the symphysis, together with the pterygoid fossa. The blood supply is also from the right external carotid. *B,* Appearance after highly selective embolization of the lesion. *C,* Completed resection of the mandible, the submandibular triangle, and the pterygoid fossa. *D,* Radiograph of the excised specimen showing the relationship of the erupting tooth to the AV malformation.

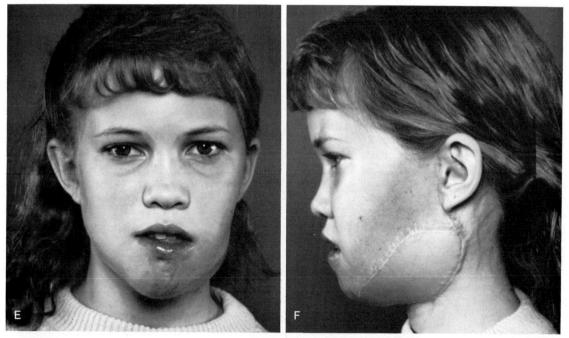

Figure 69–6 *Continued E, F,* The postsurgical defect with composite scapular microvascular flap after three years.

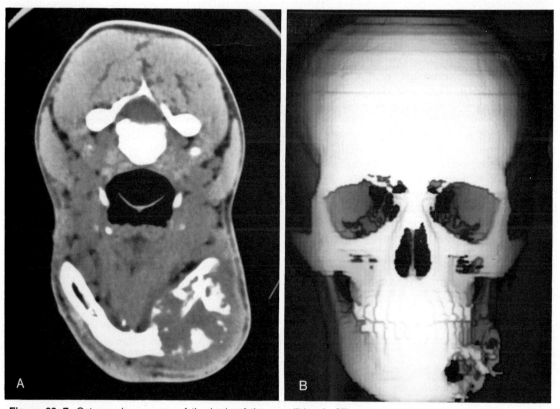

Figure 69–7. Osteogenic sarcoma of the body of the mandible. *A,* CT scan shows a destructive lesion of the left mandibular body with "bursting" appearance. *B,* Three-dimensional reformatting of CT scan shows the lesion's bony characteristics.

Surgery remains the treatment of choice (Russ and Jesse, 1980). The involved bone with surrounding soft tissue should be excised (Fig. 69–8). The resulting deformity may be considerable. Maxillectomy with orbital exenteration may be necessary for large maxillary lesions. Craniofacial surgical approaches (see below) are used for extensive lesions involving the skull base. Postoperative radiation therapy (7000 to 7500 rads) is also recommended. Preoperative radiation may be considered in large, unresectable lesions. When local disease has been controlled, surgical removal of lung metastases improves survival (Grothaus, Jackson, and Zelt, in preparation). Chemotherapy is rarely successful in the treatment of metastases (de Fries and Kornblut, 1979). If the lesion is in a favorable surgical site, the prognosis is good. Inoperable lesions are seldom cured with radiation therapy (Caron, Hajdu, and Strong, 1971). An average five year survival of 37 per cent for mandibular osteosarcoma and 27 per cent for maxillary lesions has been reported (Curtis, Elmore, and Sotereanos, 1974).

Chondrosaromas

These tumors are approximately half as common as osteosarcomas in the head and neck area. They occur most frequently in the nasoseptal region. The neoplasm is composed of fully developed cartilage formed from a sarcomatous stroma. It is important to note that chondrogenic neoplasms of the jaws are more often malignant than benign (Chaudhry and associates, 1961). Histologic differentiation between a chondrosarcoma and a benign chondroma can be extremely difficult (Miles, 1950). Benign chondrogenic lesions often recur after conservative excision and may return as more cellular or frankly malignant lesions. This supports the theory that lesions diagnosed as chondromas in this anatomic location are incipient chondrosarcomas. As with osteosarcoma, they can be peripheral, central, or juxtacortical. The tumor may be induced by radiation. Rarely, it may arise from preexisting Paget's disease (Thompson and Turner-Warwick, 1955), fibrous dysplasia (Feintuch, 1973), or bone cysts (Grabias and Mankin, 1974).

Patients range in age from the second to the ninth decade. Presenting symptoms are similar to those of osteosarcoma. Chondrosar-comas appear radiographically as large, thick-walled radiolucent areas with central areas of cotton-wool type calcifications representing medullary bone destruction (Greer, Rohrer, and Young, 1987). Cortical destruction occurs late in the disease and may result in a fuzzy peripheral shadow, extending into the adjacent soft tissues.

Treatment is radical excision, preserving an adequate margin of normal surrounding tissue (Fig. 69–9). This procedure should probably be utilized for all cartilaginous tumors of the jaws because of the difficulty in distinguishing benign and malignant lesions. Radiotherapy should be reserved for unresectable or incompletely excised lesions. There is no predictably effective chemotherapeutic agent; however, chemotherapy has been used adjunctively with surgery or for palliation.

Fibrosarcoma

Fibrosarcoma of the bone is histologically identical to fibrosarcoma of soft tissue and can be divided into well-differentiated, moderately differentiated, and undifferentiated types (Conley, Stout, and Healey, 1967). It usually originates from extragnathic sites, including the soft tissues of the face and neck, the paranasal sinuses, and the nasopharynx. When the mandible and maxilla are the primary sites, the tumor is often described as being endosteal or periosteal, the latter having a much better prognosis (Batsakis, 1979). The tumors are extremely radioresistant. After radical excision of primary jaw fibrosarcomas, the reported survival rates for the endosteal lesions are approximately 20 per cent versus 50 per cent for the periosteal type (Batsakis, 1979).

Ewing's Sarcoma

Ewing's sarcoma is a primary malignancy of bone and extraskeletal soft tissues. When located in the head and neck area, it occurs most commonly during the first and second decades of life. Metastases are commonly blood borne, lungs and bones being the most frequent sites (Telles, Rabson, and Pomeroy, 1978). Radiation (5000 to 5500 rads) is the principal form of therapy (Potdar, 1970). Small mandibular lesions, however, may be excised. Chemotherapy should be used adjunctively to improve survival rates (Pomeroy

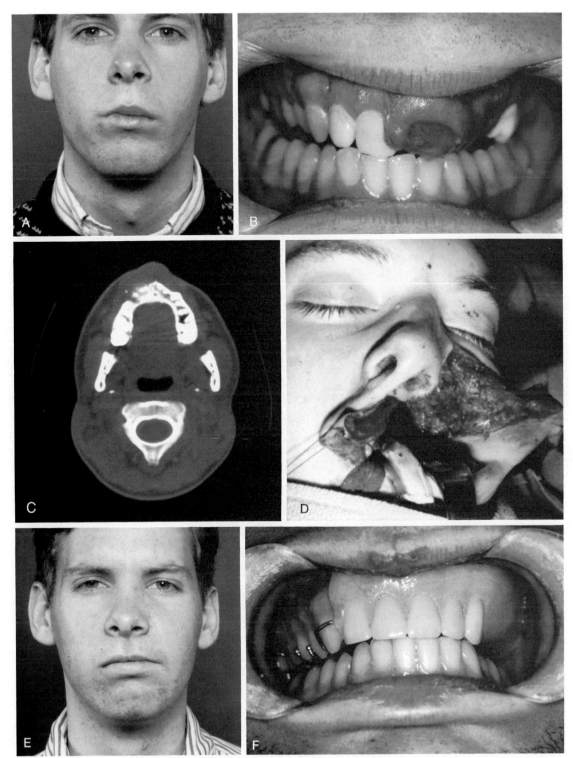

Figure 69–8. Osteogenic sarcoma of the maxilla. *A,* Patient with slight swelling of the left cheek preoperatively. *B,* Lesion clearly involving the left half of the upper alveolus. *C,* CT scan illustrating the destructive lesion of the left upper alveolus. *D,* Maxillectomy sparing the floor of the left orbit. *E,* Appearance one year after surgery. *F,* Maxillary prosthesis in place.

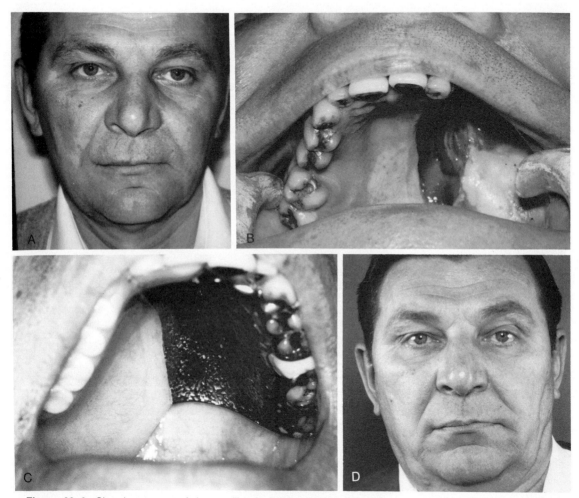

Figure 69–9. Chondrosarcoma of the maxilla. *A,* Patient has slight swelling of the left cheek preoperatively. *B,* Appearance after radical maxillectomy and skin grafting. The orbital floor is intact. *C,* Dental prosthesis in place. *D,* Appearance six years after surgery.

and Johnson, 1975); the most frequent regimen is vincristine, cyclophosphamide, dactinomycin, and doxorubicin hydrochloride. The reported five year survival rate with combination therapy is 50 per cent (Nesbit and associates, 1981).

Malignant Fibrous Histiocytoma

Malignant fibrous histiocytomas of bone are rare and are accepted as a separate entity, distinct from fibrosarcoma (Dahlin, Unni, and Matsuno, 1977). Electron microscopy shows at least two cell lines: histiocytes and fibroblastic types. Depending on the path of differentiation of the neoplastic cells, either type may predominate (Fu and associates, 1975). The clinical presentation is similar to that of other malignancies of the jaws, pain and swelling being most common (Slootweg and Muller, 1977; Webber and Wienke, 1977). The tumor usually occurs during the fourth and fifth decades of life. It is locally invasive and may metastasize to regional lymph nodes. Treatment is wide resection (Weiss and Enzinger, 1978), with lymph node dissection for clinically abnormal nodes. Radiotherapy is ineffective, and the role of chemotherapy is unclear (Weiner and associates, 1983). Five year survival rates vary from 34.5 to 67 per cent (Huvos, 1976; Ghandur-Mnaymneh, Zych, and Mnaymneh, 1982).

Non-Hodgkin's Lymphoma of Bone

Primary malignant lymphomas make up approximately 5 per cent of all malignant bone tumors (Dahlin, 1978). The most common sites are the maxillary antrum and the mandible. Most patients are in the fifth and sixth decades of life. The most common finding is pain, followed by a palpable mass, paresthesias, and tooth mobility. Male-to-female ratio is 3:1 (Boston and associates, 1974). There are osteolytic areas with less prominent areas of osteoblastic change on radiographic study (Scott and Ellis, 1987). Unlike the case with other malignancies of the jaws, destruction of the cortex and soft tissue extension are not commonly seen. The cell type varies, and both nodular or diffuse histologic patterns are seen (Rappaport, 1966). Tumor stage is determined, followed by treatment consisting of combined megavoltage radiation and chemotherapy. When treatment is begun early, the prognosis is

good. Combined chemotherapy and radiation therapy yields reported five year survival rates of 70 per cent for patients with Stage I disease and 60 per cent with Stage II disease (Scott and Ellis, 1987).

Burkitt's Lymphoma

This neoplasm of B lymphocytes is noted in African children as jaw swelling, abdominal masses, and, often, paraplegia (Burkitt, 1958). It is associated with the Epstein-Barr virus (Ziegler, 1981). A nonendemic form of the disease also occurs (Batsakis, 1979), but jaw lesions are infrequent. In the African form, maxillary involvement is most common; however, jaw lesions may be found in all four quadrants. Renal failure, attributable to abdominal involvement, is common. Radiographs of the jaws demonstrate large radiolucent defects with cortical disruption. The tumor grows extremely rapidly, and definitive treatment should be initiated early to avoid a fatal outcome (Ziegler, 1981). It does, however, respond well to alkylating agents, with remission occurring in more than 90 per cent of patients (Scott and Ellis, 1987). It is one of the few malignancies that can be cured by chemotherapy alone. Surgical debulking prior to chemotherapy may be indicated in large lesions.

Angiosarcoma

Angiosarcoma of bone is an extremely rare jaw malignancy. Histologic evaluation shows neoplastic vascular proliferation within a loose connective tissue stroma. Angiosarcoma of bone behaves less aggressively than its soft tissue counterpart, and the prognosis is significantly better. Treatment is radical excision. Well-differentiated lesions demonstrate a five year survival rate of 95 per cent. Patients with undifferentiated tumors are reported to have a 20 per cent survival rate (Wold and associates, 1982).

Primary Salivary Gland Tumors

Intraosseous salivary gland neoplasms are rare. They may arise from embryonic salivary gland inclusions (Bhaskar, 1963) or from mucous metaplasia of the lining of odontogenic cysts (Marano and Hartman, 1974). The vast majority of primary salivary gland tumors of bone are of the mucoepidermoid type (Browand and Waldron, 1975). The most common presentation is a painless swelling in the posterior aspect of the mandible. Treatment consists of wide excision. Maxillary tumors are best treated by maxillectomy (Smith, Dahlin, and Waite, 1968). The tumors do not readily metastasize but, on occasion, may involve regional lymph nodes.

TUMORS OF NASAL CAVITY AND PARANASAL SINUSES

The paranasal sinuses are diverticula of the nasal cavity. They are lined by respiratory mucosa that is derived from ectoderm (schneiderian mucosa) (Batsakis, 1980), as opposed to the epithelium of the lower airway, which is derived from foregut (see also Chap. 68). The sinus mucosal lining contains pseudostratified columnar ciliated cells, basal cells, and mucous secretory cells. Thus it can give rise to epithelial neoplasms of an epidermoid (squamous cell lesions) and a nonepidermoid origin (primarily salivary gland adenocarcinomas). The lateral nasal wall and the septum, craniad to the superior turbinate, are lined by specialized nonciliated olfactory mucosa containing modified nerve elements; thus olfactory neuroblastomas (esthesioneuroblastomas) arise in this area. Melanoma and teratomatous lesions compose the rest of the primary tumors of the sinus areas. Other soft tissue sarcomas that may secondarily involve these regions are discussed below under Soft Tissue Sarcomas of Head and Neck.

The lymphatic drainage of the frontal, ethmoid, and sphenoid sinuses is transosseous via the ostium of the individual sinus to the lymphatic network of the posterior nasal cavity, as well as via the meningeal lymphatics. The maxillary sinus lymphatics drain into the submandibular and upper cervical chains; the remainder of the drainage from this sinus is via its ostium to the lymphatics of the posterior nasal cavity and via channels penetrating the nasopharyngeal region to the deep cervical fascia and nodes around the carotid and internal jugular veins. The posterior nasal cavity lymphatic drainage is to the retropharyngeal nodes and subsequently to the superior deep cervical nodes. The vestibular skin and the anterior-most nasal mucosa drain to the periparotid and submaxillary nodes and then to the superior deep

cervical chain (Moss-Salentijn, 1985). The majority of malignancies in this area affect the surgically inaccessible retropharyngeal nodes first. Thus, elective neck dissection is futile for prophylactic control of lymphatic spread of these malignancies.

Papillomas

These lesions, also known as schneiderian papillomas (Batsakis, 1981b), arise from the respiratory mucosa of the nasal cavity and paranasal sinuses. They are uncommon, being much less frequent than the common nasal polyp. They are not allergic in type, and they occur mainly in the fifth decade of life. The lesions arise from a proliferation of cells located at the basement membrane of the mucosa; the overlying epithelium is transitional, with a tendency toward squamous cell differentiation. Occasionally, multilayered, columnar cells may predominate, and the papillomas are then termed cylindric cell. The latter group may be confused histologically with a papillary adenocarcinoma. Schneiderian papillomas are described according to their anatomic location as lateral wall and septal types. This distinction is important because the septal variety tends to remain localized and is rarely associated with squamous cell carcinoma. In contrast, the lateral wall variety may involve multiple sites, including the sinuses, and may contain squamous cell carcinoma. The carcinoma arises as an in situ focus within the papilloma or within the same anatomic region. Papillomas may grow in two patterns, inverted and exophytic. The inverted type is most commonly associated with lesions of the lateral wall or sinuses. The inverted form grows into the underlying stroma, whereas the exophytic or fungiform type exhibits surface proliferation most commonly on the septum. Extensive keratinization in a papilloma is atypical and should arouse suspicion of an early squamous cell carcinoma. Treatment consists of conservative excision. Papillomas have a tendency to recur (Hyams, 1971), and, in diagnosing lesions of the lateral wall, squamous cell carcinoma must be considered.

Squamous Cell Carcinoma

This neoplasm arises from metaplastic epithelium of the respiratory mucosa and makes up approximately 75 to 90 per cent of malignancies in this site. Primary squamous cell carcinoma restricted to the nasal cavity is uncommon. Most lesions arise from the turbinates or the nasal septum (Batsakis, 1980). Bony invasion occurs in more than one-third of cases. Regional nodal metastases occur in 10 per cent of patients (Batsakis, 1980). Surgical excision and irradiation appear to be equally effective for treatment of early lesions.

Since the paranasal sinuses are a clinically silent area, diagnosis of sinus tumors is frequently delayed (Batsakis, 1980) (see Chap. 68). The majority are moderately well differentiated and are usually keratinizing; nonkeratinizing and anaplastic carcinomas make up the remainder (Batsakis, 1987). Although the anaplastic variety may progress more rapidly, the prognosis is mainly related to the size of the tumor at diagnosis; 80 per cent of paranasal squamous cell carcinomas arise in the maxillary antrum (Frazell and Lewis, 1963). Squamous cell carcinoma of the ethmoid sinuses is the next most common, followed by rare primary lesions of the frontal and sphenoid sinuses (Robin, Powell, and Stansbie, 1979). Tumors may have oral, nasal, ocular, or neurologic signs and symptoms. These include a palatal mass or erosion, trismus, dental pain, epistaxis or nasal stuffiness, nasal mass, exophthalmos, eye dystopia, blindness, facial deformity, pain, paresthesia, or anesthesia in the distribution of the trigeminal nerve or one of its branches. Maxillary antral tumors may mimic chronic sinusitis in their early phase and may be diagnosed at the time of the drainage procedure. There is an increased incidence of carcinomas of the maxillary sinus in patients with exposure to heavy metals, particularly nickel (Pedersen, Hogetveit, and Andersen, 1973). Ninety per cent of sinus lesions have invaded through at least one wall at the time of diagnosis, and this will be evident on radiographic evaluation (Batsakis, 1980).

Combined treatment with surgery and irradiation gives a 45 per cent five year survival rate for patients with resectable lesions (Rice and Stanley, 1987). Surgical treatment consists of maxillectomy, sometimes in combination with ethmoid sinus and anterior cranial fossa resection, depending on the location and extent of the tumor at the time of diagnosis. Criteria for unresectability, when the cavernous sinus or the trigeminal ganglion is invaded, are discussed below. Invasion of the trigeminal ganglion occurs by infiltration along the first or second division of the nerve. Patients with unresectable lesions treated by radiation therapy alone have five year survival rates of 12 to 19 per cent (Hamberger, Martensson, and Sjorgren, 1967).

Nonepidermoid Carcinoma

These tumors arise from the glandular elements of the sinus mucosa and ductal epithelium; adenocarcinomas predominate. The most common site is the ethmoid region (Batsakis, 1980). Adenocarcinomas are described as papillary, sessile, or alveolar-mucoid in type. Less frequently, well-differentiated adenocarcinomas can occur as nasal polyps (Heffner and associates, 1982). They resemble gastrointestinal adenocarcinomas histologically. Wood dust, mustard gas, and isopropanol are all thought to be environmental factors causing these tumors (Rousch, 1979). Treatment is the same as that suggested for squamous cell carcinoma.

Adenoid cystic carcinomas are the most common of the salivary gland tumors occurring in the paranasal sinuses. Delayed diagnosis is the rule, and fixation or extension to adjacent structures is noted in nearly 75 per cent of patients (Spiro, Huvos, and Strong, 1974). Perineural spread is common, occurring along the frontal and maxillary divisions of the trigeminal nerve. Lymphatic spread occurs in 14 per cent of patients; hematogenous dissemination is much more common, occurring in up to 40 per cent. The lungs and the bones are the most frequent sites of metastases, and this spread is usually associated with failure of local control. Treatment is similar to that proposed for squamous cell carcinoma.

Melanoma

Approximately 1 per cent of all melanomas are primary to the nasal cavity and paranasal sinuses (Batsakis and associates, 1982). Sixteen per cent are found in blacks (Holdcraft and Gallagher, 1969). They originate from melanocytes in the mucosa and the submucosa of the nasal cavity and the paranasal sinuses. The most common sites of occurrence are the anterior part of the nasal septum, the middle and inferior turbinates, and the maxillary antrum (Batsakis and associates, 1982). Epistaxis is the most frequent initial sign, followed by nasal obstruction, pain, and swelling. Melanomas may be heavily pigmented or amelanotic; in the latter case, they are often misdiagnosed as anaplastic carcinoma or sarcoma. Regional lymph node metastases are rare at the initial presentation (Shah, Huvos, and Strong, 1977). Treatment consists of radical excision (Fig. 69–10). Ten year survival rates range from 17 to 38 per cent (Batsakis, 1987).

Esthesioneuroblastoma

This is a rare tumor of the olfactory epithelium, occurring in the most superior portion

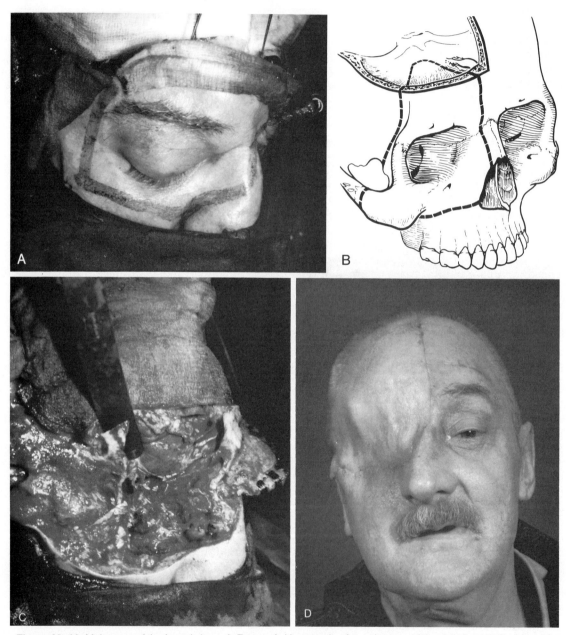

Figure 69–10. Melanoma of the frontal sinus. *A,* Extent of skin resection for melanoma of the right frontal sinus involving the right orbit and the floor of the anterior cranial fossa. *B,* Outline of the bony resection. *C,* Resection completed. Radical neck dissection also performed. *D,* Postoperative result after coverage with a large scalp flap.

of the nasal cavity, the nasal septum, the turbinates, the ethmoid sinuses, or the cribriform plate; it forms exophytic or sessile masses. The tumor is found in patients from the first to the ninth decades (Silva and associates, 1982). It behaves aggressively and has symptoms ranging from epistaxis and nasal obstruction to ocular pain and headaches (Jackson, 1985). Metastases may occur, the most common sites being the cervical lymph nodes, lungs, and bone. Approximately 50 per cent of patients die from uncontrolled intracranial extension. The most useful preoperative examinations are CT and magnetic

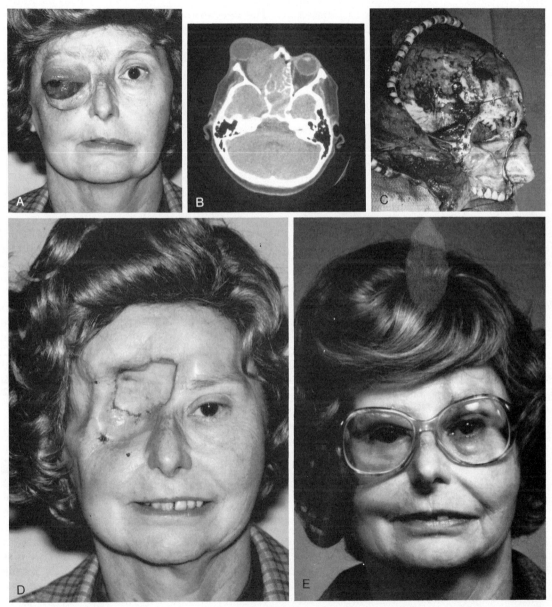

Figure 69–11. Esthesioneuroblastoma of the anterior cranial fossa. *A,* Recurrent esthesioneuroblastoma of the right orbit, the anterior skull base, the left orbit, and the right maxilla. Previous maxillectomy and radiotherapy were unsuccessful. *B,* CT scan shows the extent of the recurrent esthesioneuroblastoma. *C,* Resection completed. There was removal of the right orbit and its contents together with the anterior skull base, the medial wall of the left orbit, and the remainder of the maxilla. The skull base was covered with a galeal frontalis flap and a temporalis flap. Note the insertion of the patient's previous denture, which was built up with a stent covered with a split-thickness skin graft. *D,* Six months after surgery, there was erosion of a portion of the skull through radiotherapy-damaged skin. This was treated by debridement and application of a split-thickness skin graft to the dura. *E,* External prosthesis in place three years after resection.

resonance imaging (MRI). Treatment should be aggressive, using if necessary a combined extra- and intracranial approach with total surgical extirpation. After radical resection, galeal frontalis myofascial flaps or temporalis muscle flaps are used to separate the oral cavity and the nasopharynx from the extra-dural space; this is frequently necessary to prevent postoperative ascending infection in this region (Fig. 69–11) (Jackson, 1985). A full tumoricidal dose of radiation therapy is given postoperatively. Inadequate surgical resection or radiotherapy alone results in a high incidence of recurrence.

Malignant Teratomas

These are extremely rare tumors characterized by a combination of epithelial and connective tissue elements. Sarcomatous components are a prominent finding. Malignant teratoma commonly occurs as a nasal cavity mass (Heffner and Hyams, 1984). The ethmoid and maxillary sinuses are frequently involved. Wide excision seems to be the only effective method of treatment (Fig. 69–12).

Metastatic Tumors

Renal tumors are by far the most common tumor of infraclavicular origin to metastasize to the paranasal sinuses (Batsakis, 1981b). Tumors of the lungs, the breasts and the gastrointestinal tract may also metastasize to this area, the maxillary antrum and the nasal cavity being the most common sites. Treatment depends on the resectability and the histologic features of the primary tumor.

TUMORS OF ORBITS

Orbital tumors originate from the contents of the orbit, the skeleton of the orbit, or the surrounding structures (by invasion). Tumors that are totally contained within the periorbitum are not considered here, since these require standard exenteration from an external approach. Only tumors that frequently require craniofacial surgical resection are discussed; treatment is presented below.

In adults, the majority of orbital cancers are lymphomas, invasive eyelid or sinus tumors, and metastatic lesions (Dutton and Anderson, 1987). In children, rhabdomyosar-

coma accounts for up to 75 per cent of orbital malignancies, with metastatic neuroblastoma, lymphoid tumors, and extraocular retinoblastomas composing the remainder (Porterfield and Zimmerman, 1962).

The unique anatomy of the orbit often allows for early diagnosis. The most common presentations include proptosis, disturbances in ocular motility and vision, displacement of the eye, orbital pain, and headache. Rarely, infiltration by cicatrizing lesions may lead to enophthalmos (Pindborg, Kramer, and Torloni, 1971). The most valuable noninvasive investigations are high resolution CT and MRI; ultrasonography can also be used. Selective angiography is of value in vascular lesions. High resolution CT scan shows the margins as smooth or infiltrative (Pindborg, Kramer, and Torloni, 1971). Erosion of bone suggests an aggressive lesion, whereas excavation and expansion imply a long-standing, noninfiltrative process (Rootman and Allen, 1987). With contrast enhancement, it is often possible to differentiate vascular lesions, mucoceles, and solid tumors (Pindborg, Kramer, and Torloni, 1971). The site of origin and the degree of extension can also be defined. With these diagnostic techniques and a careful evaluation of the patient's clinical history, a preoperative confirmatory biopsy may not be necessary. When the diagnosis remains in doubt, aspiration biopsy under CT control can be of value (Pindborg, Kramer, and Torloni, 1971); however, MRI scanning may reduce the need for such procedures (Pindborg, Kramer, and Torloni, 1971).

Lymphoma

Lymphomas compose 8 per cent of all orbital tumors and need to be differentiated from benign lymphoid infiltrations, which occur twice as often (Henderson, 1980). The most common type is the lymphocytic lymphoma. The lesion is noted as a palpable mass with or without proptosis and occurs most commonly during the fifth and sixth decades (Knowles and Jakobiec, 1980). The treatment of choice is radiation therapy.

Rhabdomyosarcoma

This tumor is the most common primary orbital malignancy in childhood (Dutton and Anderson, 1987). The management and prog-

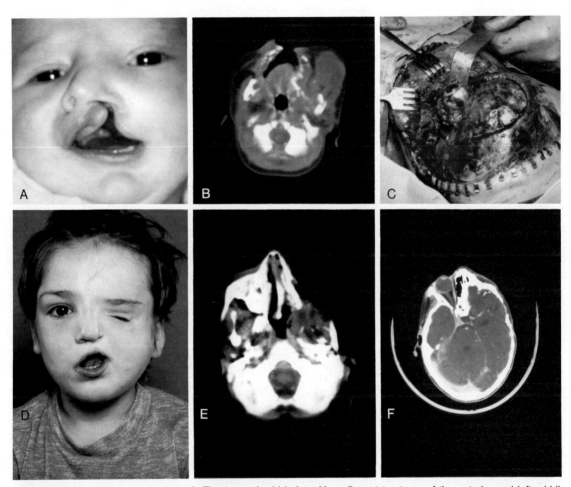

Figure 69–12. Malignant teratoma. *A,* Three month old baby with malignant teratoma of the anterior and left middle cranial fossae, the orbit, and the maxilla. Note the swelling of the left cheek and slight proptosis of the left eye. There is also a cleft lip and palate. *B,* CT scan showing the extent of the tumor in the maxilla, the orbit, the skull base, and the infratemporal fossa area. *C,* Resection of the anterior and middle cranial fossae and the skull base, together with the orbital contents, the maxilla, and the infratemporal fossa. *D,* The patient's appearance six years after surgery. *E,* CT scan one year after surgery. *F,* CT scan six years after reconstruction of the bony defect.

nosis vary depending on the site of the tumor. Those within the orbit have the best prognosis, probably because the orbital skeleton and periorbita act as a barrier to tumor spread. The diagnosis should be confirmed by biopsy. The tumors may grow rapidly, and a delay in diagnosis may have dire consequences. Rhabdomyosarcomas usually metastasize to lungs and bones (Porterfield and Zimmerman, 1962), and regional lymph node involvement may occur. In orbital rhabdomyosarcoma, radiation therapy with adjuvant chemotherapy, rather than surgical enucleation, is recommended (Albright and associates, 1937; Reichart and Ries, 1983). Vision may be retained, although, with doses greater than 5000 rads, useful vision is preserved in only 25 per cent of patients. In children less than 6 years of age, a total of 4000 to 4500 rads is given; older children receive 4500 to 5500 rads. The neck should be included if it is clinically involved. The chemotherapy regimen usually includes vincristine, actinomycin D, and cyclophosphamide. With combined radiation and chemotherapy, prognosis has improved dramatically with overall survival rates of approximately 70 per cent (Maurer and associates, 1977). Recurrent tumors require extensive resection, usually with orbital exenteration (Fig. 69–13).

Other Malignant Tumors

Invasion of the orbit from surrounding areas, such as the paranasal sinuses and eyelids, accounts for 20 per cent of orbital malignancies. Squamous cell carcinoma is the most common, followed by basal cell carcinoma, sebaceous cell carcinoma, and soft tissue sarcoma (Dutton and Anderson, 1987). Treatment of these lesions is radical surgery, often with adjunctive local radiotherapy and chemotherapy.

Extension of intraocular retinoblastomas and malignant melanomas accounts for approximately 15 per cent of orbital neoplasms (Dutton and Anderson, 1987). Treatment usually consists of orbital exenteration with or without orbital bone resection, in association with adjunctive radiotherapy and chemotherapy.

Hemangiopericytomas are aggressive vascular orbital tumors, producing signs associated with a growing mass lesion; pain is a frequent feature. More than 75 per cent of

these tumors originate in the superior orbit (Croxatto and Font, 1982). The treatment is radical surgical excision.

Malignant optic nerve gliomas are rare tumors occurring almost exclusively in adults. Treatment is surgical excision. For tumors involving the base of the skull or those located superiorly and posteriorly, a transcranial approach is advocated. Schwannomas, fibrous dysplasia, and neurofibromatosis of the orbit, although not malignant, frequently require a craniofacial approach for adequate surgical exposure and resection.

Lacrimal Gland Tumors

The most common lacrimal gland malignancy is the adenoid cystic carcinoma, followed in frequency by adenocarcinomas, malignant mixed tumors, and mucoepidermoid carcinomas (Dutton and Anderson, 1987). The tumors can occur at any age and have symptoms of a mass lesion in the orbit and pain due to perineural invasion. They are aggressive and generally have a poor prognosis (Font and Gamel, 1978). En bloc radical intra- and extracranial resection is recommended for extensive tumors in this area. Radiotherapy has not proved to be effective adjuvant therapy.

Metastatic Neoplasms

Metastatic tumors to the orbit represent approximately 5 per cent of all solid orbital masses (Henderson, 1980). In adults, the primary lesion is most frequently in the breast and lung (Font and Ferry, 1976). In children, metastases from abdominal or thoracic neuroblastomas are more common. Management is determined by the primary tumor. Surgical intervention is usually not indicated, but it may be considered for control of intractable pain.

SOFT TISSUE SARCOMAS OF HEAD AND NECK

These lesions are considered briefly, since they may require combined intra- and extracranial resection for complete removal. These tumors are rare, and they frequently involve the facial skeleton and skull base. Craniofa-

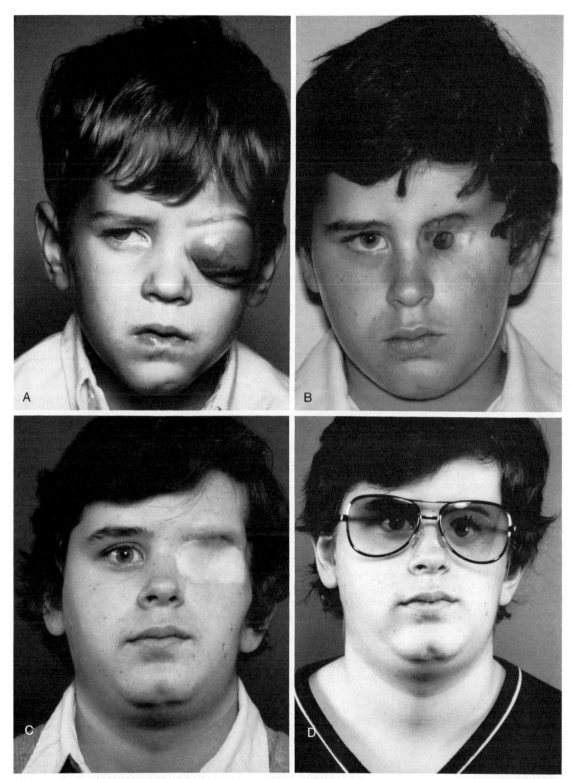

Figure 69–13. Rhabdomyosarcoma. *A,* Rhabdomyosarcoma of the left orbit, which recurred after chemotherapy and radiotherapy. *B,* Appearance six years after resection and skin grafting. *C,* A pectoralis major musculocutaneous flap was applied after resection of the ethmoid sinuses and closure of the defect into the nose. The orbit was reconstructed with cranial bone grafts. *D,* Appearance after placement of the orbital prosthesis.

cial surgery for congenital deformity correction has stimulated the development of new surgical approaches that provide excellent exposure, which is the key to safe en bloc resection.

The incidence of sarcomas in the head and neck region is less than that in other parts of the body. It is difficult to compare childhood and adult sarcomas, since each group develops different types; however, the management is similar. After a histopathologic diagnosis has been established by biopsy, a treatment plan is selected. Therapy includes surgery, radiotherapy, and chemotherapy, as indicated. Virtually all treatment of head and neck sarcomas is based on experience gained in treating similar tumors elsewhere. In surgical resection, the first procedure undoubtedly has the best chance for success. Local recurrence due to inadequate resection has been a frequent cause of treatment failure. Node dissection is generally indicated only for clinically involved nodes or because of the need for exposure of the vascular anatomy before skull base resection. Radiotherapy may be administered pre-, intra-, or postoperatively. Chemotherapy has been useful in the treatment of rhabdomyosarcomas, and it has been reported to be of value in other sarcomas (Glenn and associates, 1985). Immunotherapy is controversial. Preoperative chemotherapy and radiotherapy may be used to reduce the size of large, inaccessible sarcomas. Experience, however, shows this to be a rare event.

Preoperative evaluation should define the extent of local as well as distant disease; the treatment can be planned and the prognosis established. Radiographic examinations should include plain x-ray films of the skull and facial bones, high resolution axial and coronal CT scans of the skull and facial bones, high resolution axial and coronal CT scans of the skull and face, and, when indicated, MRI scans. In some orbital tumors, ultrasound scanning can be helpful. Radioactive scanning of the brain, skeleton, liver, and spleen is performed, if indicated. Other investigations may include fine needle aspiration, bone marrow aspiration and biopsy, and lumbar puncture.

Rhabdomyosarcoma

This is the most common head and neck sarcoma of childhood. Management and prognosis vary depending on the site of origin. In 1972, the Intergroup Rhabdomyosarcoma Study was established to evaluate treatment modalities. Three groups were identified depending on anatomic location of the rhabdomyosarcoma: (1) eyelid and orbital, (2) parameningeal, and (3) other. Those in the orbit had the best prognosis. Parameningeal tumors (those of the middle ear, mastoid, ear canal, nasal cavity, paranasal sinuses, nasopharynx, and infratemporal fossa) had an increased risk of meningeal extension and, therefore, the poorest prognosis. Lesions in other locations were intermediate in prognosis.

Orbital rhabdomyosarcoma was discussed above. Parameningeal lesions frequently have bony or meningeal involvement, and central nervous system treatment may be of benefit, either craniospinal axis irradiation or intrathecal chemotherapy. Treatment of the remainder of the rhabdomyosarcomas is surgical excision of as much tumor as possible without causing mutilating defects. If tumor remains, surgery is followed by radiation therapy and chemotherapy. Neck dissection should be performed for clinically abnormal nodes. Radiotherapy dose is a total of 4000 to 4500 rads in children under 6 years; older children receive 4500 to 5500 rads. The usual chemotherapy regimen is vincristine, actinomycin D and cyclophosphamide.

Staging of rhabdomyosarcoma is based on postsurgical findings: Group I, completely resected without residual tumor; Group II, resected with histologic evidence of microscopic residual tumor; Group III, gross residual tumor; and Group IV, documented metastatic disease. Except for Group I lesions, triple chemotherapy and radiotherapy are given according to a strict protocol. For Group IV patients, adriamycin can be added. With this treatment survival rates have improved significantly; however, patients with parameningeal tumors or distant metastases still have a poor prognosis.

Fibrosarcoma

This is the most common soft tissue head and neck sarcoma in adults (Greager and associates, 1985) and the second most common in children. Radical surgery is the recommended treatment. Radiotherapy and chemotherapy are not curative but should be used in recurrent or metastatic disease (Das

Gupta, 1983). The prognosis is excellent in infantile fibrosarcoma (in children under 5 years of age) with five year survival rates reported as 85 per cent or greater.

Neuroblastoma

This is an uncommon primary tumor of the head and neck area, which may be congenital. Metastases are frequent and should be looked for carefully prior to commencement of therapy. Staging of the disease is important (Evans, D'Angio, and Randolph, 1971). In Stage I and II disease, complete excision results in 90 per cent survival in patients under 1 year of age (Fig. 69–14). In Stage II disease with residual tumor, and Stage III disease with postoperative irradiation, satisfactory results have been reported (Breslow and McCann, 1971). Older patients and those with Stage IV disease have a uniformly poor prognosis. Patients under 1 year of age with Stage IV lesions also have a good survival rate, probably because of activation of the immune system. Metastatic disease is treated with chemotherapy.

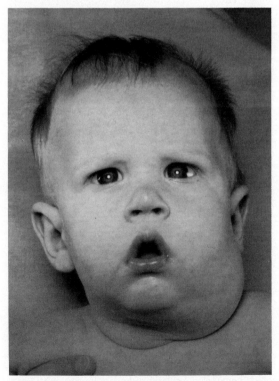

Figure 69–14. Large neuroblastoma involving the left side of the neck in a 2 month old child.

Neurofibrosarcoma (Malignant Schwannoma)

This is a rare neoplasm, which may arise independently or in association with generalized neurofibromatosis (von Recklinghausen's disease). Twelve per cent of neurofibrosarcomas occur in the head and neck. It is difficult to determine the exact incidence because of varying institutional criteria (Enzinger and Weiss, 1983). A malignant transformation in neurofibromatosis can occur, but the true incidence is probably not known because patients are lost to follow-up. Staging with the tumor, nodes, and metastases (TNM) classification and histopathologic grading of the malignancy correlate well with the outcome. Patients with Stage I tumors have an 80 per cent five year survival, whereas with Stage III tumors it is less than 20 per cent. Treatment is radical excision. If the nerve from which the tumor is arising can be found, it should be removed and the remaining cut end examined intraoperatively by frozen section to rule out tumor infiltration. Spread is usually blood borne, and therefore node dissection is not indicated. The role of adjuvant radiotherapy has not been evaluated in a prospective manner. Radiotherapy may, however, decrease local recurrence. Since most patients die of systemic disease, adjuvant chemotherapy may be warranted.

Malignant Fibrous Histiocytoma

This is a rare tumor in the head and neck region. Primary malignant fibrous histiocytoma of the jaws is discussed above. Treatment consists of wide, local excision. The place of regional lymph node dissection is unclear; however, some centers have reported satisfactory results in a small group of patients with clinically involved nodes. Adjuvant chemotherapy may decrease the recurrence rate. Factors influencing the prognosis are the depth of invasion, the size, and the histologic grade of the tumor. Overall five year survival rate is reported as 65 per cent (Enzinger and Weiss, 1983).

Hemangiopericytoma

This tumor is uncommon and only 1 per cent occur in the head and neck region. There are benign and malignant varieties; histologic differentiation is difficult. They most often occur in the sixth to seventh decades, and sex distribution is equal. Local excision is recommended for benign histiotypes and radical excision for malignant ones (Fig. 69–15). Neck dissection is performed for clinical involvement of nodes. Radiotherapy may be useful in large tumors, but the value of chemotherapy is unproved. The reported recurrence rates have decreased as the apprecia-

tion of malignant potential and the need for wide resections have become better understood. Histologic study showing high mitotic activity, necrosis, and hemorrhage indicates a poor prognosis, the ten year survival rate being 29 per cent. In lesions with low mitotic activity without necrosis, the ten year survival rate is approximately 80 per cent. The superior survival rate is probably related to more aggressive primary resection. The malignant potential of the tumors may become

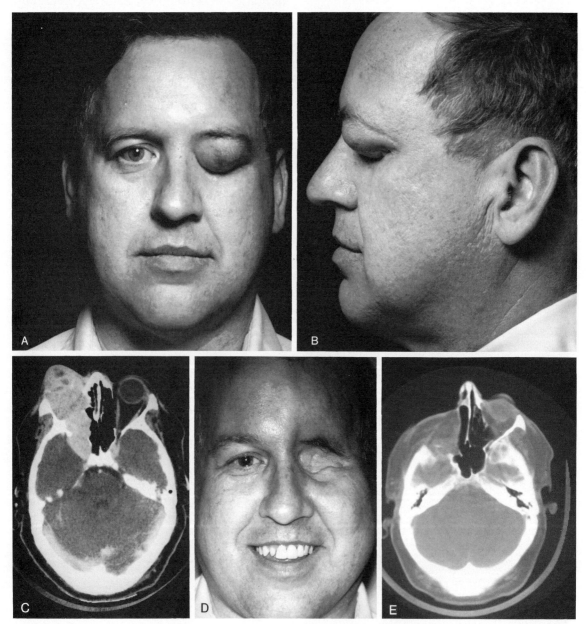

Figure 69–15. *A,* Malignant hemangiopericytoma. *A, B,* Malignant hemangiopericytoma involving the left orbit and the anterior skull base. *C,* CT scan showing extension of the tumor throughout the orbit and the middle cranial fossa. *D,* Appearance after radical resection of the anterior cranial fossa, the middle cranial fossa, and the left orbit. *E,* Postoperative CT scan.

evident only after some time has elapsed; metastases may occur ten years or more after primary excision.

Angiosarcoma

Angiosarcoma of the jaws is discussed above. When it originates in the soft tissues, wide surgical excision is the treatment of choice. Radiotherapy is useful for recurrences, but the effectiveness of chemotherapy is unknown. The prognosis is generally considered poor.

Liposarcoma

Liposarcomas rarely occur in the head and neck region, the reported incidence being 2 to 6 per cent (Spittle, Newton, and Mackenzie, 1970; Enzinger and Weiss, 1983; Barnes, 1985). Radical excision is the recommended primary treatment. The tumors are radiosensitive, but few cures have been reported with radiotherapy alone. Combination chemo- and radiotherapy is recommended for tumors that are recurrent or incompletely excised. Chemotherapy has not proved useful to date. The prognosis is dependent on the type and grade. Five year survival is reported as over 80 per cent for myxoid types and well-differentiated tumors but less than 50 per cent for round cell and pleomorphic types (Barnes, 1985).

Less than 15 cases have been reported in patients under the age of 18 years. In one series, seven of eight tumors recurred locally after incomplete excision. With complete removal, 8 of 24 cases recurred. Overall survival was 80 per cent for patients followed for at least 18 months (Saunders and associates, 1979).

Synovial Cell Sarcoma

Of these tumors only 1 per cent occur in the head and neck region. Primary treatment is wide excision. The tumor is moderately sensitive to radiotherapy and chemotherapy, and these may prove useful as adjunctive therapy. The prognosis depends on the size and grade of the tumor; the larger the tumor and higher the grade, the worse is the prognosis. The overall five year survival rate is reported as 47 per cent.

Leiomyosarcoma

This tumor is rarely found in the head and neck. Treatment consists of wide local excision, followed by chemotherapy and possibly radiotherapy. After adequate surgical resection, the prognosis is relatively good.

Desmoplastic Melanoma

Desmoplastic malignant melanoma represents a type of cutaneous melanoma that is characterized histologically by spindle cell morphology and an associated production of fibrous connective tissue (Constanzo and associates, 1987). It is locally aggressive and has a poor prognosis. It frequently occurs as an enlarging lentigo maligna with an underlying palpable subcutaneous element; 7 per cent occur in the head and neck area, usually in the older patient. Histologic recognition is difficult, especially in differentiating it from spindle cell squamous carcinoma and benign and malignant fibrous histiocytoma. Junctional activity may be indicative of its true origin. Local invasion is present as a fibrous plaque, which ultimately penetrates bone, muscle, and nerve. What appears to be adequate local excision is often followed by multiple local recurrences. Spread to regional nodes may be late but is common. Hematogenous spread may be present at the time of diagnosis. Less than 40 per cent of patients are disease free at five years, and mortality approaches 100 per cent at ten years (Constanzo and associates, 1987). Treatment is by wide local resection (Fig. 69–16). Careful and frequent follow-up is necessary. Any areas of induration, particularly those associated with pain, require biopsy. It is advised that reconstruction be performed only for functional reasons. The area should be left as accessible as possible for examination and biopsy after the initial excision. Regional nodes should be removed if palpable adenopathy is present, or if the primary lesion is close to an area of lymph node drainage.

SURGICAL TREATMENT OF TUMORS INVOLVING JAWS AND CRANIOFACIAL SKELETON

The majority of tumors affecting the craniofacial skeleton and their treatment are

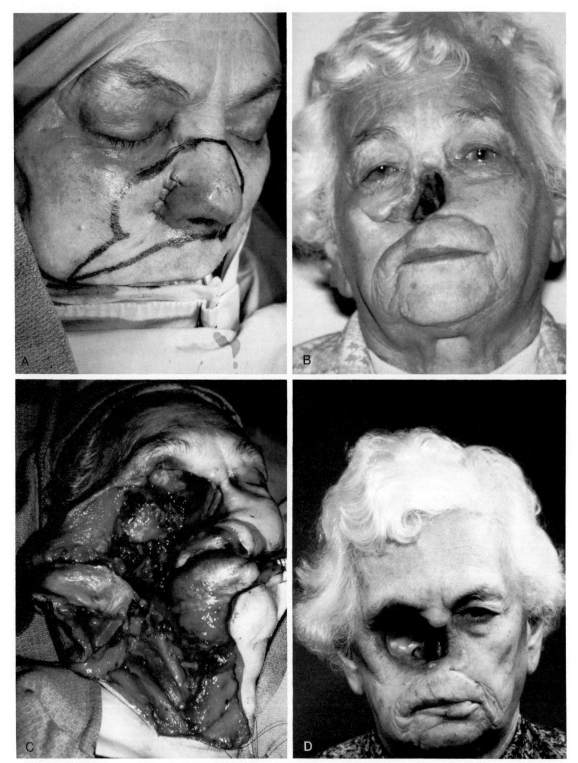

Figure 69–16. Desmoplastic melanoma. *A,* Biopsy proven desmoplastic melanoma involving the tip of the nose and the nasolabial area. The extent of the planned resection is outlined. *B,* Recurrence in the right maxilla after six months. *C,* Radical resection of the orbit, the maxilla, the base of the middle cranial fossa, and the infratemporal fossa and modified radical neck dissection using a mandibular swing exposure. *D,* Postoperative appearance six months later. The patient died within three years of the first resection.

described above. The planning and execution of surgical procedures necessary to excise malignancies or aggressive "benign" lesions is presented here. Although a relatively localized malignancy of the mandible or the maxilla can be adequately treated by segmental mandibulectomy or maxillectomy, local extension to the orbit, the sinuses, the infratemporal fossa, or the cranial base increases the complexity of the problem. If this is discovered intraoperatively, it requires a departure from the original surgical plan. It should be appreciated that these procedures progress from the simple to the complex in a graduated fashion, and they should not be thought of as separate unrelated operations. Application of craniofacial surgical techniques allows excellent exposure, permitting relatively safe, total tumor removal in lesions previously considered unresectable. In this region, local recurrence due to inadequate excision has traditionally been a cause of treatment failure.

Tumors of Mandible

As described above, tumors of the mandible fall into three groups: *benign, slow-growing, limited lesions; benign, locally aggressive lesions;* and *malignant neoplasms.*

Treatment of *benign, slow-growing, limited lesions* is relatively simple. Using an intraoral approach, a buccal or lingual mucoperiosteal flap is raised, depending on the location of the lesion. A portion of the mandibular cortex is removed, and the tumor is enucleated or curetted and cauterized. Examination of an intraoperative biopsy specimen confirms the benign nature of the lesion. The mucoperiosteal flap is sutured in place.

Locally aggressive and *frankly malignant tumors* require more extensive resections, which can be divided into four categories: (1) marginal resection; (2) segmental resection; (3) hemimandibulectomy, preserving the condyle; and (4) disarticulation. In rare circumstances, a near-total mandibulectomy may be required. If the tumor has perforated the mandibular cortex to involve the surrounding soft tissue, a generous margin of soft tissue is resected. Nasotracheal intubation is preferred. A prophylactic tracheostomy is usually not necessary, except when the symphyseal area is removed with resulting tongue instability. Hypotensive anesthesia facilitates dissection and reduces blood loss.

When planning the incision for mandibular resections, several factors should be considered. First, the size and location of the tumor determines whether an intraoral or an extraoral approach will suffice. Although many segmental mandibular resections can be achieved by an intraoral approach, the lip should be split to obtain adequate exposure if the tumor is large or in a posterior location. Second, a decision has to be made as to whether a simultaneous elective or therapeutic neck dissection is indicated. The upper incision of the Hayes-Martin technique or the McFee incision allows access to the mandible. The lip-splitting incision, when used, is extended to the transverse lip crease and is curved around the chin mound toward the affected side, ending in the center of the submental area, where it continues into the upper neck dissection incision. Third, if there has been previous irradiation or if there is poor intraoral hygiene, an intraoral approach should not be used.

After the segment of mandible to be excised is isolated, with or without a cuff of soft tissue, it is advisable to extract a tooth at the osteotomy site. In hemimandibulectomies, it is desirable to preserve the condyle, if at all possible, since this greatly improves the quality of functional rehabilitation. In all mandibular resections for malignancy, whether they be segmental or hemimandibular, biopsy should be performed on the proximal end of the inferior dental nerve. The nerve is the direct route to the cranial cavity by intraneural spread of tumor. Abnormal biopsy results can indicate unresectability or need for a more extensive procedure.

DISARTICULATION OF MANDIBLE

To disarticulate the mandible, the lip is split and the incision is carried transversely across the neck inferior to the lower border of the mandible. The lip and soft tissues of the cheek are retracted to determine the site and extent of the tumor. An incision is made along the buccal sulcus, and the soft tissue is dissected from the mandible, leaving the periosteum in situ. If the cortex is invaded by tumor, a margin of soft tissue is left around the mandible in that area. A frozen section of the deep surface of the cheek flap is obtained and examined to ensure absence of tumor. The masseter attachment is divided, and the external surface of the mandible is exposed up to the mandibular notch. The tooth lying in the area of the anterior body section is extracted, and the mandible is divided with a microsagittal, reciprocating, or Gigli's saw or a side-cutting bur. The mandible can be retracted laterally, and the attachments to the floor of the mouth can be divided. The incision is carried parallel to the mandible, opening the sublingual space. The mylohyoid muscle is detached and the pterygomandibular ligament is divided from the buccinator crest externally, allowing easy division of the temporalis muscle from the coronoid. The specimen can now be retracted inferiorly and laterally, allowing the coronoid process to be freed from beneath the zygomatic arch. If the condyle is invaded by tumor, the zygomatic arch may need to be resected. With further mandibular retraction, the pterygoid muscles are divided under direct vision. The lingual nerve and the maxillary artery are protected. The inferior alveolar neurovascular bundle is clamped and divided. After the insertion of the external pterygoid muscle is divided, the joint capsule is opened and the specimen is removed. The remaining soft tissue attachments are divided at this point. Brisk bleeding may occur during resection of the pterygoid muscle or freeing of the mandibular head. This is due to injury of the pterygoid plexus of veins and maxillary artery.

MANDIBULAR RECONSTRUCTION

When mandibular resection is performed, the question of immediate versus delayed reconstruction arises. If the operating time is prolonged and wound healing is a cause for concern or if there is large, aggressive tumor, delayed reconstruction may be advisable. In this situation, a space-maintaining appliance should be employed to prevent postoperative collapse of the remaining mandibular segments. Kirschner wires have been used; however, telescoping may occur and with time the wires can loosen and may ultimately erode through the skin (Cohen and Schultz, 1985). A custom designed metallic prosthesis with or without a condylar head is preferred. This is securely fixed to the remaining mandible and, if possible, to the condyle or the condylar area. The teeth are placed in intermaxillary fixation. Failure to do this usually results in malocclusion and a later eating problem. Extensive soft tissue resection, if performed, should be immediately replaced

with a regional musculocutaneous flap, the pectoralis major being the flap of choice in most instances, although platysma, sternomastoid, and trapezius flaps have all been used.

Some segmental resections do not necessarily require reconstruction. Unilateral resection of the ramus and the posterior portion of the body is one example. Immediate reconstruction in this situation may be complicated by significant trismus. If there has been extensive soft tissue resection, primary replacement is indicated to avoid mandibular drift resulting from contracture of the remaining soft tissues. A dental glide bar may be useful in reestablishing occlusal contact after resection of the mandibular ramus without reconstruction.

Immediate mandibular reconstruction after tumor surgery does offer definite advantages in selected cases, especially when the tumor has been adequately excised, the nutritional status is satisfactory, and the patient is able to tolerate an extended operating time. The first decision is whether a nonvascularized bone graft is adequate, or whether a vascularized reconstruction is preferable. Factors that favor the latter procedure include inadequate residual soft tissue cover (necessitating flap reconstruction), previous tumor dose irradiation, or plans for irradiation soon after the resection. Vascularized bony reconstructions can be achieved by using pedicled flaps or free microvascular transfers. In the former group, a pectoralis major muscle flap incorporating a rib (Cuono and Ariyan, 1980; Little, McCulloch, and Lyons, 1983; Lam, Wei, and Siu, 1984), a sternocleidomastoid muscle flap with clavicle (Siemssen, Kirkby, and O'Connor, 1978), a serratus anterior flap with rib, and a trapezius flap with the spine of the scapula (Panje and Cutting, 1980; Guillamondegui and Larson, 1981) have been described, but only the latter two are consistently reliable. However, the trapezius flap may not be possible because of sacrifice of the transverse cervical vessels in the neck dissection. Donor site morbidity and flap bulk are other disadvantages. Several microvascular free osseous transfers, with or without soft tissue, have been described, including rib (Serafin, Villarreal-Rios, and Georgiade, 1977), iliac crest (Taylor, 1982), scapula, and metatarsal bone. Procedures for mandibular reconstruction are discussed in greater detail in Chapter 29.

Tumors of Maxilla

The surgical treatment of benign lesions of the maxilla is described above. The extent of maxillary resection for sinus malignancies is related to tumor extensions, but it should, if possible, be an en bloc procedure. The malignancies may extend into several areas: (1) the nasal cavity, (2) the nasopharynx, (3) the oral cavity and alveolus, (4) the orbit, (5) the soft tissues of the face, (6) the infratemporal fossa, (7) the paranasal sinuses, (8) the base of the skull, and (9) multiple other regions. The procedures of total maxillectomy and subtotal maxillectomy are described in Chapter 68.

Medial maxillectomy is reserved for low grade malignant and benign lesions of the lateral nasal wall such as the inverted papilloma (Rice and Stanley, 1987). A Weber-Fergusson incision is used to raise a broad laterally based cheek flap. Alternatively, for anterior lesions, the upper lip may be left intact and a lateral rhinotomy incision with a Caldwell-Luc exposure used in combination. With either approach, access to the medial maxilla is obtained, and, after an inferior and medial subperiosteal orbital dissection, orbital contents are retracted. This gives adequate exposure to perform the necessary osteotomies to free and remove the medial orbital wall and the ethmoid sinuses in an en bloc fashion. If necessary, the medial canthal ligament attachment, the nasal mucosa, and any overlying involved skin are included. No reconstruction is performed as part of this procedure. The decision to perform a total or a subtotal maxillectomy is made during the preoperative clinical assessment. The extent of the procedure may have to be increased because of tumor infiltration into surrounding areas.

Several important points about maxillectomy need to be emphasized. If complete resection is to be obtained, it may be necessary in some cases to alter the preoperative plan during the procedure. Preoperative high resolution CT scans and MRI scans are invaluable aids in estimating the likely extent of the procedure. The patient should always be informed that removal of the eye may be necessary if the tumor has invaded the orbital floor. It is advisable that facilities for performing intraoperative frozen section examinations be available, although ideally no visual evidence of the lesion should be seen during the surgery if the resection is adequate. If possible, the nasolacrimal duct and the eustachian tube and its pharyngeal ostium should be excluded from the resection. If the infratemporal fossa is extensively invaded, it may be necessary to use an additional lateral approach and to remove the ascending ramus of the mandible, the parotid gland, or both, with facial nerve preservation, to achieve satisfactory exposure. This approach is described in greater detail below. Medial extension into the ethmoid sinuses necessitates ethmoid sinus resection and, in some cases, en bloc removal of the floor of the anterior cranial fossa (see below). Involvement of the overlying soft tissue necessitates excision of cheek or nasal skin.

There can be significant complications of maxillectomy (e.g., profuse bleeding from the maxillary artery; failure of the skin graft, which will result in cavity contracture; and facial deformity). Occasionally, trismus may result from pterygoid muscle scarring. The temporary obturator may fit poorly and cause ulceration. Conductive deafness may result from stenosis or blockage of the eustachian tube. Pneumonia can occur from aspiration of food or wound secretions. If the soft palate must be sacrificed, there will be resulting difficulties with eating and speech. If Lockwood's suspensory ligament, which is, in effect, the periorbita of the floor of the orbit, is kept intact, there should be little if any globe dystopia or enophthalmos. Diplopia may be minimal or absent. Resection of the periorbita will inevitably lead to eye displacement; this problem will be ameliorated by a prosthesis that fits high into the cavity. If the patient remains tumor free, the floor can be reconstructed and the intraorbital volume adjusted with a nonvascularized or vascularized calvarial bone transfer.

Tumors of Skull Base

These tumors may have an extracranial origin and subsequently involve the cranial base, or they may initially be intracranial and exit through one of the skull base foramina to involve the sub–skull base soft tissue; alternatively, but rarely, they may invade a sinus. In the past, surgical ablation was often incomplete, and recurrence was frequent. Radiation therapy and chemotherapy did little to alter the outcome. Attempts

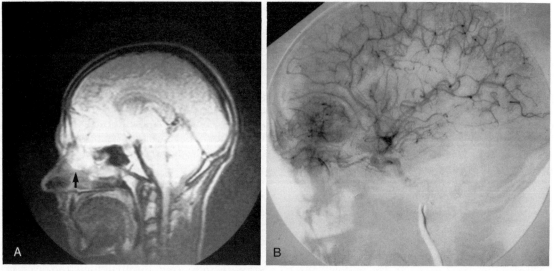

Figure 69–17. Scanning examinations of skull base tumors. *A,* MRI scan showing an anterior skull base esthesioneuroblastoma *(arrow). B,* Angiography demonstrating the vascularity of the lesion.

to achieve total resection were associated with significant complications, particularly extradural abscesses and meningitis.

By using approaches developed for the correction of congenital craniofacial anomalies, considerable advances in the surgical extirpation of the lesions have been attained. Exposure is satisfactory; en bloc resection is usually possible; and morbidity and operative mortality are greatly decreased.

These tumors have frequently been treated by resection, radiation therapy, and chemotherapy. The tumors can be nonmalignant or malignant. The variety of tumor involvement is considerable because of the many differing structures in this area. In most cases, the treatment choice is surgery with adjuvant radiation therapy or chemotherapy as indicated. In selected orbital rhabdomyosarcomas and reticuloendothelial tumors, the latter two modalities represent the first line of treatment. The most useful preoperative examinations have been CT and MRI and carotid angiography (Fig. 69–17). High resolution CT scans (axial, coronal, and sagittal) show the extent of the tumor (e.g., involvement of bone or invasion of sinuses). Three-dimensional reformatting may be of help in some cases. MRI scans may supply more accurate information about the extent of soft tissue infiltration of areas such as the infratemporal and temporal fossae. Carotid angiography is essential in evaluation of extensive tumors, especially when the CT scan suggests tumor involvement of the cavernous sinus or evidence of tumor approximating or displacing the carotid artery. At this time, there is opportunity to check the status of crosscerebral blood flow by compression of the carotid artery on the involved side. This preoperative information is important in case the carotid artery has to be resected. If the tumor is vascular (e.g., neurofibroma or meningioma), it can be embolized at this time to reduce the amount of intraoperative bleeding. If these investigations reveal invasion of the cavernous sinus or extensive cerebral involvement, the tumor is judged unresectable. However, the practical approach to the majority of tumors in this region is to consider most to be operable and to classify them as inoperable only after an unsuccessful attempt has been made to remove them.

ANATOMY OF SKULL BASE

In planning the surgical approach, it is useful to divide the skull base into an *anterior area,* consisting of the anterior cranial fossa, and a *posterior area,* which consists of the remainder of the skull base (Jackson, 1985). The posterior area can be further subdivided into thirds consisting of anterior, central, and posterior segments (Fig. 69–18). The anterior segment lies between the greater wing of the sphenoid and the anterior margin of the petrous bone; the central segment is the petrous bone itself; and the posterior segment is

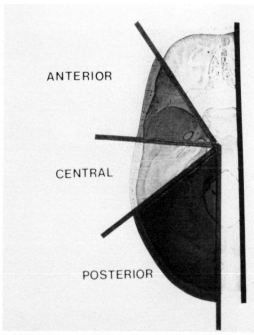

Figure 69–18. Anatomic division of the posterior area of the skull base. The posterior area, or the middle and posterior cranial fossae, is subdivided into anterior, central, and posterior segments.

bounded by the posterior margin of the petrous bone and the posterior fossa midline.

The foramina in these areas are the routes by which tumor enters or leaves the cranium. In the anterior cranial fossa area, the foramina are in the cribriform plate. In the anterior segment of the posterior area there are the optic nerve foramen, the foramen rotundum (maxillary nerve), foramen ovale (mandibular nerve), foramen lacerum (internal carotid artery), foramen spinosum (middle meningeal artery), and the vidian canal (deep petrosal and greater superficial petrosal nerves). In the central segment within the petrous bone there are the internal carotid canal, the facial nerve canal and its foramen, and the internal auditory meatus. In the posterior segment, the jugular foramen contains the internal jugular vein. The intracranial end of long foramina may not lie in the same position as the extracranial end, an important surgical consideration particularly in relation to the carotid canal.

ANTERIOR AREA OF SKULL BASE

Any tumor involving the frontal bone, the frontal or ethmoid sinuses, the medial can-

thus, the orbit, the orbital contents, or the nasopharynx can directly invade the anterior cranial fossa (Jackson and Marsh, 1983). Indirect involvement by skin, maxilla, or muscle tumors can occur, usually via the ethmoid sinuses or the orbit. Tumors arising in the brain or meninges can also involve the skull base. Tumors in the upper face should always arouse suspicion of skull base involvement, and this can be confirmed or refuted by CT scan.

Nonmalignant Tumors

Fibrous dysplasia is a nonmalignant tumor requiring fronto-orbital resection (Jackson and associates, 1982a). In this region, it often behaves differently from the more common type of fibrous dysplasia of the maxilla and the mandible. In the cranio-orbital area, it can cause eye displacement, proptosis, diplopia, diminution of visual acuity, and, in some cases, blindness. The latter is attributable to compression of the nerve by optic canal involvement. The tumor does not usually resolve in adolescence and may continue to grow. If resection is not complete, there may be recurrence, which can be extensive. Lesions may be multiple or may arise elsewhere on the skull after resection of the main lesion. This behavior suggests malignant change, but this has been seen only after radiation therapy (Fig. 69–19). Radiographs show the affected bone to be thickened, dense, and granular; occasionally, cystic changes are present.

Treatment is total resection and immediate reconstruction (Fig. 69–20). The true contours and extent of the condition are well shown on the reformatted three-dimensional CT images.

A bicoronal flap is elevated to expose the frontal area, the orbit, and the nasal skeleton until healthy bone is identified. If necessary, the temporal periosteum and temporalis muscle are elevated. The orbital contents are dissected in the subperiosteal plane. A craniotomy is performed; this should include all involved bone, which is discarded. All areas of the orbit and the nose affected by the process are resected. Frequently, only the orbital floor is spared. If necessary, the optic canal is deroofed to decompress the optic nerve. If the temporoparietal area is affected, it is also removed. It is not always possible to remove all of the involved cranial base,

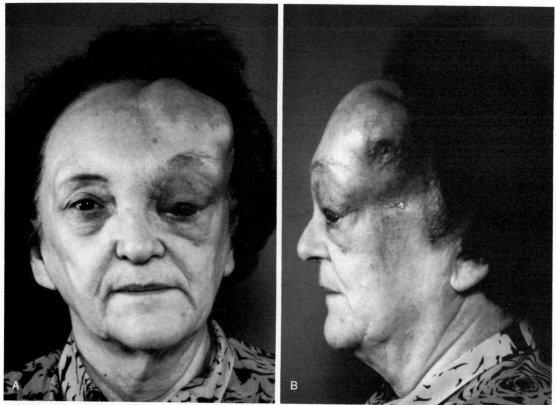

Figure 69–19. Malignant change in fronto-orbital fibrous dysplasia. *A, B,* Fifty-two years after radiotherapy for fibrous dysplasia, the patient developed an osteogenic sarcoma involving the frontal area, the nasal bones, the ethmoid sinuses, the sphenoid sinus, the floor of the anterior cranial fossa and orbit, and the maxilla.

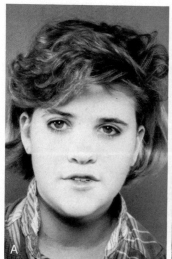
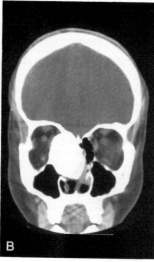
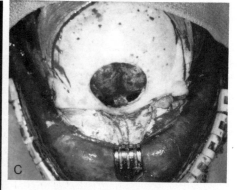

Figure 69–20. Fibrous dysplasia of the skull base. *A,* Patient with fibrous dysplasia of the right orbit and the anterior skull base. *B,* CT scan showing the extent of the lesion. *C,* Bicoronal approach with frontal trephination.

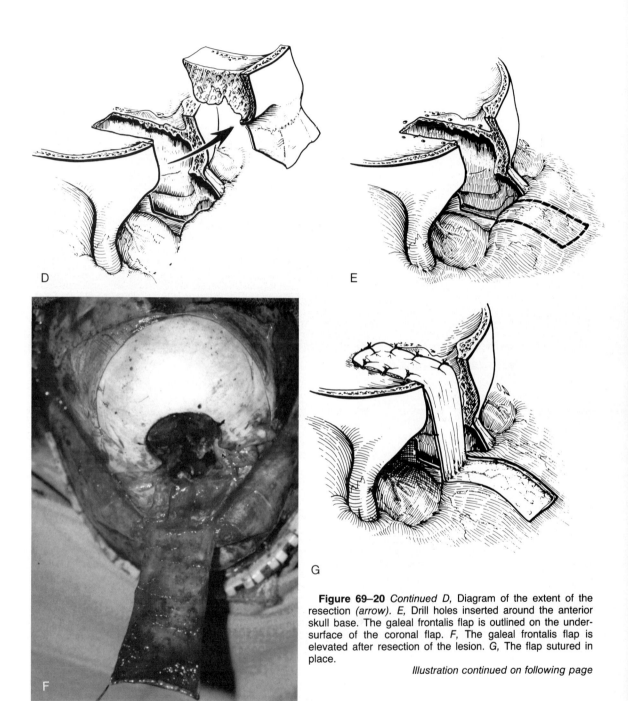

Figure 69–20 *Continued D,* Diagram of the extent of the resection *(arrow). E,* Drill holes inserted around the anterior skull base. The galeal frontalis flap is outlined on the undersurface of the coronal flap. *F,* The galeal frontalis flap is elevated after resection of the lesion. *G,* The flap sutured in place.

Illustration continued on following page

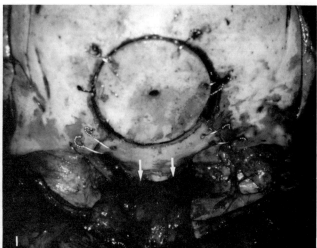

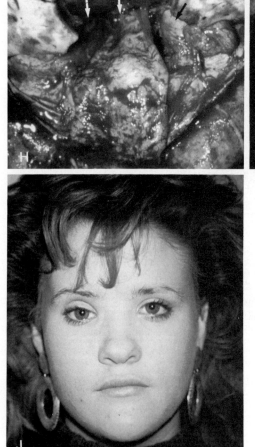

Figure 69–20 *Continued H,* Galeal frontalis flap in position *(arrows). I,* Nasoglabellar osteotomy and trephine segment wired back in position. The galeal frontalis flap is "mailed" under the nasoglabellar osteotomy *(arrows). J,* Postoperative result two years after resection.

but with increased experience, this goal becomes more feasible. The margins of resection are sent for frozen section examination to ensure that excision has been adequate. The dura may be torn, and, if so, it is repaired by direct suture, autogenous fascia lata, or rarely lyophilized cadaveric dura. The temporal region, the orbital roof, and the lateral orbital wall are best reconstructed with split cranial bone grafts. Split rib grafts are usually employed for the orbital and frontal reconstruction. Bone dust harvested with the craniotome is used to contour concavities between grafts; a surprisingly smooth surface can be obtained with this technique. The coronal flap is replaced, and the incision is sutured. A suction drain is placed, and a light pressure dressing is applied.

Other nonmalignant tumors in this area that may require a craniofacial approach are rare and include osteomas and intradiplopic epidermoid cysts.

Complications are few if surgery is performed in a careful and efficient manner. Appropriate antibiotics are given before, during, and after surgery. The importance of closing any connections between the extradural space and the nasopharynx cannot be overemphasized. Failure to do so results in ascending infection and possible extradural abscess formation and meningitis. Closure of this area can be effected in various ways; the optimal method is the *galeal frontalis myofascial flap* (Jackson and associates, 1986a). The flap is based on the supraorbital and supratrochlear vessels, and it can be made as long as necessary. After the flap is elevated, it is transposed, packed, and sutured into the defect.

Malignant Tumors

Malignant tumors may be extra- or intracranial. The pathologic changes vary considerably, and the lesions are recurrent after surgery, radiotherapy, and chemotherapy. Because of their biologic behavior, limited reconstruction after radical resection is usually indicated to avoid masking later recurrence. If complete reconstruction is performed and there is recurrence, the diagnosis is delayed, the patient is reluctant to undergo additional surgery, and the resection has removed what was probably the best reconstructive option. In general, immediate reconstruction after craniofacial resections should

be reserved for coverage of vital structures and separation of the oronasopharynx from the extradural space. In patients in whom complete resection has not been possible, immediate reconstruction, usually with a microvascular free flap, will improve the quality of whatever life the patient has left.

Orbital Tumors

The orbit may be involved by tumors arising from its contents, its bony architecture, or extraorbital structures. Extraorbital tumors may arise in the anterior or middle cranial fossae; the frontal, ethmoid, and maxillary sinuses; the nose; and the temporal or infratemporal fossae. Indirect invasion occurs when tumors such as meningiomas escape from the middle cranial fossa by way of a skull base foramen. Assessment and treatment of orbital tumors are more secure if they are considered as anterior cranial fossa tumors until proved otherwise. If they are seen to encroach on or to invade the skull base on high resolution CT scans and MRI scan, a transcranial orbitectomy should be planned. A less aggressive approach will result in inadequate resection.

Procedures utilized for treatment of these tumors fall into one of several types: (1) orbitectomy and replacement (exposure osteotomy); (2) partial orbitectomy with preservation of the orbital contents without reconstruction; (3) partial orbitectomy with sacrifice of the orbital contents without reconstruction; (4) total transcranial orbitectomy with preservation of the orbital contents and reconstruction; and (5) total transcranial orbitectomy with resection of the orbital contents without reconstruction (Jackson, 1986).

Orbitectomy and replacement (exposure osteotomy) is a fairly new technique in skull base surgery. A portion of the orbit is removed to gain access for resection of the lesion. After this has been accomplished and after any bony defect resulting from tumor excision has been reconstructed, the removed portion of the orbit is reinserted. The procedure is applicable in many situations. Benign tumors such as neurofibromas, schwannomas, hemangiomas, selected meningiomas, and nonspecific granulomas involving the superior half of the orbit, particularly if they lie behind the meridian of the globe, may be approached in this way, as can deep lateral tumors. The approach is not advised for malignant tumors for which exenteration is the treatment of choice.

In all orbitectomies, only the bicoronal flap approach is used. After a subperiosteal dissection of the orbital contents has been performed and if a transcranial resection is planned, the neurosurgeon performs a hemifrontal craniotomy, leaving the supraorbital area intact. The frontal lobe is elevated from the orbital roof area; the orbital contents are dissected from the roof and protected with a malleable retractor. A power drill or a sagittal saw is used to perform the osteotomy. The supraorbital rim is cut medially and laterally. If more exposure is required, the osteotomy can be made farther down the lateral orbital wall. The block of supraorbital rim and roof is removed, and the orbital contents are well displayed (Fig. 69–21). With the frontal lobe retracted, an incision can be made through the periorbita and the orbital tissues can be retracted to expose the tumor under direct

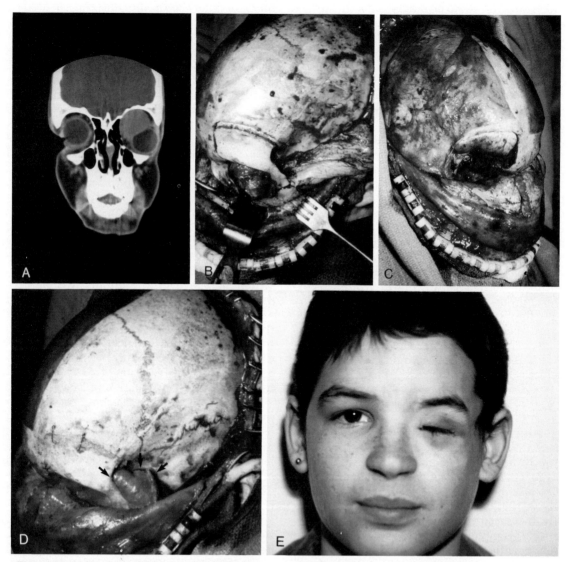

Figure 69–21. Exposure osteotomy (supraorbital). *A,* Coronal CT scan showing rhabdomyosarcoma, which recurred after radiotherapy and chemotherapy, involving the anterior skull base, the orbit, the ethmoid sinuses, and the nasal cavity. *B,* Through a bicoronal flap, the left supraorbital osteotomies have been made. *C,* The supraorbital segment removed. Resection of the anterior skull base, the medial orbital wall, and the orbital contents was accomplished. *D,* The supraorbital segment was replaced. The temporalis muscle was "mailed" through the lateral orbital wall defect to resurface the orbital cavity *(arrows). E,* Postoperative appearance after 18 months.

vision. After repair of the orbital layers, the partial orbitectomy segment is replaced and osteosynthesis is performed with wires or miniplates.

If the tumor is in the middle cranial fossa (e.g., a meningioma), the osteotomy includes more of the lateral orbital wall, and the cranial bone flap is raised in the temporal region (Fig. 69–22). For subcranial tumors (i.e., deep lateral tumors), the exposure osteotomy consists of the lateral wall and lateral orbital rim, a portion of the maxilla, the infraorbital rim, and the orbital floor. Removal of this segment allows for satisfactory exposure and tumor removal. The osteotomy

segment is subsequently replaced and stabilized.

If the tumor involves the orbital wall, a partial orbitectomy and exenteration may be necessary. The need for an intracranial approach is determined by the position of the tumor. Any malignant osseoinvasive tumor in the upper lateral roof or upper medial portion of the orbit should be approached in this way. The amount of orbit removed is that which is necessary to obtain total tumor resection.

Extensive or aggressive tumors in or around the orbit occasionally require total resection of the orbit and its contents. The

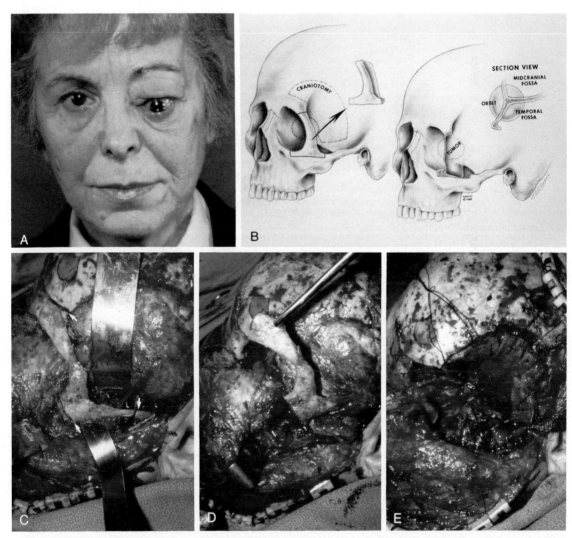

Figure 69–22. Exposure osteotomy (orbitozygomatic). *A,* Sphenoid ridge meningioma involving the middle cranial fossa and the left orbit with proptosis and downward displacement of the left eye. *B,* Outline of the orbitozygomatic osteotomy. *C,* Osteotomy lines outlined *(arrows)* after the bicoronal flap has been turned down. *D,* Removal of the osteotomized segment of bone. *E,* Exposure and resection of the meningioma.

Illustration continued on following page

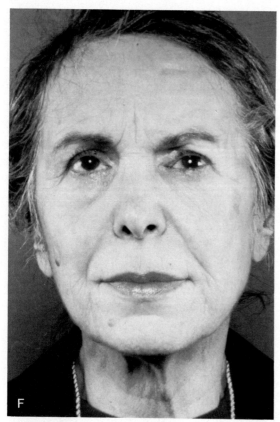

Figure 69–22 *Continued F,* Postoperative appearance after three years.

osteotomy resembles that used for hypertelorism correction but is more extensive. The osteotomies are taken across the orbital roof, along the lateral wall, horizontally across the maxilla below the infraorbital nerve, and vertically up the medial wall far enough posteriorly to include the ethmoid sinuses. The nasopharynx is sealed off with a galeal frontalis myofascial flap, and skin cover is achieved with scalp rotation, a forehead flap, or a distant flap, such as the pectoralis major or deltopectoral flap. Free tissue transfer may also be used.

Penetrating Midface Tumors

The tumors that penetrate the midface area are usually recurrent, aggressive basal cell carcinomas or squamous cell carcinomas; less frequently, adenoid cystic or mucoepidermoid carcinomas, adenocarcinomas, sarcomas, or esthesioneuroblastomas are seen (Jackson, Somers, and Marsh, 1985). The previously used treatment modalities included multiple excisions, curettage, Mohs micrographic resection, radiation therapy, and chemotherapy. Resection should be performed with frozen section examination of the remaining defect (Fig. 69–23). Removal of extensive portions of the facial soft tissues and skeleton is usually necessary: the nose or its remnants, parts of the orbit, the orbital contents, the maxilla, the palate, a varying amount of the nasopharynx, the base of the anterior cranial fossa, the overlying dura, the frontal bone, and the frontal, ethmoid, and sphenoid sinuses.

A combined transcranial orbitectomy approach greatly facilitates removal of these lesions. In selected cases, the exposure osteotomy method is applicable (Fig. 69–24) (Jackson and associates, 1986a). A bicoronal flap is used for exposure. If the anterior cranial base is not extensively involved, this incision may not be necessary, especially if glabellar skin is to be resected. This gives adequate exposure for a trephine craniotomy. The tumor is considered inoperable if there is extensive penetration of the posterior wall of the sphenoid sinus into the cavernous sinus. With resection of the floor of the anterior cranial fossa and the frequent necessity of resecting and replacing dura with fascia lata or stored dura, the patient is exposed to ascending infection from the nasopharynx. This can result in an extradural infection or meningitis, with loss of any craniotomy or osteotomy bone and death of the patient. It is essential that this connection be securely closed. Various methods have been used: a midline forehead flap, an extended glabellar flap, and a galeal frontalis myofascial flap (Jackson and associates, 1986a). The latter method is favored because a wide, long flap can be obtained (see Fig. 69–24); if necessary, two flaps can be formed. The flap is vascular and can be molded as necessary. It is secured to the edges of the bony defect by suturing through multiple drill holes. The whole area is skin grafted, and it heals remarkably well. Others have used free tissue transfer in these cases and reported rapid healing (Jones, 1933).

Osseointegration techniques are now being utilized to improve the stability of intra- and extraoral prostheses (Fig. 69–25) (Brånemark and associates, 1969, 1977; Jackson and associates, 1986b; Jackson, French, and Tolman, 1988). This also reduces the trauma to the skin associated with adhesives. These

Text continued on page 3390

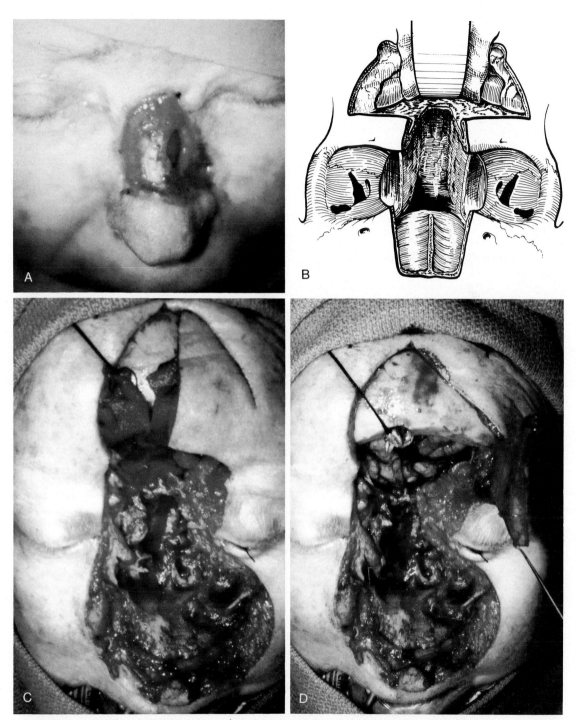

Figure 69–23. Penetrating midface tumor. *A,* Basal cell carcinoma (treated by Mohs chemosurgery) with involvement of the left orbit, the underlying nasal bones, and the base of the anterior cranial fossa. *B,* Diagram of resection of the anterior cranial base, the medial orbital walls, the palate, and the ethmoid and sphenoid sinuses. *C,* Resection completed. The extended glabellar flap has been elevated. *D,* The glabellar flap has been retracted and resection of the skull base and the dura of the frontal lobe is well displayed. The extended glabellar flap will be transferred along the floor of the middle cranial fossa and sutured to the edges of the bony defect through drill holes. Before placement of the glabellar flap, the left orbit was resected.

Illustration continued on following page

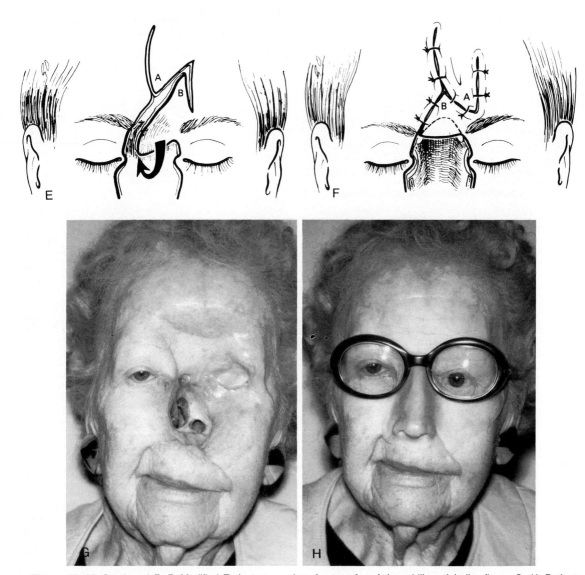

Figure 69–23 *Continued E, F,* Modified Z-plasty procedure for transfer of the midline glabellar flaps. *G, H,* Patient without and with the external prosthesis seven years after resection.

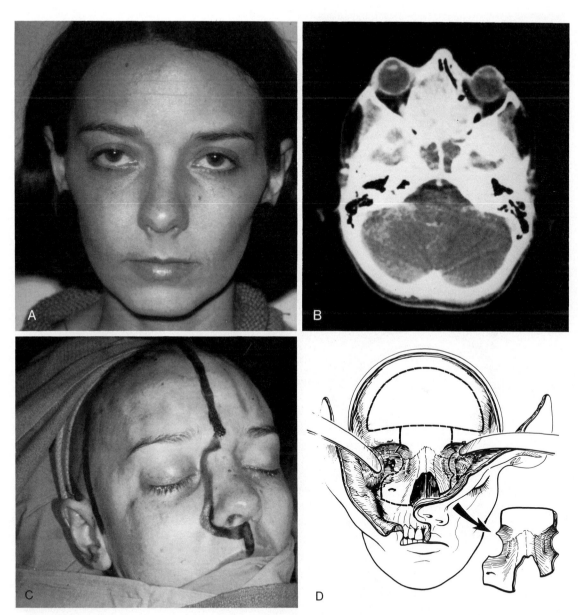

Figure 69–24. Exposure osteotomy (frontonasomaxillary). *A,* Patient with chondrosarcoma of the anterior skull base and the nasal septum. *B,* Axial CT scan showing the position of the chondrosarcoma. *C,* Bicoronal flap and face-splitting approach. *D,* Procedure for the exposure osteotomy and bony segment removal *(arrow).*

Illustration continued on following page

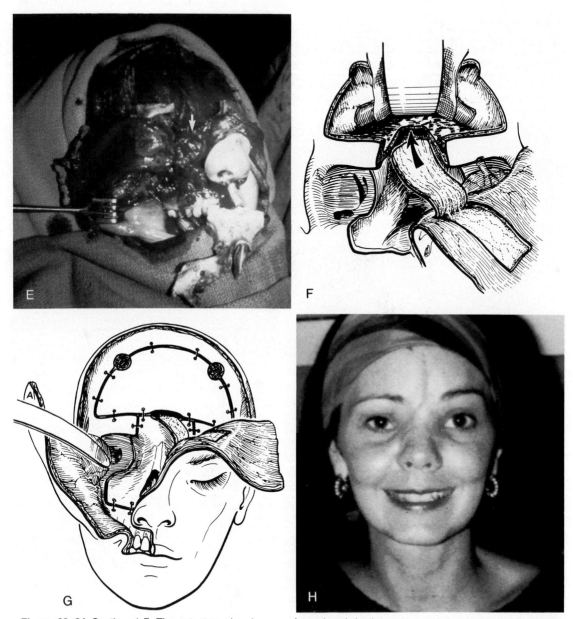

Figure 69–24 *Continued E,* The osteotomy has been performed and the bone removed, leaving the dentoalveolar segment intact. The tumor is designated by an arrow. *F,* After the resection is completed, the galeal frontalis (myofascial) flap is inserted *(arrow)* and sutured around the defect to separate the nasopharynx from the anterior cranial fossa. *G,* The osteotomized segments placed back in position. The galeal frontalis flap has been "mailed" through a slot above the nasomaxillary osteotomy. *H,* Appearance six years after surgery.

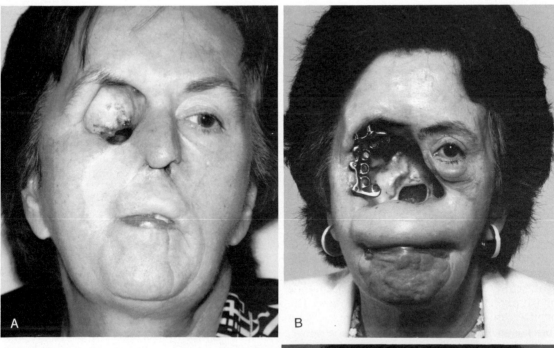

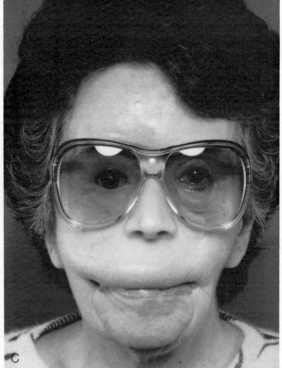

Figure 69–25. Osseointegration of external prosthesis. *A,* Patient with a recurrent basal cell carcinoma of the anterior cranial fossa, the nose, the orbit, and the maxilla after surgery and radiotherapy. *B,* After radical resection of the floor of the anterior cranial fossa, the orbit, the maxilla, the nose, and the palate, an osseointegrated framework with magnets (Brånemark prosthesis) was inserted. *C,* Patient with external prosthesis in position five years after surgery.

patients are examined every three months, and have annual CT scans. Any hidden areas are examined with the flexible endoscope or a dental mirror; biopsy of suspicious or indurated areas is performed. If there is a recurrence, additional aggressive resection should be undertaken, if possible.

Ethmoid Carcinoma

Tumors arising in or invading the ethmoid sinuses are considered anterior cranial base tumors. A bicoronal approach with a limited frontal craniotomy is used (Fig. 69–26). The glabellar bony segment is frequently removed to obtain better exposure. The frontal lobes are retracted to expose the ethmoid roof area; the osteotomies are made around this. The nose and medial orbital walls are exposed subperiosteally. The extracranial resection is determined by the position and the extent of the tumor invasion. The excision includes the nasal bone on the involved side and the medial wall of the orbit. It can also include overlying skin, the nasal septum, and the orbital contents. Maxillary involvement is an indication for partial or total maxillectomy. If the latter is necessary, the facial incision

is taken down the middle of the forehead and extended into a Weber-Fergusson approach. The resection is performed in an en bloc fashion. The communication between the nasopharynx and the extradural space is closed with a galeal frontalis myofascial flap. Any external defect is replaced with an external prosthesis. Reconstruction is undertaken at 12 to 18 months postoperatively if the area remains tumor free.

Midface Sarcoma

Chondrosarcomas and osteogenic sarcomas can arise in the nasal septum and involve the anterior cranial fossa, often in its posterior region. Nasal congestion is the usual presentation, and a mass may be seen in the nasal cavity. A biopsy confirms the diagnosis. Nasendoscopy may be necessary to detect smaller and more posterior lesions. A CT scan documents the extent of the tumor.

The preferred approach is through a bicoronal flap combined with a face-splitting incision (see above under Ethmoid Carcinoma). In some cases, the midline forehead component of the incision can be omitted. The bicoronal flap is turned down, and subperi-

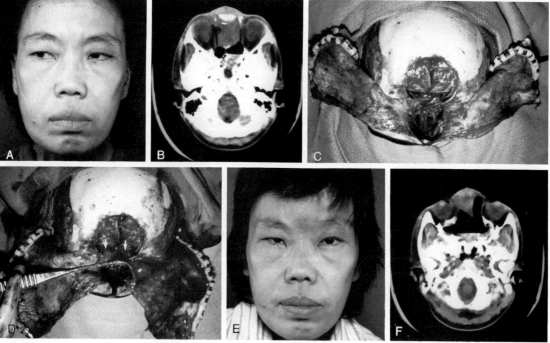

Figure 69–26. Adenocarcinoma of the ethmoid sinuses. *A,* Postradiotherapy recurrent right ethmoid adenocarcinoma. *B,* Axial CT scan showing the position and extent of the ethmoid adenocarcinoma. *C,* Resection completed using frontal flap, face-splitting incision, and frontal trephination. There was extensive resection of the skull base and the nasoethmoido-orbital area. A galeal frontalis myofascial flap was also elevated. *D,* The frontalis flap sutured in position *(arrows). E,* Result 18 months after surgery. *F,* Axial CT scan showing the extent of the resection and no evidence of recurrence.

osteal dissection is performed over the nasal bones, the medial aspects of both orbits, and the front of the maxilla. An incision is made in the upper buccal sulcus; this maneuver allows the cheek and forehead soft tissue to be elevated as a flap based laterally, similar to turning the page of a book. If wider exposure is required, the conjunctiva can be incised in the upper and lower fornices to separate the lids from the globe. The lids are then included in the face flap. An eye exposed in this way must be protected and covered with ointment at all times. Through a limited craniotomy, the frontal lobes are elevated and any intracranial involvement can be evaluated.

The exposure osteotomy is planned. When the tumor is extensive and posteriorly located, it may be necessary to remove the glabellar area, the nasal skeleton, the medial orbital wall, and the inferior orbital rim and floor, in association with the maxilla above the tooth roots as a single segment. The lower segment can be bilateral, if necessary. Excellent exposure is obtained, and an en bloc resection of the medial orbital walls, the nasal septum, the anterior cranial fossa floor, and the ethmoid and sphenoid sinuses is accomplished. The previously removed bony complex, if not involved, may later be replaced and plated or wired back into position, together with the frontal bone flap. Two galeal frontalis myofascial flaps are raised. One is used to cover the portion of the osteotomy that is exposed into the nose; the other separates the anterior cranial fossa from the nasopharynx. The nasopharynx area can be skin grafted or left to heal spontaneously. The graft is held in place with sutures and a pack of iodoform gauze, which can later be removed through the nostril. The facial flap is returned and sutured in position, and the bicoronal flap is closed. In this way, primary healing is achieved, and the area can be observed for recurrence using a nasendoscope.

POSTERIOR AREA OF SKULL BASE

Anterior Segment of Posterior Area

Nonmalignant Tumors. The two most commonly encountered are *neurofibroma* and *fibrous dysplasia*.

Neurofibroma. An orbital neurofibroma without bony involvement can cause proptosis, but typically the lesion is present in the temporal area and within the orbit (orbito-temporal). The greater wing of the sphenoid is absent to a varying degree. There is a resulting defect between the orbit and the middle cranial fossa, allowing herniation of the temporal lobe, which in turn causes a pulsating proptosis (Jackson, Laws, and Martin, 1983). The orbit is expanded, the floor is depressed, and there is hypoplasia of the malar and zygomatic arch. Occasionally, there may be an arachnoid cyst of the temporal lobe. The eyelids are nonfunctional in severe cases owing to neurofibroma infiltration of the orbicularis muscle. If the bony defect is in an inferior position in the greater wing, there is a connection into the temporal fossa with enophthalmos but without pulsation.

In the other type of neurofibroma, there is generalized unilateral involvement of the face with infiltration into the orbit, causing some degree of proptosis. This will frequently be associated with other stigmata of neurofibromatosis. The diffuse type of neurofibromatosis is difficult to resect and has a tendency to recur.

The orbitotemporal form can be divided into three groups: (1) orbital soft tissue involvement with a seeing eye, (2) orbital soft tissue and bony involvement with a seeing eye, and (3) orbital soft tissue and bony involvement with a blind eye. In addition to the clinical examination, facial bone radiographs and CT scan with three-dimensional formatting are extremely useful for treatment planning.

If there is orbital soft tissue involvement and a seeing eye, the neurofibroma can often be exposed and removed through an upper or lower eyelid incision.

If there is soft tissue and bony involvement with a seeing eye, the orbit is approached using the bicoronal flap (Fig. 69–27). The orbital contents are liberated laterally and inferiorly. The temporalis muscle is elevated from the lateral orbital wall. Orbital osteotomies are performed through the lateral orbital rim, vertically down the lateral orbital wall, horizontally across the maxilla, and vertically through the medial part of the infraorbital rim. The fragment is removed, and wide exposure of the posterior orbital area and the defect on the posterior orbital wall is obtained. The periorbitum is incised, and the tumor is exposed and removed with as little disruption of the normal anatomy as possible. The orbital bony defect is reconstructed with a split calvarial graft; split ribs may also be used. A portion of the lateral

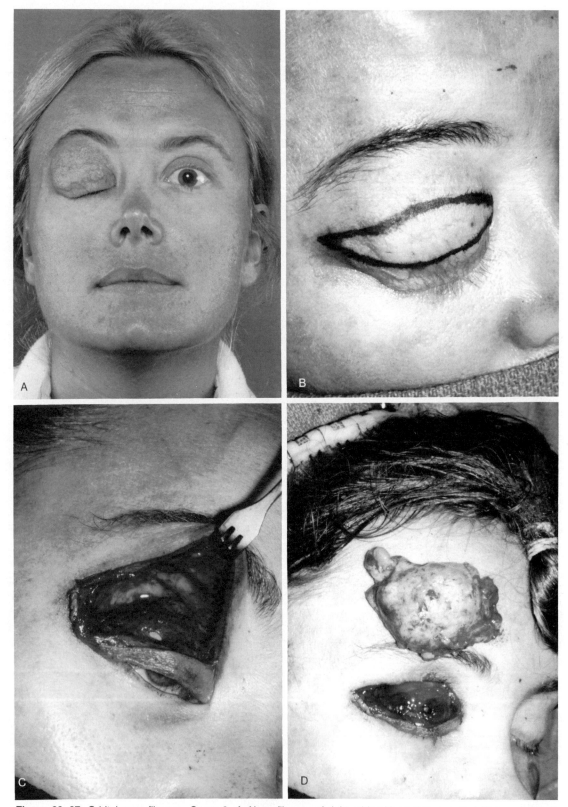

Figure 69–27. Orbital neurofibroma, Group 2. *A,* Neurofibroma of right orbit with seeing eye. *B,* Initial approach by excision of excess skin and entry through the orbital septum. *C,* Tumor exposed. *D,* Tumor resected.

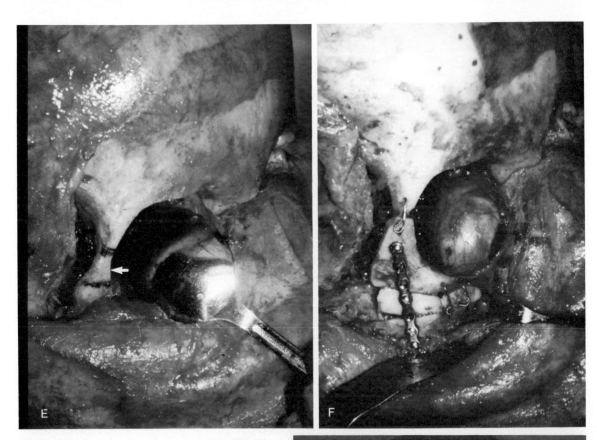

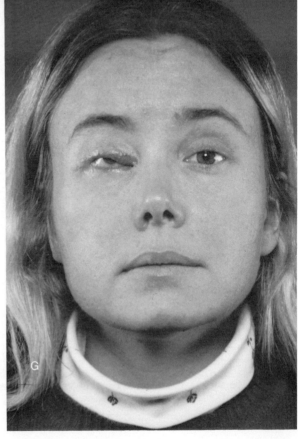

Figure 69–27 *Continued E,* Bicoronal flap for exposure of the orbit and reduction osteotomy. Precalculated amount of orbit will be resected on the lateral wall *(arrow). F,* Result after orbital osteotomy and ostectomy and lateral orbital osteosynthesis with wire. Definitive osteosynthesis of segment using miniplate and skull bone graft to fill the maxillary defect. *G,* Postoperative result prior to corrective surgery on the upper eyelid.

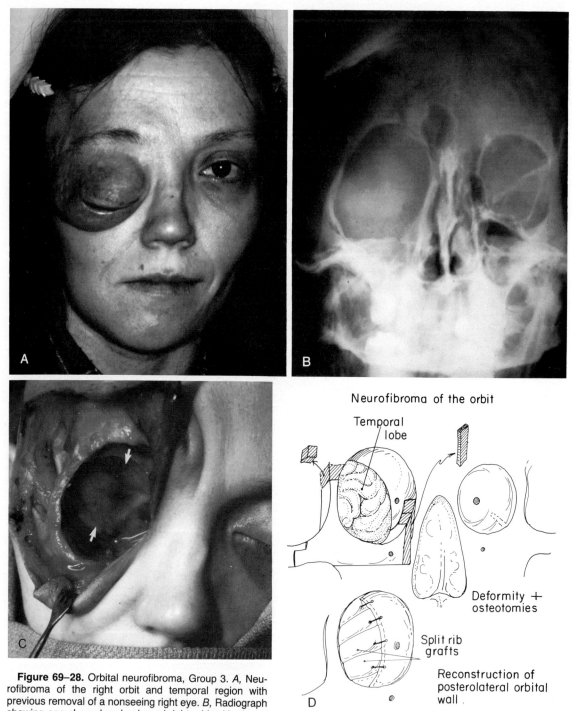

Figure 69–28. Orbital neurofibroma, Group 3. *A,* Neurofibroma of the right orbit and temporal region with previous removal of a nonseeing right eye. *B,* Radiograph showing egg-shaped and enlarged right orbit with absence of the greater wing of the sphenoid and a hypoplastic maxilla and zygoma. *C,* Resection of the temporo-orbital neurofibroma with preservation of orbital skin. The posterior orbital wall defect can be seen *(arrows). D,* Procedure for the osteotomies and the reconstruction of the posterior orbital wall with split rib grafts. Cranial bone grafts can also be used.

Neurofibroma of the orbit

Temporal lobe

Deformity + osteotomies

Split rib grafts

Reconstruction of posterolateral orbital wall

orbital wall is removed; the extent is precalculated from the reformatted three-dimensional CT scan, which gives the correct orbital volume. The orbital segment is replaced. Osteosynthesis is achieved with wires and miniplates. The temporalis muscle is relocated on the lateral orbital rim and skull. Through drill holes, the lateral canthal ligament is reattached, and the bicoronal flap is closed over suction drainage.

The third group, with soft tissue and bony involvement with a blind eye, contains the most severe cases. In this group, the most satisfactory results have been obtained by sacrificing the nonseeing eye (Fig. 69–28). The area of temporal involvement is outlined. This is excised down to the temporal fascia,

and if this layer is involved, it is removed. Incisions are continued along the edge of the lids to preserve the eyelid skin. The skin is elevated from the orbicularis oculi muscles. Orbital exenteration is performed by excising everything deep to the subdermal plexus of the eyelids. The temporal lobe is reduced, and the posterior orbital wall defect is reconstructed with cranial bone grafts. Split ribs can also be used. The orbit is osteotomized and reduced as described for the previous group. The supraorbital rim and maxilla are augmented with onlay bone grafts as indicated. The eyelid skin, which is never involved with the neurofibroma, is sutured together and used to line the new orbit.

After healing is achieved, the defect is

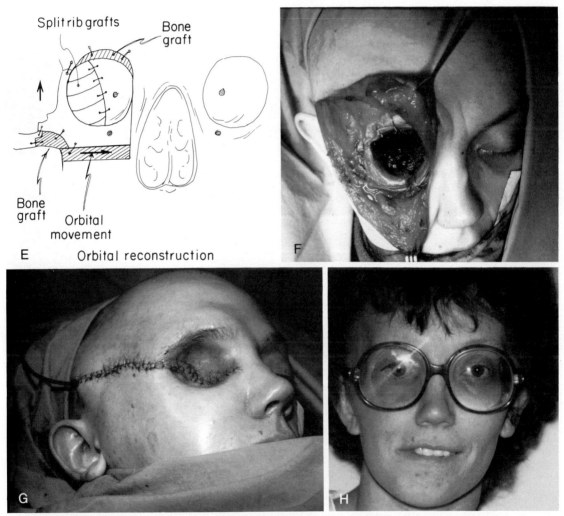

Figure 69–28 *Continued E,* Diagram of completed osteotomies and bone grafts. Arrows show the direction of movement of the osteotomized segment. *F,* Appearance of the orbit at the end of the procedure. The bone grafts have been placed in the supraorbital rim and wired in position. *G,* Soft tissue reconstruction by suturing the edges of the eyelid skin together. *H,* Appearance five years after surgery without recurrence of the neurofibroma. External prosthesis in place.

reconstructed with a total eye and eyelid prosthesis. When there is extensive intracranial disease, a two-stage operation is performed. At the first stage, the lesion is removed from the middle cranial fossa and the posterior wall defect is bone grafted. In the second stage, the orbital contents are removed and the orbital reconstruction is performed. If possible, the eyelids are maintained and fixed in an open position. In the radically treated cases, followed for five years, the cosmetic result has been satisfactory, and there have been no recurrences.

Fibrous Dysplasia. This process can involve the posterolateral area of the orbit and the related craniofacial skeleton. It can cause proptosis and progressive reduction of visual acuity owing to narrowing of the optic canal.

Using a bicoronal flap, the surgeon can dissect the orbital contents and temporalis muscle in a subperiosteal plane to expose the lesion in the temporal fossa and the orbit. If the anterior orbit is uninvolved, an orbitomaxillotemporal exposure osteotomy is performed (Fig. 69–29). The frontal and temporal lobes are elevated, and the involved area is resected with a margin of unaffected bone. Immediate reconstruction is with split calvarial bone grafts. If the defect is extensive, split ribs are also used. The osteotomized segments and cranial bone flap are replaced, and the bicoronal flap is closed.

Superior and Low Infratemporal Tumors. The remainder of the tumors affecting the anterior segment of the posterior area are divided into superior and low infratemporal

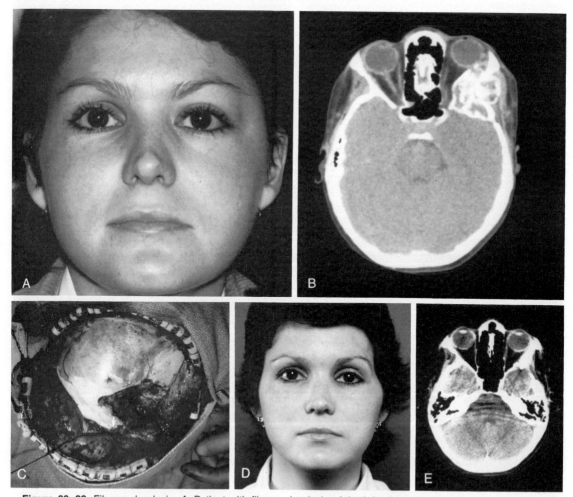

Figure 69–29. Fibrous dysplasia. *A,* Patient with fibrous dysplasia of the left orbit and the middle cranial fossa base. Note the left proptosis. *B,* Axial CT scan showing the extent of the fibrous dysplasia. *C,* Orbitomaxillotemporal exposure osteotomy performed *(arrow)* with a temporoparietal craniotomy for exposure after resection of the fibrous dysplasia. The exposure osteotomy segment was replaced, and the bony defects were reconstructed with split cranial grafts. *D,* Appearance three years after surgery. *E,* Axial CT scan three years after surgery.

fossa tumors. This classification refers to the site of extension or the origin of the tumor and dictates the surgical approach.

Superior Infratemporal Fossa Tumors. Tumors of the superior region of the infratemporal fossa may be meningiomas, fibrous dysplasia, or neurofibromas. They often involve the lateral orbital wall, resulting in proptosis, dystopia, and visual problems. The invasion occurs directly through the posterior or lateral wall or indirectly through the superior orbital fissure. CT, MRI, and carotid angiography are recommended for preoperative planning.

Meningiomas compose 14 to 18 per cent of all primary intracranial tumors. The male-to-female ratio is 1:3 or 1:4; they occur on average at age 45 years. Approximately 20 per cent of intracranial meningiomas have an extracranial extension; this follows anatomic pathways. The orbit is involved through the optic canal or the superior orbital fissure. Entry into the nasopharynx and nasal cavity may occur when a tumor erodes through the cribriform plate. Extension into the paranasal sinuses and pterygoid space is through the floor of the middle cranial fossa. Involvement of the cranial vault and scalp is by extension through the cranial suture lines. Intracranial meningiomas are generally thought of as locally limited neoplasms, usually having a relatively favorable prognosis. This view is significantly altered by recognition of meningiomas with extracranial spread. These have a different, more aggressive behavior, and they are referred to as invading meningiomas.

The surgical approach is similar to that described for fibrous dysplasia (see Fig. 69–29). Through a bicoronal flap, the skull, the temporal fossa, the orbits, and the upper maxilla are exposed. If a maxillectomy is to be performed, the face-splitting incision is made. A frontotemporal craniotomy provides intracranial access; an exposure osteotomy of the superior orbital rim and the lateral orbital wall, the malar bone, and the zygomatic arch allows entry to the orbit and infratemporal area. The tumor and involved bone are removed intra- and extracranially in en bloc fashion, if possible. Any dural tears are repaired; dural reconstruction is performed with fascia lata. Any connections into the nasopharynx or frontal sinus are closed with a galeal frontalis myofascial flap. Bony defects are reconstructed with split calvarial grafts, and the noninvolved removed bone is replaced. In vascular lesions, bleeding can be significantly reduced by preoperative selective embolization of the external carotid artery, performed 24 to 48 hours prior to the planned resection. When there is extensive intraorbital infiltration, an orbital exenteration is advised. Complete resection is often not possible without unacceptable neurologic consequences. This is particularly the case in recurrent lesions. Extensive debulking can, however, provide prolonged symptom free periods and allow subsequent resection of recurrences. This approach has improved results, particularly for primary tumors.

Low Infratemporal Fossa Tumors. These tumors consist of meningiomas, neurofibromas, and extracranial tumors, including squamous cell carcinomas, adenocarcinomas, adenoid cystic carcinomas, and various types of sarcomas. The primary tumor may originate from the orbit, the maxilla, the tonsillar area, or the parotid or retromaxillary region with superior extension to the skull base. Symptoms include visual disturbances, dysphagia, or dyspnea. Proptosis and tonsillar, retromandibular, and temporal swelling may be seen. Anesthesia, or more rarely hyperparesthesia, indicating involvement of the trigeminal nerve, is a significant clinical finding, as is facial weakness (suggesting facial nerve invasion). CT and MRI scans are helpful in planning surgery. A carotid angiogram should be done to show the position of the artery in relation to the tumor and to assess cerebral crossflow. The latter must be established in case it becomes necessary to resect the carotid artery.

In the past, it was difficult to obtain sufficiently satisfactory exposure to perform an en bloc resection. The incision begins in the midcoronal area and extends inferiorly to the front of the ear and continues into the neck (Fig. 69–30) (Jackson and associates, 1982a). If only the carotid artery and internal jugular vein are to be exposed, the incision ends in the midneck; for a neck dissection, it is extended to the clavicle. The skin flap, consisting of the forehead, cheek, and neck, is elevated based anteriorly. This gives exposure to the frontotemporal, zygomatic, and mandibular areas and to the neck. A frontotemporal craniotomy is performed, and the temporal lobe is elevated until the tumor comes into view. The resectability of the lesion can be assessed at this point either by seeing

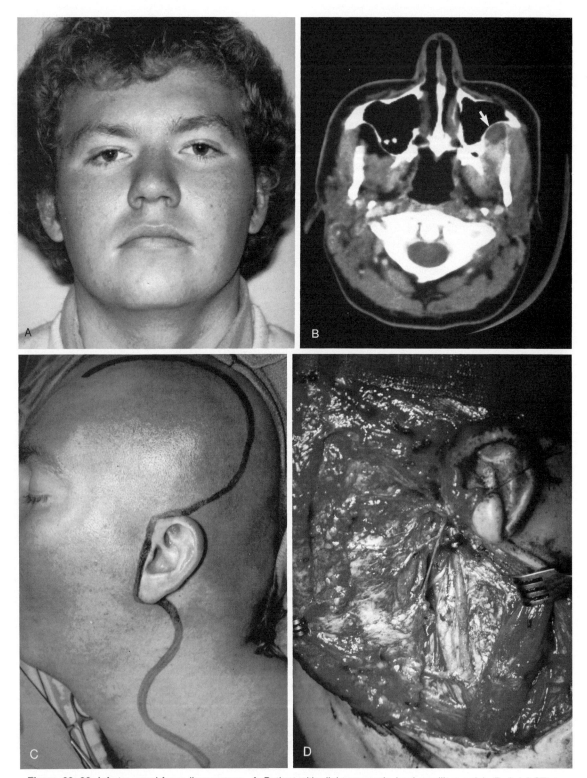

Figure 69–30. Infratemporal fossa liposarcoma. *A,* Patient with slight proptosis (and maxillary pain). *B,* Axial CT scan showing a lesion in the infratemporal fossa with displacement of the posterior wall of the maxilla *(arrow). C,* Surgical approach through a temporoparietal preauricular neck incision. *D,* Total parotidectomy with preservation of the facial nerve and a modified radical neck dissection.

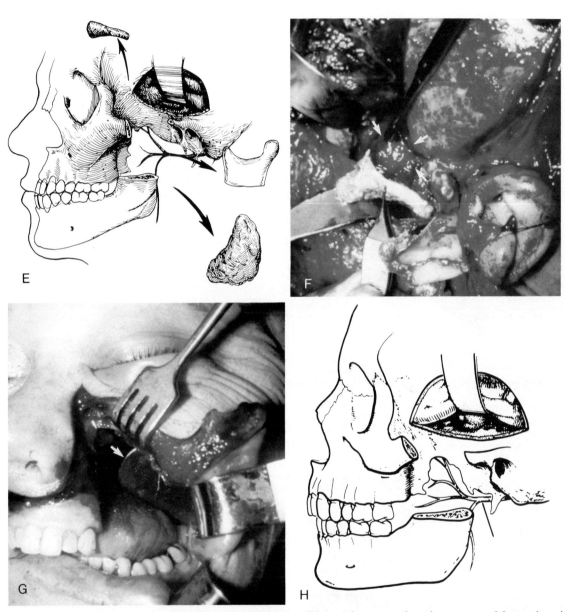

Figure 69–30 *Continued E,* The ascending ramus of the mandible and the zygomatic arch are removed *(arrows),* and a temporal craniotomy is carried out. The facial nerve is preserved. *F,* Excision of the zygomatic arch and exposure of the tumor in the infratemporal fossa *(arrows). G,* Through a Weber-Fergusson incision, the maxilla was resected and was removed in continuity with the tumor from the lateral approach. The malleable retractor can be seen in the maxillary area, having been inserted from the lateral approach *(arrow). H,* The osteotomies required for tumor exposure.

Illustration continued on following page

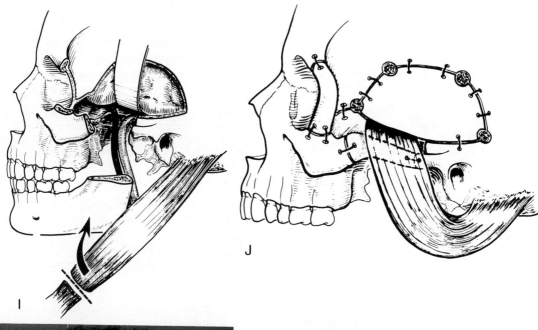

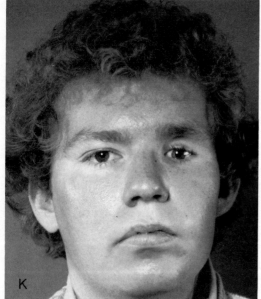

Figure 69–30 *Continued I,* The skull base resection. Note the division of the sternocleidomastoid muscle inferiorly in preparation for transfer *(arrow). J,* The sternocleidomastoid muscle has been transferred on its superior pedicle to provide padding and cover for the dural repair in the middle cranial fossa base. The muscle may be taken over or under the zygomatic arch. *K,* Eighteen months after surgery. Note the slight enophthalmos of the left globe. The patient died after 2½ years of spinal metastases.

gross tumor invasion or by exposing the trigeminal ganglion as it lies in Meckel's cave and performing a biopsy of the ganglion. If the biopsy results are positive, the tumor is judged inoperable and resection is not attempted, but local irradiation can be given by using radioactive implants. The patient thus preserves quality of life for the few remaining months of life rather than having function and appearance severely disturbed.

A preliminary upper neck dissection is performed to identify the internal carotid artery and the internal jugular vein, particularly in the skull base area. A therapeutic dissection is performed when cervical lymph nodes contain tumor. After this procedure, a total parotidectomy with preservation of the facial nerve is carried out. The ascending ramus of the mandible and the zygomatic arch are removed to expose the infratemporal fossa. The intra- and extracranial position of the mass can now be assessed. The temporal lobe is elevated, and the periosteum is raised from the undersurface of the skull base toward the tumor. The skull base is removed piecemeal until the involved foramen or area of skull is reached.

At this point, the position of the tumor relative to the carotid artery is assessed. The styloid process is the key; lateral to this reference marker it is safe to dissect; medial lies the carotid artery. The tumor is isolated above and below as extensively as possible with as much surrounding bone and soft tissue as is judged necessary. In nonmalignant tumors, only an amount of skull base sufficient to excise the tumor is removed. In malignant lesions, the bone surrounding the tumor is resected. Invasion of the cavernous sinus indicates probable inoperability. If the orbit is invaded, an orbital osteotomy is performed; occasionally the orbital contents must be removed. If the tumor arises from behind or invades the maxilla, depending on its extent, an anterior approach using the Weber-Fergusson incision may be necessary to perform a partial or a total maxillectomy (see Fig. 69–30). In this type of case, there can be extension from the orbit to the ethmoid sinuses. The latter also require resection. In some infratemporal tumors, there may be no evidence of involvement of the cranial base. Usually this is well shown on preoperative CT scan. In these cases, an intracranial approach is not indicated unless there is evidence of trigeminal nerve invasion.

Central Segment of Posterior Area

Tumors of the central segment of the posterior area include basal cell and squamous cell carcinomas of the external ear region growing medially to involve the petrous bone. Other lesions are advanced primary, but more often recurrent, malignant parotid tumors and squamous cell carcinomas arising in the middle ear. Glomus tumors are not discussed in this chapter.

Partial petrosectomy (Fig. 69–31) does not involve entry into the cranial cavity. The external ear is resected when indicated. If skin cover is required, this can be obtained with a temporal muscle transposition and the application of a split-thickness skin graft. More extensive tumors require subtotal or total petrosectomy (Fig. 69–32) (Jackson and associates, 1982a). The incision is similar to that described for tumors of the deep infratemporal fossa. In cancers of the middle ear, the ear may be left attached to the anterior flap with transection of the external canal. If the ear is to be resected, an ellipse of skin is taken. Again, a neck dissection is advised to locate the vessels at the skull base. The facial nerve is sacrificed during the resection. In less extensive tumors, the nerve can be preserved by removing the bone using a micro air drill under magnification. This maneuver requires considerable experience and judgment. A temporal craniotomy is performed to assess tumor resectability; tumor extension into the temporal lobe dura, the trigeminal ganglion, or the area beyond the apex of the petrous bone into the cavernous sinus indicates unresectability. If the tumor is believed to be resectable, the neck dissection is performed. The internal carotid artery is identified, and the internal jugular vein is preserved intact. If the vein is ligated early in the procedure, this results in considerable distention of the lateral sinus, which can bleed profusely if traumatized. In extensive lesions, it is necessary to remove the ascending ramus of the mandible and a portion of the zygomatic arch for better exposure. The temporal lobe is retracted, and the periosteum is stripped from the skull base anterior to the petrous bone. The muscle attachments are incised posteriorly. Resection of the skull base is performed anterior and posterior to the petrous bone. The extent of the osteotomies is determined by the size of the tumor. The temporal lobe is retracted farther, and

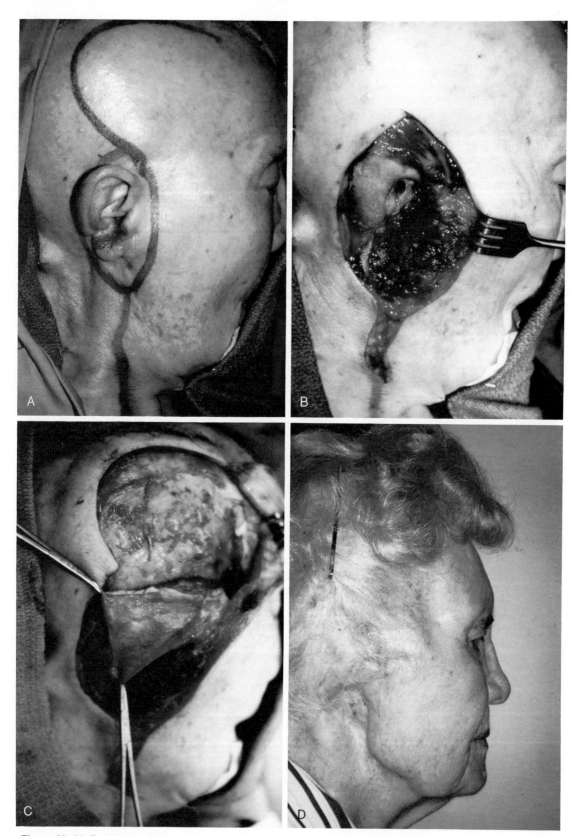

Figure 69–31. Partial petrosectomy. *A,* Patient with recurrent basal cell carcinoma of the right ear. The incision extends from the temporoparietal area around the ear into the neck. *B,* Resection completed with a superficial parotidectomy, partial petrosectomy, and biopsy of the facial nerve canal. *C,* Use of the temporalis muscle to cover the defect. The muscle was covered with a split-thickness skin graft. *D,* The patient died five years after surgery without evidence of recurrence.

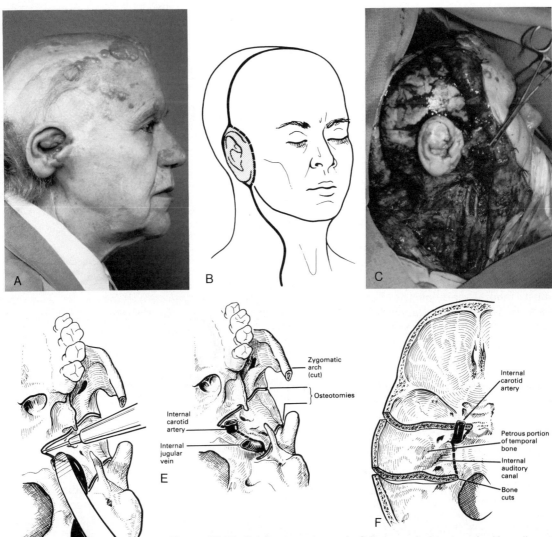

Figure 69–32. Total petrosectomy. *A,* Cylindroma (turban tumor) with malignant degeneration in the region of the right ear after previous resection. There was extensive involvement of the middle ear. *B,* The incision line extending from the temporoparietal area around the ear and into the neck for a modified radical neck dissection. *C,* A modified radical neck dissection has been performed and an in-continuity petrosectomy may be carried out. The carotid vessels and the internal jugular vein were exposed for ease of dissection in the cranial base. *D,* Approach to the base of the middle cranial fossa after the infratemporal fossa dissection has been performed with prior removal of the zygomatic arch and the ascending ramus of the mandible as necessary. *E,* Relationship of the osteotomies to the internal carotid artery and the internal jugular vein (undersurface of the middle cranial fossa). *F,* Relationship of the osteotomies to the internal carotid artery (internal surface of middle cranial fossa base).

Illustration continued on following page

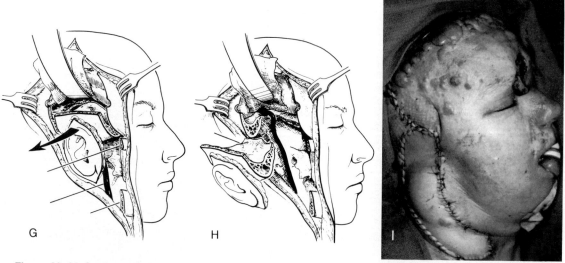

Figure 69–32 *Continued G,* Following these osteotomies, the bony segment is mobilized *(arrow). H,* After removal of the bony segment, the position of the carotid artery can be visualized. *I,* Closure of the defect with a large pectoralis major musculocutaneous flap. Note the other area of malignant degeneration in the glabellar region, which has been resected and will be covered with a local flap.

the osteotomies continued medially until the most medial part of the tumor has been passed. The lateral sinus can be lacerated at this point, and, if so, it is packed with absorbable cellulose gauze (Surgicel). Ligation of the internal jugular vein should be postponed as long as possible and may even be unnecessary in some cases. The carotid artery is freed from its bony canal from above and below using an air drill. Extracranial osteotomies are completed, corresponding to the intracranial osteotomies. The petrous bone can be freed medially by gentle rocking movements. At this point in the procedure, there is definite danger of tearing the internal carotid artery. If this occurs, depending on results of the preoperative crossflow studies, it can be ligated or repaired. Any dural tear is repaired or reconstructed with autogenous fascia lata. The temporal bone flap is replaced. There may be no skin defect, and the ear is returned to its former position and sutured. Any skin defect can be closed by using a scalp rotation flap or, if the defect is more extensive, a pectoralis major musculocutaneous flap. This is a convenient technique since repositioning of the patient is not required. If these alternatives are not available, latissimus and trapezius musculocutaneous flaps have been used.

The potential complications of this procedure are considerable: death usually from hemorrhage, stroke, deafness, blindness, im-mobile eye, facial palsy, vertigo, and nausea. The latter two problems occur more frequently when the patient is given postoperative radiation. In basal cell carcinomas and squamous cell carcinomas, the results are usually good if the resection is adequate. Middle ear carcinomas are rarely cured, even with postoperative radiotherapy. Mixed results are obtained in recurrent parotid tumors; adenoid cystic carcinoma, in particular, tends to recur.

Posterior Segment of Posterior Area

Tumors of the posterior cranial fossa include acoustic neuroma, neurofibroma, meningioma, and fibrous dysplasia; sarcoma and carcinoma in the posterior neck can invade the posterior fossa. Presenting symptoms are headache or dizziness. Palsies of the last four cranial nerves are caused by compression or direct invasion. The resulting symptoms and signs are wasting and weakness of the trapezius, sternocleidomastoid, and tongue muscles, hoarseness, and occasionally dysphagia. Intracranial tumors escape through the jugular foramen and can present behind the mandibular ramus as a deep lobe parotid tumor. Skull base CT scans often demonstrate an enlarged jugular foramen. Angiography may show displacement of the carotid artery when the tumor extends into the neck.

The standard neurosurgical posterior fossa

approach is used. A posterior scalp flap is raised; its position is determined by the location of the occipital vessels. The anterior incision is extended into the neck to allow exposure as required by the position of the tumor. In the occipital area, several layers of muscle must be stripped from the skull base until the transverse processes of the atlas and axis are reached; the vertebral artery is preserved. A posterior craniotomy allows exposure of the tumor. The neck incision provides exposure to the extracranial part of the tumor, which is dissected from the carotid gland, the facial nerve, and the internal carotid artery. The jugular foramen is reached by following the internal jugular vein up to the skull base. The posterior lobe and cerebellum are retracted, and the cranial base is

resected to the jugular. Tumor removal can be performed under direct vision. No reconstructive measures are performed, except a dural repair, if necessary.

Principles of Reconstruction After Craniofacial Tumor Resection

After extensive resections of cranial base tumors, reconstruction may be immediate or delayed, depending on the biologic behavior of the tumor (Jackson, 1987). Extensive immediate reconstruction is performed after resection of benign lesions such as fibrous dysplasia or neurofibromatosis in which local recurrence after adequate resection is unusual. If total resection of malignant tumors is not possible, immediate reconstruction

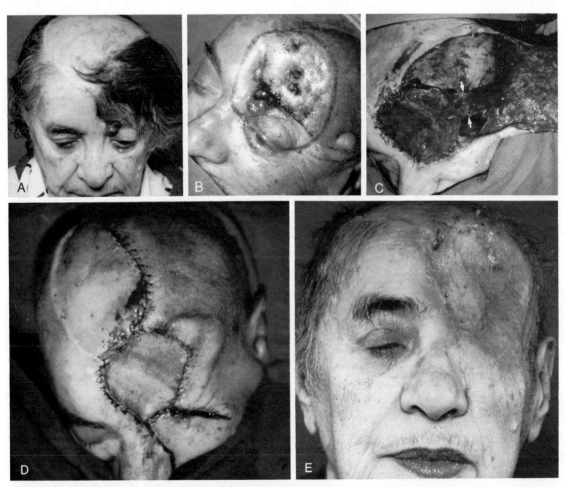

Figure 69–33. Temporalis muscle flap. *A,* Patient with squamous cell carcinoma of the left frontal and orbital areas after surgical resection and radiotherapy. *B,* Proposed resection of the recurrent tumor with exenteration of the orbit and removal of the frontal bone and the underlying dura. *C,* After resection, a temporalis myogaleal flap was elevated to cover the dural repair and close the nasopharynx from the extradural space. The temporalis muscle pedicle is shown *(arrows).* *D,* The myofascial flap was covered wtih a split-thickness skin graft. *E,* Four years after surgical resection the patient had no evidence of recurrence.

should be carried out to return the patient to as close to normal form and function as possible to retain some element of quality of life. Although immediate reconstruction, often with microvascular free tissue transfer, after extensive resection of aggressive or recurrent tumors has been recommended, this is not routinely practiced for several reasons: First, extensive immediate reconstruction may ultimately lead to delay in detection of early recurrence, which when detected may be amenable to further resection. Second, the first major reconstruction usually employs the optimal method of reconstruction. If there is a recurrence, the ideal reconstructive option may have to be sacrificed. This has been seen frequently with forehead nasal reconstruction after resections of basal and squamous cell carcinoma. Many of the facial and orbital defects are amenable to prosthetic rehabilitation after extensive resection (see Chap. 72). As experience with osseointegration techniques increases, more satisfactory external prostheses are becoming available (Jackson and associates, 1986b; Jackson, French, and Tolman, 1988). In this procedure, titanium implants are placed, and these eventually become integrated within the bone. The external prosthesis is stabilized using magnets or attachments to a framework of metal struts (see Fig. 69–25).

There are two indications for immediate reconstruction. The first is to prevent ascending infection from an open nasopharynx or to close the frontal sinus. The most useful technique for this is the galeal frontalis myofascial flap procedure (see Fig. 69–26); in some cases the temporalis muscle flap or fascial flap can be used (Fig. 69–33). The second indication is to prevent exposure of brain, fascia lata grafts, or bone. The options for this are again galeal or temporalis muscle flaps and skin grafting. Local skin or scalp flaps are ideal in some instances, whereas distant flaps (e.g., pectoralis musculocutaneous flaps) are indicated in others. Free tissue transfer may be occasionally necessary.

REFERENCES

Adekeye, E. O., Edwards, M. B., and Goubran, G. F.: Ameloblastic fibrosarcoma. Oral Surg. Oral Med. Oral Pathol., 46:254, 1978.

Albright, F., Butler, A. M., Hampton, A. O., et al.: Syndrome characterized by osteitis fibrosa disseminata, areas of pigmentation and endocrine dysfunction, with precocious puberty in females; report of five cases. N. Engl. J. Med., 16:727, 1937.

Altini, M., and Farman, A. G.: The calcifying odontogenic cyst. Eight new cases and a review of the literature. Oral Surg. Oral Med. Oral Pathol., 40:751, 1975.

Anderson, H. C., Kim, B., and Minkowitz, S.: Calcifying epithelial odontogenic tumor of Pindborg. An electron microscopic study. Cancer, 24:585, 1969.

Austin, L.T., Jr., Dahlin, D. C., and Royer, R. O.: Giant-cell reparative granuloma and related conditions affecting the jawbones. Oral Surg. Oral Med. Oral Pathol., 12:1285, 1959.

Baden, E., Moskow, B. S., and Moskow, R.: Odontogenic gingival epithelial hamartoma. J. Oral Surg., 26:702, 1968.

Banerjee, S. C.: Juxtacortical osteosarcoma of mandible: review of the literature and report of a case. J. Oral Surg., 39:535, 1981.

Barnes, L.: Tumors and tumorlike lesions of the soft tissues. In Barnes, L. (Ed.): Surgical Pathology of the Head and Neck. New York, Marcel Dekker, 1985, p. 809.

Batsakis, J. G. (Ed.): Tumors of the Head and Neck. Clinical and Pathological Considerations. 2nd Ed. Baltimore, Williams & Wilkins Company, 1979.

Batsakis, J. G.: The pathology of head and neck tumors: nasal cavity and paranasal sinuses, part 5. Head Neck Surg., 2:410, 1980.

Batsakis, J. G.: The pathology of head and neck tumors: the occult primary and metastases to the head and neck, part 10. Head Neck Surg., 3:409, 1981a.

Batsakis, J. G.: Pathology consultation. Nasal (schneiderian) papillomas. Ann. Otol. Rhinol. Laryngol., 90:190, 1981b.

Batsakis, J. G.: Pathology of tumors of the nasal cavity and paranasal sinuses. In Thawley, S. E., and Panje, W. R. (Eds.): Comprehensive Management of Head and Neck Tumors. Philadelphia, W. B. Saunders Company, 1987.

Batsakis, J. G., Regezi, J. A., Solomon, A. R., and Rice, D. H.: The pathology of head and neck tumors: mucosal melanomas, part 13. Head Neck Surg., 4:404, 1982.

Batsakis, J. G., Rice, D. H., and Solomon, A. R.: The pathology of head and neck tumors: squamous and mucous gland carcinomas of the nasal cavity, paranasal sinuses, and larynx, part 6. Head Neck Surg., 2:497, 1980.

Bhaskar, S. N.: Central mucoepidermoid tumors of the mandible. Report of 2 cases. Cancer, 16:721, 1963.

Bhaskar, S. N.: Oral surgery–oral pathology conference No. 13, Walter Reed Army Medical Center. Gingival cyst and keratinizing ameloblastoma. Oral Surg. Oral Med. Oral Pathol., 19:796, 1965.

Bhaskar, S. N.: Oral surgery–oral pathology conference No. 17, Walter Reed Army Medical Center. Periapical lesions—types, incidence, and clinical features. Oral Surg. Oral Med. Oral Pathol., 21:657, 1966.

Biesecker, J. L., Marcove, R. C., Huvos, A. G., and Mike, V.: Aneurysmal bone cysts. A clinicopathologic study of 66 cases. Cancer, 26:615, 1970.

Boston, H. C., Jr., Dahlin, D. C., Ivins, J. C., and Cupps, R. E.: Malignant lymphoma (so-called reticulum cell sarcoma) of bone. Cancer, 34:1131, 1974.

Brånemark, P-I., Breine, U., Adell, R., Hansson, B. O., Lindström, J., and Ohlsson, A.: Intraosseous anchorage of dental prostheses. I. Experimental studies. Scand. J. Plast. Reconstr. Surg., 3:81, 1969.

Brånemark, P-I, Hansson, B. O., Adell, R., Breine, U., Lindström, J., et al.: Osseointegrated implants in the treatment of the edentulous jaw. Experience from a 10-year period. Scand. J. Plast. Reconstr. Surg., *16*:1, 1977.

Brannon, R. B.: The odontogenic keratocyst. Part I. Oral Surg. Oral Med. Oral Pathol., *42*:54, 1976.

Breslow, N., and McCann, B.: Statistical estimation of prognosis for children with neuroblastoma. Cancer Res., *31*:2098, 1971.

Browand, B. C., and Waldron, C. A.: Central mucoepidermoid tumors of the jaws. Report of nine cases and review of the literature. Oral Surg. Oral Med. Oral Pathol., *40*:631, 1975.

Browne, R. M.: Metaplasia and degeneration in odontogenic cysts in man. J. Oral Pathol., *1*:145, 1972.

Browne, R. M.: The pathogenesis of odontogenic cysts: A review. J. Oral Pathol., *4*:31, 1975.

Buchner, A., and Hansen, L. S.: The histomorphologic spectrum of the gingival cyst in the adult. Oral Surg. Oral Med. Oral Pathol., *48*:532, 1979.

Budnick, S. D.: Compound and complex odontomas. Oral Surg. Oral Med. Oral Pathol., *42*:501, 1976.

Burkitt, D. P.: A sarcoma involving the jaws in African children. Br. J. Surg., *46*:218, 1958.

Caron, A. S., Hajdu, S. I., and Strong, E. W.: Osteogenic sarcoma of the facial and cranial bones. A review of forty-three cases. Am. J. Surg., *122*:719, 1971.

Cataldo, E., and Berkman, M. D.: Cysts of the oral mucosa in newborns. Am. J. Dis. Child., *116*:44, 1968.

Chaudhry, A. P., Robinovitch, M. R., Mitchell, D. F., and Vickers, R. A.: Chondrogenic tumors of the jaws. Am. J. Surg., *102*:403, 1961.

Cohen, M., and Schultz, R. C.: Mandibular reconstruction. Clin. Plast. Surg., *12*:411, 1985.

Coley, B.: Neoplasms of Bone. New York, Paul B. Hoeber, 1960, p. 298.

Conley, J., Stout, A. P., and Healey, W. V.: Clinicopathologic analysis of 84 patients with an original diagnosis of fibrosarcoma of the head and neck. Am. J. Surg., *114*:564, 1967.

Constanzo, C., Jackson, I. T., McEwan, C., and Self, J. M.: Desmoplastic malignant melanoma: an aggressive tumor. Eur. J. Plast. Surg., *9*:137, 1987.

Corio, R. L., Crawford, B. E., and Schaberg, S. J.: Benign cementoblastoma. Oral Surg. Oral Med. Oral Pathol., *41*:524, 1976.

Courtney, R. M., and Kerr, D. A.: The odontogenic adenomatoid tumor. A comprehensive study of twenty new cases. Oral Surg. Oral Med. Oral Pathol., *39*:424, 1975.

Craig, G. T.: The paradental cyst. A specific inflammatory odontogenic cyst. Br. Dent. J., *141*:9, 1976.

Croxatto, J. O., and Font, R. L.: Hemangiopericytoma of the orbit: a clinicopathologic study of 30 cases. Hum. Pathol., *13*:210, 1982.

Cuono, C. B., and Ariyan, S.: Immediate reconstruction of a composite mandibular defect with a regional osteomusculocutaneous flap. Plast. Reconstr. Surg., *65*:477, 1980.

Curtis, M. L., Elmore, J. S., and Sotereanos, G. C.: Osteosarcoma of the jaws: report of case with review of the literature. J. Oral Surg., *32*:125, 1974.

Dachi, S. F., and Howell, F. V.: A survey of 3,874 routine full-mouth radiographs. II. A study of impacted teeth. Oral Surg. Oral Med. Oral Pathol., *14*:1165, 1961.

Dahl, E. C., Wolfson, S. H., and Haugen, J. C.: Central odontogenic fibroma: review of literature and report of cases. J. Oral Surg., *39*:120, 1981.

Dahlin, D. C. (Ed.): Bone Tumors. General Aspects and Data in 6,221 Cases. 3rd Ed. Springfield, IL, Charles C Thomas, 1978.

Dahlin, D. C., Unni, K. K., and Matsuno, T.: Malignant (fibrous) histiocytoma of bone—fact or fancy? Cancer, *39*:1508, 1977.

Das Gupta, T. K.: Tumors of the Soft Tissue. New York, Appleton & Lange, 1983.

Daugherty, J. W., and Eversole, L. R.: Aneurysmal bone cyst of the mandible: report of case. J. Oral Surg., *29*:737, 1971.

de Fries, H. O., and Kornblut, A. D.: Malignant disease of the osseous adnexae: osteogenic sarcoma of the jaws. Otolaryngol. Clin. North Am., *12*:129, 1979.

Dubin, B., and Jackson, I. T.: The use of liposuction to contour cherubism. Plast. Reconstr. Surg. (in press).

Dubin, B., Jackson, I. T., and Carbonell, A.: Craniofacial surgery for invading meningiomas (in press).

Dutton, J. J., and Anderson, R. L.: Treatment of tumors of the eye, orbit and lacrimal apparatus. *In* Thawley, S. E., and Panje, W. R. (Eds.): Comprehensive Management of Head and Neck Tumors. Philadelphia, W. B. Saunders Company, 1987.

El Deeb, M., Sedano, H. O., and Waite, D. E.: Aneurysmal bone cyst of the jaws. Report of a case associated with fibrous dysplasia and review of the literature (review). Int. J. Oral Surg., *9*:301, 1980.

Ellis, E., III, and Fonseca, R. J.: Management of odontogenic cysts and tumors. *In* Thawley, S. E., and Panje, W. R. (Eds.): Comprehensive Management of Head and Neck Tumors. Philadelphia, W. B. Saunders Company, 1987, p. 1483.

Elzay, R. P.: Primary intraosseous carcinoma of the jaws: Review and update of odontogenic carcinomas. Oral Surg. Oral Med. Oral Pathol., *54*:299, 1982.

Enzinger, F. M., and Weiss, S. W.: Liposarcomas. *In* Enzinger, F. M., and Weiss, S. W.: Soft Tissue Tumors. St. Louis, MO, C. V. Mosby Company, 1983.

Enzinger, F. M., and Weiss, S. W.: Soft Tissue Tumors. St. Louis, MO, C. V. Mosby Company, 1983.

Evans, A. E., D'Angio, G. J., and Randolph, J.: A proposed staging for children with neuroblastoma. Cancer, *27*:374, 1971.

Eversole, L. R., Sabes, W. R., and Rovin, S.: Fibrous dysplasia: a nosologic problem in the diagnosis of fibroosseous lesions of the jaws. J. Oral Pathol., *1*:189, 1972.

Farman, A. G., Kohler, W. W., Nortje, C. J., and Van Wyk, C. W.: Cementoblastoma: report of case. J. Oral Surg., *37*:198, 1979.

Farman, A. G., Nortje, C. J., and Grotepass, F.: Periosteal benign osteoblastoma of the mandible: report of a case and review of the literature pertaining to benign osteoblastic neoplasms of the jaws. Br. J. Oral Surg., *14*:12, 1976.

Feintuch, T. A.: Chondrosarcoma arising in a cartilaginous area of previously irradiated fibrous dysplasia. Cancer, *31*:877, 1973.

Finkelstein, J. B.: Osteosarcoma of the jaw bones. Radiol. Clin. North Am., *8*:425, 1970.

Font, R. L., and Ferry, A. P.: Carcinoma metastatic to the eye and orbit III. A clinicopathologic study of 28 cases metastatic to the orbit. Cancer, *38*:1326, 1976.

Font, R. L., and Gamel, J. W.: Epithelial tumors of the lacrimal gland: an analysis of 265 cases. *In* Jakobiec, F. A. (Ed.): Ocular and Adnexal Tumors. Birmingham, AL, Aesculapius Publishing Company, 1978.

Forbes,. G., Earnest, F., IV, Jackson, I. T., Marsh, W. R., Jack, C. R., and Cross, S. A.: Therapeutic embolization angiography for extra-axial lesions in the head. Mayo Clin. Proc., *61*:427, 1986.

Franklin, C. D., and Pindborg, J. J.: The calcifying epithelial odontogenic tumor: a review and analysis of 113 cases. Oral Surg. Oral Med. Oral Pathol., *42*:753, 1976.

Frazell, E. L., and Lewis, J. S.: Cancer of the nasal cavity and accessory sinuses: a report of the management of 416 patients. Cancer, *16*:1293, 1963.

Freedman, P. D., Cardo, V. A., Kerpel, S. M., and Lumerman, H.: Desmoplastic fibroma (fibromatosis) of the jawbones. Oral Surg. Oral Med. Oral Pathol., *46*:386, 1978.

Freedman, P. D., Lumerman, H., and Gee, J. K.: Calcifying odontogenic cyst. Oral Surg. Oral Med. Oral Pathol., *40*:93, 1975.

Fu, Y., Gabbiani, G., Kaye, G. I., and Lattes, R.: Malignant soft tissue tumors of probable histiocytic origin (malignant fibrous histiocytomas): general considerations and electron microscopic and tissue culture studies. Cancer, *35*:176, 1975.

Gardner, D. G., and Pecak, A. M.: The treatment of ameloblastoma based on pathologic and anatomic principles. Cancer, *46*:2514, 1980.

Garrington, G. E., Scofield, H. H., Cornyn, J., and Hooker, S. P.: Osteosarcoma of the jaws. Analysis of 56 cases. Cancer, *26*:377, 1967.

Ghandur-Mnaymneh, L., Zych, G., and Mnaymneh, W.: Primary malignant fibrous histiocytoma of bone: report of six cases with ultrastructural study and analysis of the literature. Cancer, *49*:698, 1982.

Giansanti, J. S., Someren, A., and Waldron, C. A.: Odontogenic adenomatoid tumor (adenoameloblastoma): survey of 3 cases. Oral Surg. Oral Med. Oral Pathol., *30*:69, 1970.

Glenn, J., Kinsella, T., Glatstein, E., Tepper, J., Baker, A., et al.: A randomized prospective trial of adjuvant chemotherapy in adults with soft tissue sarcomas of the head and neck, breast, and trunk. Cancer, *55*:1206, 1985.

Goldblatt, L. I., Brannon, R. B., and Ellis, G. L.: Squamous odontogenic tumor. Report of five cases and review of the literature. Oral Surg. Oral Med. Oral Pathol., *54*:187, 1982.

Goldstein, G., Parker, F. P., and Hugh, G. S.: Ameloblastic sarcoma: pathogenesis and treatment with chemotherapy. Cancer, *37*:1673, 1976.

Gorlin, R. J.: Odontogenic tumors. *In* Gorlin, R. J., and Goldman, H. M. (Eds.): Thoma's Oral Pathology. 6th Ed. St. Louis, MO, C. V. Mosby Company, 1970.

Gorlin, R. J., Chaudhry, A. P., and Pindborg, J. J.: Odontogenic tumors: classification, histopathology, and clinical behavior in man and domesticated animals. Cancer, *14*:73, 1961.

Gorlin, R. J., and Goltz, R. W.: Multiple nevoid basal cell epithelium, jaw cysts, and bifid rib: a syndrome. N. Engl. J. Med., *269*:908, 1960.

Gorlin, R. J., Pindborg, J. J., Clausen, F. P., and Vickers, R. A.: The calcifying odontogenic cyst—a possible analogue of the cutaneous calcifying epithelioma of Malherbe. Oral Surg. Oral Med. Oral Pathol., *15*:1235, 1962.

Grabias, S., and Mankin, H. J.: Chondrosarcoma arising in histologically proved unicameral bone cyst. A case report. J. Bone Joint Surg. [Am.], *56*:1501, 1974.

Grand, N. G., and Marwah, A. S.: Pigmented gingival cyst. Oral Surg. Oral Med. Oral Pathol., *17*:635, 1964.

Greager, J. A., Patel, H. K., Briele, H. A., Walker, M.

J., and Das Gupta, T. K.: Soft tissue sarcomas of the adult head and neck. Cancer, *56*:820, 1985.

Greer, R. O., Jr., Mierau, G. W., and Favara, B. F.: Tumors of the Head and Neck in Children. New York, Praeger Publishers, 1983, p. 125.

Greer, R. O., Jr., Rohrer, M. D., and Young, S. K.: Non-odontogenic tumors, clinical evaluation and pathology. *In* Thawley, S. E., and Panje, W. R. (Eds.): Comprehensive Management of Head and Neck Tumors. Philadelphia, W. B. Saunders Company, 1987, p. 1510.

Gross, C. W., and Montgomery, W. W.: Fibrous dysplasia and malignant degeneration. Arch. Otolaryngol., *85*:653, 1967.

Grothaus, P., Jackson, I. T.,, and Zelt, R.: Head and neck sarcomas. Part III: management in adults (in preparation).

Guillamondegui, O. M., and Larson, D. L.: The lateral trapezius musculocutaneous flap: its use in head and neck reconstruction. Plast. Reconstr. Surg., *67*:143, 1981.

Hallberg, O. E., and Bagley, J. W.: Origin and treatment of osteomas of the paranasal sinuses. Arch. Otolaryngol., *51*:750, 1950.

Hamberger, C. A., Martensson, G., and Sjorgren, H A.: Treatment of Malignant Tumors of the Paranasal Sinuses in Cancer of the Head and Neck. International Workshop on Cancer of the Head and Neck, Washington, DC, Butterworth, 1967.

Hamner, J. E., III, Scofield, H. H., and Cornyn, J.: Benign fibro-osseous jaw lesions of periodontal membrane origin. Cancer, *22*:861, 1968.

Hartman, K. S.: Granular-cell ameloblastoma. Oral Surg. Oral Med. Oral Pathol., *38*:241, 1974.

Hayward, J. R.: Cysts of bone and soft tissue lesions. *In* Hayward, J. R. (Ed.): Oral Surgery. Springfield, IL, Charles C Thomas, 1976.

Heffner, D. K., and Hyams, V. J.: Teratocarcinosarcoma (malignant teratoma?) of the nasal cavity and paranasal sinuses. A clinicopathologic study of 20 cases. Cancer, *53*:2140, 1984.

Heffner, D. K., Hyams, V. J., Hauck, K W., and Lingeman, C.: Low-grade adenocarcinoma of the nasal cavity and paranasal sinuses. Cancer, *50*:312, 1982.

Heimdal, A., Isacsson, G., and Nilsson, L.: Recurrent central odontogenic fibroma. Oral Surg. Oral Med. Oral Pathol., *50*:140, 1980.

Henderson, J. W. (Ed.): Orbital Tumors. 2nd Ed. New York, B. C. Decker, 1980.

Hinds, E. C., Kent, J. N., and Fechner, R. E.: Desmoplastic fibroma of the mandible: report of case. J. Oral Surg., *27*:271, 1969.

Hirschl, S., and Katz, A.: Giant cell reparative granuloma outside the jaw bone: diagnostic criteria and review of the literature with the first case described in the temporal bone. Hum. Pathol., *5*:171, 1974.

Hodgkinson, D. J., Woods, J. E., Dahlin, D. C., and Tolman, D. E.: Keratocysts of the jaw. Cancer, *41*:803, 1978.

Holdcraft, J., and Gallagher, J. C.: Malignant melanomas of the nasal and paranasal sinus mucosa. Ann. Otol. Rhinol. Laryngol., *78*:5, 1969.

Howell, R. M., and Burkes, E. J., Jr.: Malignant transformation of ameloblastic fibro-odontoma to ameloblastic fibrosarcoma. Oral Surg. Oral Med. Oral Pathol., *43*:391, 1977.

Huvos, A. G.: Primary malignant fibrous histiocytoma of bone; clinicopathologic study of 18 patients. N. Y. State J. Med., *76*:552, 1976.

Huvos, A. G. (Ed.): Bone Tumors: Diagnosis, Treatment, and Prognosis. Philadelphia, W. B. Saunders Company, 1979.

Hyams, V. J.: Papillomas of the nasal cavity and paranasal sinuses. A clinicopathologic study of 315 cases. Ann. Otol. Rhinol. Laryngol., 80:192, 1971.

Jackson, I. T.: Craniofacial approach to tumors of the head and neck. Clin. Plast. Surg., 12:375, 1985.

Jackson, I. T.: Transcranial orbitectomy. In Smith, B. C., Della Rocca, R. C., Nesi, F. A., and Lisman, R. D. (Eds.): Ophthalmic Plastic and Reconstructive Surgery. Vol. 2. St. Louis, MO, C. V. Mosby Company, p. 1100.

Jackson, I. T.: Craniofacial tumors. In Georgiade, N. G., Georgiade, G. S., Riefkohl, R., and Barwick, W. J. (Eds.): Essentials of Plastic Maxillofacial, and Reconstructive Surgery. Baltimore, Williams & Wilkins Company, 1987.

Jackson, I. T., Adham, M. N., and Marsh, W. R.: Use of the galeal frontalis myofascial flap in craniofacial surgery. Plast. Reconstr. Surg., 77:905, 1986.

Jackson, I. T., French, D. J., and Tolman, D. E.: A system of osseointegrated implants and its application to dental and facial rehabilitation. Eur. J. Plast. Surg., 11:1, 1988.

Jackson, I. T., Grothaus, P., and Zelt, R.: Head and neck sarcomas. Clinical and pathological features. Plast. Reconstr. Surg. (in press).

Jackson, I. T., Hide, T. A. H., Gomuwka, P. K., Laws, E. R., Jr., and Langford, K.: Treatment of cranio-orbital fibrous dysplasia. J. Maxillofac. Surg., 10:138, 1982a.

Jackson, I. T., Jack, C., Aycock, B., Dubin, B., and Irons, G. B.: The management of interosseous AV malformation in the head and neck. Plast. Reconstr. Surg. (in press).

Jackson, I. T., Laws, E. R., Jr., and Martin, R. D.: The surgical management of orbital neurofibromatosis. Plast. Reconstr. Surg., 71:751, 1983.

Jackson, I. T., and Marsh, W. R.: Anterior cranial fossa tumors. Ann. Plast. Surg., 11:479, 1983.

Jackson, I. T., Marsh, W. R., Bite, U., and Hide, T. A. H.: Craniofacial osteotomies to facilitate skull base tumour resection. Br. J. Plast. Surg., 39:153, 1986a.

Jackson, I. T., Munro, I. R., Salyer, K. E., and Whitaker, L. A. (Eds.): Atlas of Craniomaxillofacial Surgery. St. Louis, MO, C. V. Mosby Company, 1982b, p. 752.

Jackson, I. T., Somers, P., and Marsh, W. R.: Esthesioneuroblastoma: treatment of skull-base recurrence. Plast. Reconstr. Surg., 76:195, 1985.

Jackson, I. T., Tolman, D. E., Desjardins, R. P., and Brånemark, P-I.: A new method for fixation of external prostheses. Plast. Reconstr. Surg., 77:668, 1986b.

Jaffe, H. L.: Osteoid-osteoma. A benign osteoblastic tumor composed of osteoid and atypical bone. Arch. Surg., 31:709, 1935.

Jaffe, H. L.: Giant-cell reparative granuloma, traumatic bone cyst, and fibrous (fibro-osseous) dysplasia of the jawbones. Oral Surg., 6:159, 1953.

Jones, W. A.: Familial multilocular cystic disease of the jaws. Am. J. Cancer, 17:946, 1933.

Killey, H. C., and Kay, L. W.: Fibromyxomata of the jaws. Br. J. Oral Surg., 2:124, 1965.

Knowles, D. M., II, and Jakobiec, F. A.: Orbital lymphoid neoplasms. A clinicopathologic study of 60 patients. Cancer, 46:576, 1980.

LaBriola, J., Steiner, M., Bernstein, M. L., Verdi, G. D., and Stannard, P. F.: Odontoameloblastoma. J. Oral Surg., 38:139, 1980.

LaLonde, E. R.: A new rationale for the management of periapical granulomas and cysts: an evaluation of histopathological and radiographic findings. J. Am. Dent. Assoc., 80:1056, 1970.

LaLonde, E. R., and Luebke, R. G.: The frequency and distribution of periapical cysts and granulomas. Oral Surg. Oral Med. Oral Pathol., 25:861, 1968.

Lam, K. H., Wei, W. I., and Siu, K. F.: The pectoralis major costomyocutaneous flap for mandibular reconstruction. Plast. Reconstr. Surg., 73:904, 1984.

Lawson, W., Abaci, I. F., and Zak, F. G.: Studies on melanocytes. V. The presence of melanocytes in the human dental primordium: an explanation for pigmented lesions of the jaws. Oral Surg. Oral Med. Oral Pathol., 42:375, 1976.

Leider, A. S., Nelson, J. F., and Trodahl, J. N.: Ameloblastic fibrosarcoma of the jaws. Oral Surg. Oral Med. Oral Pathol., 33:559, 1972.

Lichtenstein, L.: Aneurysmal bone cyst. A pathological entity commonly mistaken for giant-cell tumor and occasionally for hemangioma and osteogenic sarcoma. Cancer, 3:279, 1950.

Lichtenstein, L.: Histiocytosis X. Integration of eosinophilic granuloma of bone, "Letterer-Siwe disease," and "Schuller-Christian disease," as related manifestations of a single nosologic entity. Arch. Pathol., 56:84, 1953.

Lichtenstein, L.: Benign osteoblastoma: A category of osteoid and bone forming tumors other than classical osteoid osteoma which may be mistaken for giant cell tumor or osteogenic sarcoma. Cancer, 9:1044, 1956.

Lichtenstein, L.: Diseases of Bone and Joints. 2nd Ed. St. Louis, MO, C. V. Mosby Company, 1975.

Little, J. W., III, McCulloch, D. T., and Lyons, J. R.: The lateral pectoral composite flap in one-stage reconstruction of the irradiated mandible. Plast. Reconstr. Surg., 71:326, 1983.

Lovely, F. W.: Recurrent aneurysmal bone cyst of the mandible. J. Oral Maxillofac. Surg., 41:192, 1983.

Lund, B. A., and Dahlin, D. C.: Hemangiomas of the mandible and maxilla. J. Oral Surg., 22:234, 1964.

Marano, P. D., and Hartman, K. S.: Central mucoepidermoid carcinoma arising in a maxillary odontogenic cyst. J. Oral Surg., 32:915, 1974.

Marlow, C. D., and Waite, D. E.: Fibrous-osseous dysplasia of the jaws: report of case. J. Oral Surg., 23:632, 1965.

Marsh, B. W., Bonfiglio, M., Brady, L. P., and Enneking, W. F.: Benign osteoblastoma: range of manifestations. J. Bone Joint Surg. [Am.], 57:1, 1975.

Masson, J. K., and Soule, D. H.: Desmoid tumors of the head and neck. Am. J. Surg., 12:615, 1966.

Maurer, H. M., Moon, T., Donaldson, M., Fernandez, C., Gehan, E. A., et al.: The Intergroup Rhabdomyosarcoma Study: a preliminary report. Cancer, 40:2015, 1977.

McClatchey, K. D., Hakimi, M., and Batsakis, J. G.: Retrotympanic odontoma. Am. J. Surg. Pathol., 5:401, 1981.

McDaniel, R. K.: Odontogenic cysts and tumors. In Thawley, S. E., and Panje, W. R. (Eds.): Comprehensive Management of Head and Neck Tumors. Philadelphia, W. B. Saunders Company, 1987, p. 1446.

McLeod, R. A., Dahlin, D. C., and Beabout, J. W.: The spectrum of osteoblastoma. Am. J. Roentgenol., 126:321, 1976.

Mehlisch, D. R., Dahlin, D. C., and Masson, J. K.: Ameloblastoma: a clinicopathologic report. J. Oral Surg., 30:9, 1972.

Mendelsohn, D. B., Hertzanu, Y., Glass, R. B., Kassner, G., and Altini, M.: Giant complex odontoma of the maxillary antrum. S. Afr. Med. J., 63:704, 1983.

Miles, A. C.: Chondrosarcoma of the maxilla. Br. Dent. J., 88:257, 1950.

Moreillon, M. C., and Schroeder, H. E.: Numerical frequency of epithelial abnormalities, particularly microkeratocysts, in the developing human oral mucosa. Oral Surg. Oral Med. Oral Pathol., 53:44, 1982.

Moskow, B. S., and Baden, E.: The peripheral ameloblastoma of the gingiva. Case report and literature review. J. Periodontol., 53:736, 1982.

Moskow, B. S., Siegel, K., Zegarelli, E. V., Kutscher, A. H., and Rothenberg, F.: Gingival and lateral periodontal cysts. J. Periodontol., 41:249, 1970.

Moss-Salentijn, L.: Anatomy and embryology. In Blitzer, A., Lawson, W., and Friedman, W. H. (Eds.): Surgery of the Paranasal Sinuses. Philadelphia, W. B. Saunders Company, 1985.

Nesbit, M. E., Jr., Perez, C. A., Tefft, M., Burger, E. O., Jr., Vietti, T. J., et al.: Multimodal therapy for the management of primary, non-metastatic Ewing's sarcoma of bone: an Intergroup Study. Natl. Cancer Inst. Monogr., 56:255, 1981.

Newton, W. A., Jr., and Hamoudi, A. B.: Histiocytosis: a histologic classification with clinical correlation. Perspect. Pathol., 1:251, 1973.

Nilsen, R., and Magnusson, B. C.: Ameloblastic fibroma. Int. J. Oral Surg., 8:370, 1979.

Nolph, M. B., and Luikin, G. A.: Histiocytosis X. Otolaryngol. Clin. North Am., 15:635, 1982.

Oberman, H. A.: Idiopathic histiocytosis: a clinicopathologic study of 40 cases and review of the literature on eosinophilic granuloma of bone, Hand-Schüller-Christian disease and Letterer-Siwe disease. Pediatrics, 28:307, 1961.

Panje, W., and Cutting, C.: Trapezius osteomyocutaneous island flap for reconstruction of the anterior floor of the mouth and the mandible. Head Neck Surg., 3:66, 1980.

Pedersen, E., Hogetveit, A. C., and Andersen, A.: Cancer of respiratory organs among workers at a nickel refinery in Norway. Int. J. Cancer, 12:32, 1973.

Pindborg, J. J.: Calcifying epithelial odontogenic tumor (abstract). Acta Pathol. Microbiol. Scand. (Suppl.), 111:71, 1955.

Pindborg, J. J., Kramer, I. R. H., and Torloni, H.: Histological Typing of Odontogenic Tumors, Jaw Cysts, and Allied Lesions. Geneva, World Health Organization, 1971, p. 15.

Pomeroy, T. C., and Johnson, R. E.: Combined modality therapy of Ewing's sarcoma. Cancer, 35:36, 1975.

Porterfield, J. T.: Orbital tumors in children: a report on 214 cases. Int. Ophthalmol. Clin., 2:319, 1962.

Porterfield, J. T., and Zimmerman, L. E.: Rhabdomyosarcoma of the orbit: a clinicopathologic study of 55 cases. Virchows Arch. [Pathol. Anat.], 335:329, 1962.

Potdar, G. G.: Ewing's tumors of the jaws. Oral Surg. Oral Med. Oral Pathol., 29:505, 1970.

Pullon, P. A., Shafer, W. G., Elzay, R. P., Kerr, D. A., and Corio, R. L.: Squamous odontogenic tumor. Report of six cases of a previously undescribed lesion. Oral Surg. Oral Med. Oral Pathol., 40:616, 1975.

Rappaport, H.: Tumors of the hematopoietic system. In Atlas of Tumor Pathology. Sec. 3, Fasc. 8. Washington, DC, Armed Forces Institute of Pathology, 1966.

Regezi, J. A., Kerr, D. A., and Courtney, R. M.: Odontogenic tumors: analysis of 706 cases. J. Oral Surg., 36:771, 1978.

Reichart, P. A., and Ries, P.: Considerations on the classification of odontogenic tumours. Int. J. Oral Surg., 12:323, 1983.

Rice, D. H., and Stanley, R. B., Jr.: Surgical therapy of nasal cavity, ethmoid sinus, and maxillary sinus tumors. In Thawley, S. E., and Panje, W. R. (Eds.): Comprehensive Management of Head and Neck Tumors. Philadelphia, W. B. Saunders Company, 1987, p. 368.

Robin, P. E., Powell, D. J., and Stansbie, J. M.: Carcinoma of the nasal cavity and paranasal sinuses: incidence and presentation of different histological types. Clin. Otolaryngol., 4:431, 1979.

Rootman, J., and Allen, L. H.: Clinical evaluation and pathology of tumors of the eye, orbit and lacrimal apparatus. In Thawley, S. E., and Panje, W. R. (Eds.): Comprehensive Management of Head and Neck Tumors. Philadelphia, W. B. Saunders Company, 1987.

Rousch, G. C.: Epidemiology of cancer of the nose and paranasal sinuses: current concepts. Head Neck Surg., 2:3, 1979.

Russ, J. E., and Jesse, R. H.: Management of osteosarcoma of the maxilla and mandible. Am. J. Surg., 140:572, 1980.

Saunders, J. R., Jacques, D. A., Casterline, P. F., Percarpio, B., and Goodloe, S., Jr.: Liposarcoma of the head and neck: a review of the literature and addition of four cases. Br. J. Cancer, 43:162, 1979.

Scott, R. F., and Ellis, E., III: Surgical treatment of nonodontogenic tumors. In Thawley, S. E., and Panje, W. R. (Eds.): Comprehensive Management of Head and Neck Tumors. Philadelphia, W. B. Saunders Company, 1987, p. 1559.

Serafin, D., Villarreal-Rios, A., and Georgiade, N.: Rib-containing free flap to reconstruct mandibular defects. Br. J. Plast. Surg., 30:263, 1977.

Shafer, W. G., Hine, M. K., and Levy, B. M. (Eds.): A Textbook of Oral Pathology. 4th Ed. Philadelphia, W. B. Saunders Company, 1983.

Shah, J. P., Huvos, A. G., and Strong, E. W.: Mucosal melanomas of the head and neck. Am. J. Surg., 134:531, 1977.

Shear, M.: Primary intra-alveolar epidermoid carcinoma of the jaw. J. Pathol., 97:645, 1969.

Shear, M.: Cysts of the Oral Regions. 2nd Ed. Boston, Wright-PSG Publishing Company, 1983, p. 3, 4, 56, 79, 114.

Shiffman, M. A.: Familial multiple polyposis associated with soft and hard tissue tumors. J.A.M.A., 182:514, 1962.

Siemssen, S. O., Kirkby, B., and O'Connor, T. P.: Immediate reconstruction of a resected segment of the lower jaw, using a compound flap of clavicle and sternocleidomastoid muscle. Plast. Reconstr. Surg., 61:724, 1978.

Silva, E. G., Butler, J. J., Mackay, B., and Goepfert, H.: Neuroblastomas and neuroendocrine carcinomas of the nasal cavity. Cancer, 50:2388, 1982.

Slootweg, P. J.: An analysis of the interrelationship of the mixed odontogenic tumors—ameloblastic fibroma, ameloblastic fibro-odontoma, and the odontomas. Oral Surg. Oral Med. Oral Pathol., 51:266, 1981.

Slootweg, P. J., and Muller, H.: Malignant fibrous histiocytoma of the maxilla. Oral Surg. Oral Med. Oral Pathol., 44:560, 1977.

Slootweg, P. J., and Muller, H.: Malignant ameloblastoma or ameloblastic carcinoma. Oral Surg. Oral Med. Oral Pathol., 57:168, 1984.

Slow, I. N., and Friedman, E. W.: Osteogenic sarcoma

arising in a preexisting fibrous dysplasia: report of a case. J. Oral Surg., 29:126, 1971.

Small, I. A., and Waldron, C. A.: Ameloblastomas of the jaws. Oral Surg. Oral Med. Oral Pathol., 8:281, 1955.

Smith, R. A., Hansen, L. S., Resnick, D., and Chan, W.: Comparison of the osteoblastoma in gnathic and extragnathic sites. Oral Surg. Oral Med. Oral Pathol., 54:285, 1982.

Smith, R. L., Dahlin, D. C., and Waite, D. E.: Mucoepidermoid carcinomas of the jawbones. J. Oral Surg., 26:387, 1968.

Spiro, R. H., Huvos, A. G., and Strong, E. W.: Adenoid cystic carcinoma of salivary origin: a clinicopathologic study of 242 cases. Am. J. Surg., 128:512, 1974.

Spiro, R. H., Huvos, A. G., and Strong, E. W.: Adenoid cystic carcinoma: factors influencing survival. Am. J. Surg., 138:579, 1979.

Spittle, M. F., Newton, K. A., and Mackenzie, D. H.: Liposarcoma: a review of 60 cases. Br. J. Cancer, 24:696, 1970.

Standish, S. M., and Shafer, W. G.: The lateral periodontal cyst. J. Periodont., 29:27, 1958.

Stanley, H. R., Jr., Krogh, H. W., and Pannkuk, E.: Age changes in the epithelial components of follicles (dental sacs) associated wtih impacted third molars. Oral Surg. Oral Med. Oral Pathol., 19:128, 1965.

Stasinopoulos, M.: Mixed calcified odontogenic tumors. Br. J. Oral Surg., 8:93, 1970.

Steiner, G. C., and Kantor, E. B.: Ultrastructure of aneurysmal bone cyst. Cancer, 40:2967, 1977.

Stout, A. P.: Fibrosarcoma in infants and children. Cancer, 15:1028, 1962.

Stout, F. W., Lunin, M., and Calonius, P. E. B.: A study of epithelial remnants in the maxilla. Abstracts of the 46th General Meeting of the International Association for Dental Research, March 1968, San Francisco, CA. Abstracts 419, 420, 421, 1968, p. 142.

Stroncek, G. G., Dahl, E. C., Fonseca, R. J., and Benda, J. A.: Multiosseous osteosarcoma involving the mandible: metastatic or multicentric? Oral Surg. Oral Med. Oral Pathol., 52:271, 1981.

Struthers, P., and Shear, M.: Root resorption by ameloblastomas and cysts of the jaws. Int. J. Oral Surg., 5:128, 1976.

Swan, R. H., and McDaniel, R. K.: Squamous odontogenic proliferation with probable origin from the rests of Malassez (early squamous odontogenic tumor?). J. Periodontol., 54:493, 1983.

Taylor, G. I.: Reconstruction of the mandible with free composite iliac bone grafts. Ann. Plast. Surg., 9:361, 1982.

Telles, N. C., Rabson, A. S., and Pomeroy, T. C.: Ewing's sarcoma: an autopsy study. Cancer, 41:2321, 1978.

Ten Cate, A. R.: Oral Histology. Development, Structure, and Function. St. Louis, MO, C. V. Mosby Company, 1980.

Thompson, A. D., and Turner-Warwick, R. T.: Skeletal sarcomata and giant cell tumor. J. Bone Joint Surg. [Br.], 37:266, 1955.

Tillman, B. P., Dahlin, D. C., Lipscomb, P. R., and Stewart, J. R.: Aneurysmal bone cyst: an analysis of ninety-five cases. Mayo Clin. Proc., 43:478, 1968.

Trodahl, J. N.: Ameloblastic fibroma. A survey of cases from the Armed Forces Institute of Pathology. Oral Surg. Oral Med. Oral Pathol., 33:547, 1972.

Waldron, C. A., and Giansanti, J. S.: Benign fibro-osseous lesions of the jaws: a clinical-radiologic-histologic review of sixty-five cases. II. Benign fibro-osseous lesions of periodontal ligament origin. Oral Surg. Oral Med. Oral Pathol., 35:340, 1973.

Waldron, C. A., and Shafer, W. G.: The central giant cell reparative granuloma of the jaws. An analysis of 38 cases. Am. J. Clin. Pathol., 45:437, 1966.

Webber, W. B., and Wienke, E. C.: Malignant fibrous histiocytoma of the mandible. Case report. Plast. Reconstr. Surg., 60:629, 1977.

Weine, F. S., and Silverglade, L. B.: Residual cysts masquerading as periapical lesions: three case reports. J. Am. Dent. Assoc., 106:833, 1983.

Weiner, M., Sedlis, M., Johnston, A. D., Dick, H. M., and Wolff, J. A.: Adjuvant chemotherapy of malignant fibrous histiocytoma of bone. Cancer, 51:25, 1983.

Weiss, S. W., and Enzinger, F. M.: Malignant fibrous histiocytoma: an analysis of 200 cases. Cancer, 41:2250, 1978.

Wertheimer, F. W., Zielinski, R. J., and Wesley, R. K.: Extraosseous calcifying epithelial odontogenic tumor (Pindborg tumor). Int. J. Oral Surg., 6:266, 1977.

Wesley, R. K., Borninski, E. R., and Mintz, S.: Peripheral ameloblastoma: report of case and review of the literature. J. Oral Surg., 35:670, 1977.

Wold, L. E., Unni, K. K., Beabout, J. W., Ivins, J. C., Bruckman, J. E., et al.: Hemangioendothelial sarcoma of bone. Am. J. Surg. Pathol., 6:59, 1982.

Worth, H. M., and Stoneman, D. W.: Radiology of vascular abnormalties in and about the jaws. Dent. Radiogr. Photogr., 52:1, 1979.

Wysocki, G. P., Brannon, R. B., Gardner, D. G., and Sapp, P.: Histogenesis of the lateral periodontal cyst and the gingival cyst of the adult. Oral Surg. Oral Med. Oral Pathol., 50:327, 1980.

Zallen, R. D., Preskar, M. H., and McClary, S. A.: Ameloblastic fibroma. J. Oral Maxillofac. Surg., 40:513, 1982.

Zegarelli, E. V., Kutscher, A. H., Napoli, N., et al.: The cementoma—a study of 230 patients with 435 cementomas. Oral Surg. Oral Med. Oral Pathol., 17:219, 1964.

Ziegler, J. L.: Burkitt's lymphoma (review). N. Engl. J. Med., 305:735, 1981.

70

Stephan Ariyan
Zeno N. Chicarilli

Cancer of the Upper Aerodigestive System

Over the last three decades, cancer of the head and neck has been subjected to a coordinated multidisciplinary therapeutic approach in an attempt to decrease the incidence and improve survival. Through the efforts of various groups, including the American Cancer Society, the Commission on Cancer of the American College of Surgeons, and civic organizations, legislation has been passed to improve the safety of the environment of the workplace as it relates to occupational hazards. Public education programs have also been instituted to warn about the risks of the development of cancer.

These programs have enlightened the general public as to the major risks of tobacco and alcohol and their association with the development of oral and laryngeal cancers. Such formal attempts to decrease the number of new patients using tobacco products have been aided by an increasing change in social attitudes toward the use of tobacco. While most public education on the consequences of tobacco use has focused on the development of cancers of the lung and oropharynx, most campaigns against the use of alcohol have been developed in association with motor vehicle accidents rather than its association with oral cancers or liver disease.

The medical profession, on the other hand, has attempted to manage head and neck cancers by a more pragmatic approach. The work of interdisciplinary cancer teams composed of surgeons, radiotherapists, chemotherapists, dentists, prosthodontists, speech therapists, and social workers has led to the development of hospitals dedicated solely to the treatment of cancer or specialized units within general hospitals. These teams try to provide optimal clinical care and an environment for clinical and basic research within the area of head and neck cancer by consolidating the experiences and expertise of the various specialties. Despite these various attempts at cancer prevention and therapy, only modest improvements have been documented over the last 25 years in these areas. Although the statistics on the incidence and cure of oropharyngeal cancers have not revealed significant improvement, there have been certain advances in the early reconstruction and decreased disability of patients after treatment. These developments have shortened the length of hospital stay for many of these patients and improved the overall quality of life postoperatively.

Cancers of the upper aerodigestive tract account for 8 per cent of all malignancies diagnosed in men and 3 per cent of all malignancies diagnosed in women in the United States—this means that approximately 25,000 to 35,000 new patients will be diagnosed each year. While these statistics have not changed appreciably over the past quarter century, the change in the ratio of men to women developing cancer of the head and neck has shown that women have had an increase in incidence that is most likely due to their increased use of tobacco. The ratio of men to women developing oropharyngeal cancer was 9:1 three decades ago, but it is now closer to 2:1. Furthermore, while the incidence of cancer, specifically of the larynx, has changed little among white males, it has doubled among white females. The statistics have also shown a doubling within these various sites among black males and females (Dorn and Cutler, 1958; Young, Perry, and Asire, 1981; Cann and Fried, 1984). These cancers account for an annual mortality in the U.S. of approximately 16,000 males and 6000 females (Silverberg and Lubera, 1983; Silverberg, 1984, 1985). The overall five year disease-free cure rates for oropharyngeal cancers have remained in the range of 30 to 40 per cent irrespective of the site of the primary tumor (Mashberg, 1977). These poor results are influenced by the size of the primary tumor, the presence of regional lymphatic involvement, and distant metastases.

HISTORY

Surgery

Contemporary surgery had its true beginnings in 1846 with the introduction of general anesthesia, when Dr. W. Morton administered sulfuric ether to a patient while Dr. J. C. Warren ligated a vascular tumor in the patient's neck (Absolon, Rogers, and Aust, 1962). Subsequent advances in surgical therapy for patients with head and neck cancer stemmed from the observations and understanding of the nature of cancers of the upper aerodigestive tract and their mode of dissemination (Hanna, 1969). In the latter part of the nineteenth century, the surgical treatment of these cancers was directed at removing the primary tumor; later it would include the removal of the regional draining lymph nodes (Kocher, 1880; Rush, 1966).

The first successful total laryngectomy for cancer was performed by Bilroth on New Year's Eve, 1873 (Gussenbauer, 1874). Kocher advocated the "en bloc" resection of the primary tumor to include regional lymph nodes as early as 1880 (Ward and Hendrick, 1950). These pioneering surgeons performed heroic procedures in the face of significant morbidity and mortality secondary to wound infection, pulmonary compromise, and hypovolemic shock (Gluck and Sorensen, 1914). It is for these reasons that a conservative approach was chosen to treat the tonsillar cancer and cervical metastases of President Ulysses S. Grant, whose surgeons felt that the operative risks and complications were too great for the "best interests of the distinguished patient . . .," and surgery was deferred (Shrady, 1885).

Other surgeons, however, continued with a more aggressive approach. Whitehead stated in 1891: "I have operated on cases indiscriminately and . . . have never allowed the extent of the disease or the emaciated condition of the patient to deter me from operating when I have seen any reasonable prospect for prolonging life . . ." Whitehead's statement referred to his experience with 100 consecutive total glossectomies performed under ether drip anesthesia and he reported a 16 per cent mortality rate, 26 patients surviving one year or more. Crile (1903) described the advantages of endotracheal intubation during these extensive procedures to minimize the respiratory complications associated with general anesthesia and bleeding in the oropharyngeal area. In 1906 he proposed and popularized the radical neck dissection to treat the regional draining lymph nodes, because he noted that patients died of head and neck cancer as a result of regional nodal metastases rather than distant metastases.

Crile described the removal of the sternoclei-domastoid muscle not for control of the cancer but rather for access to the internal jugular vein; however, he did not remove the spinal accessory nerve. If the tumor lay adjacent to the mandible, he recommended that segmental resection should be performed because he was convinced that wide local resection and radical neck dissection of the lymphatics were the key elements for the improved curability of this disease.

Butlin (1909) in England proposed similar aggressive approaches toward these cancers. He reported the treatment of cancer of the tongue with wide excision of the primary site, segmental resection of the mandible, and removal of the lymph nodes in the upper cervical chain, rather than the complete regional lymphadenectomy in the radical neck dissection that Crile described.

Radiation Therapy

The discovery of the x-ray by Roentgen in 1895 and radium by the Curies in 1898 ushered in a new therapeutic modality for the treatment of cancers. At the turn of the century, the relative risks associated with the surgical treatment of head and neck cancer as well as the deformities that resulted following surgical removal prompted the evaluation of radiation therapy for oropharyngeal cancers. It was felt that radiation therapy would be much better tolerated and would prevent the disfigurement caused by surgery. However, this early enthusiasm was tempered by the subsequent reports of radiation dermatitis (Daniel, 1896), malignant transformations (Frieben, 1902; Conway and Hugo, 1966), and osteoradionecrosis (Coleman and Hoopes, 1963).

Radium was initially applied externally to the area of the head and neck, and later the direct application of interstitial radium implants was introduced for the treatment of cancer of the tongue. However, with the development of the 200 keV x-ray machine in 1920, external radium treatment was replaced by external beam radiation. Treatment with single dose therapy was disappointing until the appropriate doses and fractionations were identified in the 1930's (Paterson and Parker, 1934, 1938; Coutard, 1937). Coutard (1937) recommended fractionation of the doses over a three week period, while Baclesse (1949, 1953) reported administration of higher doses to the central tumor by further fractionation over six to ten weeks of treatment. Strandqvist (1944) further defined the time-dose relationships, and Paterson (1952) reported the advantages of 5500 rads administered over a period of five weeks in divided doses, as is practiced today. The development of supervoltage therapy machines generating photon energies of over 1 million electron volts (meV) provided an additional margin of safety by delivering the effects of radiation deeper into the tissues and sparing the effects on the skin (Buschke, Cantril, and Parker, 1950).

Combination Treatment

The treatment of these malignancies with radiation therapy proved disappointing, especially in the control of large tumors with extensive cervical metastases or bony invasion. Certain medical advances in the 1940's led to a resurgence of surgical management for these cancers. The improvement of anesthetic agents and techniques with endotracheal intubation, the introduction of blood banks, and the development of antibiotics led to a significant decrease in operative morbidity and mortality following resections of extensive cancers. In addition, the reconstructive techniques developed for post-traumatic deformities during World War II provided the experience to restore form and function in the cancer patient after extensive resections. In 1939 Martin (1953) began performing "en bloc resections" of primary cancers together with neck dissection in a single procedure, the "Commando procedure." The value and safety of "composite resections" were further confirmed by the concurrent work of Ward in Baltimore, (Ward and Hendrick, 1950; Martin, 1957). These aggressive approaches to the management of cancer led to the selection of some patients for radiation, some for surgery, and some for the combination of the two modalities to improve the cure rates (Martin and associates, 1951). Large tumors have a poorer response to either modality alone, while the combination of radiation and surgery appears to offer improved local and regional control if not improvement in overall survival (Hoffmeister, Macomber, and Wang, 1968; Leonard and Hass, 1970; Fayos and Lampe, 1972; Lawrence and associates, 1974; Hirata and associates, 1975; Jesse and Lindberg, 1975; Marchetta and Sako, 1975; Hamberger and associates, 1976). The attempts to improve the cure rates with the combination of preoperative radiation followed by surgery of the primary site and the neck, however, led to higher postoperative complications (Ketcham and associates, 1969; Yarington, Yonkers, and Beddoe, 1973; Joseph and Shumrick, 1973). Therefore, retrospective reviews of experiences and prospective randomized trials evaluated preoperative and postoperative radiation. These data demonstrated that the local control rates and cure rates were similar, but that planned preoperative radiation led to higher complication rates than radiation administered in the postoperative period (Lindberg, Jesse, and Fletcher, 1974; Van den Brouck and associates, 1977; Snow and associates, 1978, 1980; Arriagada and associates, 1983). These findings convinced most surgeons to prefer surgical resection of the tumor without the radiation effects in the operative field. In addition, postoperative radiation therapy can be given at much higher doses, which does not seem to have a detrimental effect on wound healing; moreover, the higher doses may indeed improve the local control rates.

The reevaluation of the classical treatment techniques has also been directed toward the neck dissection. The efficacy of a more "functional" neck dissection by preservation of the sternocleidomastoid muscle, the internal jugular vein, and the accessory nerve was described by Bocca and Pignataro (1967). There are also reports advocating the neck dissection only after the development of nodal metastases and not in continuity with the primary tumor (Marchetta, Sako, and Murphy, 1971; Spiro and Strong, 1973). In addition, the preservation of the arch of the mandible by marginal mandibular resections, rather than the traditional segmental bloc resections, has also been found to be reliable in the control of cancer (Byers and associates, 1981; Beecroft and associates, 1982). Elective irradiation of the clinically negative (N_0) neck has also been advocated (Fletcher, 1972).

Chemotherapy

Since the report by Sullivan (1971) on the clinical usefulness of methotrexate for head and neck cancers, this chemotherapeutic agent has been considered the standard against which all other agents are measured (Bertino, Boston, and Capizzi, 1975). Cisplatin has also been considered an active drug in the management of cancers of this site, with response rates varying from 20 to 40 per cent (Hong and associates, 1983). However, there are no significant data demonstrating survival benefits with a combination of various chemotherapeutic agents as compared with a single agent in patients with recurrent cancers of the head and neck (Deconti and Schoenfeld, 1981; Williams and associates, 1982; Jacobs and associates, 1983; Drelichman, Cummings, and Al-Sarraf, 1983). There have also been various trials determining the role of chemotherapy given to patients before definitive surgical treatment or radiation therapy, but these studies have yielded contradictory data as to chemotherapeutic effectiveness; further work will be required to clarify the particular roles (Knowlton and associates, 1975; Hong and associates, 1979; Perry, Davis, and Weiss, 1982; Price, MacRae, and Hill, 1983; Schuller and associates, 1983; Kies and associates, 1984; Sheetz and associates, 1984).

Reconstructive Surgery

In the past decade alone, there have been significant improvements in the quality of life of these patients as a result of developments of one-stage reconstruction with musculocutaneous flaps and microvascular free tissue transfers. The advances in surgical technique have provided well-vascularized composite tissue to improve healing, decrease wound complications, and improve the functional result. The most significant developments have resulted from the use of the pectoralis major (Ariyan and Krizek, 1977; Ariyan, 1979a), sternocleidomastoid (Ariyan, 1979b), trapezius (Demergasso and Piazza, 1979), and latissimus dorsi (Quillen, 1979) musculocutaneous flaps, and the microsurgical transfers of the jejunum (Seidenberg and associates, 1959), the radial forearm flap (Soutar and associates, 1983; Harii and associates, 1985; Chicarilli and Price, 1986; Chicarilli, Ariyan, and Cuono, 1986a,b), the scapular flap (Barwick, Goodkind, and Serafin, 1982; Swartz, Banis, and Newton, 1986), and the iliac bone composite flap (Taylor, 1982).

ANATOMY

For the purpose of classifying and staging head and neck cancers, the sites are anatomically divided into the oral cavity; the pharynx (oropharynx, nasopharynx, and hypopharynx); the larynx (supraglottis, glottis, and subglottis); and the paranasal sinuses (Table 70–1).

The *oral cavity* extends from the junction of the skin and vermilion of the lips to an imaginary vertical plane reaching from the junction of the hard and soft palate above to the circumvallate papillae of the tongue below (Fig. 70–1). This region includes the vermilion of the lips, the upper and lower alveolar ridges, the retromolar trigone, the floor of the mouth, the hard palate, and the anterior two-thirds of the tongue (oral tongue).

The *pharynx* is divided into three separate regions that take into consideration different prognoses and different therapeutic options.

The *oropharynx* continues from the posterior limit of the oral cavity, as described above, and extends posteriorly to the posterior pharyngeal wall. The cephalad boundary of the oropharynx is marked by a horizontal plane at the level of the soft palate above, and the inferior limit is a similar plane drawn

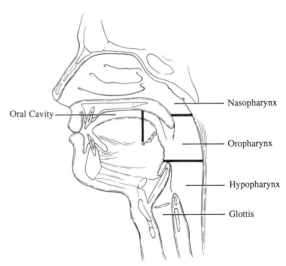

Figure 70–1. The anatomic divisions of the aerodigestive tract.

across the lingual surface of the closed epiglottis. The oropharynx includes both surfaces of the soft palate, the anterior and posterior tonsillar pillars, the tonsils, the pharyngoepiglottis, the glossoepiglottic folds, the posterior pharyngeal wall, and the posterior one-third of the tongue and the vallecula (which make up the base of the tongue).

The *nasopharynx* lies above the oropharynx and extends anteriorly along the base of the skull, which is the roof of this anatomic site. The anterior limit is the posterior choanae of the nose, and the lateral walls are bounded by the pterygoids. The nasopharynx includes the mucosal lining of the base of the skull (the basisphenoid), the torus tubarius, the eustachian tube orifice, and the fossa of Rosenmüller.

The *hypopharynx* extends from the horizontal plane of the epiglottis to the inferior border of the cricoid cartilage. The hypopharynx includes the piriform sinuses, the postcricoid area, and the posterior hypopharyngeal wall, but excludes the larynx.

The *larynx* includes the lingual surface of the epiglottis as well as the endolarynx proper. The subdivisions of the larynx are based on the biologic predisposition to regional lymph node metastases, and therefore lead to different therapeutic approaches. The *supraglottis* includes the lingual and laryngeal surfaces of the epiglottis, the aryepiglottic folds, the arytenoids, and the ventricular bands (false vocal cords). Its most inferior limit is a horizontal plane passing through the apex of the ventricles. The *glottis* extends

Table 70–1. Anatomic Sites of Tumor

Oral Cavity

Lip	Retromolar trigone
Buccal mucosa	Hard palate
Alveolar ridges	Oral tongue
Floor of mouth	(anterior to circumvallate papillae)

Pharynx
  Nasopharynx
    Posterior superior wall
    Lateral wall
  Oropharynx
    Faucial arch (includes anterior tonsillar pillar, soft palate, and uvula)
    Tonsil (and tonsillar fossa)
    Base of tongue (includes glossoepiglottic and pharyngoepiglottic folds)
    Pharyngeal walls (includes posterior tonsillar pillar)
  Hypopharynx
    Piriform sinus
    Postcricoid area
    Posterior hypopharyngeal wall
Larynx
  Supraglottis
    Epiglottis (and aryepiglottic folds)
    False cords (ventricular bands)
  Glottis
    True cords
  Subglottis

from this plane to a second horizontal plane 1 cm below the free edge of the vocal cords. The glottis includes the true vocal cords together with the anterior and posterior commissures. The *subglottis* extends from the glottis to the inferior aspect of the cricoid cartilage. The posterior limit of the larynx proper is the hypopharynx, and its anterior limit is formed by the thyrohyoid membrane, thyroid cartilage, the cricothyroid membrane, and cricoid cartilage.

The *paranasal sinuses* include the paired maxillary, ethmoid, frontal, and sphenoid sinuses. Although cancers of the paranasal sinuses are uncommon, the maxillary sinuses are the most common site for carcinoma of these structures. The maxillary sinuses are divided into an anteroinferior (infrastructure) and a superoposterior (suprastructure) based on an imaginary plane joining the medial canthus of the eye with the angle of the mandible on a lateral view of a skull radiograph (Öhngren's line) (Fig. 70–2). The ethmoid sinuses and nasal cavity may eventually be subdivided but at present are considered as a single unit. Cancers of the frontal and sphenoid sinuses are so infrequent that no classification or subdivision is warranted.

The lymphatic drainage of cancers of the upper aerodigestive tract is primarily to the region of the neck. Within this region, the

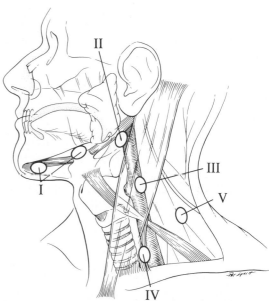

Figure 70–3. The location of potential metastases to lymph nodes at various levels of the cervical chain: submandibular/submental (I), subdigastric (II), midjugular (III), low-jugular (IV), and posterior triangle (V).

lymph nodes are divided into Levels I to V as follows (Fig. 70–3):

   I. Submandibular, submental.
  II. Subdigastric (jugulodigastric).
 III. Midjugular.
 IV. Low-jugular.
  V. Posterior cervical triangles.

ETIOLOGIC FACTORS

The data on the relationship between smoking and oral cancer are voluminous, and although direct cause and effect is not confirmed, most of the findings point to a significant association. It is often difficult, however, to separate the effects of smoking alone from other risk factors. In studying the risk of cigarette smoking alone, Mashberg, Garfinkel, and Harris (1981) reported an incremental increase of the incidence of cancer from three to five times control as there was an increase in the consumption of tobacco from 10 to 40 cigarettes per day. Wynder, Bross, and Feldman (1957) described the additive effects of smoking and alcohol, demonstrating a threefold risk for patients who smoked 40 or more cigarettes a day and who also consumed 7 oz or more of alcohol per day. Graham and associates (1977) reported that poor oral hygiene and poor dentition in addition

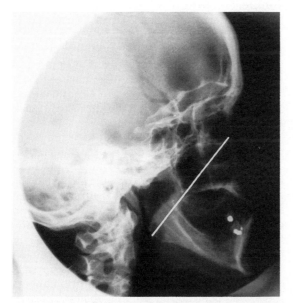

Figure 70–2. Öhngren's line, drawn from the medial canthus of the eye to the angle of the mandible on a lateral view, divides the location of maxillary sinus tumors into infrastructure *(below)* and suprastructure *(above)*.

to the consumption of tobacco and alcohol increased the risk eightfold. Rothman (Rothman and Keller, 1972; Rothman, 1978a,b) demonstrated the synergistic effect of many of these factors (Table 70–2).

The association of various forms of smokeless tobacco with oral cancer is also well known (Ackerman, 1948). In certain regions of the southeastern United States there is an unusual female preponderance in the habit of "snuff dipping," which leads to a mucosal cancer of the buccal region (Brown and associates, 1965; Winn and associates, 1981). The practice of "betel nut chewing," commonplace in India, has also led to oral cancers. In this practice, tobacco may be blended with lime and rolled in a betel nut leaf to form a "quid" and held in the mouth's cheek pouch for prolonged periods. This addition of tobacco to the quid is known as "pan" and has been shown by Khadim (1977) to increase the risk of oral cancer sevenfold.

To isolate the risk of alcohol alone is just as difficult as in tobacco studies. Reports of alcohol leading to a three- to 20-fold increase of the risk of oral cancer have been published by Keller and Terris (1965), Wynder, Bross, and Feldman (1957) and Vincent and Marchetta (1963). Mashberg, Garfinkel, and Harris (1981) felt that consumption of more than 6 oz or more of whiskey a day carries a higher risk than smoking 40 or more cigarettes per day. Fischman and Martinez (1977) suggested that the higher incidence of oral cancer in Puerto Rico, as contrasted with the mainland of the U.S., is related to a greater consumption of home-distilled spirits on the island. Masse (1972) offered a similar explanation for variations in the incidence of esophageal cancers following the consumption of wines in France. Others have alluded to the possibility that alcohol acts as a solvent, altering the mucosal penetration of these carcinogens (e.g., tobacco) and facilitating their deleterious effects (Wynder, Mushinski, and Spivak, 1977; McCoy, 1978; Rothman, 1978b).

While tobacco and alcohol rank as the most common inciting factors associated with the increased risk of oral cancers, two less common systemic illnesses have also been implicated: syphilis and Plummer-Vinson syndrome. Tertiary syphilis is rare today, but it has in the past resulted in atrophic glossitis that was strongly associated with cancer of the tongue (Fry, 1929). This cancer had a particular predisposition to the dorsum of the tongue, as opposed to the more common occurrence today along the lateral and ventral surfaces. Plummer-Vinson (Paterson-Kelly) syndrome, a complex of chronic dysphagia and mucosal atrophy of the upper gastrointestinal tract among middle-aged women in the Scandinavian countries, leading to chronic anemia and low stores of iron, was initially noted to have a high association with esophageal cancers (Paterson, 1919). Further studies also demonstrated the increased incidence of buccal mucosa and tongue cancers among these patients (Ahlbom, 1936; Wynder and Fryer, 1958; Watts, 1961).

Other factors that have been considered to play a role in the development of oral cancers have been chronic candidiasis (Cawson and Binnie, 1980) and repeated herpes simplex virus infections (Lehner and associates, 1973; Silverman and associates, 1976). Although conclusive evidence is not available for herpesvirus, there appears to be a specific and constant relationship between Epstein-Barr virus (EBV) and carcinoma of the nasopharynx among the Chinese (deThe and associates, 1975).

Occupational exposure to repeated episodes of toxic irritants has also been reported to lead to malignancies of the head and neck area. An increased incidence of cancers of the nasopharynx and paranasal sinuses has been identified among workers in the nickel and chromium industry (Doll, Morgan, and Speizer, 1970; Pedersen, Hogetveit, and Andersen, 1973) and among factory workers in the boot and shoe industry (Acheson, Pippard, and Winter, 1982). Paranasal sinus cancers have also been found among woodworkers in the furniture industry (Acheson, Hadfield, and MacBeth, 1967; Hausen, 1981), and there appear to be variations in incidence and anatomic location of these cancers on the basis

Table 70–2. Synergy of Tobacco and Alcohol on Oral Cancer*

Alcohol (oz/day)	Cigarette Consumption/Day (Packs)			
	0	1	1–2	2
0	1.00	1.5	1.4	2.4
0.1–0.4	1.4	1.7	3.2	3.2
0.4–1.5	1.6	4.4	4.5	8.2
>1.5	2.3	4.1	9.6	15.5

*Risk expressed relative to an abstinent nonsmoker (1.00).

Modified from Rothman, K. J., and Keller, A. Z.: The effect of joint exposure to alcohol and tobacco on risk of cancer of the mouth and pharynx. J. Chronic Dis., 25:711, 1972.

of the various types of woods used in the furniture industry in different countries.

LEUKOPLAKIA AND ERYTHROPLAKIA

Leukoplakia, "white patch or plaque," is a clinical description of white lesions in the oral cavity for which no definitive etiology is known. Most of these lesions are benign, and histopathologic examination demonstrates hyperkeratosis; however, some have demonstrated atypical changes, carcinoma in situ, or invasive squamous cell carcinoma. Erythroplakia (erythroplasia) is a clinical diagnosis of a flat or slightly raised red, velvety, or slightly granular lesion without a known precipitating cause. Shear (1972) described three clinical variations: (1) homogeneous erythroplakia, (2) erythroplakia interspersed with patches of leukoplakia, and (3) granular or speckled erythroplakia.

Most oral cancers present without clinically apparent precancerous lesions (Silverman, 1981). In a study of oral cancers, Chierici, Silverman, and Forsythe (1968) found that only 15 per cent had associated leukoplakia. Prospective studies of the incidence of malignant transformation of leukoplakia yielded a variable incidence ranging from 0.13 to 17.5 per cent (Pindborg and associates, 1968; Kramer, 1969; Roed Petersen, 1971; Silverman and associates, 1976; Banoczy, 1977; Kramer, El-Labban, and Lee, 1978; Gupta and associates, 1980; Silverman, Gorsky, and Lozada, 1984). The site at which the leukoplakia is discovered may affect the likelihood of malignant transformation; Silverman, Gorsky, and Lozada (1984) found leukoplakia of the tongue, lip, floor of mouth, and gingiva to be twice as likely to develop malignant degeneration than leukoplakia detected on the palatal or buccal mucosa. Kramer, El-Labban, and Lee (1978), on the other hand, found that the incidence in sublingual sites was five times that in other sites. However, these findings may simply reflect more common sites for the development of oral cancers, rather than an influence by the presence of leukoplakia.

Many authors reported the greater likelihood of the development of malignancy in the presence of erythroplakia (a four- to sevenfold increase in incidence) (Roed Petersen, 1971; Banoczy, 1977; Kramer, El-Labban, and Lee,

1978; Silverman, Gorsky, and Lozada, 1984). Shafer and Waldron (1975) reported that biopsies of lesions with a clinical diagnosis of erythroplakia yielded invasive carcinoma in 51 per cent, carcinoma in situ or severe dysplasia in 40 per cent, and moderate dysplasia in 9 per cent. The likelihood of microscopic dysplasia in a leukoplakic lesion converting to a malignancy has been estimated to be two to six times greater than when the histologic examination reveals only hyperplasia (Shafer and Waldron, 1975; Banoczy and Csiba, 1976; Pindborg, Daftary, and Mehta, 1977; Silverman, Gorsky, and Lozada, 1984).

CLINICAL EVALUATION

The most common presentation of oral and oropharyngeal cancers is a painless ulceration. However, it also is not uncommon for patients to complain of vague symptoms of soreness in the gingiva, tongue, or throat, which on casual examination could be attributed to an aphthous ulcer, irritation from the teeth, or a common sore throat. Benign conditions should resolve within a short time or in response to appropriate therapy. Persistence of the symptoms should lead to further diagnostic considerations. Tumors of the posterior oral cavity, particularly in the area of the tonsil or the base of the tongue, may invade deeper structures and produce pain referred to the ear by way of the glossopharyngeal nerve and the vagus nerve, both of which have sensory distribution in the ear through the nerve of Jacobson (glossopharyngeal nerve) and the nerve of Arnold (vagus nerve). Odynophagia (painful swallowing) and dysphagia (difficulty in swallowing) are also common complaints of patients with tumors of the oropharynx and the base of the tongue.

Hoarseness is the most frequent complaint of patients with cancer of the vocal cords, and this symptom occurs relatively early, requiring indirect laryngoscopy to determine the cause. On the other hand, tumors of the supraglottic larynx and hypopharynx may remain silent for long periods, thereby permitting considerable growth of the tumor before the patients complain of dysphagia or hoarseness. Hemoptysis and respiratory compromise may occasionally be noted, particularly with large tumors of the supraglottis and subglottis that are friable and bulky.

When the tumor has grown with relatively few symptoms or if the patient has neglected the presenting symptoms, the patient may first be seen with a mass in the neck as the only complaint. This is most notable in cancers of the nasopharynx, base of tongue, supraglottis, and hypopharynx, which notoriously are subject to early metastases to regional lymph nodes with only a small primary tumor.

Patients with nasal and paranasal cancers may present with nasal obstruction, epistaxis, pain and swelling of the cheeks (secondary to direct nerve invasion or sinusitis), diplopia, or limited ocular movement secondary to orbital invasion. They may also have dental symptoms secondary to involvement of the alveolar process and dental roots from growth of the tumor in the maxillary sinus. Occasionally, a patient may report only the sensation of having one ear "plugged," and examination may reveal a serous effusion as a result of obstruction of the eustachian canal from a tumor of the nasopharynx.

Symptoms from cancers of the maxillary sinus often are not present until the tumor has grown sufficiently to invade the adjacent structures. This is why most maxillary sinus tumors are not detected early, unless an abnormality is identified from an examination of the head and neck area for other reasons. Unilateral maxillary sinusitis or opacification detected on radiographic study of a patient without a history of trauma or sinusitis and with a history of exposure to toxic materials should raise suspicion of this diagnosis.

Physical Examination

The oral and pharyngeal examination is carried out by direct examination of the mucous membranes, and it should include digital palpation of the floor of the mouth and the base of the tongue. With the use of a tongue blade, a systematic examination should include evaluation of the labial and buccal mucosa, gingiva, tongue, floor of the mouth, hard and soft palate, tonsillar fossa, and pharyngeal walls. The dental alveolar structures should be assessed for diseases of the gums as well as for the level of dental repair. If the teeth are in poor repair, the patient should be referred for examination and treatment by a dentist to minimize complications during surgery or radiation therapy, if that should become necessary.

Laryngopharyngeal evaluation requires a mirror and topical anesthesia. With the patient's tongue immobilized by the examiner's fingers, a mirror is placed against the posterior pharynx barely touching the soft palate in a single deliberate motion, so that the examination may be carried out with minimal contact of the mirror to the pharyngeal structures in order to prevent the gagging response. The vocal cords are evaluated for movement by asking the patient to phonate. The mirror examination should also evaluate the base of the tongue, vallecula, and epiglottis in addition to the aryepiglottic folds and cords. The piriform sinuses of the hypopharynx, including the apices, may also be evaluated by mirror examination in some cooperative patients.

Intranasal evaluation requires a nasal speculum and a headlight. The mucosa should be shrunk with the application of a vasoconstrictor (ephedrine or cocaine atomizer). Suspicious lesions may be biopsied with an alligator cup forcep, and cautery with silver nitrate is usually adequate for hemostasis.

A flexible nasopharyngoscope can be helpful in viewing the nasopharynx as well as the laryngopharynx directly when the mirror examination proves inadequate or if the epiglottis is retrodisplaced. As an office procedure, the rigid Hopkins endoscope (Fig. 70–4) allows examination of the nasopharynx through the mouth. Direct visualization of the laryngopharynx and cervical esophagus can also be accomplished with the rigid endoscope under local or general anesthesia. The examination can determine the extent of the primary lesion, permit biopsy, and allow a search for secondary synchronous primaries before staging of the patient.

Examination of the neck should include both the anterior and posterior cervical triangles, as well as the pretracheal region, to detect regional lymphadenopathy. Bimanual palpation of the submental and submandibular areas should be performed with one finger of one hand in the floor of the mouth and the opposite hand in the submental or submandibular area. Lymph nodes that are less than 1 to 2 cm in diameter may be extremely difficult to detect, especially when they are located deep to the sternocleidomastoid muscle.

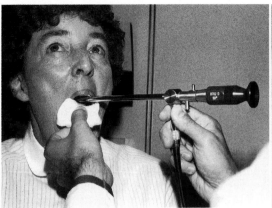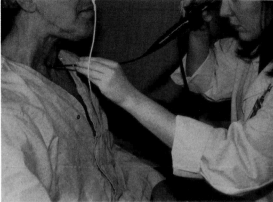

Figure 70–4. The Hopkins endoscope *(left)* is rigid and has an angled lens to view the nasopharynx or hypopharynx. The fiberoptic endoscope *(right)* is flexible and can be used to view the nasopharynx, larynx, and trachea transnasally, or directly as illustrated.

Tissue Sampling

The site and size of all lesions should be recorded accurately in a diagram placed in the patient's file. At this point a biopsy of lesions in the *oropharyngeal* area should be performed. The biopsy should consist of an excision of the small lesion or an incision of deeper and more extensive lesions.

Cancers of the *hypopharynx, piriform sinuses,* and *maxillary sinus* should not be biopsied before radiographic examination because such biopsies may alter the radiographic appearance of these structures, confuse the extent of the malignancy, and make the clinical staging difficult. Therefore, at these sites the diagnostic evaluation of a highly suspicious lesion should precede the biopsy. In addition, although rigid endoscopy

is routinely used to biopsy hypopharyngeal and laryngeal lesions, it is advisable to perform triple endoscopy under anesthesia in these patients to search for a second primary. The triple endoscopy includes nasopharyngoscopy, laryngobronchoscopy (with bronchial washings), and esophagoscopy (the esophagus being the most common site for a synchronous second primary).

A lesion in the oral cavity may occasionally appear indistinct and not readily visualized on inspection. In these cases, toluidine blue dye can be applied to delineate the area of involvement more clearly. Toluidine blue stains the nucleus of cells in an area of ulceration but not where there is intact normal mucosa (Fig. 70–5). The dye is not specific for malignant cells but it stains areas of ulceration with increased cell turnover, or

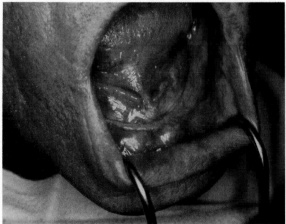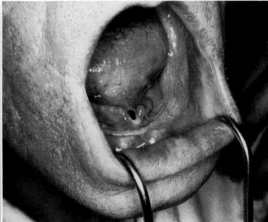

Figure 70–5. Early or superficial lesions of the oral cavity *(left)* can be more readily identified by the use of toluidine blue stain *(right)*.

with aberrant cells. The technique therefore is also useful in staining the mucosa of individuals with suspected field cancerizations in order to select suspicious sites to be biopsied (Mashberg, 1980, 1981).

Neck Node Biopsy

Open biopsy of a suspicious neck node is contraindicated until all other diagnostic techniques have been exhausted. If the diagnosis cannot be confirmed and the patient is suspected of having an "unknown primary," the lymph node can be biopsied by a fine needle aspiration (FNA). The FNA can be performed with a 22 gauge needle (Fig. 70–6) to aspirate a minute amount of tissue and tissue fluid to prepare cytologic slides and provide samples for preparation of a cell block (Goldberg and associates, 1981). The technique has a 90 per cent accuracy in determining the histopathology when an adequate sample is obtained and is not associated with spread of tumor through the needle tract, as with large needle biopsy. Fine needle aspiration can be performed as an office procedure, is cost effective, and makes open neck biopsy unnecessary in all but a few exceptional cases. In the rare patient in whom an open biopsy is indicated, the procedure should be performed by the physician who will be performing the definitive surgical procedure if it should be indicated. At that time, the biopsy scar should be excised together with the specimen of the neck resection to remove any residual tumor cells that may have been entrapped at the time of the open biopsy.

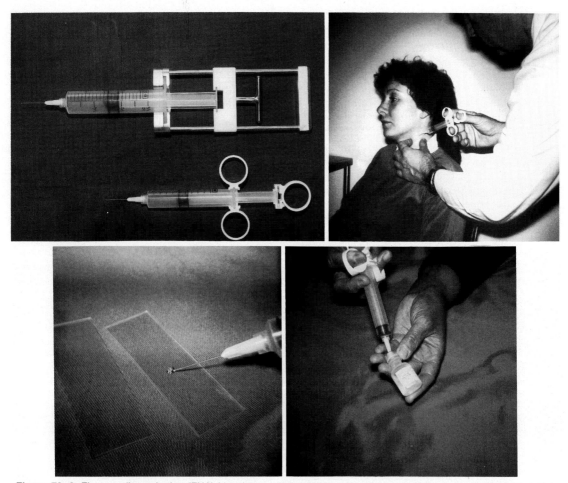

Figure 70–6. Fine needle aspiration (FNA) biopsies can be obtained with disposable syringe-needles *(above, left)* by immobilizing the mass and direct passage *(above, right)*. A small drop of the aspirate can be smeared on a slide *(below, left)* and the remainder flushed into a vial of saline *(below, right)* for subsequent examination by cell block.

Radiographic Examination

Squamous cell carcinomas of the head and neck are epithelial tumors of surface origin for which radiography is limited to the detection of surface irregularities with the aid of contrast media on the mucosal surface. When the tumor progresses further, bony invasion or distortion by a mass effect may be detected by conventional radiographs, xeroradiograms, or computed tomographic (CT) scanning. Tumors of the paranasal sinuses are located in an area in which radiography is indispensable in discerning the extent of tumor involvement. Plain films should include the Waters view, the Caldwell view, and lateral and submentovertex projection for general examination of the facial bony structures (Fig. 70–7). The Waters view is most helpful in visualizing the maxillary sinus, and the lateral view allows superimposition of Öhngren's line (see Fig. 70–2) to locate the tumor for staging purposes. The Caldwell view permits an undisturbed projection of the ethmoid and frontal sinuses, but the maxillary antrum has superimposition of the petrous ridge. The floor of the orbit, however, can be evaluated as laminae representing the anterior and posterior orbital floors. The CT scan has proved indispensable in detecting the extent of tumor size and local invasion (Fig. 70–8). The other anatomic areas for which radiography can be helpful are the tonsillar fossa and the lateral pharyngeal wall. CT scanning provides an accurate assessment of the proximity of the primary tumor to the deeper structures, including the carotid or the base of the skull.

A nasopharyngeal tumor may be visualized as a soft tissue density on a plain lateral skull film, and gross destruction at the base of the skull may be seen. However, a more refined image of the tumor of the skull base can be seen with CT scanning (Fig. 70–9) and may allow early detection of bony destruction.

While the oral cavity and oropharynx are usually best evaluated by direct clinical examination, tumors may grow deeply and invade the adjacent mandible. In these cases, a *Panorex* view allows assessment of the mandible for bone destruction (Fig. 70–10).

The laryngohypopharynx can usually be assessed fairly accurately by indirect and direct examination, but radiography may be useful in several areas. The *barium swallow* with *cineradiography* helps to visualize the extent of hypopharyngeal tumors by expanding the hypopharynx. The barium swallow is also a back-up study in detecting a second primary lesion in the esophagus. *Polytomography* of the larynx, with and without contrast medium (laryngography), may be helpful in assessing endolaryngeal disease, particularly when conservation laryngectomy is being considered. *Xeroradiography* can also be utilized to determine inferior extension of the tumor (Fig. 70–11). The identification of infiltration or destruction of the thyroid cartilage or preepiglottic space on xeroradiog-

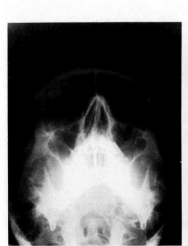 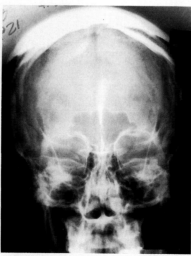 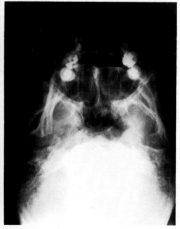

Figure 70–7. The Waters view *(left)* visualizes the maxillary sinuses best and detects involvement of the floor of the orbit through the roof of the sinus. The Caldwell view *(center)* visualizes the frontal and ethmoid sinuses best. The submentovertix view *(right)* determines the anterior and posterior extent of tumors in the maxillary sinuses.

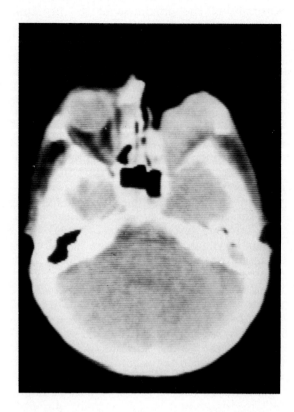

Figure 70–8. A CT scan demonstrating a tumor of the ethmoid sinus extending into the orbital cavity.

Figure 70–9. A tumor of the nasopharynx *(arrowheads)* can be seen to extend along the base of the skull on CT scan.

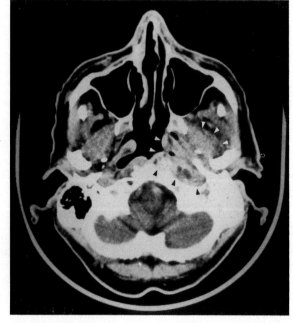

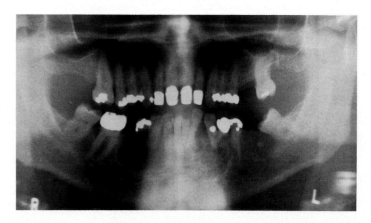

Figure 70–10. A Panorex view demonstrating tumor invasion of the symphyseal region of the mandible.

raphy would change the staging of a tumor from a T_1 or T_2 to a T_3, even though there is no limitation of movement of the vocal cord. However, the evaluation is not as accurate as CT scanning with coronal cuts of the larynx. If conservation surgery is contemplated, a CT scan should be obtained if there is any doubt of the extent of the tumor. Finally, diagnostic imaging is also necessary in certain cases to evaluate the possibility of distant metastases. These tests include routine chest radiography, chest tomography, and nuclear scans of the liver, bone, or brain.

STAGING

After the diagnosis of malignancy has been confirmed by biopsy and all diagnostic studies

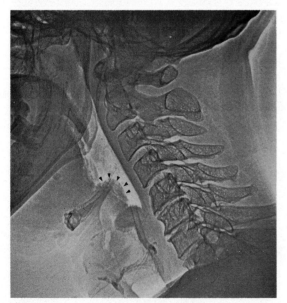

Figure 70–11. Xeroradiograph showing the irregular surface of a tumor of the hypopharynx *(arrowheads)*.

have been performed to determine the extent of the tumor, the clinical diagnostic staging (TNM) is assigned. The classification system is based on the clinical evaluation before any definitive major therapy is instituted, and should not be altered after treatment has begun, despite findings contrary to the original assessment. In this manner, the system becomes useful as a prognostic tool to determine an optimal treatment course based on past experience. It also allows orderly communication between treatment centers to discuss and compare end results of various treatment methods.

The uniformly accepted staging system is the TNM system popularized by the International Union Against Cancer (UICC) and the American Joint Committee for Cancer Staging and End Results Reporting (AJC). For purposes of uniformity, the AJC classification is used in this chapter. The TNM classification is based on data from retrospective analysis of group tumors that have similar statistical chances for cure. The AJC continually reviews and assigns task forces to update the staging system on the basis of experience with its clinical use and retrospective studies to assess its prognostic accuracy. The latest revision of this task force of the AJC was published in 1976 for all head and neck sites (Chandler and associates, 1976). The data base gathered on examination is assigned to three subsets: (1) the primary tumor size and extent (T), (2) clinical regional lymph node involvement (N), and (3) the presence or absence of distant metastases (M).

PRIMARY TUMOR (T)

The local extent of the primary tumors is assessed on absolute size, specific sites in-

Table 70–3. T Categories of Oral Cavity

T_{is}	Carcinoma in situ
T_1	Tumor 2 cm or less in greatest diameter
T_2	Tumor more than 2 cm but not more than 4 cm in greatest diameter
T_3	Tumor more than 4 cm in greatest diameter
T_4	Massive tumor more than 4 cm in diameter with invasion of antrum, pterygoid muscles, base of tongue, or skin of neck

volved within a particular region, or dysfunction within the region. The classification varies with respect to the particular region involved and it is assigned a subset from T_1 to T_4. The specific classification for each region involved is listed in Tables 70–3, 70–4, and 70–5. In general, lesions of the oral cavity and oropharynx are based on measurable size, whereas those of the remainder of the pharynx and larynx are based on extension and dysfunction.

CERVICAL NODES (N)

This portion of the classification has undergone changes in the latest revision to include only those nodes that are felt to be involved by tumor; the criterion of fixation of a lymph node or nodal mass to underlying or adjacent structures has been eliminated (Table 70–6). The nodes are assessed primarily by size and

Table 70–4. Definition of T Categories of Pharynx

Nasopharynx

T_{is}	Carcinoma in situ
T_1	Tumor confined to one site of nasopharynx or no tumor visible (positive biopsy only)
T_2	Tumor involving two sites (both posterosuperior and lateral walls)
T_3	Extension of tumor into nasal cavity or oropharynx
T_4	Tumor invasion of skull and/or cranial nerve involvement

Oropharynx

T_{is}	Carcinoma in situ
T_1	Tumor 2 cm or less in greatest diameter
T_2	Tumor more than 2 cm but not more than 4 cm in greatest diameter
T_3	Tumor more than 4 cm in greatest diameter
T_4	Massive tumor more than 4 cm in diameter with invasion of bone, soft tissues of neck, or root (deep musculature) of tongue

Hypopharynx

T_{is}	Carcinoma in situ
T_1	Tumor confined to site of origin
T_2	Extension of tumor to adjacent site or region without fixation of hemilarynx
T_3	Extension of tumor to adjacent site or region with fixation of hemilarynx
T_4	Massive tumor invading bone or soft tissues of neck

Table 70–5. Definition of T Categories of Larynx

Supraglottis

T_{is}	Carcinoma in situ
T_1	Tumor confined to site of origin with normal mobility
T_2	Tumor involves adjacent supraglottic site(s) or glottis without fixation
T_3	Tumor limited to larynx with fixation and/or extension to involve postcricoid area, medial wall of piriform sinus, or preepiglottic space
T_4	Massive tumor extending beyond larynx to involve oropharynx or soft tissues of neck, or destruction of thyroid cartilage

Glottis

T_{is}	Carcinoma in situ
T_1	Tumor confined to vocal cord(s) with normal mobility (includes involvement of anterior or posterior commissures)
T_2	Supraglottic and/or subglottic extension of tumor with normal or impaired cord mobility
T_3	Tumor confined to larynx with cord fixation
T_4	Massive tumor with thyroid cartilage destruction and/or extension beyond confines of larynx

Subglottis

T_{is}	Carcinoma in situ
T_1	Tumor confined to subglottic region
T_2	Tumor extension to vocal cords with normal or impaired cord mobility
T_3	Tumor confined to larynx with cord fixation
T_4	Massive tumor with cartilage destruction or extension beyond confines of larynx

location. Allowance is given to any intervening soft tissues for this measurement, and it is generally assumed (although not necessarily correct) that nodes greater than 3 cm in diameter are either multiple and confluent, or there has been tumor spread outside of the capsule into adjacent tissues.

DISTANT METASTASES (M)

The classification for distant metastases is based on whether or not distant metastases are absent (M_0) or have been confirmed during the evaluation (M_1). At times, confirmation of distant metastases may require needle or open biopsy (e.g., solitary lung nodules or

Table 70–6. Cervical Node (N) Classification

N_0		No clinically positive nodes
N_1		Single clinically positive homolateral node, less than 3 cm in diameter
N_2	2a	Single clinically positive homolateral node, 3–6 cm in diameter
	2b	Multiple clinically positive homolateral nodes, none greater than 6 cm in diameter
N_3	3a	Clinically positive homolateral node(s), one greater than 6 cm in diameter
	3b	Bilateral clinically positive nodes (each side should be staged separately, e.g., N_{3b}—right N_{2a}, left N_1)
	3c	Contralateral clinically positive node(s) only

bony radiolucency) particularly if this finding would alter the treatment.

CLINICAL DIAGNOSTIC STAGING

There are four clinical stages that represent increasing extent of disease, and as such, decrease in likelihood of curability (Table 70–7). Owing to the large number of combinations within each stage, it can be seen that stage alone is not always as meaningful as the individual TNM descriptive classification from which it is derived. For example, a $T_4N_{3b}M_1$ and a $T_1N_2M_0$ are both Stage IV disease, and yet the former probably represents an unresectable tumor whereas the latter may be controlled with surgical resection and radiation therapy. As a general rule, however, one can assume a five year cancer cure rate with no evidence of disease (NED) in the following general ranges: Stage I ≥ 75 per cent; Stage II, 50 to 75 per cent; Stage III, 25 to 50 per cent; Stage IV, 25 per cent or less.

MANAGEMENT OF NECK

The intention of the treatment of neck nodes in a patient with head and neck cancer is to "eradicate" the tumor within these nodes. While the prophylactic treatment of cervical lymph nodes may be successful with either surgical resection or radiation therapy, the management of palpable lymph nodes suggestive of metastases is generally surgical. The goal of an operation for cancer of the neck is to remove all the tissue that potentially harbors the cancer cells. In 1906 Crile advocated the systematic removal of the lymphatic contents of the neck, as he realized that upper aerodigestive tract tumors spread primarily to the lymph nodes. The therapeu-

tic advantages of this procedure were reemphasized by the work of Martin and associates in 1951. In more recent years, the decision regarding the management of the palpable cervical nodes is centered mostly around the method of treatment, either classical radical neck dissection or functional radical neck dissection, with or without radiation.

The decision between a functional or classical radical neck dissection is often dependent on the extent of regional disease or evidence of extracapsular spread of the tumor into the adjacent structures. Initially, the functional neck dissection was selected mostly for prophylactic lymphadenectomy (N_0 neck), and later for selected N_1 and N_2 necks. It later became apparent that the true limitation of the functional neck dissection is related to the extracapsular spread of the tumor beyond the lymph nodes. Nevertheless, the principle of complete extirpation of all the neck contents based on classification alone is not warranted. An example of this is a patient with an N_{2b} or one 2 cm lymph node located in the posterior triangle, and another 4 cm lymph node located over the midjugular chain adherent to the jugular vein. Although removal of the jugular vein en bloc with resection may facilitate removal of the lymph node in the anterior triangle, a similar en bloc resection of the sternocleidomastoid muscle and the spinal accessory nerve for the lymph node in the posterior triangle may not be necessary. In this case, with the addition of postoperative radiation to the neck as an adjuvant to "clear any residual microscopic tumor," the risk of recurrence in the neck would be expected from the anterior triangle lymph node because of its local spread before the resection. Therefore, the decision whether functional or classical radical neck dissection is appropriate should be made according to the clinical and surgical judgment of the surgeon in evaluating each case individually.

Although Crile (1906) advocated the radical resection of all the neck contents for squamous cell carcinoma, he did not remove the spinal accessory nerve, and he included the sternocleidomastoid muscle merely to provide better exposure of the anatomy during the dissection. Suarez (1963) demonstrated that the cervical lymph nodes lie within the space enveloped by the superficial and the deep layers of the cervical fascia and are not found in vessel walls nor on the muscles overlying the vessels. Since the internal jugular vein and the sternocleidomas-

Table 70–7. Stage Groupings

Stage I	$T_1N_0M_0$
Stage II	$T_2N_0M_0$
Stage III	$T_3N_0M_0$
	T_1 or T_2 or T_3, N_1, or M_0
Stage IV	T_4, N_0 or N_1, M_0
	Any T, N_2 or N_3, M_0
	Any T, any N, M_1

	N_0	N_1	N_2	N_3
T_1	I	III	IV	IV
T_2	II	III	IV	IV
T_3	III	III	IV	IV
T_4	IV	IV	IV	IV

toid muscle are outside of the fascial enve-lopes, there is little rationale for their removal unless there is extranodal spread of the tumor to include these structures. On the other hand, the spinal accessory nerve does course through the periphery of this space. It does not appear to be at greater risk of tumor involvement than is the hypoglossal nerve or the lingual nerve, both of which are routinely preserved in the neck dissection. Therefore, the type of resection of the spinal accessory nerve, internal jugular vein, or sternocleido-mastoid muscle should be determined by po-tential tumor involvement and not in terms of the facilitation of the dissection. Few would argue against the classical radical neck dis-section in a patient in whom there is spread of tumor through the capsule of the lymph nodes and adherence to the surrounding soft tissues, but there appears to be little justifi-cation for the entire removal of all the neck structures in every case.

Bocca and Pignataro (1967) and Bocca, Pig-nataro, and Sasaki (1980) reported their ex-perience with several hundred cases of neck dissections in which they spared the internal jugular vein and the sternocleidomastoid muscle during the neck dissection without altering the disease-free rates. When the in-volvement of the cervical nodes with tumor is more extensive (N_3), a more classical radi-cal neck dissection is indicated with the re-moval of the internal jugular vein, the ster-nocleidomastoid muscle, and any other structures or nerves that may be involved with the tumor. A more difficult decision is raised when the tumor invades the common carotid artery, vagus nerve, phrenic nerve, or brachial plexus. In general, tumors that have extended beyond the fascial planes of the regional neck dissection are rarely cured by surgery or by a combination of treatment modalities. In these cases, the value of the resection must be weighed against the com-plications, which are generally high. Marti-nez and associates (1975) reported a 14 per cent mortality rate with elective resection of the carotid artery, as contrasted with 64 per cent mortality when the carotid resection was necessary because of hemorrhage. Kennedy, Krause, and Loevy (1977) documented a com-plication rate of 57 per cent and no difference in the recurrence rate or survival rate be-tween palliative (incomplete) tumor removal, curative (complete) resection of gross tumor from the preserved carotid artery, and carotid

resection. In this series, the authors reported a 46 per cent incidence of neck recurrence, a 67 per cent incidence of distant metastases, and only a 14 per cent five year survival.

Radiation therapy also plays a role in the management of clinically positive cervical lymph nodes. Million, Fletcher, and Jesse (1963), Fletcher (1962), and others (Meoz-Mendez and associates, 1978; Lindberg and Fletcher, 1978) reported the use of radiation therapy for selected patients with cervical lymph node involvement (N_1, N_{2a}), particu-larly when radiation was chosen for the treat-ment of the primary tumor site. However, it is difficult to ascertain the true control rates in these cases, since there was no histologic documentation of the incidence of microscopic tumor in the lymph nodes. Since therapeutic lymphadenectomies for palpable nodes in the neck have yielded an incidence of 20 to 25 per cent false-positive diagnosis, it would be expected that a similar percentage of the patients treated with radiation would have been treated for inflammatory responses or reactive lymph nodes.

In general, the treatment of the N_0 neck is based on the statistical likelihood of finding occult positive tumor within the nodes on the basis of the size and location of the primary tumor. Stage I tumors of the oropharyngeal area, regardless of the site of origin, have less than a 20 per cent incidence of regional lymph node disease, and therefore elective lymphadenectomy usually is not indicated. On the other hand, Stage II disease has a wide variation in the incidence of regional node involvement (up to 36 per cent), depend-ing on the site of the primary tumor. The controversy over the management of the N_0 neck is complicated by the 20 per cent false-negative rate in the assessment of the neck by clinical evaluation. Mendelson, Woods, and Beahrs (1976) demonstrated that in pa-tients with clinically negative necks (N_0) who did not subsequently develop regional nodal metastases there was a 90 per cent five year survival rate, while in those who eventually had enlargement of the cervical nodes requir-ing a lymphadenectomy the five year survival rate was 21 per cent. Furthermore, the pa-tients with N_0 necks who were treated with prophylactic lymphadenectomy and who were found to have histologically positive nodes did not have an improvement in their five year survival rates (29 per cent). Ferrara and associates (1982) also demonstrated no difference in five year survival rates between patients treated with prophylactic lymphadenectomy (64 per cent) and those treated with resection of the primary tumor, who underwent lymphadenectomy only when the neck subsequently became clinically positive (69 per cent).

One argument in favor of prophylactic treatment of the N_0 neck relates to the early detection of metastases to the neck (e.g., N_1 as opposed to N_2 or N_3). Although the overall effect on five year survival is small, the lymphadenectomy performed when the neck metastases are small results in a better regional control rate. Roux-Berger, Baud, and Courtial (1949) demonstrated an improved five year survival rate of 36 per cent with prophylactic lymphadenectomy as contrasted with a 19 per cent rate with a delayed therapeutic dissection for patients who converted to clinically palpable nodes.

Therefore, in those patients whose follow-up may be difficult or who may be noncompliant, treatment of the N_0 neck with surgery or radiation is indicated when the probability of nodal disease is greater than 20 per cent (Jesse and associates, 1970; Southwick, 1971; Jesse, 1977). Radiation to the neck (5000 to 5500 rads in five to six weeks) has been shown to be equally effective as surgery in treating subclinical tumor deposits, with a 95 per cent control rate if the primary tumor is also controlled (Bagshaw and Thompson, 1971; Rabuzzi, Chung, and Sagerman, 1980). The selection of surgery or radiation for the treatment of the neck should take into consideration the patient's general health and the risk of surgical morbidity, the patient's compliance and reliability, the choice of treatment of the primary tumor (whether surgery or radiation), and finally the experience of the physicians on the treatment team.

Classical Radical Neck Dissection

The technique of neck dissection begins with the selection of the skin incision, of which there are many variations. The most commonly used are illustrated in Figure 70–12, of which the "Y" and its many variations have been the most popular because they provide excellent exposure and permit easy dissection. However, they are also the most likely to result in flap necrosis at the distal

ends, and if the sternocleidomastoid muscle has been removed in a previously irradiated neck, necrosis of the flaps usually results in exposure of the vascular structures. The MacFee (1960) bipedicle flap incision is more reliable because this flap has a better blood supply and the scars are esthetically more acceptable, but its proper elevation with the underlying platysma muscle may be more tedious. A dissection of the neck structures beneath this bipedicle flap requires continuous manipulation and traction of the structures and the skin flap in order to maintain exposure during the procedure.

The authors have found that the hockey-stick incision provides excellent exposure and the healed scars are esthetically acceptable

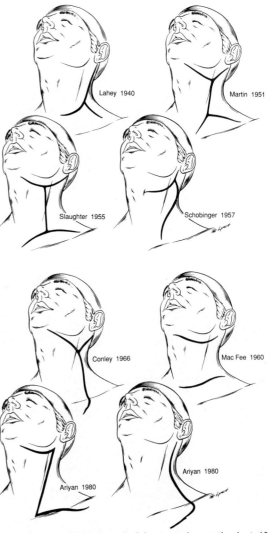

Figure 70–12. Various incisions used over the last 40 years for access to the cervical lymph nodes.

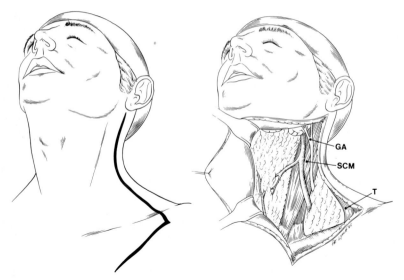

Figure 70–13. Technique of the hockeystick incision *(left)*. Elevation begins from the mastoid prominence to the shoulder traversing 2 cm posterior to the anterior border of the trapezius muscle *(T)*. It turns obliquely along the infraclavicular area. The flap is elevated with the underlying platysma muscle *(right)* to expose the sternocleidomastoid muscle *(SCM)*, the superficial veins, and the sensory nerves including the greater auricular nerve *(GA)*.

(Ariyan, 1980a). The incision is made from the mastoid to the shoulder, running approximately 2 cm behind the anterior border of the trapezius muscle before extending medially below the clavicle. If the incision is placed anterior to the border of the muscle, the eventual contraction of the healing wound can result in a linear web from the mastoid to the shoulder; on the other hand, an incision placed behind the edge of the muscle allows the scar to heal by adherence to the underlying trapezius muscle without contracture or webbing in the neck (Fig. 70–13).

The apron flap (Fig. 70–14) is used selectively for tumors requiring laryngectomy, with or without a posteroinferior extension for access to the contents of the neck. The flap is well vascularized, and after its elevation the neck dissection on either or both sides can be performed without vascular compromise to the distal end of the flap. The incision extends from mastoid to mastoid, passing along the posterior border of the sternocleidomastoid muscle, with a slight inferior curve to the midline located 2 to 3 fingerbreadths above the suprasternal notch. The flap has also been used for resections of the floor of the mouth in which the distal portion of the flap may be used as a platysma myocutaneous flap for reconstruction of the defect.

The elevation of the flaps can be performed at a plane deep to the platysma muscle but above the superficial layer of the investing cervical fascia, in order to incorporate the platysma muscle and its blood supply with the skin flap. Regardless of the individual flaps chosen, the flaps are elevated to the

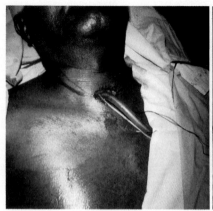
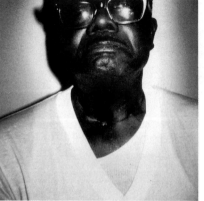
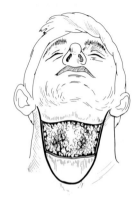

Figure 70–14. The apron flap is an extension of a bilateral neck incision extending from mastoid to mastoid into the lower neck *(left)* to provide access to the larynx and both necks while maintaining circulation to the skin for healing without tissue loss *(center)*. The flap can also be deepithelized at its base to transfer the distant skin paddle for reconstruction of intraoral defects *(right)*.

limits of the proposed neck dissection: anteriorly to the sternohyoid muscle, inferiorly to the clavicle, posteriorly to the trapezius, and superiorly to the mandible. During the elevation of the flap to the superior margin, care must be taken to avoid injury to the marginal mandibular branch of the facial nerve, which curves as much as 2 to 4 cm below the mandible at the level of the antigonial notch. The branches of this nerve are best identified at this point of the dissection as they course over the anterior facial vein below the mandible.

The authors preference is to dissect the cervical contents from below and posterior in a direction anteriorly and superiorly (Fig. 70–15). The fascia is incised along the anterior border of the trapezius and above the clavicle, and the inferior belly of the omohyoid muscle is identified and transected (or alternatively clamped and its origin avulsed from the scapula). As the deep cervical fascia overlying the brachial plexus is reached, the cervical contents can be "peeled" and swept forward by means of an operative sponge. The spinal accessory nerve is identified and transected as it enters the trapezius muscle along its anterior border.

With further dissection along the anterior aspect of the clavicle, the two heads of the sternocleidomastoid muscle are transected from the sternum and clavicle, and the specimen is swept forward toward the internal jugular vein. The vagus nerve is identified, dissected, and preserved before the jugular vein is transected and suture ligated. Dissection along this area of the internal jugular vein may reveal clear fluid, which is an indication that there has been disruption of the thoracic duct. This lymphatic duct can usually be seen as it takes a C-shaped loop cephalad and returns on itself to its junction with the internal jugular vein. It usually needs to be clamped and transected and ligated twice as it takes the turn. This maneuver avoids the postoperative complication of a chylous leak.

As the dissection proceeds in a cephalad direction, the branches of the internal jugular vein are ligated and transected, the sensory cutaneous nerves of the cervical plexus are transected, and a block dissection is continued toward the submandibular area. Along this direction, the transverse scapular vessels (suprascapular) may be ligated, but the deeper transverse cervical artery and vein are preserved.

In the midportion of the neck, the spinal accessory nerve exits behind the sternocleidomastoid muscle into the posterior triangle within a 2 cm area of Erb's point. Erb's point is the site of confluence of the superficial sensory nerves, including the great auricular nerve, as they exit behind the sternocleidomastoid muscle. The often thick sensory branches from the cervical plexus need to be transected and occasionally ligated because of the accompanying vessels.

At this point, the dissection returns to the internal jugular vein, which is dissected free of the vagus nerve and the carotid artery as the specimen is elevated cephalad. The phrenic nerve is identified deep to the fascia, crossing obliquely and inferomedially over the scalenus anterior muscle, and is preserved.

As the dissection proceeds cephalad, the middle thyroid and superior thyroid veins are ligated and transected. The marginal mandibular branch of the facial nerve is again identified and preserved as it crosses the facial vessels. The anterior belly of the omohyoid muscle is detached from the hyoid and the dissection is continued to the carotid bifurcation. The carotid sinus is blocked by infiltration of 1 per cent lidocaine (Xylocaine) (without epinephrine) by means of a 27 to 30 gauge needle into the loose adventitia over the bifurcation of the artery. This maneuver blocks the carotid sinus reflex to avoid bradycardia as a result of manipulation of the carotid artery during the dissection.

Further dissection identifies the hypoglossal nerve as it crosses the carotid artery, and preserves it. The contents of the submandibular triangle, including the submaxillary gland, are removed after the lingual nerve is identified and preserved. As the dissection continues along the angle of the mandible, the tail of the parotid gland is transected at the anterior border of the sternocleidomastoid muscle. The jugular vein is doubly ligated at the base of the skull, transected, and suture ligated. The sternocleidomastoid muscle is transected from its attachment at the mastoid, and the block dissection of the cervical contents is completed.

The neck is irrigated with sterile water to lyse the blood clots and to identify any sites of small bleeding vessels that should be cauterized. Large suction catheters are placed in the neck, not so much to drain blood as to apply suction to the neck flaps to bring the flap into contact with the bed of the wound

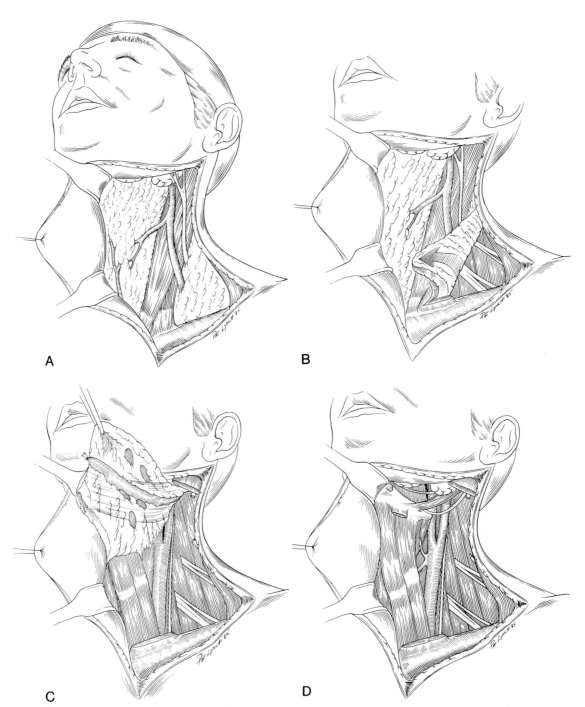

Figure 70–15. The classical neck dissection. *A,* A hockeystick incision is used to gain exposure to the neck contents. *B,* The dissection of the cervical contents begins with the posterior triangle and moves anterior and superior. *C,* The dissection includes the internal jugular vein as well as the sternocleidomastoid muscle. *D,* All the contents of the neck have been removed while preserving the carotid artery, vagus nerve, phrenic nerve, hypoglossal nerve, and lingual nerve. (From Ariyan, S.: Radical neck dissection. Surg. Clin. North Am., *66:*133, 1986.)

to obliterate dead space. If the neck wound were to bleed actively at the time of the closure, the suction catheters would not be able to remove the blood effectively. The clots in the neck elevate the flap and cause further bleeding and formation of a large hematoma. The most common cause of bleeding in the neck at the time the patient is awakened from anesthesia is gagging on the endotracheal tube, which causes a Valsalva maneuver, increases the venous pressure, and leads to venous bleeding under the neck flaps.

Functional Radical Neck Dissection

As stated earlier, Crile (1906) did not sacrifice the spinal accessory nerve routinely, and he resected the sternocleidomastoid muscle merely to provide better exposure of the anatomy. Therefore, the functional neck dissection removes the lymphatic contents of the neck while selectively preserving the spinal

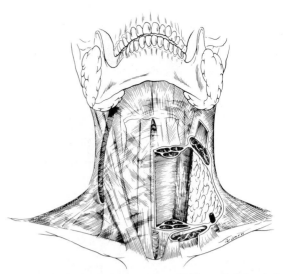

Figure 70–17. The sternocleidomastoid muscle is located outside of the cervical fascia covering the lymphatics and lymph nodes in the neck. (From Ariyan, S.: Radical neck dissection. Surg. Clin. North Am., 66:133, 1986.)

accessory nerve, the internal jugular vein, and the sternocleidomastoid muscle when these structures are not involved intimately with the tumor. Previous radiation treatment to the neck is not a contraindication, and in fact may represent a proper indication when one considers the fact that preservation of the sternocleidomastoid muscle decreases the likelihood of carotid exposure.

The sternocleidomastoid muscle has three blood supplies (Fig. 70–16) (Ariyan, 1979b). Inferiorly, the blood supply is from the thyrocervical trunk, in the midportion from the superior thyroid artery, and superiorly from the branches of the occipital artery. In addition, the investing layer of the superficial cervical fascia extends across the posterior triangle, splits to envelop the sternocleidomastoid muscle by its two layers, and reforms as a single layer to extend across the anterior cervical triangle (Fig. 70–17). If the sternocleidomastoid muscle is dissected and elevated from the neck, the deeper half of the split cervical fascia would remain in continuity with the cervical fascia covering the anterior and posterior cervical triangles. This maneuver permits the same composite dissection of the lymphatics and lymph nodes as in a classical lymphadenectomy in the neck (Fig. 70–18).

The carotid sheath, which encloses the carotid artery, the vagus nerve, and the inter-

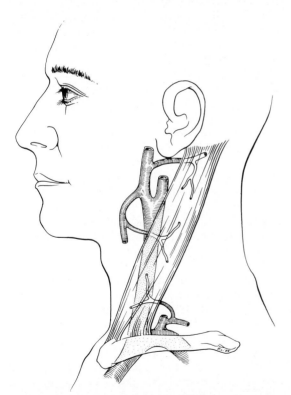

Figure 70–16. The three blood supplies to the sternocleidomastoid muscle are from the occipital artery above, the thyrocervical trunk below, and the superior thyroid artery in the midportion. (From Ariyan, S.: Radical neck dissection. Surg. Clin. North Am., *66*:133, 1986.)

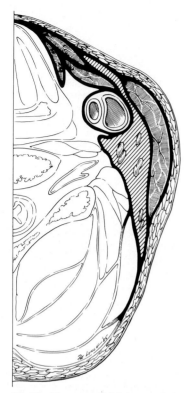

Figure 70–18. The superficial layer of the investing cervical fascia extends across the posterior triangle, splits to envelop the sternocleidomastoid muscle, and reforms into a single layer to extend across the anterior cervical triangle. The contents of the cervical lymphatics and lymph nodes are superficial to the carotid sheath and the vessels within the sheath. (From Ariyan, S.: Radical neck dissection. Surg. Clin. North Am., *66*:133, 1986.)

nal jugular vein, is composed of a confluence of fascial layers including the superficial and deep layers of the investing cervical fascia and the prevertebral fascia, and as such the contents of the sheath may be excluded from the dissection. However, some arguments have been offered for including the carotid sheath with the dissection because of its intimate association with the midjugular lymph nodes. Moreover, its removal and inclusion with the bloc dissection is easy to perform.

The technique for the functional neck dissection begins after the elevation of the skin flaps with the underlying platysma muscle (Fig. 70–19). The authors prefer to use the hockeystick incision because of its exposure and reliability, and the excellent cosmetic result (Ariyan, 1980a). The superficial cervical fascia is incised along the entire length of both the posterior border and anterior borders of the sternocleidomastoid muscle

(SCM). At this point, the origins of the two heads of the sternocleidomastoid muscle are transected; the muscle is elevated by sharp dissection from the deeper split layer of the superficial cervical fascia, maintaining its superior blood supply from branches of the occipital artery (Ariyan, 1980a). It is helpful to place small tagging silk sutures at the tendinous origins on the clavicle and sternum in order to identify the proper locations of the two heads of the sternocleidomastoid muscle for reinsertion at the end of the dissection. An alternative method reported by Bocca, Pignataro, and Sasaki (1980) leaves the origin and insertion of the muscle undisturbed but retracts the muscle with wide Penrose drains to permit dissection of the neck contents underneath the elevated and retracted muscle.

The spinal accessory nerve (SAN) is identified as it enters the anterior border of the trapezius muscle, usually between the midportion and the junction of the middle and lower thirds of the anterior border of this muscle. The contents of the posterior cervical triangle are incised and the spinal accessory nerve is dissected along its length between the trapezius and the sternocleidomastoid muscles. On occasion, the spinal accessory nerve is found not to pass through the sternocleidomastoid muscle but rather to traverse along the undersurface of this muscle to give a motor branch to the sternocleidomastoid muscle (Fig. 70–20).

The removal of the lymphatic contents is begun from the inferior posterior aspect of the neck, as described earlier for the radical neck dissection. As the dissection proceeds in an anterior and cephalad direction, the carotid sheath is incised along the entire length of the carotid artery and stripped posteriorly over the vagus nerve and internal jugular vein. The sheath is included with a block dissection of the cervical lymphatics. The remainder of the dissection is essentially the same as in the radical neck dissection. After completion of the block dissection, the sternocleidomastoid muscle is returned to its original position and the sternoclavicular heads are sutured to their sites of origin (Fig. 70–21). The flaps are closed over large suction catheters placed in the operative wound. It is critical, however, to obtain meticulous hemostasis since the repositioning of the SCM does not permit the dead space to be as easily conformed by the cutaneous flap after the application of suction to the catheters.

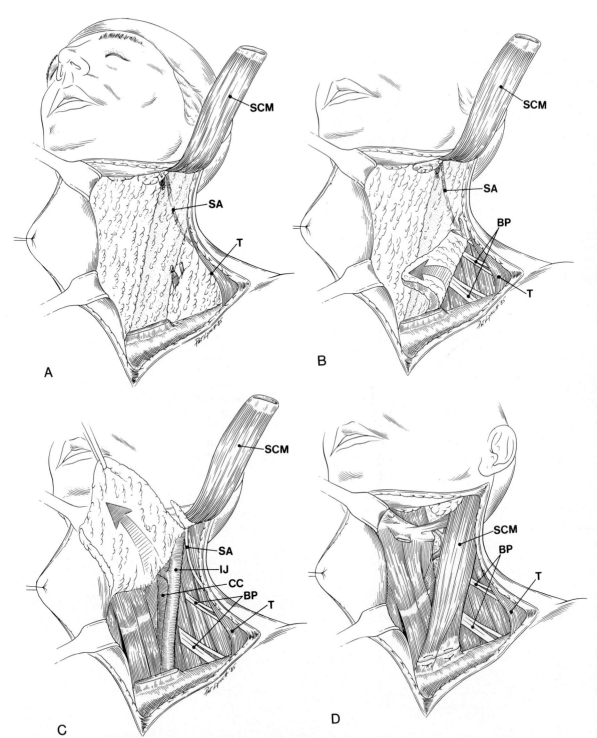

Figure 70–19. The functional radical neck dissection. *A,* The sternocleidomastoid muscle *(SCM)* is elevated from the cervical fascia, and the spinal accessory *(SA)* nerve is identified as it enters the anterior border of the trapezius (T) muscle. *B,* The cervical fascia is incised to dissect and preserve the spinal accessory nerve. The neck dissection begins in the posterior triangle and moves anteriorly and superiorly, preserving the brachial plexus *(BP)*. *C,* As the dissection continues cephalad, the internal jugular *(IJ)* vein is preserved along the carotid sheath with the common carotid *(CC)* and the two branches of the carotid. *D,* After completion of the neck dissection, the sternocleidomastoid muscle is returned to its proper sternal and clavicular origins and sutured into position. (From Ariyan, S.: Radical neck dissection. Surg. Clin. North Am., *66*:133, 1986.)

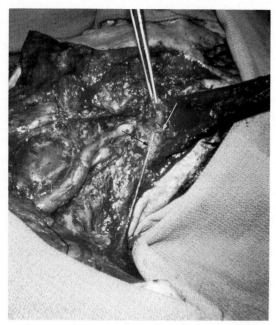

Figure 70–20. The spinal accessory nerve can occasionally be seen to travel under the sternocleidomastoid muscle *(black arrow)* on its way to the trapezius muscle, giving off a motor branch to the sternocleidomastoid *(white arrow).*

FLAP RECONSTRUCTION

Small defects of the tongue or the floor of the mouth may be closed with nasolabial flaps or tongue flaps. Larger deficits may require a sternocleidomastoid muscle flap to transfer a larger paddle of skin. If bulk is necessary with the addition of skin, the pectoralis major myocutaneous flap or trapezius myocutaneous flap may be used. Reconstructions of the mandible may be performed with nonvascularized bone grafts, which are then covered with the muscle flaps, or the bone may be brought attached to the muscle with the periosteal blood supply, as in the pectoralis major, trapezius muscle, or latissimus dorsi transfers (Chicarilli and Ariyan, 1985).

FOREHEAD

The forehead flap (McGregor, 1963) has also been a reliable flap for intraoral wounds. The flap is elevated on the superficial temporal vessels (Fig. 70–22). The flap is elevated by incising along the hairline superiorly and at the upper limit of the eyebrows inferiorly, and incorporating the entire forehead esthetic unit. The flap can be deepithelized at its base in order that it can be transferred into the oral cavity in one stage. The flap can be passed either superficially or deep to the zygomatic arch. The donor site is skin grafted. The advantage of this flap is that it provides thin, pliable tissue for reconstruction of the buccal mucosa, floor of the mouth, or tongue. The disadvantage is that it leaves an unesthetic skin graft on the forehead, and it is too

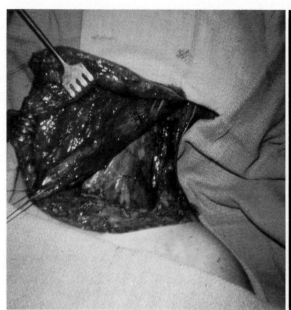
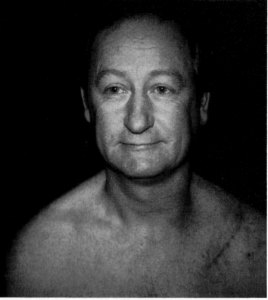

Figure 70–21. The sternocleidomastoid muscle, which had been elevated with traction sutures, is returned to the sternal and clavicular origins *(left)* and sutured into position *(right).* The wound heals with a well-vascularized flap, and the suture line is easily covered by most open-neck shirts.

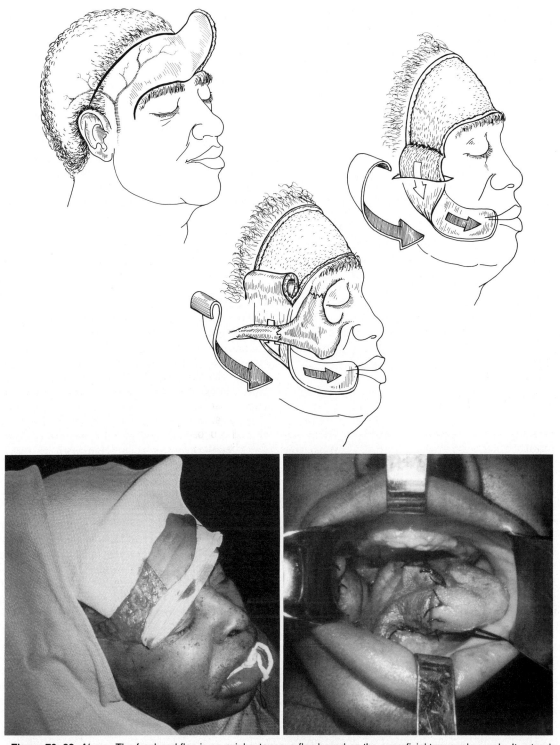

Figure 70–22. *Above,* The forehead flap is an axial cutaneous flap based on the superficial temporal vessels. It extends across the midline to incorporate the skin of the opposite side. The flap can be passed over or under the zygoma for intraoral positioning. *Below,* The base of the flap can be deepithelized *(left)* to transfer the skin into the oral cavity in one stage *(right).*

thin for reconstruction of significant losses of the tongue. Because of the absence of bulk, it acts as a funnel and causes fluid to pool anteriorly or directs it toward the larynx posteriorly. Although this flap is not used often in present-day reconstructions, it is still one to be considered in the surgical armamentarium.

NASOLABIAL

Nasolabial flaps are more effectively used for intraoral reconstruction if they are based inferiorly. A long, tapered flap may be designed on the hairless skin edge along the nasolabial fold and is dissected as a flap incorporating the thick portion of the underlying subcutaneous tissues to provide its blood supply from branches of the facial artery (Fig. 70–23). The flap is deepithelized at the base, tunneled through the cheek, and sutured in position in the oral cavity. If the patient has teeth, the base need not be deepithelized, but the flap is then divided and inset at 10 to 14 days.

TONGUE

Tongue flaps can be used effectively to resurface the lateral or anterior floor of mouth defects (see also Chap. 71). With the tongue retracted, the flap is elevated from the lateral aspect of the tongue, equal amounts covering the dorsal and the ventral surfaces (Fig. 70–24). The incision should be wedged in toward the depth of the tongue to excise the muscle with the flap to permit closure of the donor site while providing bulk and blood supply to the flap. The flap should be dissected wider as the incision proceeds posteriorly in order to ensure a more vascular base to the flap.

APRON

The apron flap can provide an adequate size of thin tissue to resurface a significant defect in the floor of the mouth. This is a musculocutaneous flap incorporating the platysma muscle. The paddle of skin necessary for the reconstruction is outlined in the lower portion of the neck (Fig. 70–25). The base of the flap may be deepithelized in order to turn it under the mandible and into the floor of the mouth in one stage, eliminating the need for division and inset of the flap. The donor

site of the flap in the neck may then be closed by advancement of the margins of the cervical skin and a small skin graft.

STERNOCLEIDOMASTOID

The sternocleidomastoid (SCM) muscle may be incorporated in a flap on either its superior or inferior attachment. As mentioned earlier, the sternocleidomastoid has three blood supplies (superiorly, inferiorly, and from the midportion of the muscle) (see Fig. 70–16). The skin paddles may be outlined on the lower portion of the muscle and transferred on the superior blood supply, or alternatively a skin paddle in the inframastoid region can be transferred on the inferior blood supply (Fig. 70–26). However, the disadvantage of transferring the flap on the inferior blood supply is that it requires sacrifice of the 11th nerve in most cases.

The skin paddle is outlined over the selected portion of the muscle, and after the incision is made to the underlying musculature, the skin paddle is sutured from the dermis to the muscle fascia to prevent traction damage to the thin and delicate perforating vessels from the muscle to the skin. This maneuver is particularly important over the supraclavicular area where there is abundant loose areolar tissue between the skin and the underlying musculature. Traction sutures are placed at the end of the muscle pedicle, and the cervical fascia is incised along the anterior and posterior borders of the muscle (Fig. 70–27). The flap is elevated from the deeper layer of the investing cervical fascia that roofs the anterior and posterior cervical triangles. The dissection of the muscle pedicle should proceed only as far as is necessary to mobilize the flap sufficiently to transfer the skin paddle to the intraoral defect. After the flap is transferred under the mandible and into the intraoral defect, the muscle must be securely anchored to whatever structure is of substance in the margin of the wound, to prevent traction on the suture line postoperatively. The donor site in the neck can be closed by advancement of cervical flaps without the need for skin grafts.

PECTORALIS MAJOR

The pectoralis major (PM) muscle can provide more significant amounts of skin and muscle for bulk to fill defects and cavities.

Text continued on page 3444

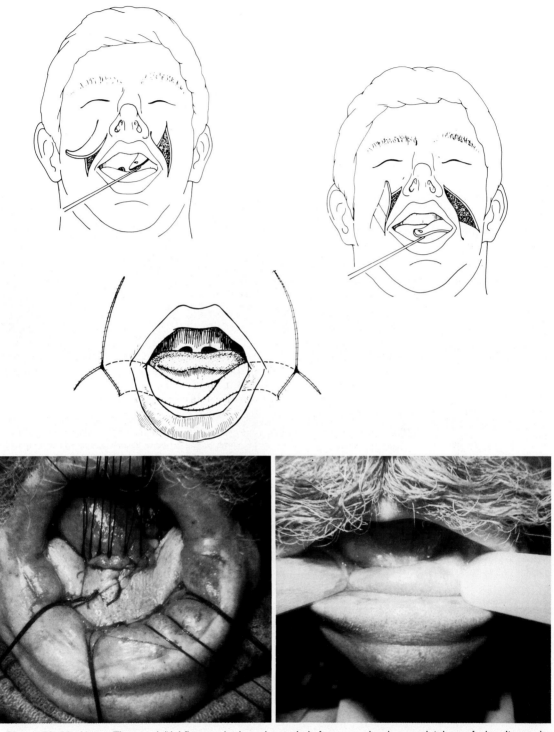

Figure 70–23. *Above,* The nasolabial flap can be based superiorly for upper alveolar or palatal resurfacing. It can also be based inferiorly for resurfacing the anterior floor of the mouth. *Below, left,* The flaps lie side by side to provide coverage over a wide area of the anterior floor of the mouth as well as the mandibular alveolus *(below, right).*

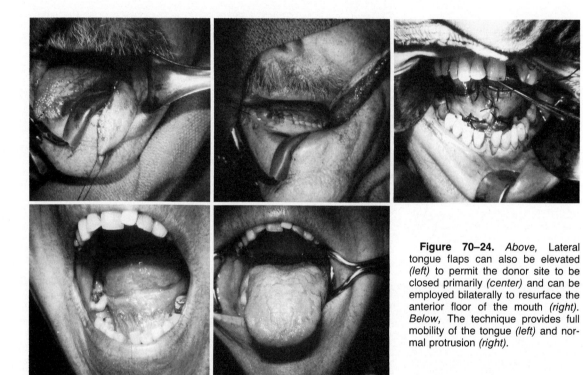

Figure 70–24. *Above,* Lateral tongue flaps can also be elevated *(left)* to permit the donor site to be closed primarily *(center)* and can be employed bilaterally to resurface the anterior floor of the mouth *(right).* *Below,* The technique provides full mobility of the tongue *(left)* and normal protrusion *(right).*

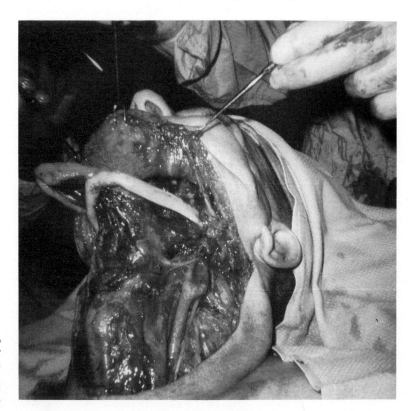

Figure 70–25. The apron flap can be elevated to gain access for resection of a floor of the mouth lesion, marginal mandibulectomy, and neck dissection *(above)* and then draped over the mandible. The base of the flap can be deepithelized *(center)* and the inferior portion of this apron flap can be turned and rolled under the mandible. The distal tip can resurface the floor of the mouth *(below, left).* This reconstruction provides a thin lining to the remaining mandible and reconstructed floor of a mouth *(below, right).*

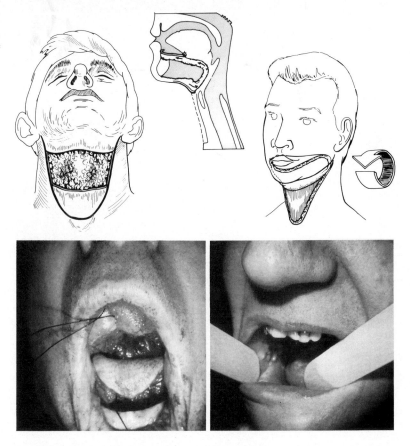

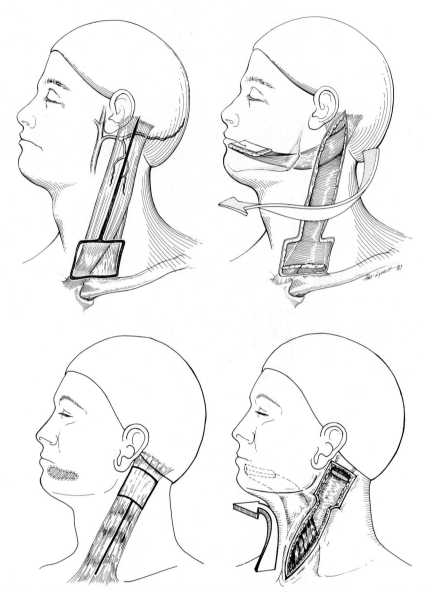

Figure 70–26. The sternocleidomastoid muscle may be elevated on its superior blood supply *(above)* to transfer a paddle of skin at the distal portion of the muscle to the anterior floor of the mouth. The muscle can also be elevated on its inferior blood supply *(below)* to transfer a paddle of skin to the floor of the mouth or the tonsillar region.

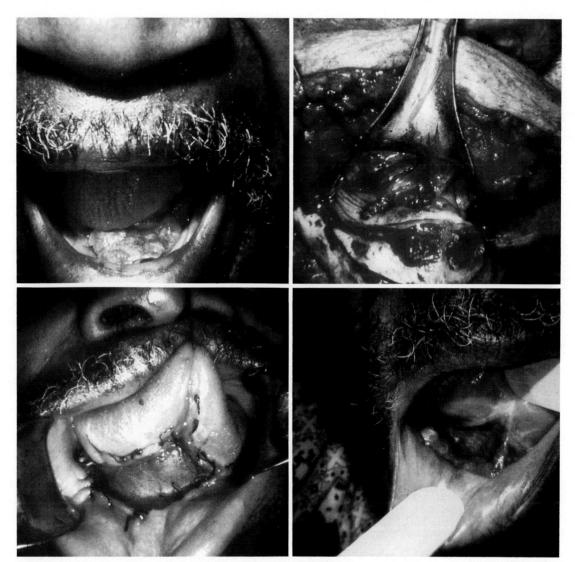

Figure 70–27. *Above,* Cancer of the anterior floor of the mouth *(left)* can be resected together with a horizontal rim of the mandible *(right). Below,* The surgical defect can be resurfaced with a paddle of skin on the sternocleidomastoid muscle *(left)* to provide thin and pliable covering to permit full motion of the tongue *(right).*

This muscle is a flat, fan-shaped structure covering the upper chest, and has its dominant blood supply from the thoracoacromial artery, which leaves the subclavian artery at the midportion of the clavicle. This vessel perforates the clavipectoral fascia and travels along the undersurface of the fascia of the pectoralis major along an axis from the shoulder to the xiphoid (Fig. 70–28). There are also secondary sources of blood supply from the intercostal perforators of the internal mammary artery (medially) as well as the lateral thoracic artery (laterally). The flap is particularly suited for large resections of the floor of the mouth that include removal of a portion of the tongue and require additional bulk in reconstruction.

The skin paddle is outlined along the inferomedial aspect of the muscle and elevated with a narrow pedicle of only that portion of

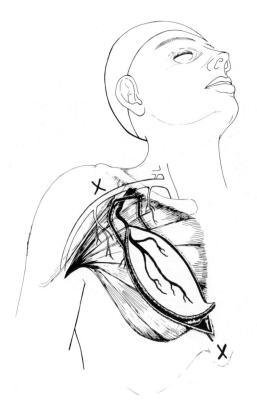

Figure 70–28. Pectoralis major muscle flap. The thoracoacromial vascular axis exits from the subclavian artery at the level of the middle third of the clavicle, on a line drawn from the shoulder to the xiphoid (marked "X"), and turns along this axis to travel inferomedially under the pectoralis major muscle. A skin paddle can be outlined on the vascular axis and elevated with a narrow segment of only a portion of the muscle. The infraclavicular portion of the muscle can then be resected to leave the flap attached only by its vascular pedicle.

the muscle that is necessary to include the underlying vascular pedicle (Fig. 70–29). The muscle is dissected to the clavicle, at which point the infraclavicular portion of the muscle is removed from the vascular pedicle, leaving the flap attached only by its arteriovenous pedicle in the subpectoral fascia. With this maneuver, the flap can be transposed over the clavicle and only the vessels lie over this bone, rather than the bulk of the muscle at its base. The flap can be passed under the neck skin and mandible to reach the intraoral wound. The muscle must be securely sutured to the margins of the wound in the oral cavity to prevent any traction injury to the skin paddle in the postoperative period. The skin paddle can be sutured to the mucosal margins of the wound without any tension. The chest donor site is closed by liberal undermining of chest skin flaps and primary closure following advancement of these flaps.

If a segment of mandible has been resected, it is possible to transfer a portion of the fourth or fifth rib to which the muscle fibers are attached (Fig. 70–30). It has been demonstrated (Ariyan and Finseth, 1978; Ariyan, 1980b) that vascularized ribs can be transferred by microsurgery on the anterior blood supply from the intercostal vessels through the periosteum. With the documentation of periosteal blood supply, Cuono and Ariyan (1980) showed the feasibility of transferring vascularized rib with blood supply from the pectoralis major muscle to the periosteum of the rib. Therefore, the segment of the rib is meticulously dissected incorporating the attached periosteum. The rib can be brought into the intraoral defect with either a single skin paddle for intraoral covering of the surgical defect (Fig. 70–31) or two skin paddles, one for intraoral lining and one for external coverage.

TRAPEZIUS

The trapezius muscle has also been useful in intraoral and external reconstructions. In addition, the trapezius may be transferred with a segment of attached bone from either the transverse spine or the acromion (Demergasso and Piazza, 1979; Dufresne and associates, 1987). The trapezius is a flat, triangular muscle of the neck and back. The fibers, which originate from the occiput of the skull and the spinous process of all the thoracic vertebrae, insert on the lateral third of the

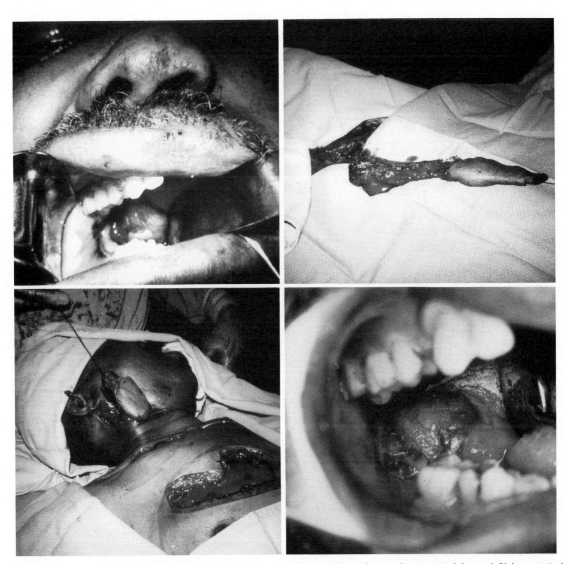

Figure 70–29. A cancer of the retromolar trigone, floor of the mouth, and posterior tongue *(above, left)* is resected widely and reconstructed with a paddle of skin on a segment of pectoralis major muscle completely detached except for the vascular pedicle *(above, right)*. The paddle is brought underneath the chest and neck skin *(below, left)* to pass under the mandible into the area of resection, where it provides adequate tissue to the tongue and floor of the mouth *(below, right)* and permits the swallowing of liquids without aspiration.

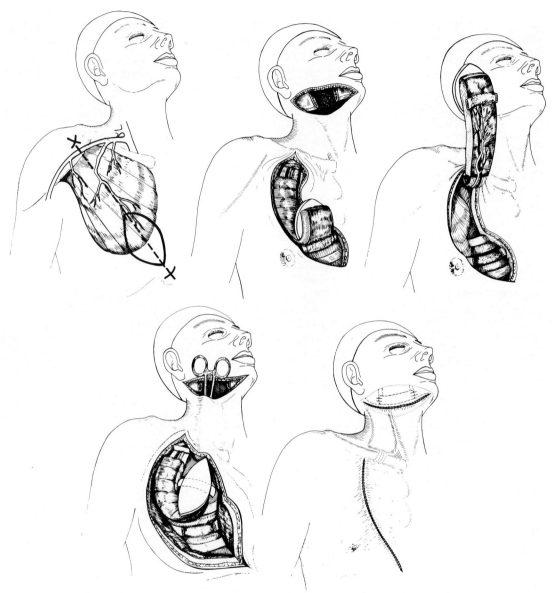

Figure 70–30. The pectoralis major flap can also be utilized to incorporate a segment of underlying attached rib (fourth or fifth and occasionally the sixth) for transfer to the oropharyngeal area to reconstruct a segment of missing mandible as well as provide skin lining for the intraoral defect.

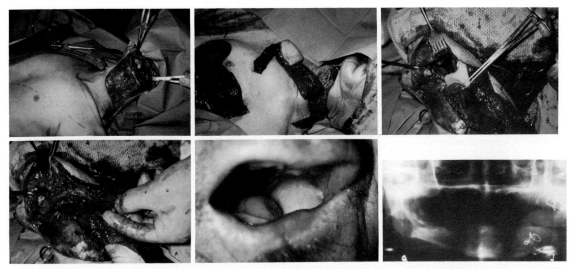

Figure 70–31. *Above,* A missing segment of the mandible *(left)* was reconstructed using a segment of the rib attached to the origins of the pectoralis major muscle *(center)* while the skin paddle was used for intraoral lining *(right). Below,* More rib was harvested than was necessary and then resected to size *(left).* The late follow-up demonstrates proper lining of the intraoral defect *(center)* and stabilization of the mandible *(right).*

clavicle, the acromion, and the scapular spine. The skin paddle that is required is outlined over the trapezius muscle as distally as is necessary, depending on the length of pedicle required. The skin paddle can be placed inferiorly over the descending posterior portion of the transverse cervical artery, or transversely over the shoulder (Fig. 70–32). The flap is elevated with only a portion of the muscle that is necessary for the transfer, and is dissected together with the under-lying muscle fascia to preserve the blood supply. If the acromion or the scapular spine is to be included in the flap for composite reconstruction (Fig. 70–33), the segment of bone is cut with an oscillating saw. An additional 1 or 2 cm of bone is taken to be trimmed at the site of the reconstruction. In the dissection of the flap, the transverse cervical artery and vein are identified at the neck between the trapezius and levator scapulae muscles and are incorporated with the flap.

Figure 70–32. The trapezius muscle may be used to transfer skin overlying the muscle along the descending portion of the transverse cervical artery *(left)* or in a transverse direction *(right),* using the upper portion of the muscle on the transverse cervical artery The latissimus dorsi muscle flap is also outlined.

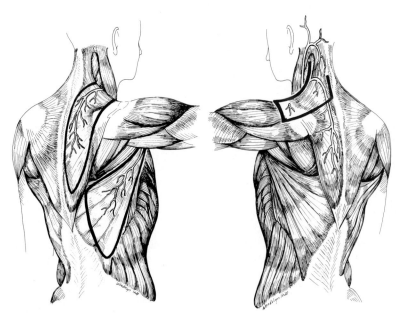

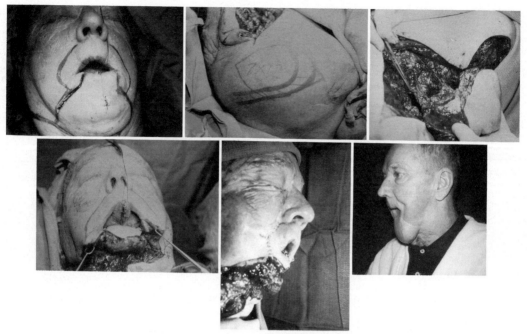

Figure 70–33. *Above,* A tumor of the floor of the mouth eroding through the symphysis of the mandible and the overlying skin required complete resection of the entire segment *(left)*. A paddle of skin overlying the acromion was incorporated *(center)* on a segment of the transverse portion of the trapezius *(right)* for the reconstruction. *Below,* The skin paddle was used for intraoral lining of the floor of the mouth *(left)* while the acromion was used for the reconstruction of the symphysis of the mandible *(left* and *center)*. The flap was resurfaced with a pectoralis major myocutaneous flap *(right)*. (From Ariyan, S.: Cancer of the Head and Neck. St. Louis, MO, C. V. Mosby Company, 1987.)

It is also advantageous to identify and preserve the suprascapular vessels as they approach the acromion along the clavicle. If the latter vessels are incorporated in the flap, they further increase the circulation to the bone. The flap can be elevated on a pedicle of muscle, or it can be completely freed on the vessels alone as a true vascular island flap. The donor site can often be closed by advancement skin flaps without the need for grafts.

LATISSIMUS DORSI

The latissimus dorsi muscle may be used for reconstruction if other regional flaps are inadequate or unavailable (Quillen, 1979). This is a triangular muscle arising from a broad aponeurosis attached to the spinous processes of the lower six thoracic, lumbar, and sacral vertebrae and the iliac crest, and inserting on the humerus. The muscle is supplied by the thoracodorsal artery and vein. A skin paddle (see Fig. 70–32) is outlined on the inferolateral portion of the muscle and the segment of the muscle is elevated with a thoracodorsal vascular pedicle. It can be tunneled beneath the pectoralis major muscle

and brought anteriorly into the neck and then under the neck flaps through the pharyngeal region for reconstruction (Fig. 70–34). This myocutaneous flap is helpful in posterior cervical or occipital reconstructions, but less useful for anterior floor of mouth defects.

MICROVASCULAR (FREE)

Microvascular (free) flaps may also be employed to resurface defects of the intraoral region. The most versatile are either jejunal free flaps (Seidenberg and associates, 1959) or radial forearm free flaps (Soutar and associates, 1983; Harii and associates, 1985; Chicarilli, Ariyan, and Cuono, 1986b). The jejunal free flap is useful to reconstruct the cervical esophagus following laryngopharyngectomies and it has also been used as a "patch flap" to resurface intraoral lining after resections.

Since the jejunal free flap requires an intra-abdominal procedure, the radial forearm free flap is becoming more popular for thin flap reconstruction of defects in the oropharyngeal area. An Allen test is employed to ensure proper circulation and perfusion of

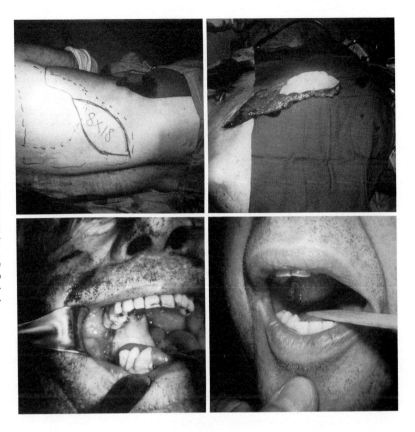

Figure 70–34. Latissimus dorsi flap. *Above,* Reconstruction of an oropharyngeal defect can be accomplished with a latissimus dorsi flap by outlining the skin paddle along the inferolateral aspect of the muscle *(left).* The flap is elevated with a portion of the muscle on the thoracodorsal blood supply and passed under the pectoralis major to the anterior chest *(right). Below,* The flap is transferred under the neck skin to the oropharynx *(left)* to provide reliable coverage of the tonsillar fossa, lateral pharynx, and hypopharynx *(right).*

the fingers through the ulnar artery when the radial artery is digitally occluded. If the radial forearm flap is used, the skin paddle is outlined over the distal portion of the radial artery to incorporate the vessel and a cutaneous vein of the forearm (Fig. 70–35). With tourniquet control of an exsanguinated arm, the skin paddle is elevated with the underlying vascular fascia. The free flap is transferred to the primary resection site where the radial artery and the cutaneous vein are anastomosed to a properly selected artery and vein in the neck. After the flap is observed for proper circulation, the skin is positioned in the oropharyngeal region and sutured securely to the wound margins.

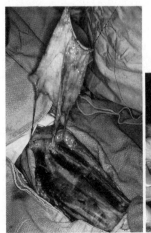
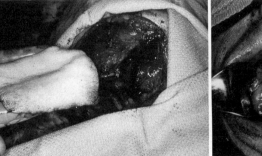
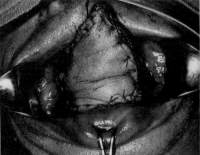

Figure 70–35. The skin overlying the distal forearm can be elevated on the radial artery and cutaneous veins *(left)* for reconstruction of the oral cavity. The flap can be revascularized by anastomosis to an artery or vein in the neck *(center)* to provide thin skin lining to the floor of the mouth and the portion of tongue that was resected *(right).*

Table 70–8. Five Year Survival Rates for Oral Cancers (Percentages)

Site	Stage			
	I	II	III	IV
Anterior tongue	35–85	25–75	10–50	0–25
Floor of mouth	60–75	40–65	20–40	0–15
Gingival	75	40	20	0–10
Buccal	75–85	45–65	20–25	0–20

MANAGEMENT OF PRIMARY TUMOR

Oral Cavity

The most common sites of squamous cell carcinoma of the oral cavity and their order of frequency are the tongue, 36 per cent; floor of the mouth, 35 per cent; mandibular gingiva, 16 per cent; buccal mucosa, 10 per cent; and hard palate and maxillary gingiva, 3 per cent (O'Brien, 1982). The overall five year survival rate in the oral cavity ranges from 31 to 66 per cent (Table 70–8).

ORAL TONGUE (ANTERIOR TWO-THIRDS)

Sqamous cell carcinoma of the oral or mobile tongue covers that area from the posterior circumvallate papillae to the anterior tip. Tumors of this area have a predilection for lymphatic drainage to the subdigastric, submaxillary, and midjugular lymph node groups, in that descending order of frequency. Spread to the submental, lower jugular, or posterior triangle lymph nodes is uncommon. The probability of nodal metastases is based on the size of the primary tumor and ranges as follows: T_1, 15 per cent; T_2, 30 per cent; T_3, 50 per cent; and T_4, 75 per cent. The incidence of regional nodal metastases at the time of initial clinical evaluation is 35 per cent (Lindberg, 1972). Of patients who have an N_0 neck and whose necks are not treated electively (either by radiation or surgery), 25 per cent subsequently develop metastases to the neck nodes, and 11 per cent also have either a synchronous or a metachronous second primary tumor (Ildstad, Bigelow, and Remensnyder, 1983).

Patients classified as Stage I or Stage II may be treated equally effectively with radiation therapy or surgical resection. The dose of radiation for cure is generally 6000 to 6500 rads of external beam radiation in six to seven weeks, although interstitial implantation with radioactive seeds may also be used to deliver a greater concentration to the center of the tumor. Surgical management of the tumor requires radical excision with at least a 1 to 2 cm margin around the tumor. At the time of resection of the primary tumor, it is essential that all the gross tumor and the microscopic extensions are removed. If there is any question of submucosal spread of the tumor, the margins should be checked by frozen section examination in the operating room. The best chance of cure is after complete resection at the first operation rather than at subsequent salvage procedures. The treatment of a neck node requires complete neck dissection (either a classical radical or functional neck dissection) (Donegan, Gluckman, and Crissman, 1982).

Stage I tumors (no clinically evident neck metastases) do not require a prophylactic lymphadenectomy. However, in Stage II tumors there is a significant incidence of occult cervical neck metastases. As such, more advanced tumors even without palpable nodes should be treated with either a neck dissection or prophylactic radiation to the neck. Stages III and IV cancers of the anterior tongue are best treated with resection of the tumor together with a therapeutic neck dissection. In these more advanced cases, postoperative radiation therapy may also be considered as part of the initial treatment plan.

The surgical reconstruction of the resected site is based on the extent of the wound. T_1 tumors can usually be closed primarily or with local flaps without producing any significant functional deficit (Hovey, 1983; Chicarilli, 1987). Larger primary tumors leaving significant surgical defects require regional or more distant flap reconstruction, or free flaps to restore bulk and preserve motion of the remaining tongue musculature without tethering it. Larger resections of the tongue or the floor of the mouth require more tissue for the reconstruction, particularly if the mandible needs to be resected with the tumor. However, the authors believe that the mandible has all too often been resected unnecessarily either for surgical exposure or for the belief that this maneuver improves the cure rate. It must be remembered that the tumor usually is attached to or involves the alveolar portion of the mandible, and therefore this portion can be resected with the primary tumor leaving the lower (cortical) portion of the mandible intact to maintain the arch.

This maneuver obviates the need for reconstruction with bone grafts. On the other hand, the occasional far-advanced tumors that invade and destroy the mandible and do need to be resected segmentally may not need reconstruction if the mandibulectomy includes the body alone, preserving the opposite portion of the mandible as well as the entire symphysis and parasymphyseal area.

Results. The overall five year survival rates in patients with cancers of the mobile tongue and anterior floor of the mouth range between 30 and 60 per cent. In general, Stages I and II tumors of both sites do well by either surgical resection or radiation therapy. The decision for selecting one or the other modality is generally based on an assessment of the patient's individual needs and the clinical judgment and experience of the treating physicians at various centers. The dose of radiation therapy is usually in the range of 6000 to 6500 rads to the primary site. Interstitial radiation therapy has also been used for these tumors. Stages III and IV tumors do relatively poorly with either modality alone. Therefore, in most cases a combination of the two should be considered for proper treatment of the more advanced tumors. The primary tumor should be excised radically, and the neck nodes should be removed at the same time. In the postoperative period the patient should be treated with a course of radiation to the site of the primary and also to the neck if tumor is found in the lymph nodes after pathologic examination. The treatment of choice in the author's institution is postoperative radiation because it is associated with a lower complication rate of wound breakdown and infection. In significant tumors grouped in Stage IV, intraoperative radiation therapy is occasionally administered by the implantation of iodine seeds or iridium (Fig. 70–36). The use of intraoperative radiation has been reported by Son and Ariyan (1985) to provide significant control of advanced tumors.

LOWER ALVEOLUS (MANDIBULAR GINGIVA)

Cancers of the lower alveolar gingiva are the third most common type in the oral cavity and include the retromolar trigone. The lymphatic drainage is commonly to the jugulodigastric lymph nodes as well as to the submaxillary and midjugular chain. The probability of spread to cervical nodes is dependent on the extent of the primary tumor as follows: T_1, 10 to 15 per cent; T_2, 40 per cent; T_3, 50 per cent; and T_4, 70 per cent; also, 30 to 50 per cent of patients may demonstrate clinically positive nodes at the time of the initial examination (Lindberg, 1972; Byers and associates, 1981). Among these patients, 10 to 15 per cent are diagnosed as having a second primary, and 15 to 20 per cent of the patients are eventually found to have distant metastases. The most significant indicator of the patients' prognosis appears to be evidence of invasion of the tumor into the mandible. The two year survival rate for T_1 tumors is 83 per cent if the bone is not involved but drops to 66 per cent with bone invasion; for T_3 and T_4 tumors the prognosis falls from 67 to 20 per cent if bone is involved (Wald and Calcaterra, 1983).

The preferred treatment for Stages I and II tumors of the lower alveolus is surgical because of the proximity of tumor to bone, even if the mandible is not involved. Resection of

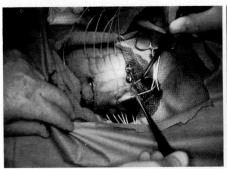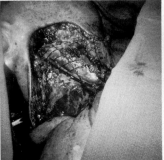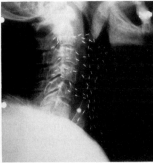

Figure 70–36. Intraoperative radiation may be applied either by iridium needles through Teflon catheters *(left)* or by radioactive iodine seeds incorporated within Vicryl suture *(center)*. The placement of the seeds can be calculated postoperatively to determine the proper dosage *(right)*.

the primary tumor with a marginal mandibulectomy and coverage of the defect with local flaps has been shown to be equally efficacious and far less deforming than segmental resection of the mandible (Wald and Calcaterra, 1983).

Selected patients with Stage III tumors may be treated with marginal mandibulectomy and postoperative radiation after the reconstruction (Wald and Calcaterra, 1983), but more advanced (Stage IV) tumors with gross invasion of bone should be managed by segmental resection of the mandible (Wald and Calcaterra, 1983; Ildstad, Bigelow, and Remensnyder, 1984). While reconstruction of the symphysis of the mandible is more complicated, it is necessary to avoid the significant deformity and disability caused by salivary leakage from an incontinent anterior floor of the mouth. The procedure may be carried out with conventional bone grafting or a secondary stage procedure with metal trays to avoid the high rate of complications of fistulas and infections. However, there can be a significant amount of wound contraction while the secondary reconstruction is awaited. At present, therefore, the availability of the vascularized composite flaps with bone (pectoralis major, trapezius, radial forearm, or iliac crest with deep circumflex vessels) has provided significant improvement in the ability to reconstruct these patients. The flaps can be transferred as single-stage procedures with minimal morbidity and significant restoration of the resected structures (see Fig. 70–33).

The overall five year survival rates for patients with cancers of the lower alveolus range from 50 to 65 per cent, with a significant drop in more advanced cases.

BUCCAL MUCOSA

Although cancers of the buccal mucosa account for only 10 per cent of malignant lesions of the oral cavity, they appear to have a higher distribution in the southeastern United States where "snuff dipping" is a common practice. While the overall incidence of oropharyngeal cancers is more common among men, the incidence of carcinoma of the buccal mucosa appears to be equally distributed among men and women (Ildstad, Bigelow, and Remensnyder, 1985). This is probably because of the frequent and common practice of "snuff dipping" among women in the Southeast. The lesions tend to occur frequently along the occlusal plane or just below it, and commonly involve the mandible more than the maxilla.

The lymphatic drainage of cancers of the buccal mucosa is primarily to the submaxillary nodes, followed in frequency by the jugulodigastric, preparotid, and jugular nodes. At the time of the initial presentation, lymph nodes are palpable in 40 to 50 per cent of the patients, and this frequency of nodal metastases is associated with the size of the primary tumor: T_1 to T_2, 30 to 35 per cent; T_3, 50 to 60 per cent (Vegers, Snow, and van der Waal, 1979; Bloom and Spiro, 1980; Ildstad, Bigelow, and Remensnyder, 1985). In these various studies, distant metastases were found in only 2 per cent of the patients but 11 per cent had developed metastases at the time of subsequent follow-up examination. Furthermore, second primaries were subsequently diagnosed in 14 to 29 per cent of the patients.

Cancers of the buccal mucosa are readily treated with surgical resection and reconstruction. Although local flaps and buccal flaps can be incorporated in the reconstruction of smaller lesions, resection of larger tumors requires reconstruction with more substantial flaps. The buccal mucosa requires thin flaps for reconstruction, and the deltopectoral flap is ideal for this purpose (Fig. 70–37). This technique requires a two-stage operation but gives a significantly better reconstruction than the bulkier myocutaneous flaps. In addition, microvascular transfer of jejunum as a "patch" flap or a radial forearm flap can also accomplish a similar type of thin flap reconstruction.

Stages III and IV cancers usually require a full-thickness cheek resection and more substantial reconstructions such as two flaps, one for lining and one for external coverage (Fig. 70–38) or double skin paddles on a single flap (Fig. 70–39).

Mandibulectomies and partial or total maxillectomies may also be necessary because of local invasion. Postoperative radiation should be incorporated to improve the local control rates. The overall five-year cure rates range from 40 to 60 per cent, with a significant decrease in Stages III and IV cancers (see Table 70–8).

HARD PALATE AND SUPERIOR ALVEOLUS

Cancers of the hard palate and superior alveolus are rare in the United States. As

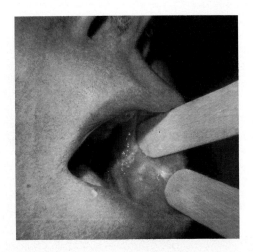

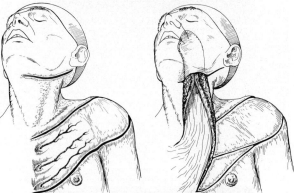

Figure 70–37. *Above,* Cancer of the buccal mucosa can be resected and the cheek resurfaced with a deltopectoral flap *(center, left* and *right)* that has been brought intraorally through a submandibular incision used for the neck dissection. *Below,* After division and inset of the flap there is thin, pliable coverage of the cheek.

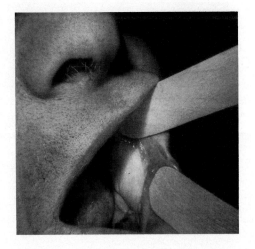

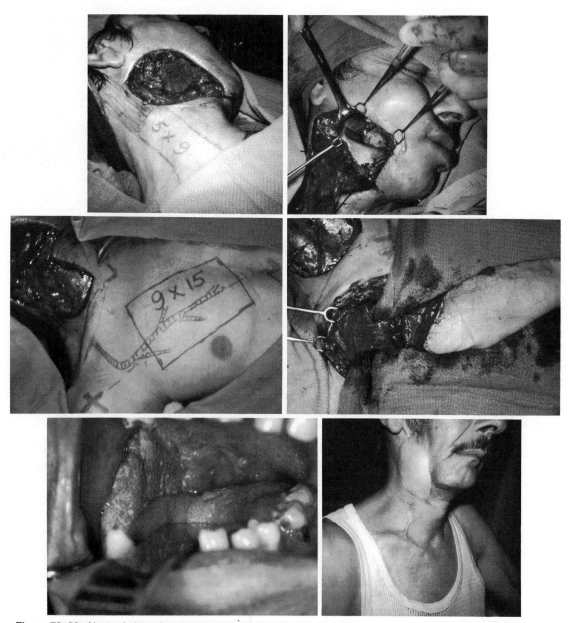

Figure 70–38. *Above,* A through and through defect of the cheek *(left)* is resurfaced intraorally with a superiorly based sternocleidomastoid *(SCM)* muscle flap *(right). Center,* The external coverage is provided with a pectoralis major *(PM)* myocutaneous flap *(left)* attached only by its vascular pedicle *(right). Below,* Late follow-up demonstrates the intraoral lining with the SCM flap *(left)* and the external coverage with the PM flap *(right).*

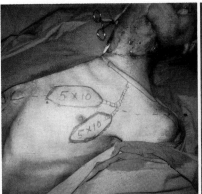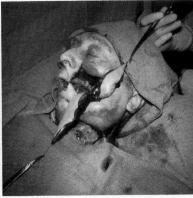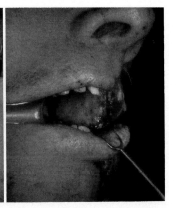

Figure 70–39. Two side by side paddles of skin on separate branches of the thoracoacromial artery of the pectoralis major can also be elevated *(left)* for reconstruction of a cheek. One paddle can be used for intraoral lining while the other can be employed for external coverage *(center)*. Later revision of the commissure shows the intact, thin cheek reconstruction *(right)*.

with buccal carcinomas, half of the cases occur among women. Lymphatic drainage is predominantly to the submaxillary and jugulodigastric lymph nodes; however, posterior palatal lesions frequently drain to the retropharyngeal lymph nodes. On initial examination, regional lymph nodes are clinically involved in one-third of the patients, and 10 to 15 per cent of patients develop distant metastases (Ratzer, Schweitzer, and Frazell, 1970; Konrad, Canalis, and Calcaterra, 1978; Ildstad, Bigelow, and Remensnyder, 1984). Because of the close proximity of the tumors to the facial bones and frequent skeletal involvement, radiation therapy is not the treatment of choice. Surgical resection requires local excision including alveolectomy or palatal resection to obtain adequate margins. More advanced tumors often require wider resections with total or hemimaxillectomies, and they are often treated with postoperative radiation. The reconstruction of the ablative sites is accomplished with large myocutaneous flaps or free flaps to provide adequate bulk. If a total maxillectomy is required, the globe should be preserved; this is often achieved by preservation of Lockwood's ligament. If there is no support to the globe, this can be provided with fascial slings or bone grafts to reconstruct the orbital floor. Alternatively, prosthodontists can employ prosthetic obturators to provide skeletal support to the soft tissue structures after these bony resections.

Because of the infrequent observation of cancers of this region, the data on survival rates and recurrences are limited. However,

it appears that the overall five year survival rate for palatal and superior alveolar tumors is between 20 and 55 per cent (Ratzer, Schweitzer, and Frazell, 1970; Konrad, Canalis, and Calcaterra, 1978; Mazzarella and Friedlander, 1982; Ildstad, Bigelow, and Remensnyder, 1984).

MANAGEMENT OF CANCERS OF PHARYNX

The pharynx is composed of three sites: the oropharynx, the nasopharynx, and the hypopharynx. Because of its proximity to the oral cavity, the oropharynx is also staged according to the measurement of the anatomic size of the tumor, as is the oral cavity. It is therefore appropriate to discuss this portion of the pharynx first.

Oropharynx

The most common sites of cancers of the oropharynx are the tonsillar fossa (43 per cent), soft palate (26 per cent), base of the tongue (20 per cent), and pharyngeal walls (11 per cent) (Zhang and associates, 1983).

TONSIL

Tonsillar cancers are the most common in the oropharynx. Because this anatomic area is rich with lymphatic tissue, metastases to cervical nodes occur frequently (70 to 90 per cent for all stages), and three-fourths of the patients already have metastases at the time of the diagnosis. The metastases of these cancers are most commonly to the submandibular, jugulodigastric, midjugular, or lower jugular lymph nodes. Bilateral metastases are seen in 11 per cent of cases (Lindberg, 1972).

The tumor frequently extends to adjacent structures, including the soft palate, pharyngeal wall, and tongue (Tong and associates, 1982). As the size of the tumors increases, the incidence of involvement of the tongue base increases, 60 to 90 per cent of the T_3 to T_4 lesions having tongue involvement. This is believed to be the major cause of failure to control the primary lesion with radiation therapy alone (Mantravadi, Liebner, and Ginde, 1978; Tong and associates, 1982). Second primary tumors occur in approximately 15 to 35 per cent of the patients, and distant metastases have been reported in as many as 20 per cent (Edstrom, Jeppsson, and Lindstrom, 1978; Givens, Johns, and Cantrell, 1981).

The results of treatment by surgery or radiation are the same for Stages I and II disease. Although surgical treatment of Stage I can be accomplished by local excision of the lesion through an intraoral approach and by leaving the wound to heal secondarily as in a tonsillectomy, Stage II lesions require more extensive exposure and resection. For this reason, most of these lesions are generally treated initially with radiation therapy. In addition, the neck should be treated because of the high incidence of metastases.

Stages III and IV cancers of the tonsil require wide resections, often including the soft palate, the pharyngeal walls, the base of the tongue, and occasionally the mandible. After the surgical resection, the operative site is reconstructed with distant myocutaneous flaps or free flaps to provide restoration of lining and bulk. Various attempts at reconstruction of the soft palate with flaps have uniformly failed because this is a unique structure with diminutive muscles and exceptionally thin mucosal lining. Therefore, restoration of velopharyngeal function after resection of the soft palate is best accomplished with a dental prosthesis (Fig. 70–40).

Although radiation therapy is less reliable for Stages III and IV cancers because of tumor extension to the base of the tongue, it should be considered as a postoperative adjuvant to increase the potential for local control. In addition, cervical lymphadenectomy or radiation therapy to the neck should be incorporated as part of the management because of the high incidence of nodal metastases, even in clinically negative necks.

The overall five year survival rates for patients with tonsillar cancers range from 25 to 60 per cent with further breakdown by Stage according to Table 70–9 (Wang, 1972; Shukovsky and Fletcher, 1973; Maltz and associates, 1974; Whicker, DeSanto, and Devine, 1974; Johnston and Byers, 1977; Mantravadi, Liebner, and Ginde, 1978; Edstrom,

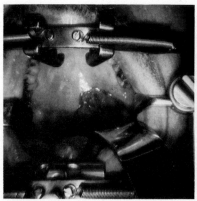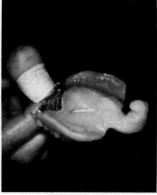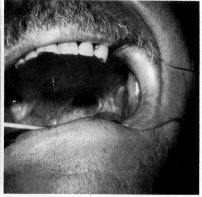

Figure 70–40. A cancer of the soft palate *(left)* was resected using frozen section controls. The resection included the entire soft palate, the left tonsillar fossa, the lateral pharyngeal wall, and two-thirds of the posterior pharyngeal wall. Because of the difficulty in reconstructing this site, the area was allowed to heal by secondary intention. To prevent nasal escape of air and fluids, a Silastic extension was fabricated to an upper denture *(center)* around which the wound contracted and epithelized *(right).* This permitted normal speech without nasal emission, and proper swallowing without nasal leakage.

Table 70–9. Five Year Survival Rates for Oropharyngeal Cancers (Percentages)

Site	\multicolumn{4}{c}{Stage}
	I	II	III	IV
Posterior tongue	55–70	50	30–40	0–20
Tonsil	65–90	40–85	25–50	5–35
Soft palate	50	25	30	30
Pharyngeal wall	75	70	40	25

Jeppsson, and Lindstrom, 1978; Givens, Johns, and Cantrell, 1981; Perez and associates, 1982; Tong and associates, 1982; Baris, van Andel, and Hop, 1983; Fayos and Morales, 1983; Garrett and Beale, 1983; Oreggia and associates, 1983; Remmler and associates, 1985).

SOFT PALATE

Cancers of the soft palate are the second most frequent type in the oropharynx. On initial examination 44 per cent of the patients present with palpable cervical lymph nodes, distributed as follows: T_1, 8 per cent; T_2, 37 per cent; T_3, 65 per cent; and T_4, 67 per cent (Lindberg, 1972). The tumors commonly drain to the jugulodigastric and midjugular lymph nodes, but on occasion may also spread to the retropharyngeal nodes, posterior triangle nodes, and lower jugular nodes. Bilateral lymph node metastases are found in 16 per cent of the patients, and second primaries are identified in subsequent follow-up in up to 24 per cent (Russ, Applebaum, and Sisson, 1977).

Either surgical treatment or radiation therapy is equally efficacious with early lesions (T_1, T_2) of the soft palate. For Stages III and IV disease, however, surgical resection requires removal of the tumor in the soft palate as well as extensions along the pharyngeal walls, along the base of the retromolar trigone, or cephalad to the pterygoid region. Therapeutic neck dissection and postoperative radiation should be incorporated as part of the treatment of these advanced cancers.

The overall five year survival rates range from 27 to 36 per cent (Ratzer, Schweitzer, and Frazell, 1970; Perussia, 1970; Russ, Applebaum, and Sisson, 1977; Snow and associates, 1977; Henk, 1978; Fee and associates, 1979) and can be further broken down by stage as noted in Table 70–9.

POSTERIOR TONGUE

Cancers of the base of the tongue (the posterior one-third) often present in more advanced stages because they remain asymptomatic until they are quite large. It is for this reason that three-fourths of the patients already have evidence of cervical lymph node metastases at the time of diagnosis. The tumors drain commonly to the jugulodigastric and midjugular nodes, and less frequently to the submaxillary regions. The frequency of lymph node metastasis according to tumor size is as follows: T_1 to T_2, 70 per cent; T_3, 75 per cent; and T_4, 85 per cent. Bilateral lymph nodes are diagnosed at the time of initial examination in 29 per cent of the cases (Lindberg, 1972). The tumor may spread to the larynx in 25 per cent of the patients and to the opposite half of the tongue in 50 per cent (Harrold, 1967). Second primary tumors are identified in up to 22 per cent (Whicker, DeSanto, and Devine, 1972).

As already mentioned, Stages I and II tumors of the base of the tongue are infrequent. They may be resected and closed primarily or with local flaps (Schechter and associates, 1980). However, larger tumors require extensive resection and larger flaps for the reconstruction (Fig. 70–41) to avoid aspiration. Occasionally, total glossectomy is necessary, frequently with total laryngectomy to prevent aspiration. However, the advent of the large myocutaneous flap has permitted the reconstruction of these ablative sites without the need for laryngectomy. Many of these patients have been able to eat without aspiration and to speak without difficulty. Five year survival rates for the base of the tongue range from 17 to 42 per cent.

PHARYNGEAL WALLS

Cancers of the pharyngeal walls are not common primary tumors, although they are often involved as secondary extensions from primary lesions of the oropharyngeal region or the larynx. The lymphatic drainage is commonly to the jugulodigastric and midjugular lymph nodes, and it occurs bilaterally in 15 to 20 per cent of the cases. At the time of the initial diagnosis, 60 per cent of the patients were found to have clinically palpable nodes, and this incidence increases with the size of the primary tumor as follows: T_1, 25 per cent; T_2, 30 per cent; T_3, 67 per cent; and

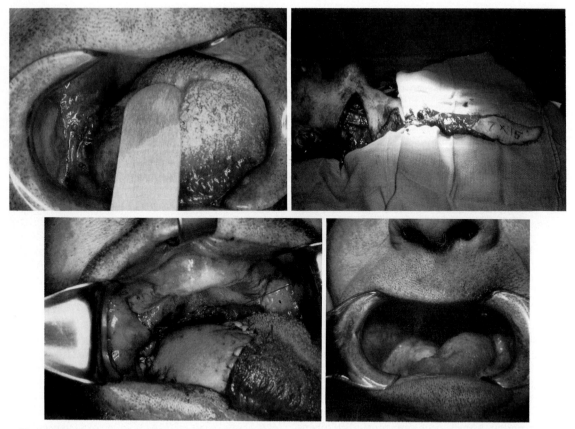

Figure 70–41. *Above,* A tumor of the retromolar trigone and base of the tongue *(left)* was resected and reconstructed with a pectoralis major flap *(right). Below,* The flap was used along the floor of the mouth and mid- to posterior tongue *(left)* to provide bulk and prevent leakage into the larynx. Normal mobility of the tongue was permitted *(right).*

T_4, 76 per cent (Henk, 1978; Guillamondegui, Meoz, and Jesse, 1978).

The therapeutic management of the early lesions of this site can be equally successful with either surgery or radiation therapy. While small lesions in Stage I can be surgically excised through the intraoral approach, the larger lesions require lateral pharyngotomy or a mandibular split to gain access to the tumor in order to perform the surgical resection with proper control of the margins. The extensive defects that result from the wide resections of the more advanced cancers can be reconstructed by any of the regional myocutaneous flaps. However, the jejunal free flap and the radial forearm free flap are ideally suited to provide a thin lining of well-vascularized tissue to the area without fear of subsequent contraction. Treatment of the neck nodes should be considered because of the high probability of regional spread with tumors classified as T_2 or greater. In the more advanced metastases to the neck, postoperative radiation therapy should be part of the adjuvant treatment following the neck dissection.

Nasopharynx

Nasopharyngeal carcinoma is an unusual tumor of the head and neck region that is associated with environmental and viral factors or with a genetic predisposition. There has been a consistent relationship with Epstein-Barr virus (EBV) among the Chinese. In addition, an increased incidence has been documented among workers in the nickel and chromium industry, woodworkers, and factory workers in the boot and shoe industry (Henderson and associates, 1976; Lin and associates, 1979; Neel, 1985).

The genetic predilection among the Chinese is seen with a distribution of 18 per cent of all the malignant neoplasms in the Chinese, as opposed to the Caucasian population in the U.S. where this disease makes up only 0.25 per cent of the malignancies (Hsu and associates, 1982). While native-born Chinese have a 118-fold incidence compared with Caucasians, the North America–born Chinese demonstrate only a sevenfold increase (Dickson, 1981), suggesting an influence by environmental factors on the genetic predisposition.

Tumors of the nasopharynx are classified by the World Health Organizaton (WHO) into three histologic types:

Type 1: Squamous cell carcinomas.

Type 2: Nonkeratinizing carcinomas or transitional cell carcinomas.

Type 3: Undifferentiated carcinomas including lymphoepitheliomas, anaplastic carcinomas, clear cell carcinomas, and spindle cell variants (Batsakis, Solomon, and Rice, 1981).

Squamous cell carcinomas (Type 1) account for 25 per cent of those in Caucasian patients in North America (Neel and associates, 1983).

In addition, elevated titers of antibodies to Epstein-Barr virus have been identified not only among people of Asian or African descent with primary recurrent nasopharyngeal carcinoma, but also among Americans with active nasopharyngeal carcinoma (Neel and associates, 1980). Analysis of the EBV titers has shown a greater association of the antibody with WHO Types 2 and 3 (85 per cent) than with Type 1 (15 per cent). Further studies using an antibody dependent cellular cytotoxicity assay have demonstrated a prognostic correlation with WHO Types 2 and 3 nasopharyngeal carcinoma (irrespective of Stage), with lower titers indicating a poor prognosis within each staging category (Neel, Pearson, and Taylor, 1984).

The nasopharynx is generally inaccessible to surgical resection because of its location at the skull base, making this tumor one generally treated with radiation therapy. The nasopharynx is a cuboidal space in the posterior nasal fossa that measures 3 by 5 cm. It is bounded posteriorly by the arch of the atlas and laterally by the mucosal walls that cover the palatine arches and the carotid artery; it is roofed by the base of the skull. The most frequent location of these tumors is along the lateral wall in the fossa of Rosenmüller (see Fig. 70–9), which is a slitlike mucosal fold posterior to the opening of the eustachian canal. Although the TNM staging of nasopharyngeal carcinoma is similar to that of other head and neck neoplasms, the T stage is based on local extension of the tumor rather than on measured size (see Table 70–4).

The lymphatic drainage most commonly involves the upper jugulodigastric lymph nodes and posterior cervical triangle nodes. Lymph nodes are palpable at the time of initial diagnosis in 60 per cent of the cases and the overall incidence of spread is in the range of 80 to 90 per cent (Lindberg, 1972; Baker, 1980). There appears to be no difference in the distribution of cervical metastases among the different T stages, since they are all between 80 and 90 per cent. However, lymph node metastases to both necks are seen in up to 50 per cent of the patients during the course of the disease, and this fact should be taken into consideration in planning treatment.

The treatment of choice is external beam radiation therapy in a dose of 6000 to 7000 rads over six to seven weeks, through bilateral opposing ports to the nasopharynx. Both necks should also be treated with radiation therapy to cover the micrometastases to these lymphatics. However, the increasing doses of radiation increase the risk of complications to the cranial base including necrosis, cranial nerve dysfunction, demyelinization, hypopituitarism, and transverse myelitis (Wang and Schulz, 1966; Ballantyne, 1975; Samaan and associates, 1982; Fogel, Weissberg, and Fischer, 1984). The dose of radiation to the neck may be lower (in the range of 5000 to 6000 rads by direct anterior fields) and should include the retropharyngeal lymph nodes because they are also a site of drainage.

The role of surgical therapy is limited to those patients with persistent involvement of the neck nodes after primary radiation therapy despite control of the tumor at the nasopharynx. In addition to cervical lymphadenectomy for recurrences, brachytherapy may be applied to recurrences in the primary site, using [192]iridium in a molded prosthesis placed in the nasopharynx. Alternatively, and in addition to surgical treatment radioactive seeds may also be implanted into the area by means of applicator needles.

The overall five year survival rates range from 35 to 50 per cent. Most studies also demonstrate a difference in the overall survival between the histologic types. The five year survival rate for WHO Type 1 range from 10 to 24 per cent, and those for Types 2 and 3 from 25 to 59 per cent (Urdaneta and associates, 1976; Tokars and Griem, 1979; Bedwinek, Perez, and Keys, 1980; Baker, 1980; Mesic, Fletcher, and Goepfert, 1981; Neel, 1985). Although early detection of disease in the nasopharynx is rare, in patients with disease limited to the nasopharynx (Stages I and II) the five year survival is 45 to 75 per cent; in those with regional distant disease (Stages III and IV), there is only a 14 to 43 per cent survival rate.

Hypopharynx

Squamous cell carcinoma of the hypopharynx is one of the most aggressive malignant tumors of the head and neck region since the diagnosis is rarely made early. Most patients present with extensive tumors of this region with little symptomatology, and often because of a large fixed mass in the neck. The hypopharynx is anatomically divided into three components. The *piriform sinus* is the most common site (68 to 81 per cent) of hypopharyngeal tumor in the U.S. It is bounded superiorly by the pharyngoepiglottic fold and inferiorly by its apex at the cricopharyngeal sphincter. The second most common site of these cancers is the *posterior pharyngeal wall* (15 to 18 per cent) and this is usually limited to the mucosal wall covering the prevertebral fascia. The *postcricoid region* is the third and least common area (4 to 15 per cent) and includes the mucosal covering of the posterior cricoid lamina.

The incidence of cervical lymph node metastases is as high as 80 per cent because of the rich lymphatics of this region. The primary sites of drainage are the jugulodigastric and midjugular node chains, and bilateral involvement is not unusual. The incidence of nodal metastases increases with the size and extent of the primary site as follows: T_1 to T_2, 60 to 70 per cent; T_3 to T_4, 75 to 80 per cent (Bakamjian, 1965; Marchetta, Sako, and Holyoke, 1967; Ballantyne, 1967; Lindberg, 1972). Furthermore, tumor invasion of the piriform region may also result in metastases to the retropharyngeal lymph nodes in 25 to 40 per cent of cases, and it is associated with a poor prognosis.

The most common presenting complaints in descending order of frequency are dysphagia, sore throat, neck mass, hoarseness, and hemoptysis (Keane, 1982). The symptoms often reflect an advanced stage of disease with involvement of the thyroid, cricoid, or arytenoid cartilages (Kirchner, 1975; Kirchner and Owen, 1977; Driscoll and associates, 1983). A thorough endoscopic examination is essential to determine the extent of the tumor, and part of the evaluation should also include a barium swallow and CT scans in the more extensive lesions. Furthermore, cancers of the hypopharynx are also notorious for submucosal spread and "skip lesions," in which the tumor may spread submucosally to adjacent sites with intact and normal-appearing intervening mucosa.

Cancers of the hypopharynx have been treated by surgery alone, radiation therapy alone, or a combination of the two. Treatment with radiation therapy alone has proved the least effective, with five year survival rates of 15 to 25 per cent (Son and Habermalz, 1979; Keane, 1982; Bataini and associates, 1982). Treatment with surgery alone has not proved much more effective, with survival rates of only 15 to 25 per cent (Razack and associates, 1977). However, the treatment combination of planned surgery and radiation therapy has provided the best control with five year survival rates of 30 to 55 per cent (Razack and associates, 1977; Son and Habermalz, 1979; El Badawi and associates, 1982; Arriagada and associates, 1983). Furthermore, controlled randomized prospective trials have shown that postoperative radiation therapy may clearly be better than preoperative radiation, with five year survival rates of 56 per cent versus 20 per cent (Van den Brouck and associates, 1977). The use of postoperative radiation has improved the clinical management by decreasing the postoperative complications of infection, wound dehiscence, fistulas, and carotid exposure (Son and Habermalz, 1979; El Badawi and associates, 1982). This is consistent with the experimental data demonstrating that irradiated tissue tolerates bacterial contamination poorly, leading to high infection rates (Ariyan and associates, 1980), and the delivery of parenteral antibiotics is significantly lower to the radiated tissue than to nonradiated tissues (Cruz and associates, 1984). An additional advantage of postoperative radiation is the ability to deliver a much larger dose to the postoperative site than is generally given preoperatively for fear of increased postoperative complications.

Early lesions of the piriform sinus at the lateral wall and those of the posterior pharyngeal wall that have not invaded the prevertebral fascia are most amenable to surgical resection while preserving the patient's voice. The surgical approach to the lesion is from an area uninvolved by tumor, in order to provide visual inspection of the resection with generous margins of 2 to 3 cm. This approach is best performed through a lateral pharyngotomy or a median lip-splitting incision to approach the hypopharynx. Frozen section examination should be made of the margins of the resection to detect occult mucosal spread. Reconstruction of small, ablative defects may be accomplished by local mucosal flaps. More extensive defects resulting from larger resections need to be closed with regional myocutaneous flaps, or microvascular free flaps to avoid tension while maintaining an adequate pharyngeal lumen. When it is determined that the closure has resulted in a tight pharynx, a cricopharyngeal myotomy may assist the passage of food and liquids. Otherwise, the piriform sinus reservoir is diminished and this leads to overflow into the larynx.

Early lesions of the medial anterior wall of the piriform sinus that did not extend to the apex and did not encroach upon the cricoid or posterior larynx may be treated by an extended hemilaryngectomy and partial pharyngectomy to preserve the voice (Ogura and Mallen, 1965). In this technique, the ipsilateral one-third to one-half of the larynx may be removed with the involved pharyngeal wall to obtain adequate surgical margins. The reconstruction is performed by mobilizing mucosal flaps from the lateral and posterior pharynx. Some surgeons have extended this technique to selected T_2 and T_3 lesions of the piriform wall, using hemicricolaryngopharyngectomy (Krespi and Sisson, 1984).

None of the lesions of the postcricoid larynx offers the option of surgical resection with preservation of the voice. Radiation is not a recommended option because of the intimate association of the tumor with the cartilage of the cricoid. Although on rare occasions some small lesions may be resected and the defect reconstructed with the remaining anterior larynx and trachea as an autograft, these are generally unusual cases (Som, 1956). For

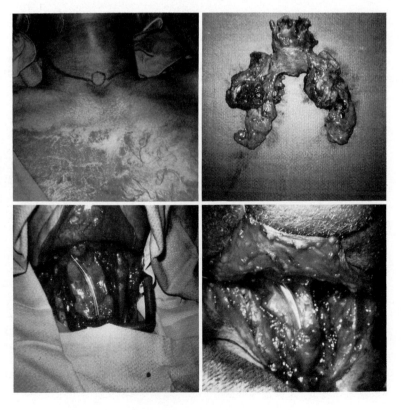

Figure 70–42. *Above,* An advanced (T_2N_2) carcinoma of the larynx *(left)* was treated with total laryngectomy and bilateral neck dissections *(right). Below,* The remaining cervical esophagus *(left)* was sutured over a nasogastric tube *(right)* to reestablish continuity between the pharynx and the esophagus.

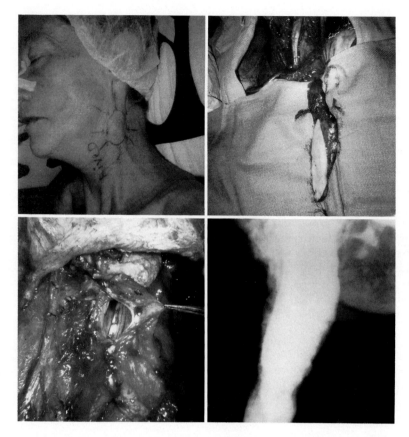

Figure 70–43. *Above,* A large tumor of the piriform region *(left)* required a laryngopharyngectomy. The cervical esophagus was reconstructed with a pectoralis major flap with skin from the medial aspect of the chest *(right). Below,* The skin paddle was used to reconstruct the esophagus over a nasogastric tube *(left).* Flow of food and fluids was demonstrated on a barium swallow *(right).*

most postcricoid tumors, the treatment of choice is a total laryngectomy and partial or total pharyngectomy, depending on the extent of tumor invasion into the pharyngeal walls. After the partial pharyngectomy, if there is sufficient mucosa for primary closure, this is performed over a soft feeding tube to provide an adequate lumen (Fig. 70–42). Since the healed mucosa can expand, this does not present a difficulty to the patient in swallowing food. If there is not sufficient mucosa to close over a No. 16 French catheter without tension, the missing tissue may be replaced with the pectoralis major myocutaneous flap (Fig. 70–43) (Theogaraj and associates, 1980; Ariyan, 1983). Other alternatives are the gastric pull-up (Krespi, Wurster, and Sisson, 1985), the free jejunal flap (Fig. 70–44) (Nahai and associates, 1984), and the microvascular free radial forearm flap (Fig. 70–45) (Harii and associates, 1985; Chicarilli and Price, 1986; Chicarilli, Ariyan, and Cuono, 1986b). Treatment of the neck is indicated for all stages of hypopharyngeal carcinoma because of the high incidence of metastases. Postoperative radiation therapy should be administered to the primary site as well as to both sides of the neck.

MANAGEMENT OF CANCERS OF LARYNX

The larynx is the most common site of squamous cell carcinoma in the head and neck area, making up 2 to 6 per cent of all the malignancies diagnosed in the U.S. (Shumrick, 1969; National Cancer Institute, 1974). The structure of the larynx extends from the vallecula to the inferior aspect of the cricoid cartilage lying anterior to the hypopharynx (see Fig. 70–1). It is divided into three regions: supraglottis, glottis, and subglottis. The *supraglottis* is embryologically derived from the buccopharyngeal remnant, whereas the *glottis* and *subglottis* originate from the tracheobronchial tree. This difference accounts for the poor prognosis of supraglottic tumors because of the higher predilection for lymphatic spread as in oropharyngeal tumors. On the other hand, glottic and subglottic tumors have a sparsity of

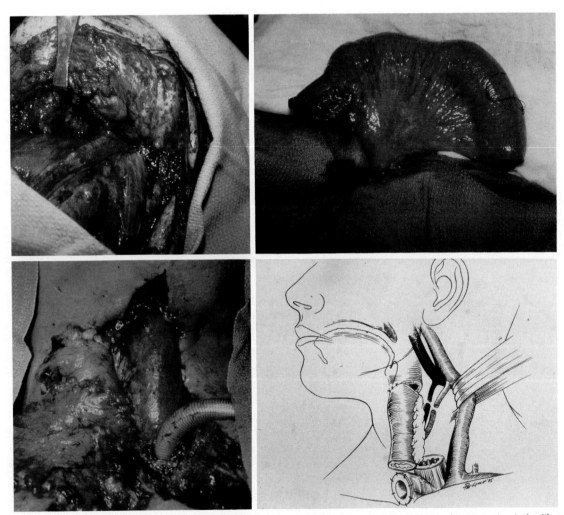

Figure 70–44. *Above,* The cervical esophagus following laryngopharyngectomy *(left)* can be reconstructed with a segment of jejunum *(right)*. *Below,* The segment of intestine can provide an excellent conduit between the pharynx and the esophagus *(left)* and the vessels can be anastomosed to an artery and vein in the neck *(right)*. (From Stahl, R. S.: Microvascular bowel transfer. *In* Ariyan, S.: Cancer of the Head and Neck. St. Louis, MO, C. V. Mosby Company, 1987.)

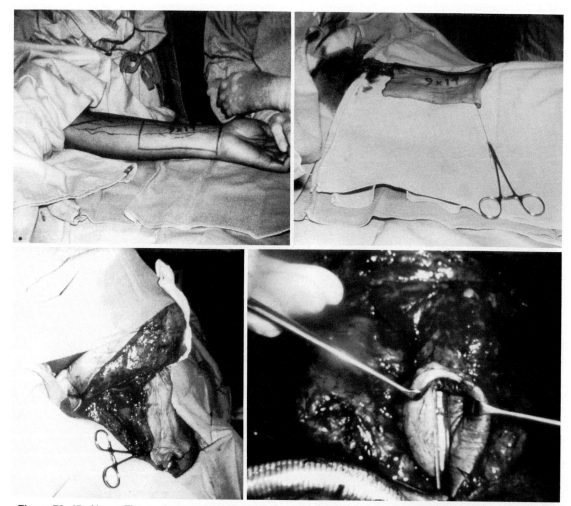

Figure 70–45. *Above,* The cervical esophagus can be reconstructed after laryngopharyngectomy with a radial forearm free flap *(left, right). Below,* The thin skin of the forearm can be sutured into a tube for the conduit between the pharynx and esophagus, and vascularized to an artery and vein in the neck *(left, right).* (From Chicarilli, Z. N., and Price, G.: Free forearm flap reconstruction of the esophagus. Plastic Surgery Educational Foundation Videotape Library, Chicago, 1987.)

lymphatics, and therefore tend to remain localized to their primary site until quite late in their growth phase.

The supraglottic larynx is further divided into the vallecula, the epiglottis, aryepiglottic folds, arytenoid, ventricular bands (false vocal cords), and ventricular cavities. Some surgeons further differentiate the supraglottis into the suprahyoid or infrahyoid portions. The suprahyoid portion appears to have a greater degree of lymphatic dissemination, and these tumors are more likely to extend to the adjacent oropharynx or hypopharynx. The infrahyoid region does not have as great a degree of lymphatic spread, and the tumors tend to be confined to the laryngeal framework with transglottic extension or invasion into the preepiglottic and paraglottic spaces to the thyroid cartilage. The glottic tumors are limited to the vocal cords and the commissures. The subglottic larynx is anatomically defined as that portion beginning 0.5 cm below the free edge of the true vocal cord and extending to the inferior aspect of the cricoid cartilage ring.

The cardinal sign of laryngeal cancer is a change in the character and quality of the voice of the patient, particularly with glottic tumors (up to 90 per cent of the cases) (English, 1976). Supraglottic and subglottic tumors are less likely to produce hoarseness until late in their course, since it requires a large bulk to muffle the pattern of the voice, or direct tumor extension into the vocal cords to affect abduction and adduction of the cords. Additional findings are sore throat (odynophagia), otalgia (referred pain to the ear), or dysphagia (difficulty in swallowing) (Daly and Strong, 1975). Patients who experience these symptoms for more than several weeks should undergo an indirect examination of the laryngopharynx.

The distribution of tumors in the larynx is most commonly in the glottic region (60 per cent) and less commonly in the supraglottic region (30 to 50 per cent). Although it is rare to have a primary tumor of the subglottic area (1 to 4 per cent of cases), it is not uncommon to find subglottic extension from tumors in the other areas of the larynx (Norris, 1969; Lee, 1974; Ogura and associates, 1975; Taskinen, 1975; Spector, 1978). The difficulty in staging the cancers of the larynx is in assessing the preepiglottic space (supraglottic), the thyroid cartilage (glottic), and submucosal spread to the glottic and subglot-

tic areas (Kirchner and Owen, 1977). It is also hard to assess the difference between an impaired cord and actual fixation.

The classification of the primary tumor of the larynx is based on involvement limited to one regional site, extension to adjacent structures within the larynx, and extension beyond the confines of the larynx (see Table 70–5). This also takes into consideration the mobility of the cord or the impairment of its motion. Laryngograms (with and without contrast), xeroradiograms, and CT scans of the larynx have been used to define the extent of the tumor for classification purposes.

The location of the tumor determines the probability of lymphatic spread. Supraglottic tumors confined to the epiglottis have a 20 per cent probability of lymphatic spread, whereas epiglottic tumors and tumors of the false cord have a lymph node metastatic rate of 50 to 55 per cent (Spector, 1978). True glottic tumors confined to the mobile vocal cord have a low incidence of metastases (0.4 to 2 per cent), while involvement of the anterior commissure or subglottis increases this incidence to 5 to 16 per cent (O'Keefe, 1959; Kirchner, 1970). Tumors originating in the subglottis or extending into the subglottis have an incidence of lymphatic spread of 23 per cent, while transglottic tumors have been shown to spread to cervical nodes in 30 to 55 per cent of cases (McGavran, Bauer, and Ogura, 1961; Bauer, Edwards, and McGavran, 1962; Spector, 1978).

The glottic tumors rarely spread to cervical nodes, the percentages being: T_1, 5 per cent; T_2, 8 per cent; and T_3, 15 per cent. Since the risk of cervical metastases is low, only transglottic and T_4 lesions require elective treatment of the neck (Daly and Strong, 1975; Spector, 1978). In these cases, the most common nodes involved are the midjugular lymph nodes, and the pretracheal (Delphian) and paratracheal nodes when subglottic extension is extensive.

SUPRAGLOTTIC TUMORS

Treatment of *supraglottic* tumors includes an attempt to preserve the voice. Stages I and II tumors are irradiated, and because of the high risk of occult nodal disease, the area for radiation therapy includes the neck within the ports. An alternative management for these tumors is horizontal (supraglottic) laryngectomy to remove the diseased portion of the larynx above the true vocal cords, in order to preserve the voice (Ogura, 1958; Som, 1959; Bocca, Pignataro, and Mosciaro, 1968). Aspiration, however, is a significant problem associated with supraglottic laryngectomy in the postoperative period, and therefore patients with preexisting impaired pulmonary function are not candidates for this conservation procedure. Furthermore, involvement of the ventrical or true vocal cords is another contraindication to the horizontal laryngectomy, whereas involvement of the arytenoids may permit this operation (Ogura, Sessions, and Ciralsky, 1975). The five year control rates and cure rates are similar for either surgery or radiation (including successful salvage with total laryngectomy) (Fu and associates, 1977). Some surgeons believe that surgical treatment of the early supraglottic tumors is better than primary irradiation, especially with ulcerated epiglottic involvement (Coates and associates, 1976). Therefore, irradiation is usually the treatment of choice for Stage I or II tumors because of the minimal morbidity, while Stages III and IV disease is best treated with laryngectomy with or without postoperative radiation to improve the local control rates. The overall five year determinate survival rate for supraglottic tumors is 37 to 57 per cent, and it is distributed by Stage: I, 69 to 88 per cent; II, 73 to 78 per cent; III, 50 to 68 per cent; and IV, 10 to 50 per cent (Norris, 1969; Coates and associates, 1976; Fu and associates, 1977; Spector, 1978).

GLOTTIC TUMORS

Glottic tumors have a number of therapeutic options, usually defined by the extent of the tumor. Tumors that are staged as T_1 respond equally well to treatment by radiation or by surgery (excision through the mouth or a vertical laryngectomy); both yield five year survival rates of up to 90 per cent. The determination of the proper choice of treatment modality is based on several considerations including the patient's choice. Radiation treatment is generally recommended, and often selected, because it preserves the voice with a minimum of morbidity (Kirchner and Fischer, 1975; Fayos, 1975), even though it has the disadvantage of a longer period of treatment. Vertical hemilaryngectomy (Ogura and Biller, 1969) is not usually recommended as the primary treatment for

T_1 lesions owing to the significant alteration in the voice it causes, despite the most successful of reconstructions. The one exception is for the treatment of verrucous carcinoma of the true vocal cord, because radiation therapy has not been found to be very effective for this disease (Myers, Sobol, and Ogura, 1980). In general, hemilaryngectomy is reserved for the salvage of T_1 tumors that have not responded to treatment by radiation, and the success of this treatment for recurrences is in the range of 60 to 70 per cent (Nichols, Stine, and Greenwald, 1980; Srensen, Hansen, and Thomsen, 1980). On the other hand, selective T_1 lesions of the true vocal cords that are limited to the mucosa or the membranous free edge may be chosen for endoscopic excision with microsurgical instruments or CO_2 laser with good success (Strong and Jako, 1972; Silver, 1981; Blakeslee and associates, 1984). If clear surgical margins cannot be obtained without deformity of the vocal cords, radiation can be given subsequently without compromise to cure.

Tumors staged as T_2 have lesser cure rates, ranging from 37 to 90 per cent, which are related to the depth of tumor invasion (Kirchner and Owen, 1977; Wang, 1983; Kaplan and associates, 1983). Nevertheless, radiation therapy is often chosen for primary treatment, reserving vertical hemilaryngectomy (or total laryngectomy) to salvage those tumors that resist a therapeutic dose of radiation. Vertical hemilaryngectomy is considered for primary treatment of tumors that invade the anterior commissure or extend subglottically beyond 5 mm of the cord, and those associated with involvement of the vocal process of the arytenoid; the alternative to radiation failure in these cases necessitates total laryngectomy and total loss of voice (Ogura and Biller, 1969; Ogura and Thawley, 1980; Karim and associates, 1980). More extensive tumors of the cord require total laryngectomy for cure. Partial vertical laryngectomy is not as successful because of the unpredictable submucosal extension and cartilage invasion (Kirchner, 1977, 1984). Radical radiation therapy is another option that preserves voice, but this has a significantly lower survival rate compared with total laryngectomy (30 to 50 per cent versus 60 per cent). The latter is reserved for salvage of recurrent tumors (Harwood, Bryce, and Rider, 1980). Nevertheless, some patients may elect to preserve the voice with primary treatment by radiation therapy, reserving laryngectomy for salvage in persistent tumors and accepting a lower survival rate (McNeil, Weichselbaum, and Pauker, 1981). Elective treatment of the neck should be considered for tumors with subglottic extension greater than 5 mm and transglottic tumors, since otherwise there is a relatively low incidence of occult metastases in T_3 lesions (7 to 15 per cent) (Daly and Strong, 1975; Spector, 1978; Ogura and Thawley, 1980).

Treatment of Stages III and IV tumors requires a total laryngectomy and postoperative radiation to the primary tumor as well as to both necks to improve local control rates (Yuen and associates, 1984).

SUBGLOTTIC TUMORS

Primary tumors of the subglottic region are too rare to gather meaningful statistical information. When the tumor is limited to less than one-half the circumference of the cricoid, extensive hemilaryngectomy may be performed to preserve function of the vocal cord. Larger lesions are treated with either radiation therapy or total laryngectomy plus radiation therapy for the paratracheal and upper mediastinal lymph nodes.

MANAGEMENT OF PARANASAL SINUS CANCERS

Cancers of the paranasal sinuses represent only 3 per cent of all malignancies of the head and neck region. There are four pairs of paranasal sinuses: maxillary, ethmoid, frontal, and sphenoid. The most common tumors are located in the maxillary antrum (75 to 80 per cent), followed by ethmoid cancers (15 to 20 per cent), while tumors of the frontal and sphenoid sinuses account for less than 1 per cent. Eighty per cent of the tumors are squamous cell carcinomas, and the remaining 20 per cent are adenocarcinomas (Badib and associates, 1969; Tabb and Barranco, 1971).

The greatest difficulty in managing tumors of the paranasal sinuses is making the initial diagnosis at an early stage. Tumors of this region are often silent or may mimic common inflammatory disorders until the tumor is sufficiently extensive to invade adjacent structures. Therefore, the clinician must have a high degree of suspicion to make the diagnosis in a patient with a persistent unilateral opacified sinus unresponsive to medical management (Eichel, 1977). Patients commonly present with the clinical symptoms and signs of local pressure or pain of the sinus, epistaxis, or toothache. As the tumor invades adjacent structures, there are additional symptoms of facial numbness and swelling, epiphora (tearing), diplopia, and proptosis (Weymuller, Reardon, and Nash, 1980). Metastases of the tumor to regional lymph nodes are rare except late in the course, and this finding generally carries an extremely poor prognosis. The lymphatic drainage of the maxillary sinuses and the anterior and middle ethmoid cells is to the submandibular lymph nodes. The posterior ethmoid cells have a predilection for the retropharyngeal lymph nodes.

When a tumor of the maxillary sinus is suspected, a diagnostic biopsy is required. Tumor may occasionally be seen in the nasal vault on intranasal examination and a biopsy may be performed. More commonly the Caldwell-Luc approach to the sinus must be employed for biopsy purposes. After the tissue diagnosis is made of a malignancy, the extent of the tumor must be further assessed with radiographs and CT scans. A lateral skull radiograph demonstrating the maxillary sinus can localize the tumor into the infrastructure (anterior and inferior) or suprastructure (posterior and superior to Öhngren's line) (Öhngren, 1933), a line drawn from the medial canthus of the orbit to the angle of the mandible (see Fig. 70–2). It was recognized that the tumors above this line were more likely to invade critical structures (e.g., pterygomaxillary space, orbital contents, or nasal base). They are associated with a poor prognosis and are therefore included in the criteria for classification of maxillary tumors (Table 70–10). The ethmoid, frontal,

Table 70–10. Primary Tumor (T) Classification of Maxilla

T_x	Tumor cannot be assessed
T_1	Tumor confined to infrastructure (with no bone erosion)
T_2	Tumor confined to suprastructure (with no bone erosion) or tumor of infrastructure with destruction of bone (medial or inferior walls only)
T_3	More extensive tumor invading anterior ethmoid sinuses, orbit, skin of cheek, or pterygoid muscles
T_4	Massive tumor with invasion of posterior ethmoid sinuses, cribriform plate, sphenoid, nasopharynx, pterygoid plates, or base of skull

and sphenoid sinuses are too infrequently involved for a meaningful classification to be devised for therapeutic management. While the plain radiographs provide a rough estimate of tumor volume (Robin and Powell, 1981), CT scans provide a higher degree of correlation of the actual extent of disease and invasion of bordering structures (Kondo and associates, 1982). The scans are critical to evaluating the extent of disease (Fig. 70–46), especially at the skull base, and to planning the appropriate surgical procedure (Lund, Howard, and Lloyd, 1983). The treatment of tumors limited to the infrastructure with subtotal or total maxillectomy alone has been associated with good results (60 per cent) (Becker and Atiyah, 1985). However, the same treatment for larger tumors has considerably poorer results at five years (35 per cent) (Lewis and Castro, 1972). The tumors treated with radiation alone have had poor survival rates (12 to 15 per cent) (Larsson and Martensson, 1953; Marchetta and associates, 1969; Bataini and Ennuyer, 1971).

The early cancers of the maxillary antrum (T_1 and T_2) are treated with a maxillectomy (see also Chap. 68). A Weber-Ferguson incision is made along the lower eyelash line, the paranasal fold, and the alar base; it splits the lip to expose the maxilla in the subperiosteal plane (Fig. 70–47), if the tumor has not invaded through the bony wall. If the tumor has eroded through the anterior maxillary wall, a cuff of soft tissue must be left on the maxilla at the time of elevation of the flap. Final assessment for preservation of the orbit is made by exploring the orbital floor and determining the possibility of extension of tumor into the orbital contents. If the orbital floor is intact and the tumor is limited and

localized to the infrastructure, a subtotal maxillectomy may be carried out. If the tumor erodes through the orbital floor, the periosteum of the orbit should be included with the specimen. If the periosteum is invaded with tumor, orbital exenteration is indicated. Tumors that are well localized to the medial maxillary wall can be considered for medial maxillectomy, which includes the medial half of the maxilla and the ethmoid sinuses to achieve adequate surgical margins.

More extensive tumors of the antrum (T_3 to T_4) require accurate assessment of the extent of disease along the cranial base to determine those patients who require a combined craniofacial resection (Ketcham and associates, 1963, 1966). These more extensive tumors require a craniotomy to determine the resectability (see also Chap. 69). If the tumor does not involve the intracranial base and the sinus can be resected, the osteotomies can be performed from both exposures (intracranial and extracranial) to remove the involved structures. If the intracranial dura needs to be resected, this can be resurfaced with a pericranial flap (Johns and associates, 1981), while the external defects following the maxillectomy may be repaired with myocutaneous flaps and microvascular free flaps to cover the wounds and to minimize cerebrospinal fluid leaks and meningitis (Ariyan, 1983; Sasaki and associates, 1985; Swartz and associates, 1986; Chicarilli and Davey, 1987). Postoperative radiation therapy is given to the primary site and to the neck in the more extensive cases (Jesse, 1965).

The overall five year survival rates for cancers of the maxillary sinus, with the combination of surgery and radiation, range from 40 to 50 per cent (Sisson, 1970; Ketcham and associates, 1973; Schramm, Myers, and Maroon, 1979; Terz, Young, and Lawrence, 1980). The cure rates for early tumors (T_1 and T_2) are better (45 to 60 per cent) than for patients with advanced disease (T_3 and T_4), which are sufficiently low (28 to 38 per cent) to indicate the need for early diagnosis. Neck dissection is considered for the tumors that grossly extend to the oral cavity and hard palate, and those that are found to be associated with subsequent nodal involvement (seen in 30 to 40 per cent of cases) (Harrison, 1971; Larsson and Martensson, 1972; Lee and Ogura, 1981). Despite these reports, the treatment of antral cancers usually fails because of local wound recurrence. Patients who have lymph node involvement usually do not

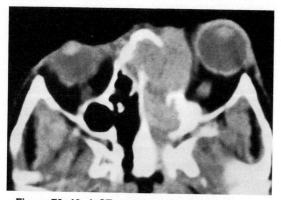

Figure 70–46. A CT scan demonstrating a tumor in the right ethmoid region penetrating the medial orbital wall and causing pressure on the globe and proptosis.

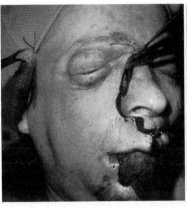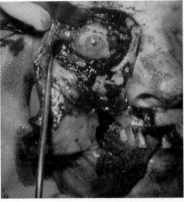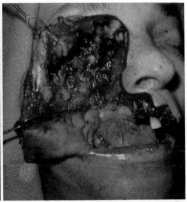

Figure 70–47. A Weber-Ferguson incision *(left)* is used to elevate a cheek flap by splitting the lip and folding under the lower lid margin. The approach provides access to the maxilla *(center)* to perform a complete orbitomaxillary resection *(right)*.

survive five years, a finding that may support treating the neck nodes only when they subsequently become positive after the primary tumor has remained under control (Öhngren, 1933; Norris, 1963; Sisson, 1970; Harrison, 1971; Hyams, 1971; Larsson and Martensson, 1972; Ketcham and associates, 1973; Vrabec, 1975; Suh and associates, 1977; Schramm, Myers, and Maroon, 1979; Terz, Young, and Lawrence, 1980; Weymuller, Reardon, and Nash, 1980; Lee and Ogura, 1981; Robin and Powell, 1981; Kondo and associates, 1982; Lund, Howard, and Lloyd, 1983).

THE UNKNOWN PRIMARY

Patients occasionally present with palpable lymph nodes or masses in the neck, and yet a primary tumor cannot be identified. In children and adolescents, persistent lymphadenopathy is probably due to benign disease (85 per cent), most commonly representing inflammatory lymph nodes. The remaining 15 per cent are malignant tumors of lymphatic origin, or are due to rhabdomyosarcomas (Southwick, Slaughter, and Majarakis, 1959; Moussatos and Baffes, 1963; Jaffe, 1973).

On the other hand, 80 to 85 per cent of cervical masses in adults represent malignant disease, and this figure rises to 90 per cent in patients over the age of 50 (Winegar and Griffin, 1973). A thorough examination of the upper aerodigestive tract usually reveals a primary carcinoma that originates from the oropharynx in 40 per cent, the lar-yngopharynx in 40 per cent, the thyroid in 10 per cent, and other sites in the remaining 10 per cent (Montgomery, 1973).

Certain tumors of the head and neck area have predilection for different cervical nodal chains. Cancer of the mid- and upper jugular or high posterior triangle nodes are most likely to be metastatic from the upper aerodigestive tract or the thyroid gland, while tumors presenting in nodes in the supraclavicular or lower posterior triangle are usually metastatic from organs in the infraclavicular site (breast, lung, gastrointestinal tract). Lymphomas and cutaneous melanomas may also present as cervical masses, but these have a less predictable pattern (Comess, Beahrs, and Dockerty, 1957; Batsakis, 1981; Johnson and Newman, 1981).

The appropriate work-up of patients who present with a cervical mass without a known primary following a thorough clinical evaluation includes indirect nasopharyngeal and laryngopharyngeal mirror examination. This should be followed by a thin needle aspiration biopsy of the mass for cytology and cell block examination under the microscope. If the diagnosis of a carcinoma is made, direct endoscopic examination should be performed under anesthesia and should include random biopsies of Waldeyer's ring to include the common sites of early metastases (tonsils, base of the tongue, hypopharynx) as well as biopsies of the nasopharynx. If the primary site is not identified, therapy should be directed toward the lymphatics in the neck with either a cervical lymphadenectomy, radiation therapy to the neck, or a combination of the two (Jose and associates, 1979; Simpson, 1980; Roseman and James, 1982; Spiro, DeRose, and Strong, 1983; Yang and associates, 1983). Five year survival rates with treatment to the neck range from 25 to 50 per cent (Barrie, Knapper, and Strong, 1970; Leipzig, Winter, and Hokanson, 1981; Schwarz, Hamberger, and Jesse, 1981; Spiro, DeRose, and Strong, 1983; Yang and associates, 1983), and no significant differences in survival have been noted if the primary site eventually becomes evident.

The variable that seems to affect both recurrence and survival rates is an open biopsy of the neck mass combined with a delay in the definitive therapy for the neck. Regional recurrence rates and distant metastases have been reported in 20 per cent of the patients who have been treated definitively without open biopsy, while those treated with an open biopsy have a 50 per cent increase in recurrent neck disease and twice the incidence of distant metastases (McGuirt and McCabe, 1977). However, there was no difference in the number of recurrences and distant metastases if the open biopsy was performed at the time of the definitive treatment. Therefore, if a needle biopsy is inconclusive or negative for tumor and an open biopsy is considered after a thorough work-up, this should be performed under general anesthesia, with the patient prepared for a formal neck dissection if cancer is found.

In summary, adult patients who present with a neck mass of unknown etiology should undergo a systematic search for the possible site of a primary malignancy so that appropriate staging and therapy can be initiated. Fine needle aspiration and random endoscopic biopsies may aid in the diagnosis and localization of the tumor. Open biopsies of the neck mass should be avoided unless needle biopsy is equivocal or negative; definitive therapy with neck dissection should be performed concomitantly if carcinoma is identified at the time of the open biopsy.

REFERENCES

Absolon, K. B., Rogers, W., and Aust, J. B.: Some historical developments of the surgical therapy of tongue cancer from the seventeenth to the nineteenth century. Am. J. Surg., *104*:686, 1962.

Acheson, E. D., Hadfield, E. H., and Macbeth, R. G.: Carcinoma of the nasal cavity and accessory sinuses in woodworkers. Lancet, *1*:311, 1967.

Acheson, E. D., Pippard, E. C., and Winter, P. D.: Nasal cancer in the Northamptonshire boot and shoe industry: is it declining? Br. J. Cancer, *46*:940, 1982.

Ackerman, L. V.: Verrucous carcinoma of the oral cavity. Surgery, *23*:670, 1948.

Ahlbom, H. E.: Simple achlorhydric anaemia, Plummer-Vinson syndrome, and carcinoma of the mouth, pharynx, and oesophagus in women. Br. Med. J., *2*:331, 1936.

Ariyan, S.: The pectoralis major myocutaneous flap. A versatile flap for reconstruction in the head and neck area. Plast. Reconstr. Surg., *63*:73, 1979a.

Ariyan, S.: One-stage reconstruction for defects of the mouth using the sternomastoid myocutaneous flap. Plast. Reconstr. Surg., *63*:618, 1979b.

Ariyan, S.: Functional radical neck dissection. Plast. Reconstr. Surg., *65*:768, 1980a.

Ariyan, S.: The viability of rib grafts transplanted with the periosteal blood supply. Plast. Reconstr. Surg., *65*:140, 1980b.

Ariyan, S.: The pectoralis major for single-stage reconstruction of difficult wounds of the orbit and pharyngoesophagus. Plast. Reconstr. Surg., *72*:468, 1983.

Ariyan, S., and Finseth, F. J.: The anterior chest approach for obtaining free osteocutaneous rib grafts. Plast. Reconstr. Surg., *62*:676, 1978.

Ariyan, S., and Krizek, T. J.: Reconstruction after resection of head and neck cancer. Cine Clinics. Clinical Congress of the American College of Surgeons, Dallas, TX, October, 1977.

Ariyan, S., Marfuggi, R. A., Harder, G., and Goodie, M. M.: An experimental model to determine the effects of adjuvant therapy on the incidence of postoperative wound infection. I. Evaluating preoperative radiation therapy. Plast. Reconstr. Surg., *65*:328, 1980.

Arriagada, R., Eschwege, F., Cachin, Y., and Richard, J. M.: The value of combining radiotherapy with surgery in the treatment of hypopharyngeal and laryngeal cancers. Cancer, *51*:1819, 1983.

Baclesse, F.: Carcinoma of the larynx. Br. J. Radiol., Suppl. *3*, 1949.

Baclesse, F.: L'étalement ou le "fractionment" dans la roentgen therapie seule des epitheliomas du pharynx et du larynx, de l'uterus et du vagin, du sien. Acta Union Internationales Contra le Cancrum, *9*:29, 1953.

Badib, A. O., Kurohara, S. S., Webster, J. H., and Shedd, D. P.: Treatment of cancer of the paranasal sinuses. Cancer, *23*:533, 1969.

Bagshaw, M. A., and Thompson, R. W.: Elective irradiation of the neck in patients with primary carcinoma of the head and neck. J.A.M.A., *217*:456, 1971.

Bakamjian, V. Y.: A two-stage method for pharyngoesophageal reconstruction with a primary pectoral skin flap. Surgery, *36*:173, 1965.

Baker, S. R.: Nasopharyngeal carcinoma: clinical course and results of therapy. Head Neck Surg., *3*:8, 1980.

Ballantyne, A. J.: Principles of surgical management of cancer of the pharyngeal walls. Cancer, *20*:663, 1967.

Ballantyne, A. J.: Late sequelae of radiation therapy in cancer of the head and neck with particular reference to the nasopharynx. Am. J. Surg., *130*:433, 1975.

Banoczy, J.: Follow-up studies in oral leukoplakia. J. Maxillofac. Surg., *5*:69, 1977.

Banoczy, J., and Csiba, A.: Occurrence of epithelial dysplasia in oral leukoplakia. Oral Surg., *42*:766, 1976.

Baris, G., van Andel, J. G., and Hop, W. C.: Carcinoma of the tonsillar region. Strahlentherapie, *159*:138, 1983.

Barrie, J. R., Knapper, W. H., and Strong, E. W.: Cervical node metastases of unknown origin. Am. J. Surg., 120:466, 1970.

Barwick, W. J., Goodkind, D., and Serafin, D.: The free scapular flap. Plast. Reconstr. Surg., 69:779, 1982.

Bataini, J. P., Brugere, J., Bernier, J., Jaulerry, C. H., Picot, C., and Ghossein, N. A.: Results of radical radiotherapeutic treatment of carcinoma of the pyriform sinus: experience of the Institut Curie. Int. J. Radiat. Oncol. Biol. Phys., 8:1277, 1982.

Bataini, J. P., and Ennuyer, A.: Advanced carcinoma of the maxillary antrum treated by cobalt teletherapy and electron beam irradiation. Br. J. Radiol., 44:590, 1971.

Batsakis, J. G.: The pathology of head and neck tumors. The occult primary and metastases to the head and neck, Part 10. Head Neck Surg., 3:409, 1981.

Batsakis, J. G., Solomon, A. R., and Rice, D. H.: The pathology of head and neck tumors: carcinoma of the nasopharynx, Part II. Head Neck Surg., 3:511, 1981.

Bauer, W. C., Edwards, D. L., and McGavran, M. H.: A critical analysis of laryngectomy in the treatment of epidermoid carcinoma of the larynx. Cancer, 15:263, 1962.

Becker, S. P., and Atiyah, R. A.: Nasal and paranasal malignancies. Carcinoma of the paranasal sinuses. Otolaryngol. Clin. North Am., 18:491, 1985.

Bedwinek, J. M., Perez, L. A., and Keys, D. J.: Analysis of failures after definitive irradiation for epidermoid carcinoma of the nasopharynx. Cancer, 45:2725, 1980.

Beecroft, W. A., Sako, K., Razack, M. S., and Shedd, D. P.: Mandible preservation in the treatment of cancer of the floor of the mouth. J. Surg. Oncol., 19:171, 1982.

Bertino, J. R., Boston, B., and Capizzi, R. L.: The role of chemotherapy in the management of cancer of the head and neck: a review. Cancer, 36:752, 1975.

Blakeslee, D., Vaughan, C. W., Shapshay, S. M., Simpson, G. T., and Strong, M. S.: Excisional biopsy in the selective management of T₁ glottic cancer. A three-year follow-up study. Laryngoscope, 94:488, 1984.

Bloom, N. D., and Spiro, R. H.: Carcinoma of the cheek mucosa. Am. J. Surg., 140:556, 1980.

Bocca, E., and Pignataro, O.: A conservation technique in radical neck dissection. Ann. Otol. Rhinol. Laryngol., 76:975, 1967.

Bocca, E., Pignataro, O., and Mosciaro, O.: Supraglottic surgery of the larynx. Ann. Otol. Rhinol. Laryngol., 77:1005, 1968.

Bocca, E., Pignataro, O., and Sasaki, C. T.: Functional neck dissection. A description of operative technique. Arch. Otolaryngol., 106:524, 1980.

Brown, R. L., Suh, J. M., Scarborough, J. E., Wilkins, S. A., and Smith, R. R.: Snuff dippers' intraoral cancer: clinical characteristics and response to therapy. Cancer, 18:2, 1965.

Buschke, F., Cantril, S. T., and Parker, H. M.: Supervoltage Roentgen Therapy. Springfield, IL, Charles C Thomas, 1950.

Butlin, H. T.: On early diagnosis of cancer of the tongue and on the results of operations in such cases. Br. Med. J., 1:462, 1909.

Byers, R. M., Newman, R., Russell, N., and Yue, A.: Results of treatment for squamous cell carcinoma of the lower gum. Cancer, 47:2236, 1981.

Cann, C. I., and Fried, M. P.: Determinants and prognosis of laryngeal cancer. Otolaryngol. Clin. North Am., 17:139, 1984.

Cawson, R. A., and Binnie, W. H.: Candida leukoplakia and carcinoma: a possible relationship. In MacKensie, I. C., Dabelsteen, E., and Squier, C. A. (Eds.): Oral Premalignancy. Iowa City, University of Iowa Press, 1980, p. 59.

Chandler, J. R., Guillamondegui, O. M., Sisson, G. A., Strong, E. W., and Baker, H. W.: Clinical staging of cancer of the head and neck: a new "new" system. Am. J. Surg., 132:525, 1976.

Chicarilli, Z. N.: Sliding posterior tongue flap. Plast. Reconstr. Surg., 79:697, 1987.

Chicarilli, Z. N., and Ariyan, S.: Physiology, anatomy, and application of musculocutaneous flaps. In Condon, R. E., and DeCosse, J. J. (Eds.): Surgical Care II. Philadelphia, Lea & Febiger, 1985, p. 351.

Chicarilli, Z. N., Ariyan, S., and Cuono, C. B.: Single-stage repair of complex scalp and cranial defects with the free radial forearm flap. Plast. Reconstr. Surg., 77:577, 1986a.

Chicarilli, Z. N., Ariyan, S., and Cuono, C. B.: Free radial forearm flap versatility for the head and neck and lower extremity. J. Reconstr. Microsurg., 2:221, 1986b.

Chicarilli, Z. N., and Davey, L.: Free rectus abdominis reconstruction of a radical cranio-orbito-maxillary resection for neurofibrosarcoma. Plast. Reconstr. Surg., 80:726, 1987.

Chicarilli, Z. N., and Price, G.: Immediate free radial forearm flap reconstruction of the esophagus following laryngopharyngoesophagectomy. Videotape Sessions. American Society of Reconstructive Microsurgery, New Orleans, LA, February, 1986.

Chierici, G., Silverman, S., Jr., and Forsythe, B.: A tumor registry study of oral squamous carcinoma. J. Oral Med., 23:91, 1968.

Coates, H. L., DeSanto, L. W., Devine, K. D., and Elveback, L. R.: Carcinoma of the supraglottic larynx. Arch. Otolaryngol., 102:686, 1976.

Coleman, C. C., Jr., and Hoopes, J. E.: The treatment of radionecrosis with persistent cancer of the head and neck. Am. J. Surg., 106:716, 1963.

Comess, M. S., Beahrs, O. H., and Dockerty, M. B.: Cervical metastases from occult carcinoma. Surg. Gynecol. Obstet., 104:607, 1957.

Conway, H., and Hugo, N. E.: Radiation dermatitis and malignancy. Plast. Reconstr. Surg., 38:255, 1966.

Coutard, H.: Results and methods of treatment of cancer by radiation. Ann. Surg., 106:584, 1937.

Crile, G.: Excision of cancer of the head and neck with special reference to plan of dissection based on 132 operations. J.A.M.A., 47:1780, 1906.

Crile, G. W.: Tubage of the pharynx for facilitating the administration of anesthetics and preventing the inhalation of blood in certain operations on the mouth and face. Ann. Surg., 37:859, 1903.

Cruz, N. I., Ariyan, S., Miniter, P., and Andriole, V. T.: An experimental model to determine the level of antibiotics in irradiated tissue. Plast. Reconstr. Surg., 73:811, 1984.

Cuono, C. B., and Ariyan, S.: Immediate reconstruction of a composite mandibular defect with a regional osteomusculocutaneous flap. Plast. Reconstr. Surg., 65:477, 1980.

Daly, C. J., and Strong, E. W.: Carcinoma of the glottic larynx. Am. J. Surg., 130:489, 1975.

Daniel, J.: The x-rays. New Science, 3:562, 1896.

Deconti, R. C., and Schoenfeld, D.: A randomized prospective comparison of intermittent methotrexate, methotrexate with leucovorin, and a methotrexate combination in head and neck cancer. Cancer, 48:1061, 1981.

Demergasso, F., and Piazza, M. V.: Trapezius myocutaneous flap in reconstructive surgery for head and neck cancer. An original technique. Am. J. Surg., 138:533, 1979.

deThe, G., Ho, J. H., Ablashi, D. V., Day, N. E., Macario, A. J., et al.: Nasopharyngeal carcinoma. IX. Antibodies to EBNA and correlation with response to other EBV antigens in Chinese patients. Int. J. Cancer, 16:713, 1975.

Dickson, R. I.: Nasopharyngeal carcinoma: an evaluation of 209 patients. Laryngoscope, 91:333, 1981.

Doll, R., Morgan, L. G., and Speizer, F. E.: Cancer of the lung and nasal sinuses in nickel workers. Br. J. Cancer, 24:623, 1970.

Donegan, J. O., Gluckman, J. L., and Crissman, J. D.: The role of suprahyoid neck dissection in the management of cancer of the tongue and floor of the mouth. Head Neck Surg., 4:209, 1982.

Dorn, H. F., and Cutler, S. J.: Morbidity from cancer in the United States. Part I: Variation in incidence by age, sex, marital status, and geographic region. Public Health Monograph 56, 1958.

Drelichman, A., Cummings, G., and Al-Sarraf, N.: A randomized trial of the combination of cis-platinum, oncovin, and bleomycin (COB) versus methotrexate in patients with advanced squamous cell carcinoma of the head and neck. Cancer, 52:399, 1983.

Driscoll, W. G., Nagorsky, M. S., Cantrell, R. W., and Johns, M. E.: Carcinoma of the pyriform sinus: analysis of 102 cases. Laryngoscope, 93:556, 1983.

Dufresne, C., Cutting, C., Valauri, F., Klein, M., Colen, S., and McCarthy, J. G.: Reconstruction of mandibular and floor of mouth defects using the trapezius osteomyocutaneous flaps. Plast. Reconstr. Surg., 79:687, 1987.

Edstrom, S., Jeppsson, P. H., and Lindstrom, J.: Carcinoma of the tonsillar region. Laryngoscope, 88:1019, 1978.

Eichel, B. S.: The medical and surgical approach in management of the unilateral opacified antrum. Laryngoscope, 187:737, 1977.

El Badawi, S. A., Goepfert, H., Herson, J., Fletcher, G. H., and Oswald, M. J.: Squamous cell carcinoma of the pyriform sinus. Laryngoscope, 92:357, 1982.

English, G. M.: Malignant neoplasms of the larynx. In English, G. M. (Ed.): Otolaryngology. Hagerstown, MD, Harper & Row, 1976.

Fayos, J. V.: Carcinoma of the endolarynx: results of irradiation. Cancer, 35:1525, 1975.

Fayos, J. V., and Lampe, I.: Treatment of squamous cell carcinoma of the oral cavity. Am. J. Surg., 124:493, 1972.

Fayos, J. V., and Morales, P.: Radiation therapy of carcinoma of the tonsillar region. Int. J. Radiat. Oncol. Biol. Phys., 9:139, 1983.

Fee, W. E., Jr., Schoeppel, S. L., Rubenstein, R., Goffinet, D. R., Goode, R. L., et al.: Squamous cell carcinoma of the soft palate. Arch. Otolaryngol., 105:710, 1979.

Ferrara, J., Beaver, B. L., Young, D., and James, A. G.: Primary procedure in carcinoma of the tongue: local resection versus combined local resection and radical neck dissection. J. Surg. Oncol., 21:245, 1982.

Fischman, S. L., and Martinez, I.: Oral cancer in Puerto Rico. J. Surg. Oncol., 9:163, 1977.

Fletcher, G. H.: Radiation Therapy in the Management of Cancers of the Oral Cavity and Oropharynx. Springfield, IL, Charles C Thomas, 1962.

Fletcher, G. H.: Elective irradiation of subclinical disease in cancers of the head and neck. Cancer, 29:1450, 1972.

Fogel, T. D., Weissberg, J. B., and Fischer, J. J.: Endocrinopathy following radiation to the head and neck. Int. J. Radiat. Oncol. Biol. Phys., 10:167, 1984.

Frieben, E. A.: Cancroid des rechten Handruckens nach langdavernder Einwirkung von Roentgenstrahlen. Fortschr. Roentgenstr., 6:106, 1902.

Fry, H. J. B.: Syphilis and malignant disease: a serologic study. Br. J. Hygiene, 29:313, 1929.

Fu, K. K., Eisenberg, L., Dedo, H., and Phillips, T. L.: Results of integrated management of supraglottic carcinoma. Cancer, 40:2874, 1977.

Garrett, P. G., and Beale, E. A.: Carcinoma of the oropharynx and tonsil. J. Otolaryngol., 12:125, 1983.

Givens, C. D., Jr., Johns, M. E., and Cantrell, R. W.: Carcinoma of the tonsil. Arch. Otolaryngol., 107:730, 1981.

Gluck, T., and Sorensen, J.: Die Resektion und Extirpation des Larynx, Pharynx, und Esophagus. In Katz, L., Preysing, H., and Blumenfeld, F. (Eds.): Handbuch der Speziellen Chirugie des Ohres und der Oberen Luftwege. Vol. IV. Wurzburg, C. Kabitzsch, 1914.

Goldberg, N. H., Cuono, C. B., Ariyan, S., and Enriquez, R. E.: Improved reliability in tumor diagnosis by fine needle aspiration. Plast. Reconstr. Surg., 67:492, 1981.

Graham, S., Dayal, H., Rohrer, T., Swanson, M., Sultz, H., Shedd, D., and Fischman, S.: Dentition, diet, tobacco, and alcohol in the epidemiology of oral cancer. J. Natl. Cancer Inst., 59:1611, 1977.

Guillamondegui, O. M., Meoz, R., and Jesse, R. H.: Surgical treatment of squamous cell carcinoma of the pharyngeal walls. Am. J. Surg., 136:474, 1978.

Gupta, P. C., Mehta, F. S., Daftary, D. R., Pindborg, J. J., Bhonsle, R. B., et al.: Incidence rates of oral cancer and natural history of oral precancerous lesions in a ten year follow-up study of Indian villagers. Community Dent. Oral Epidemiol., 8:283, 1980.

Gussenbauer, C.: Über die erste durch Th. Billroth an Menschen ausgefuhrte Kehlkopf-Extirpation und die Auswendung eines kuntslichen Kehlkopfes. Arch. Klin. Chir., 17:343, 1874.

Hamberger, A. D., Fletcher, G. H., Guillamondegui, O. M., and Byers, R. M.: Advanced squamous cell carcinoma of the oral cavity and oropharynx treated with irradiation and surgery. Radiology, 119:433, 1976.

Hanna, D. C.: The composite operation. In Gaisford, J. C. (Ed.): Symposium on Cancer of the Head and Neck. Vol. 2. St. Louis, MO, C. V. Mosby Company, 1969.

Harii, K., Ebihara, S., Ono, I., Saito, H., Tervi, S., and Takato, T.: Pharyngoesophageal reconstruction using a fabricated forearm free flap. Plast. Reconstr. Surg., 75:463, 1985.

Harrison, D. F. N.: The management of malignant tumors of the nasal sinuses. Otolaryngol. Clin. North Am., 4:159, 1971.

Harrold, C. C.: Surgical treatment of cancer at the base of the tongue. Am. J. Surg., 114:493, 1967.

Harwood, A. R., Bryce, D. P., and Rider, W. D.: Management of T_3 glottic cancer. Arch. Otolaryngol., 106:697, 1980.

Hausen, B. M.: Woods Injurious to Human Health: A Manual. New York, De Gruyter, 1981.

Henderson, B. E., Louie, E., SooHoo-Jing, J., Buell, P.,

and Gardner, M. B.: Risk factors associated with nasopharyngeal carcinoma. N. Engl. J. Med., 295:1101, 1976.

Henk, J. M.: Results of radiotherapy for carcinoma of the oropharynx. Clin. Otolaryngol., 3:137, 1978.

Hirata, R. M., Jaques, D. A., Chambers, R. G., Tuttle, J. R., and Mahoney, W. D.: Carcinoma of the oral cavity; an analysis of 478 cases. Ann. Surg., 182:98, 1975.

Hoffmeister, F. S., Macomber, W. B., and Wang, M. K.: Cancer of the oral cavity, larynx, and pharynx: radiation or surgery? Am. J. Surg., 116:615, 1968.

Hong, W. K., Schaeffer, S., Issell, B., et al.: A prospective randomized trial of methotrexate versus cisplatin in the treatment of recurrent squamous cell carcinoma of the head and neck. Cancer, 52:206, 1983.

Hong, W. K., Shapshay, S. M., Bhutani, R., Craft, M. L., Ucmakli, A., et al.: Induction chemotherapy in advanced squamous head and neck carcinoma with high dose cis-platinum and bleomycin infusion. Cancer, 44:19, 1979.

Hovey, L. M.: Hemi-tongue advancement following anterior hemiglossectomy. Plast. Reconstr. Surg., 71:552, 1983.

Hsu, M. M., Huang, S. C., Lynn, T. C., Hsieh, T., and Tu, S. M.: The survival of patients with nasopharyngeal carcinoma. Otolaryngol. Head Neck Surg., 90:289, 1982.

Hyams, V. J.: Papillomas of the nasal cavity and paranasal sinuses: a clinicopathological study of 315 cases. Ann. Otol. Rhinol. Laryngol., 80:192, 1971.

Ildstad, S. T., Bigelow, M. E., and Remensnyder, J. P.: Squamous cell carcinoma of the mobile tongue. Am. J. Surg., 145:443, 1983.

Ildstad, S. T., Bigelow, M. E., and Remensnyder, J. P.: Squamous cell carcinoma of the alveolar ridge and palate. Ann. Surg., 199:445, 1984.

Ildstad, S. T., Bigelow, M. E., and Remensnyder, J. P.: Clinical behavior and results of current therapeutic modalities for squamous cell carcinomas of the buccal mucosa. Surg. Gynecol. Obstet., 160:254, 1985.

Jabaley, M. E., Clement, R. L., and Bryant, W. M.: Recognizing oral lesions. Am. Fam. Physician, 13:604, 1976.

Jacobs, C., Meyers, F., Hendrickson, C., Kohler, M., and Carter, S.: A randomized phase III study of cisplatin with or without methotrexate for recurrent squamous cell carcinoma of the head and neck. A Northern California Oncology Study Group. Cancer, 52:1563, 1983.

Jaffe, B. F.: Pediatric head and neck tumors: a study of 178 cases. Laryngoscope, 83:1644, 1973.

Jesse, R. H.: Preoperative versus postoperative radiation in the treatment of squamous cell carcinoma of the paranasal sinuses. Am. J. Surg., 110:552, 1965.

Jesse, R. H.: The philosophy of treatment of neck nodes. Ear Nose Throat J., 56:125, 1977.

Jesse, R. H., Barkely, H. T., Jr., Lindberg, R. D., and Fletcher, G. H.: Cancer of the oral cavity. Is elective neck dissection beneficial? Am. J. Surg., 120:505, 1970.

Jesse, R. H., and Lindberg, R. G.: Efficacy of combining radiation therapy with a surgical procedure in patients with cervical metastases from squamous cancer of the oropharynx and hypopharynx. Cancer, 35:1163, 1975.

Johns, M. E., Winn, H. R., McLean, W. C., and Cantrell, R. W.: Pericranial flap for the closure of defects of craniofacial resections. Laryngoscope, 91:952, 1981.

Johnson, J. T., and Newman, R. K.: The anatomic location of neck metastasis from occult squamous cell carcinoma. Otolaryngol. Head Neck Surg., 89:54, 1981.

Johnston, W. D., and Byers, R. M.: Squamous cell carcinoma of the tonsil in young adults. Cancer, 39:632, 1977.

Jose, B., Bosch, A., Caldwell, W. L., and Frias, Z.: Metastasis to neck from unknown primary tumor. Acta Radiol. Oncol. Radiat. Phys. Biol., 18:161, 1979.

Joseph, D. L., and Shumrick, D. L.: Risks of head and neck surgery in previously irradiated patients. Arch. Otolaryngol., 97:381, 1973.

Kaplan, M. J., Johns, M. E., McLean, W. C., Fitz-Hugh, G. S., Clark, D. A., et al.: Stage II glottic carcinoma: prognostic factors and management. Laryngoscope, 93:725, 1983.

Karim, A. B., Snow, G. B., Ruys, P. N., and Bosch, H.: The heterogeneity of the T2 glottic carcinoma and its local control probability after radiation therapy. Int. J. Radiat. Oncol. Biol. Phys., 6:1653, 1980.

Keane, T. J.: Carcinoma of the hypopharynx. J. Otolaryngol., 11:227, 1982.

Keller, A. Z., and Terris, M.: The association of alcohol and tobacco with cancer of the mouth and pharynx. Am. J. Public Health, 55:1578, 1965.

Kennedy, J. T., Krause, C. J., and Loevy, S.: The importance of tumor attachment to the carotid artery. Arch. Otolaryngol., 103:70, 1977.

Ketcham, A. S., Chretien, P. B., VanBuren, J., Hoye, R. C., Beazley, R. M., and Herdt, J. R.: The ethmoid sinuses: a re-evaluation of surgical resection. Am. J. Surg., 126:469, 1973.

Ketcham, A. S., Hoye, R. C., Chretien, P. B., and Brace, K. C.: Irradiation twenty-four hours preoperatively. Am. J. Surg., 118:691, 1969.

Ketcham, A. S., Hoye, R. C., VanBuren, J. M., Johnson, R. H., and Smith, R. R.: Complications of intracranial facial resection for tumors of the paranasal sinuses. Am. J. Surg., 112:591, 1966.

Ketcham, A. S., Wilkins, R. H., VanBuren, J. M., and Smith, R. R.: A combined intracranial facial approach to the paranasal sinuses. Am. J. Surg., 106:698, 1963.

Khadim, M. I.: The effects of Pan and its ingredients on oral mucosa. J.P.M.A., 27:353, 1977.

Kies, M. S., Percaro, B. C., Gordon, L. I., Hauck, W. W., Kraut, W. J., et al.: Preoperative combination chemotherapy for advanced stage head and neck cancer. Promising early results. Am. J. Surg., 148:367, 1984.

Kirchner, J. A.: Cancer at the anterior commissures of the larynx; results with radiotherapy. Arch. Otolaryngol., 91:524, 1970.

Kirchner, J. A.: Pyriform sinus cancer: a clinical and laboratory study. Ann. Otol. Rhinol. Laryngol., 84:793, 1975.

Kirchner, J. A.: Two hundred laryngeal cancers: patterns of growth and spread as seen in serial sections. Laryngoscope, 87:474, 1977.

Kirchner, J. A.: Pathways and pitfalls in partial laryngectomy. Ann. Otol. Rhinol. Laryngol., 93:301, 1984.

Kirchner, J. A., and Fischer, J. J.: Anterior commissure cancer—a clinical and laboratory study of 39 cases. Can. J. Otolaryngol., 4:637, 1975.

Kirchner, J. A., and Owen, J. R.: Five hundred cancers of the larynx and pyriform sinus. Results of treatment by radiation and surgery. Laryngoscope, 87:1288, 1977.

Knowlton, A. H., Percarpio, B., Bobrow, S., and Fischer, J. J.: Methotrexate and radiation therapy in the treatment of advanced head and neck tumors. Radiology, 116:709, 1975.

Kocher, E. T.: Ueber Radicalheilung des Krebses. Deutsche Ztschr. Chir., 13:134, 1880.

Kondo, M., Horiuchi, M., Shiga, H., Inuyama, Y., Dokiya, T., et al.: Computed tomography of malignant tumors of the nasal cavity and paranasal sinuses. Cancer, *50*:226, 1982.

Konrad, H. R., Canalis, R. F., and Calcaterra, T. C.: Epidermoid carcinoma of the palate. Arch. Otolaryngol., *104*:208, 1978.

Kramer, I. R.: Precancerous conditions of oral mucosa: a computer aided study. Ann. R. Coll. Surg. Engl., *45*:340, 1969.

Kramer, I. R., El-Labban, N., and Lee, K. W.: The clinical features and risk of malignant transformation in sublingual keratosis. Br. Dent. J., *144*:171, 1978.

Krespi, Y. P., and Sisson, G. A.: Voice preservation in pyriform sinus carcinoma by hemicricolaryngopharyngectomy. Ann. Otol. Rhinol. Laryngol., *93*:306, 1984.

Krespi, Y. P., Wurster, C. F., and Sisson, C. A.: Immediate reconstruction after total laryngopharyngoesophagectomy and mediastinal dissection. Laryngoscope, *95*:156, 1985.

Larsson, L. G., and Martensson, G.: Carcinoma of the paranasal sinuses and the nasal cavities. Acta Radiol., *42*:149, 1953.

Larsson, L. G., and Martensson, G.: Maxillary antral cancers. J.A.M.A., *219*:342, 1972.

Lawrence, W., Jr., Tera, J. J., Rogers, C., King, R. E., Wolf, J. S., and King, E. R.: Preoperative irradiation for head and neck cancer: a prospective study. Cancer, *33*:318, 1974.

Lee, F., and Ogura, J. H.: Maxillary sinus carcinoma. Laryngoscope, *91*:133, 1981.

Lee, J. G.: Detection of residual carcinoma of the oral cavity, oropharynx, hypopharynx, and larynx: a study of surgical margins. Trans. Am. Acad. Ophthalmol. Otolaryngol., *78*:49, 1974.

Lehner, T., Shillitoe, E. J., Wilton, J. M., and Ivanyi, L.: Cell mediated immunity to herpes virus Type I in carcinoma and precancerous lesions. Br. J. Cancer, *28*:128, 1973.

Leipzig, B., Winter, M. L., and Hokanson, J. A.: Cervical nodal metastases of unknown origin. Laryngoscope, *91*:593, 1981.

Leonard, J. R., and Hass, A. C.: Management of cancer of the oral cavity: the trend toward combined radiotherapy and surgery. Am. J. Surg., *120*:514, 1970.

Lewis, J. B., and Castro, E. B.: Cancer of the nasal cavity and paranasal sinuses. J. Laryngol. Otol., *86*:255, 1972.

Lin, T. M., Yang, C. S., Tu, S. M., Chen, C. J., Kuo, K. C., and Hirayama, T.: Interaction of factors associated with cancer of the nasopharynx. Cancer, *44*:1419, 1979.

Lindberg, R. D.: Distribution of cervical lymph node metastases from squamous cell carcinoma of the upper respiratory and digestive tracts. Cancer, *29*:1446, 1972.

Lindberg, R. D., and Fletcher, G. H.: The role of irradiation in the management of head and neck cancer. Analysis of results and causes of failure. Tumori, *64*:313, 1978.

Lindberg, R. D., Jesse, R. H., and Fletcher, G. H.: Radiotherapy—before or after surgery? *In* Anderson Hospital and Tumor Institute: Neoplasia of the Head and Neck. Clinical Conference on Cancer, Chicago, Year Book Medical Publishers, 1974.

Lund, V. J., Howard, D. J., and Lloyd, G. A.: CT evaluation of paranasal sinus tumours for craniofacial resection. Br. J. Radiol., *56*:439, 1983.

MacFee, W. F.: Transverse incisions for neck dissection. Ann. Surg., *151*:279, 1960.

Maltz, R., Shumrick, D. A., Aron, B. S., and Weichert, K. A.: Carcinoma of the tonsil: results of combined therapy. Laryngoscope, *84*:2172, 1974.

Mantravadi, R. V., Liebner, E. J., and Ginde, J. V.: An analysis of factors in the successful management of cancer of the tonsillar region. Cancer, *41*:1054, 1978.

Marchetta, F. C., and Sako, K.: Preoperative irradiation for squamous carcinoma of the head and neck. Does it improve five-year survival or control figures? Am. J. Surg., *130*:487, 1975.

Marchetta, F. C., Sako, K., and Holyoke, E. D.: Squamous cell carcinoma of the pyriform sinus. Am. J. Surg., *114*:507, 1967.

Marchetta, F. C., Sako, K., Mattick, W. L., and Stinziano, G. D.: Squamous cell carcinoma of the maxillary antrum. Am. J. Surg., *118*:805, 1969.

Marchetta, F. C., Sako, K., and Murphy, J. B.: The periosteum of the mandible and intraoral carcinoma. Am. J. Surg., *122*:711, 1971.

Martin, H.: Radical surgery in cancer of the head and neck; the changing trends in treatment. Surg. Clin. North Am., *33*:329, 1953.

Martin, H., Del Valle, B., Ehrlich, H., and Cahan, W. G.: Neck dissection. Cancer, *4*:441, 1951.

Martin, H. E.: Surgery of Head and Neck Tumors. New York, Hoeber-Harper, 1957.

Martinez, S. A., Oller, D. W., Gee, W., and deFries, H. O.: Elective carotid artery resection. Arch. Otolaryngol., *101*:744, 1975.

Mashberg, A.: Erythroplasia vs. leukoplasia in the diagnosis of early asymptomatic oral squamous carcinoma. Editorial. N. Engl. J. Med., *297*:109, 1977.

Mashberg, A.: Reevaluation of toluidine blue application as a diagnostic adjunct in the detection of asymptomatic oral squamous carcinoma: a continuing prospective study of oral cancer III. Cancer, *46*:758, 1980.

Mashberg, A.: Tolonium (toluidine blue) rinse—a screening method for recognition of squamous carcinoma. Continuing study of oral cancer IV. J.A.M.A., *245*:2408, 1981.

Mashberg, A., Garfinkel, L., and Harris, S.: Alcohol as a primary risk factor in oral squamous carcinoma. Cancer, *31*:146, 1981.

Masse, L.: Epidemiology of cancer of the oesophagus in Brittany. Typescript of special lecture in the University of London, 1972.

Mazzarella, L. A., Jr., and Friedlander, A. H.: Intraoral hemimaxillectomy for the treatment of cancer of the palate. Oral Surg., *54*:157, 1982.

McCoy, G. D.: A biochemical approach to the etiology of alcohol related cancers of the head and neck. Laryngoscope (Suppl. 8), *88*:59, 1978.

McGavran, M. H., Bauer, W. C., and Ogura, J. H.: The incidence of cervical lymph node metastases from epidermoid carcinoma of the larynx and their relationship to certain characteristics of the primary tumor. Cancer, *14*:55, 1961.

McGregor, I. A.: The temporal flap in intra-oral cancer: its use in repairing the post-excisional defect. Br. J. Plast. Surg., *16*:318, 1963.

McGuirt, W., and McCabe, B. F.: Correlation of wound necrosis, local recurrence, distant metastases with time of biopsy. Clin. Trends, May–June, 1977.

McNeil, B. J., Weichselbaum, R., and Pauker, S. G.: Speech and survival: tradeoffs between quality and quantity of life in laryngeal cancer. N. Engl. J. Med., *305*:982, 1981.

Mendelson, B. C., Woods, J. E., and Beahrs, O. H.: Neck dissection in the treatment of carcinoma of the anterior two-thirds of the tongue. Surg. Gynecol. Obstet., 143:75, 1976.

Meoz-Mendez, R. T., Fletcher, G. H., Guillamondegui, O. M., and Peters, L. J.: Analysis of the results of irradiation in the treatment of squamous cell carcinomas of the pharyngeal walls. Int. J. Radiat. Oncol. Biol. Phys., 4:579, 1978.

Mesic, J. B., Fletcher, G. H., and Goepfert, H.: Megavoltage irradiation of epithelial tumors of the nasopharynx. Int. J. Radiat. Oncol. Biol. Phys., 7:447, 1981.

Million, R. R., Fletcher, G. H., and Jesse, R. H., Jr.: Evaluation of elective irradiation of the neck for squamous-cell carcinoma of the nasopharynx, tonsillar fossa, and base of tongue. Radiology, 80:973, 1963.

Montgomery, W. W.: Surgery of the Upper Respiratory System. Vol. II. Philadelphia, Lea & Febiger, 1973.

Moussatos, G. H., and Baffes, T. G.: Cervical masses in infants and children. Pediatrics, 32:251, 1963.

Myers, E., Sobol, S., and Ogura, J. H.: Hemilaryngectomy for verrucous carcinoma of the glottis. Laryngoscope, 90:693, 1980.

Nahai, F., Stahl, R. S., Hester, T. R., and Clairmont, A. A.: Advanced applications of revascularized free jejunal flaps for difficult wounds of the head and neck. Plast. Reconstr. Surg., 74:778, 1984.

National Cancer Institute Third National Cancer Survey, Washington, DC, 1974.

Neel, H. B., III: Nasopharyngeal carcinoma. Clinical presentation, diagnosis, treatment, and prognosis. Otolaryngol. Clin. North Am., 18:479, 1985.

Neel, H. B., III, Pearson, G. R., and Taylor, W. F.: Antibody-dependent cellular cytotoxicity. Relation to stage and disease course in North American patients with nasopharyngeal carcinoma. Arch. Otolaryngol., 110:742, 1984.

Neel, H. B., III, Pearson, G. R., Weiland, L. H., Taylor, W. F., Goepfert, H. H., et al.: Anti-EBV serologic tests for nasopharyngeal carcinoma. Laryngoscope, 90:1981, 1980.

Neel, H. B., III, Pearson, G. R., Weiland, L. H., Taylor, W. F., Goepfert, H. H., et al.: Application of Epstein-Barr virus serology to the diagnosis and staging of North American patients with nasopharyngeal carcinoma. Otolaryngol. Head Neck Surg., 91:255, 1983.

Nichols, R. D., Stine, P. H., and Greenwald, K. J.: Partial laryngectomy after radiation failure. Laryngoscope, 90:571, 1980.

Norris, C. M.: Laryngectomy and neck dissection. Otolaryngol. Clin. North Am., 2:667, 1969.

Norris, H. J.: Papillary lesions of the nasal cavity and paranasal sinuses. II. Inverting papillomas: a study of 29 cases. Laryngoscope, 73:1, 1963.

O'Brien, J. C.: Oropharyngeal tumors. Selected Readings in Plastic Surgery Syllabus, Vol. 2, No. 10, December, 1982.

Ogura, J. H.: Supraglottic subtotal laryngectomy and radical neck dissection for carcinoma of the epiglottis. Laryngoscope, 68:983, 1958.

Ogura, J. H., and Biller, H. F.: Conservation surgery in cancer of the head and neck. Otolaryngol. Clin. North Am., 2:641, 1969.

Ogura, J. H., and Mallen, R. W.: Partial laryngopharyngectomy for supraglottic and pharyngeal carcinoma. Trans. Am. Acad. Ophthalmol. Otolaryngol., September—October, 1965.

Ogura, J. H., Sessions, D. G., and Ciralsky, R. H.: Supraglottic carcinoma with extension to the arytenoid. Laryngoscope, 85:1327, 1975.

Ogura, J. H., Sessions, D. G., Spector, G. J., Alonso, W., and Griffiths, C. M.: Long-term therapeutic results—cancer of the larynx and hypopharynx. Preliminary report. Laryngoscope, 85:1746, 1975.

Ogura, J. H., and Thawley, S. E.: Cysts and tumors of the larynx. In Paparella, M. M., and Shumrick, D. A. (Eds): Otolaryngology. Vol. III. Philadelphia, W. B. Saunders Company, 1980, pp. 2504—2527.

Öhngren, L. G.: Malignant tumors of the maxillo-ethmoidal region. Acta Otolaryngol. (Suppl.), 19:1, 1933.

O'Keefe, J. J.: Evaluation of laryngectomy with radical neck dissection. Laryngoscope, 69:914, 1959.

Oreggia, F., DeStefani, E., Deneo-Pellegrini, H., and Olivera, L.: Carcinoma of the tonsil. Arch. Otolaryngol., 109:305, 1983.

Paterson, D. R.: A clinical type of dysphagia. J. Laryngol., 24:289, 1919.

Paterson, R.: Studies in optimum dosage. Br. J. Radiol., 25:505, 1952.

Paterson, R., and Parker, H. M.: Dosage system for gamma ray therapy. Br. J. Radiol., 7:592, 1934.

Paterson, R., and Parker, H. M.: Dosage system for gamma ray therapy. Br. J. Radiol., 8:313, 1938.

Pedersen, E., Hogetveit, A. C., and Andersen, A.: Cancer of the respiratory organs among workers at a nickel refinery in Norway. Int. J. Cancer, 12:32, 1973.

Perez, C. A., Purdy, J. A., Breaux, S. R., Ogura, J. H., and von Essen, S.: Carcinoma of the tonsillar fossa. Cancer, 50:2314, 1982.

Perry, D. J., Davis, R. K., and Weiss, R. B.: Combined modality treatment with combination chemotherapy for advanced carcinoma of the head and neck. Proc. Am. Soc. Clin. Oncol., 1:193, 1982.

Perussia, A.: Quoted in Ackerman, L. V., and del Regato, J. A.: Cancer: Diagnosis, Treatment, and Prognosis. St. Louis, MO, C. V. Mosby Company, 1970, p. 279.

Pindborg, J. J., Daftary, D. K., and Mehta, F. S.: A follow-up study of sixty-one oral dysplastic precancerous lesions in Indian villages. Oral Surg., 43:383, 1977.

Pindborg, J. J., Jolst, O., Renstrup, G., and Roed Petersen, B.: Studies in oral leukoplakia: a preliminary report on the period prevalence of malignant transformation in leukoplakia based on a follow-up study of 248 patients. J. Am. Dent. Assoc., 76:767, 1968.

Price, L. A., MacRae, K., and Hill, B. T.: Integration of safe initial combination chemotherapy (without cisplatin) with a high response rate and local therapy for untreated Stage III and IV epidermoid cancer of the head and neck: 5-year survival data. Cancer Treat. Rep., 67:535, 1983.

Quillen, C. G.: Latissimus dorsi myocutaneous flaps in head and neck reconstruction. Plast. Reconstr. Surg., 63:664, 1979.

Rabuzzi, D. D., Chung, C. T., and Sagerman, R. H.: Prophylactic neck irradiation. Arch. Otolaryngol., 106:454, 1980.

Ratzer, E. R., Schweitzer, R. J., and Frazell, E. L.: Epidermoid carcinoma of the palate. Am. J. Surg., 119:294, 1970.

Razack, M. S., Sako, K., Marchetta, F. C., Calamel, P., Bakamjian, V. Y., and Shedd, D. P.: Carcinoma of the hypopharynx: success and failure. Am. J. Surg., 134:489, 1977.

Remmler, D., Medina, J. E., Byers, R. M., Meoz, R., and Pfalzgraf, K.: Treatment of choice for squamous cell carcinoma of the tonsillar fossa. Head Neck Surg., 7:206, 1985.

Robin, P. E., and Powell, D. J.: Diagnostic errors in

cancers of the nasal cavity and paranasal sinuses. Arch. Otolaryngol., *107*:138, 1981.

Roed Petersen, B.: Cancer development in oral leukoplakia: follow-up of 331 patients. J. Dent. Res., *50*:711, 1971.

Roseman, J. M., and James, A. G.: Metastatic cancers of the neck from undetermined primary sites: long-term follow-up. J. Surg. Oncol., *19*:247, 1982.

Rothman, K. J.: Epidemiology of head and neck cancer. Laryngoscope, *88*:435, 1978a.

Rothman, K. J.: The effect of alcohol consumption on risk of cancer of the head and neck. Laryngoscope (Suppl. 8), *88*:5, 1978b.

Rothman, K. J., and Keller, A. Z.: The effect of joint exposure to alcohol and tobacco on risk of cancer of the mouth and pharynx. J. Chronic Dis., *25*:711, 1972.

Roux-Berger, J. L., Baud, M., and Courtial, J.: Cancer de la partie mobile de la langue. Le curage ganglionnaire prophylactique est-il justifié? Statistique de La Fondation Curie. Mem. Acad. Chir., *75*:120, 1949.

Rush, B. F., Jr.: Combined procedures in the treatment of oral carcinoma. *In* Ravitch, M. M. (Ed.): Current Problems in Surgery. Chicago, Year Book Medical Publishers, 1966.

Russ, J. E., Applebaum, E. L., and Sisson, G. A.: Squamous cell carcinoma of the soft palate. Laryngoscope, *87*:1151, 1977.

Samaan, N. A., Vieto, R., Schultz, P. N., Maor, M., Meoz, R. T., et al.: Hypothalamic, pituitary and thyroid dysfunction after radiotherapy to the head and neck. Int. J. Radiat. Oncol. Biol. Phys., *8*:1857, 1982.

Sasaki, C. T., Ariyan, S., Spencer, D., and Buckwalter, J.: Pectoralis major myocutaneous reconstruction of the anterior skull base. Laryngoscope, *95*:162, 1985.

Schechter, G. L., Sly, D. E., Roper, A. L., II, Jackson, R. T., and Bumatay, J.: Set-back tongue flap for carcinoma of the tongue base. Arch. Otolaryngol., *106*:668, 1980.

Schramm, V. L., Jr., Myers, E. N., and Maroon, J. C.: Anterior skull base surgery for benign and malignant disease. Laryngoscope, *89*:1077, 1979.

Schuller, D. E., Wilson, H. E., Smith, R. E., Batley, F., and James, A. D.: Preoperative reductive chemotherapy for locally advanced carcinoma of the oral cavity, oropharynx, and hypopharynx. Cancer, *51*:15, 1983.

Schwarz, D., Hamberger, A. D., and Jesse, R. H., Jr.: The management of squamous cell carcinoma in cervical lymph nodes in the clinical absence of a primary lesion by combined surgery and irradiation. Cancer, *48*:1746, 1981.

Seidenberg, B., Rosenak, S. S., Hurwitt, E. S., and Som, M. L.: Immediate reconstruction of the cervical esophagus by a revascularized isolated jejunal segment. Ann. Surg., *149*:162, 1959.

Shafer, W. G., and Waldron, C. A.: Erythroplakia of the oral cavity. Cancer, *36*:1021, 1975.

Shear, M.: Erythroplakia of the mouth. Int. Dent. J., *22*:460, 1972.

Sheetz, S., O'Donoghue, G., Bromer, R., Vaughan, C., Willett, B., et al.: Response to initial chemotherapy predicts complete response to subsequent radiotherapy in advanced squamous cell carcinoma of the head and neck. Proc. Am. Soc. Clin. Oncol., *3*:183, 1984.

Shrady, G. F.: Editorial. Recent contributions to the study of cancer. Med. Rec., *27*:325, 1885.

Shukovsky, L. J., and Fletcher, G. H.: Time dose and tumor volume relationships in the irradiation of squamous cell carcinoma of the tonsillar fossa. Radiology, *107*:621, 1973.

Shumrick, D. A.: Supraglottic laryngectomy: its place in the treatment of laryngeal cancer. Arch. Otolaryngol., *89*:629, 1969.

Silver, C. E.: Surgery for Cancer of the Larynx and Related Structures. New York, Churchill Livingstone, 1981, pp. 74–79.

Silverberg, E.: Cancer statistics, 1984. Cancer, *34*:7, 1984.

Silverberg, E.: Cancer statistics, 1985. Cancer, *35*:19, 1985.

Silverberg, E., and Lubera, J. A.: A review of American Cancer Society estimates of cancer cases and deaths. Cancer, *33*:2, 1983.

Silverman, N. A., Alexander, J. C., Jr., Hollinshead, A. C., and Chretien, P. B.: Correlation of tumor border with in vitro lymphocyte reactivity and antibodies to herpes virus tumor–associated antigens in head and neck squamous carcinoma. Cancer, *37*:135, 1976.

Silverman, S., Jr.: Oral Cancer. 1st Ed. New York, American Cancer Society, 1981.

Silverman, S., Jr., Bhargara, R., Mani, N. J., Smith, L. W., and Malaowalla, A. M.: Malignant transformation and natural history of oral leukoplakia in 57,518 industrial workers in Gujarat, India. Cancer, *38*:1790, 1976.

Silverman, S., Jr., Gorsky, M., and Lozada, F.: Oral leukoplakia malignant transformation. A follow-up study of 257 patients. Cancer, *53*:563, 1984.

Simpson, G. I., II: The evaluation and management of neck masses of unknown etiology. Otolaryngol. Clin. North Am., *13*:489, 1980.

Sisson, G. A.: Symposium: 3. Treatment of malignancies of paranasal sinuses. Laryngoscope, *80*:945, 1970.

Snow, G. B., Boom, R. P., Delemarre, J. F., and Bangert, J. A.: Squamous carcinoma of the oropharynx. Clin. Otolaryngol., *2*:93, 1977.

Snow, J. B., Jr., Gelber, R. D., Kramer, S., Davis, L. W., Marcial, V. A., and Lowry, L. D.: Evaluation of randomized preoperative radiation therapy for supraglottic carcinoma. Ann. Otol. Rhinol. Laryngol., *87*:686, 1978.

Snow, J. B., Jr., Gelber, R. D., Kramer, S., Davis, L. W., Marcial, V. A., and Lowry, L. D.: Randomized preoperative and postoperative radiation therapy for patients with carcinoma of the head and neck. Preliminary report. Laryngoscope, *90*:930, 1980.

Som, M. L.: Laryngopharyngoesophagectomy: primary closure with laryngotracheal autograft. A. M. A. Arch. Otolaryngol., *63*:474, 1956.

Som, M. L.: Surgical treatment of carcinoma of the epiglottis by lateral pharyngotomy. Trans. Am. Acad. Ophthalmol. Otolaryngol., *63*:28, 1959.

Son, Y. H., and Ariyan, S.: Intraoperative adjuvant radiotherapy for advanced cancers of the head and neck. Preliminary report. Am. J. Surg., *150*:480, 1985.

Son, Y. H., and Habermalz, H. J.: Prognostic factors in pyriform sinus carcinoma. Acta Radiol. Oncol. Radiat. Phys. Biol., *18*:561, 1979.

Soutar, D. S., Scheker, L. R., Tanner, N. S., and McGregor, I. A.: The radial forearm flap: a versatile method for intraoral reconstruction. Br. J. Plast. Surg., *36*:1, 1983.

Southwick, H. W.: Elective neck dissection for intraoral cancer. J.A.M.A., *17*:454, 1971.

Southwick, H. W., Slaughter, D. P., and Majarakis, J. D.: Malignant disease of the head and neck in childhood. Arch. Surg., *78*:678, 1959.

Spector, G. J.: Diagnosis and treatment of cancer of the larynx. Am. Acad. Otolaryngology Self-Instructional Package 77700, 1978.

Spiro, R. H., DeRose, G., and Strong, E. W.: Cervical

node metastasis of occult origin. Am. J. Surg., *146*:441, 1983.

Spiro, R. H., and Strong, E. W.: Discontinuous partial glossectomy and radical neck dissection in selected patients with epidermoid carcinoma of the mobile tongue. Am. J. Surg., *126*:544, 1973.

Srensen, H., Hansen, H. S., and Thomsen, K. A.: Partial laryngectomy following irradiation. Laryngoscope, *90*:1344, 1980.

Strandqvist, M.: Studien über die kumulative Wirkung der Roentgenstrahlen bei Fraktionierung. Acta Radiol. (Suppl.), *55*:1, 1944.

Strong, M. S., and Jako, G. J.: Laser surgery in the larynx. Early clinical experience with continuous CO_2 laser. Ann. Otol. Rhinol. Laryngol., *81*:791, 1972.

Suarez, D.: El problema de las metastasis lingfaticas y alejados del cancer de laringe e hiopfaringe. Rev. Otorhinolaryngol., *23*:83, 1963.

Suh, K. W., Facer, G. W., Devine, K. D., Weiland, L. H., and Zujko, R. D.: Inverting papilloma of the nose and paranasal sinuses. Laryngoscope, *87*:35, 1977.

Sullivan, R. D.: Chemotherapy in head and neck cancer. J.A.M.A., *217*:461, 1971.

Swartz, W. M., Banis, J. C., Newton, E. D., Ramasastry, S. S., Jones, N. F., and Acland, R.: The osteocutaneous scapular flap for mandibular and maxillary reconstruction. Plast. Reconstr. Surg., *77*:530, 1986.

Tabb, H. G., and Barranco, S. J.: Cancer of the maxillary sinus. An analysis of 108 cases. Laryngoscope, *81*:818, 1971.

Taskinen, P. J.: The early case of supraglottic carcinoma. Laryngoscope, *85*:1643, 1975.

Taylor, G. I.: Reconstruction of the mandible with free composite iliac bone grafts. Ann. Plast. Surg., *9*:361, 1982.

Terz, J. J., Young, H., and Lawrence, W.: Combined craniofacial resection for locally advanced carcinoma of the head and neck. II. Carcinoma of the paranasal sinuses. Am. J. Surg., *140*:618, 1980.

Theogaraj, S. D., Merritt, W. H., Acharya, G., and Cohen, I. K.: The pectoralis major musculocutaneous flap in single-stage reconstruction of the pharyngoesophageal region. Plast. Reconstr. Surg., *65*:267, 1980.

Tokars, R. P., and Griem, M. L.: Carcinoma of the nasopharynx and optimization of radiotherapeutic management for tumor control and spinal cord injury. Int. J. Radiat. Oncol. Biol. Phys., *5*:1741, 1979.

Tong, D., Laramore, G. E., Griffin, T. W., Russell, A. H., Tesh, D. W., et al.: Carcinoma of the tonsillar region. Results of external irradiation. Cancer, *49*:2009, 1982.

Urdaneta, N., Fischer, J. J., Vera, R., and Gutierrez, E.: Cancer of the nasopharynx. Review of 43 cases treated with supervoltage radiation therapy. Cancer, *37*:1707, 1976.

Van den Brouck, C., Sancho, H., LeFur, R., Richard, J. M., and Cachin, Y.: Results of a randomized clinical trial of preoperative irradiation versus postoperative in treatment of tumors of the hypopharynx. Cancer, *39*:1445, 1977.

Vegers, J. W., Snow, G. B., and van der Waal, I.: Squamous cell carcinoma of the buccal mucosa. Arch. Otolaryngol., *105*:192, 1979.

Vincent, R. G., and Marchetta, F. A.: The relationship of the use of tobacco and alcohol to cancer of the oral cavity, pharynx or larynx. Am. J. Surg., *106*:501, 1963.

Vrabec, D. P.: The inverted Schneiderian papilloma: a clinical and pathological study. Laryngoscope, *85*:186, 1975.

Wald, R. M., Jr., and Calcaterra, T. C.: Lower alveolar carcinoma: segmental versus marginal resection. Arch. Otolaryngol., *109*:578, 1983.

Wang, C. C.: Management and prognosis of squamous cell carcinoma of the tonsillar region. Radiology, *104*:667, 1972.

Wang, C. C.: Carcinoma of the larynx. *In* Wang, C. C. (Ed.): Radiation Therapy for Head and Neck Neoplasms. Littleton, MA, John Wright PSG, 1983, pp. 165–199.

Wang, C. C., and Schulz, M. D.: Management of locally recurrent carcinoma of the nasopharynx. Radiology, *86*:900, 1966.

Ward, G. E., and Hendrick, J. W.: Diagnosis and Treatment of Tumors of the Head and Neck. Baltimore, Williams & Wilkins Company, 1950.

Watts, J. M.: The importance of the Plummer-Vinson syndrome in the aetiology of carcinoma of the upper gastrointestinal tract. Postgrad. Med. J., *37*:523, 1961.

Weymuller, E. A., Jr., Reardon, E. J., and Nash, D.: A comparison of treatment modalities in carcinoma of the maxillary antrum. Arch. Otolaryngol, *106*:625, 1980.

Whicker, J. H., DeSanto, L. W., and Devine, K. D.: Surgical treatment of squamous cell carcinoma of the base of the tongue. Laryngoscope, *82*:1853, 1972.

Whicker, J. H., DeSanto, L. W., and Devine, K. D.: Surgical treatment of squamous cell carcinoma of the tonsil. Laryngoscope, *84*:90, 1974.

Whitehead, W.: A hundred cases of entire excision of the tongue. Br. Med. J., *1*:961, 1891.

Williams, S. D., Einhorn, L. H., Velez-Garcia, E., Essessee, I., Ratkin, G., et al.: Chemotherapy of head and neck cancer: comparison of PVB vs MTX. Proc. Am. Soc. Clin. Oncol., *1*:202, 1982.

Winegar, L. K., and Griffin, W.: The occult primary. Arch. Otolaryngol., *98*:159, 1973.

Winn, D. M., Blot, W. J., Shy, C. M., Pickle, L. W., Toledo, A., and Fraumeni, J. F., Jr.: Snuff dipping and oral cancer among women in the southern United States. N. Engl. J. Med., *304*:745, 1981.

Wynder, E. L., Bross, I. J., and Feldman, R. M.: A study of the etiological factors in cancer of the mouth. Cancer, *10*:1300, 1957.

Wynder, E. L., and Fryer, J. H.: Etiologic considerations of Plummer-Vinson (Paterson-Kelly) syndrome. Ann. Intern. Med., *49*:1106, 1958.

Wynder, E. L., Mushinski, M. H., and Spivak, J. C.: Tobacco and alcohol consumption in relation to the development of multiple primary cancers. Cancer, *40*:1872, 1977.

Yang, Z. Y., Hu, Y. H., Yan, J. H., Cai, W. M., Qin, D. X., et al.: Lymph node metastases in the neck from an unknown primary. Report on 113 patients. Acta Radiol. [Oncol.], *22*:17, 1983.

Yarington, C. T., Jr., Yonkers, A. J., and Beddoe, G. M.: Radical neck dissection. Mortality and morbidity. Arch. Otolaryngol., *97*:306, 1973.

Young, J. L., Perry, C. L., and Asire, A. J. (Eds.): Surveillance, epidemiology, and end results: incidence and mortality data, 1973–77. National Cancer Institute Monograph 57. (NIH Publication No. 81–2330). Bethesda, MD, National Cancer Institute, 1981.

Yuen, A., Medina, J. E., Goepfert, H., and Fletcher, G.: Management of stage T_3 and T_4 glottic carcinomas. Am. J. Surg., *148*:467, 1984.

Zhang, Z. X., Hu, Y. H., Xu, G. Z., and Gu, X. Z.: Radiation treatment of carcinoma of the oropharynx. Acta Radiol. [Oncol.], *22*:119, 1983.

Vahram Y. Bakamjian

Lingual Flaps in Reconstructive Surgery for Oral and Perioral Cancer

ANATOMIC CONSIDERATIONS

FLAPS FROM DORSUM OF TONGUE
    Posteriorly Based Dorsal Tongue Flap
    Anteriorly Based Dorsal Tongue Flap
    Transverse Dorsal Tongue Flap

FLAPS FROM LINGUAL TIP
    Perimeter Flaps
    Dorsoventrally Disposed Flaps

FLAPS FROM VENTRAL SURFACE OF TONGUE

The tongue has always been a source of local tissue in the repair of intraoral excisional defects by the method of direct suturing. In this technique the tongue remnant is forced by advancement to play the role of a reparative flap. In contrast, there is an assortment of uncommonly used flaps that can be borrowed from the intact organ without significantly compromising its important functions.

As early as 1909, Lexer recorded two cases in which he had repaired cheek defects by advancing mucosa as a flap from the oral floor; the flap was based on the lateral edge of the tongue (Fig. 71–1). This procedure, however, had more in common with a direct closure by advancement than with a true flap from the tongue. No mention of the concept appeared in the literature for half a century thereafter. In 1956 the author began repairing moderate-sized faucial defects with a posteriorly based flap from the ipsilateral half of the lingual dorsum. In the same year there

was a report by Klopp and Schurter (1956) of their similar use of an almost identical flap from the lateral border of the tongue. The next two reports that followed dealt with labial reconstructions (Bakamjian, 1964; Guerrero-Santos and associates, 1964). Since then, varieties in design and application of lingual flaps have been sporadically expanded.

ANATOMIC CONSIDERATIONS

The mouth cavity is divided into an outer buccal portion and an inner lingual portion by the alveolar arches and the teeth. In its anterior aspect the orifice of communication is protected by the lips, which are continuous with the cheeks; posteriorly the lingual portion communicates with the pharynx by an aperture called the isthmus of the faucium. In its superior aspect the hard and soft palate constitutes the roof; inferiorly, arising from the floor and virtually filling the cavity, is the large, mobile, and stretchable mass of the tongue. The latter is capable of donating to the repair of defects at almost any position in the oral environs.

Three parts of the tongue are distinguishable. The *radix linguae,* or pharyngeal portion, is that which falls behind the V-shaped line of the circumvallate papillae. Embryologically differing in origin from the rest of the tongue, it has mucosa knobbed by numerous aggregates of lymphoid follicles—the lingual tonsil. The radix is the part that features least in lingual flap designs. The *corpus linguae,* or middle and largest portion, is attached to the oral floor by its underside. The *apex linguae,* or tip portion, is covered

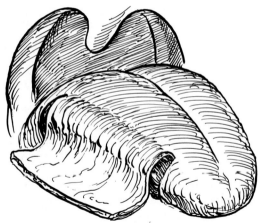

Figure 71–1. Lexer's (1909) flap for cheek repair. The flap was developed from the floor of the mouth with its base on the lateral edge of the tongue.

by mucosa on all sides and it freely projects to the inner aspect of the incisor teeth. The investing mucosa is papillary on the dorsal surface of the oral two-thirds of the tongue, and it is thick with the lamina propria or corium—a dense, submucous feltwork of connective tissue with numerous elastic fibers and penetrating vessels and nerves that supply the papillae. The mucosa is intimately adherent to the underlying musculature. At the edges and ventral side, however, the mucosa becomes smooth and delicate, making it better suited for replacing the vermilion on the lips.

The tongue consists of symmetric halves separated from each other in the midline by a fibrous septum that inferiorly attaches to the hyoid bone. Each half comprises two sets of muscles: an *extrinsic* set with origins from the skeleton (cranium, mandible, and hyoid bone) and an *intrinsic* set with origins as well as insertions within the organ (Fig. 71–2). With this anatomic arrangement it is the only structure in the body in which the muscle fibers interlace with one another in three dimensions, allowing the intricate tongue movements that are involved in articulation, mastication, and the initiation of swallowing.

The blood supply to each half is from the ipsilateral lingual artery, distributed via two branches that have practical importance in the design of tongue flaps (Fig. 71–3). A *dorsal lingual* branch ascends via the base to the dorsum of the tongue, also contributing blood supply to the vallecula, the epiglottis, the tonsil, and the neighboring part of the soft palate. A terminal branch from the for-

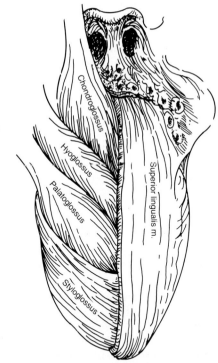

Figure 71–2. Extrinsic and intrinsic muscles of the tongue.

ward continuation of the lingual artery under the hyoglossus muscle—the *deep lingual* or *ranine* branch—courses deep to the ventral mucosa of the tongue, giving numerous offshoots vertically to the dorsum as it ascends to the tip of the organ. Thus, a distinct axiality of vascular linkages exists between the base and tip in each half of the lingual dorsum. No significant crosscirculation passes through the barrier of the median septum in

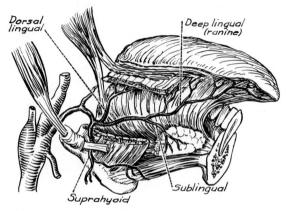

Figure 71–3. Distribution of the lingual artery branches to the tongue.

the body of the tongue, but a rich anastomotic ranine arch crosses the midline at the lingual tip. There are also transverse linkages between the dorsalis linguae arteries at the base. Thus, mucosal muscular flaps with significant viability may be designed from the dorsum, the tip, the edges, or even the ventrum of the tongue in resurfacing defects in and around the oral cavity.

FLAPS FROM DORSUM OF TONGUE

These flaps are usually designed lengthwise on one side of the midline with a posterior or an anterior base. If a transverse flap is considered, it should not cross the midline of the body of the tongue unless it is a bipedicle flap; the blood flow from one base cannot sufficiently traverse the median raphé to support the opposite end. At a thickness of approximately 8 mm, the flaps are elevated to include, with the mucosa, the adherent subjacent stratum of the superior lingual musculature. An effort is made to maintain a fairly uniform thickness so that the flap is not wedge-shaped in cross section, in order to fit better into a recipient defect. The donor wound is easily closed by direct suture, but scrupulous attention to hemostasis is essential. Two or more buried rows of interrupted

sutures are used to obliterate all possible dead space in the wound in order to prevent hematoma formation with infiltrating hemorrhage into the loose stroma of the tongue musculature. The latter can cause gigantic swelling and endanger not only the flap but also the patency of the airway.

Posteriorly Based Dorsal Tongue Flap. Relying on the dorsalis linguae artery for its survival, this longitudinally oriented flap may extend the entire length of the tongue, from the circumvallate line, or a little behind it, to near the tip of the organ. By a lateral and backward rotation it can comfortably repair a defect of moderate size in the retromolar trigone or tonsillar fossa of the ipsilateral side (Fig. 71–4A). With a lesser degree of rotation it can cover a posterior mucosal defect in the cheek (Fig. 71–4B). In the latter instance, the flap may require an edentulous space to pass safely to its buccal destination, without being compressed by the molar teeth.

In comparison with direct suturing of the unmodified tongue into an adjoining defect, the use of the tongue flap permits a freer and more equitable redistribution of available tongue tissue into the defect. The closure of a longitudinally oriented donor wound (equal in width to half that of the lingual dorsum) diminishes the girth of the remaining tongue but does not affect its length to compromise lingual function. The repair is completed in

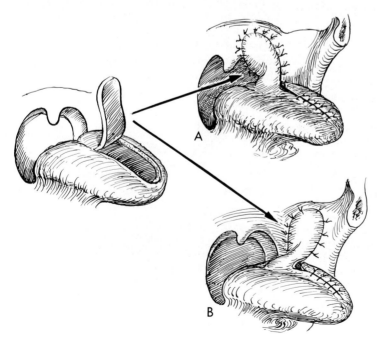

Figure 71–4. The posteriorly based dorsal tongue flap (8 mm in thickness).

one stage since division of the pedicle is not required.

Example 1. A 69 year old man presented with a squamous cell cancer in the right retromolar trigone. Through a midline lip-splitting incision a wide resection was performed that included the lesion in the trigone, the anterior tonsillar pillar, and the adjoining lateral part of the soft palate (Fig. 71–5A). A posteriorly based dorsal flap was elevated from the longitudinal right half of the oral portion of the tongue (Fig. 71–5B). With lateral and backward rotation it was transposed to cover the excisional defect, and the donor wound was closed by direct suture (Fig. 71–5C). Healing was by primary intention (Fig. 71–5D), and no appreciable impairment resulted in the function of the more slender remaining tongue (Fig. 71–5E).

Example 2. An 88 year old edentulous man presented with an extensive squamous cell cancer in the left buccal mucosa that infiltrated the cheek skin. A full-thickness cheek and commissure resection was performed (Fig. 71–6A). A posteriorly based dorsal flap was raised from the entire left half of the oral portion of the tongue, and the donor bed was closed by direct suture (Fig. 71–6B). With its raw side turned outward, it was used to replace the entire mucosa of the cheek (Fig. 71–6C). A compound flap of cervical skin with a

portion of the sternocleidomastoid muscle was used to provide external cover (Fig. 71–6D). A satisfactory outcome was achieved in a single stage in an octogenarian patient (Fig. 71–6E) whose only subsequent complaint was that he could not wear dentures to chew solid foods.

Anteriorly Based Dorsal Tongue Flap. This flap, which affords greater mobility because the pedicle is on the free end of the tongue, can be even more versatile. However, it requires greater sophistication and care in its planning and execution. As the base is approached in developing the flap toward the end of the tongue, the surgeon may feel constrained by the delicacy of the design *and* uncertain how to judge the dividing line between what is perceived as optimal freedom for the flap and danger to its blood supply. Because of the anastomotic ranine arch, however, the flap is more robust than might be imagined.

This flap can be applied to the repair of anterior cheek and commissure defects (Fig. 71–7A). With more of a rotation forward to face its raw side outward (Fig. 71–7B) it can replace lining and/or vermilion on the lips. With the same type of forward rotation, but

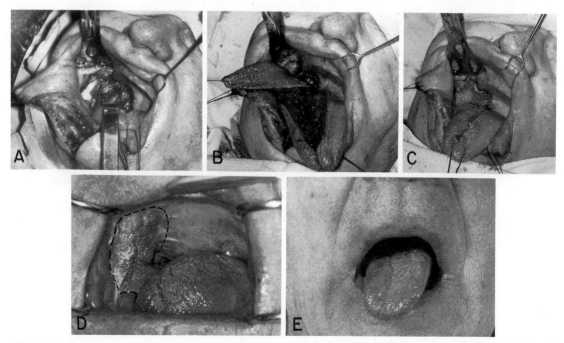

Figure 71–5. Repair of a retromolar trigone and tonsillar fossa defect with a posteriorly based dorsal tongue flap. *A,* Lesion after a lip-splitting incision. *B,* Dorsal tongue flap. *C,* Direct closure of the donor defect. *D,* Healed flap. *E,* Narrower but functional tongue. (From Bakamjian, V. Y.: Tongue flaps in cancer surgery of the oral cavity. *In* Chretien, P. B., Johns, H. E., Shedd, D. P., Strong, E. W., and Ward, P. H. (Eds.): Head and Neck Cancer. Vol. 1. Proceedings of International Conference, Baltimore, MD, July 22-27, 1984. Toronto, B. C. Decker, 1985, p. 169.)

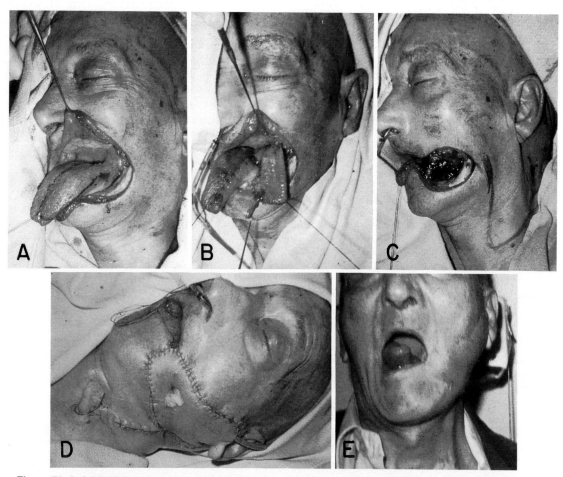

Figure 71–6. A full-thickness cheek and commissure reconstruction, using the posteriorly based dorsal tongue flap and a small sternocleidomastoid musculocutaneous flap. *A,* Excisional defects. *B,* Dorsal tongue flap. *C,* Tongue flap in place and design of cervical flap. *D,* At completion of surgery. *E,* Final result. (From Bakamjian, V. Y.: Tongue flaps in cancer surgery of the oral cavity. *In* Chretien, P. B., Johns, H. E., Shedd, D. P., Strong, E. W., and Ward, P. H. (Eds.): Head and Neck Cancer. Vol. 1. Proceedings of International Conference, Baltimore, MD, July 22-27, 1984. Toronto, B. C. Decker, 1985, p. 169.)

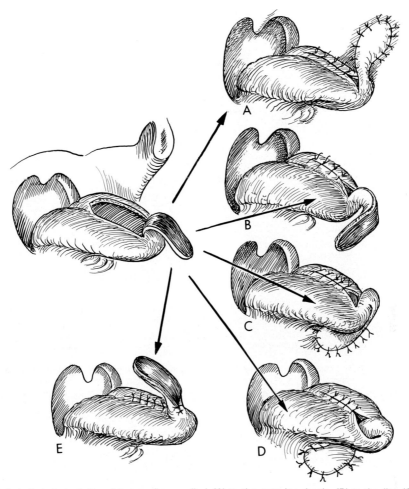

Figure 71–7. Anteriorly based dorsal tongue flap applied *(A)* to the anterior cheek, *(B)* to the lip, *(C)* to the anterior floor of the mouth, *(D)* to the anterolateral floor of mouth, and *(E)* to the palate.

with a twist to face its raw side downward (Fig. 71–7*C*), it can be used to resurface anterior defects in the floor. Turned medially, it can pass through a window created in the midline raphé (Fig. 71–7*D*) to reach an opposite anterolateral defect in the floor. It can also be used for defects in the roof. By simply reflecting it forward, it can close oronasal fistulas in patients after cleft lip repair. By a 180 degree twist at its base (Fig. 71–7*E*) it can resurface posteriorly located excisional defects in the hard palate.

In the first two of the above applications, a bite block may be required (specially prepared ahead of time) to protect the pedicle from the teeth, especially until the patient is fully recovered from anesthesia and can consciously cooperate to desist from biting on the pedicle. Unlike the posteriorly based tongue

flap, all repairs with the anteriorly based flap require a second stage for release of the tongue with division of the pedicle. It is, however, noteworthy how little speech and swallowing are inconvenienced in the interim before release of the tongue.

Example 3. A 71 year old man presented with a right anterior buccal cancer that eroded to the skin just behind the oral commissure. A full-thickness resection was performed, and an ipsilateral anteriorly based dorsal tongue flap was raised for the repair (Fig. 71–8*A*). The donor wound was closed by direct suture, and the flap was applied as lining for the reconstructed cheek (Fig. 71–8*B*). The covering layer was provided with a flap of laterally based submental skin (Fig. 71–8*C*). Three weeks later both flaps were divided, with no loss in elasticity of the cheek and no appreciable damage to tongue functions (Fig. 71–8*D,E*).

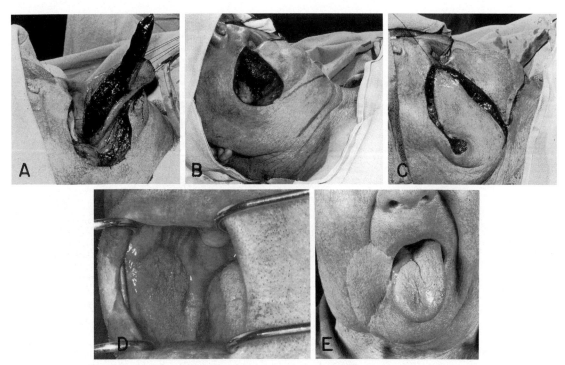

Figure 71–8. A full-thickness cheek and commissure reconstruction, using the anteriorly based dorsal tongue flap and a laterally based flap of submental skin. *A,* Excisional defect. *B,* Tongue flap in position and outline of coverage flap. *C,* Transposition of skin flap. *D,* Healed tongue flap. *E,* Final result. (From Bakamjian, V. Y.: Tongue flaps in cancer surgery of the oral cavity. *In* Chretien, P. B., Johns, H. E., Shedd, D. P., Strong, E. W., and Ward, P. H. (Eds.): Head and Neck Cancer. Vol. 1. Proceedings of International Conference, Baltimore, MD, July 22-27, 1984. Toronto, B. C. Decker, 1985, p. 169.)

Example 4. A 70 year old man presented with a spindle cell carcinoma, recurring in the lower lip several years after a previous wedge resection. A bulging mass, occupying considerably more than three-fourths of the lip, encroached onto the chin. It necessitated a total resection of the lip, including the soft tissues of the chin (Fig. 71–9*A*). An anteriorly based ipsilateral flap was developed laterally on the dorsum of the tongue (Fig. 71–9*B*). The flap was rotated laterally and forward to be used for the lining and vermilion of the reconstructed lip. Covering for the lip as well as for the chin was supplied by a bipedicle flap of upper neck skin (Fig. 71–9*C*). Healing was uneventful (Fig. 71–9*D*), and there was surprisingly little functional inconvenience while division of the tongue and skin flap pedicles was awaited (Fig. 71–9*E,F*). A satisfactory outcome was apparent some weeks later (Fig. 71–9*G,H*).

Example 5. A 59 year old man presented with squamous cell cancer in the anterior oral floor, which persisted after unsuccessful treatment with external and interstitial irradiation. A pull-through resection was performed along with a right radical neck dissection (Fig. 71–10*A*). An anteriorly based tongue flap was raised on the dorsum of the oral left half of the tongue (Fig. 71–

10*B*). After a lateral and forward rotation the raw side was turned inferiorly to the anterior defect in the oral floor under the tip of the tongue (Fig. 71–10*C*). At the end of three weeks the pedicle was divided to return the unused portion of the flap to its original position on the dorsal side (Fig. 71–10*D,E*).

Example 6. A 64 year old man presented with a squamous cell cancer located anterolaterally at the ventral junction of the tongue with the oral floor on the right side (Fig. 71–11*A*). As in Example 5, a pull-through resection was performed with a right radical neck dissection. An anteriorly based flap from the contralateral oral half of the tongue was turned medially to pass through a window in the median raphé (Fig. 71–11*B*) to the site of the defect in the oral floor. Healing was by primary intention (Fig. 71–11*C*), with division of the pedicle at three weeks and closure of the window in the median raphé (Fig. 71–11*D*).

Example 7. A 69 year old man presented with verrucous carcinoma in the right upper buccal gutter and molar portion of the hard palate. A right partial maxillectomy was performed via a Weber-Ferguson approach (Fig. 71–12*A*). An anteriorly based dorsal flap, developed from the ipsilateral half of the tongue, was turned raw side

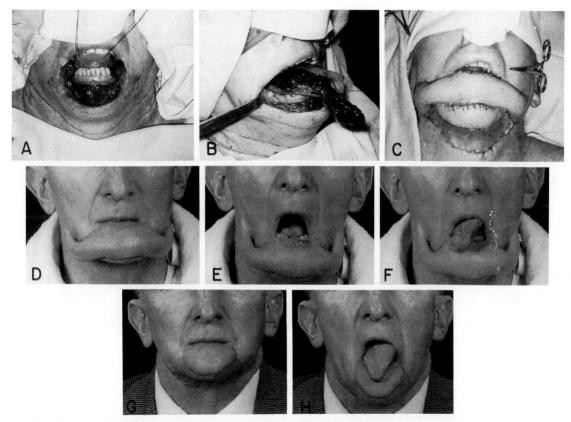

Figure 71–9. A total lower lip reconstruction, using the anteriorly based dorsal tongue flap and a bipedicle flap of skin from the upper neck. *A,* Excisional defect. *B,* Tongue flap. *C,* Bipedicle neck skin flap. *D, E, F,* Before division of the pedicles. *G, H,* Final result. (From Bakamjian, V. Y.: Tongue flaps in cancer surgery of the oral cavity. *In* Chretien, P. B., Johns, H. E., Shedd, D. P., Strong, E. W., and Ward, P. H. (Eds.): Head and Neck Cancer. Vol. 1. Proceedings of International Conference, Baltimore, MD, July 22-27, 1984. Toronto, B. C. Decker, 1985, p. 169.)

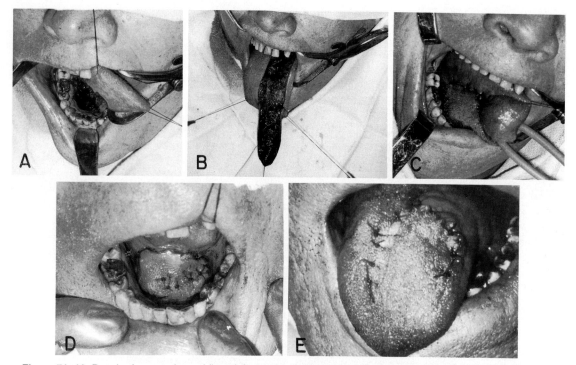

Figure 71–10. Repair of an anterior oral floor defect, using the anteriorly based dorsal tongue flap. *A,* Excisional defect. *B,* Tongue flap. *C,* Flap transposition. *D, E,* Return of the unused portion to the donor site. (From Bakamjian, V. Y.: Tongue flaps in cancer surgery of the oral cavity. *In* Chretien, P. B., Johns, H. E., Shedd, D. P., Strong, E. W., and Ward, P. H. (Eds.): Head and Neck Cancer. Vol. 1. Proceedings of International Conference, Baltimore, MD, July 22-27, 1984. Toronto, B. C. Decker, 1985, p. 169.)

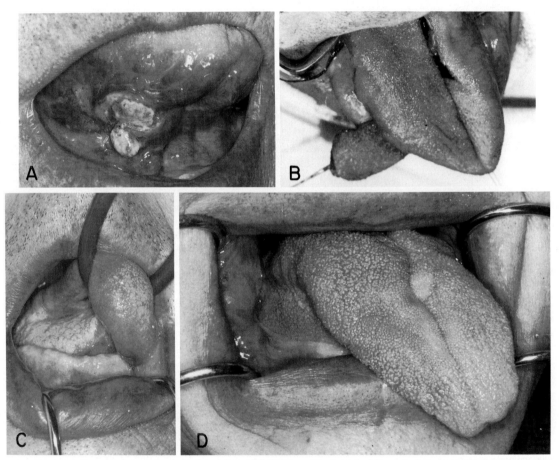

Figure 71–11. Repair of an anterolateral oral floor defect by median transit of the anteriorly based dorsal tongue flap. *A,* Lesion. *B,* Flap passing through a window in the median raphé. *C,* Healed recipient site. *D,* Healed donor site. (From Calamel, P. M.: The median transit flap. Plast. Reconstr. Surg., *51*:315, 1973.)

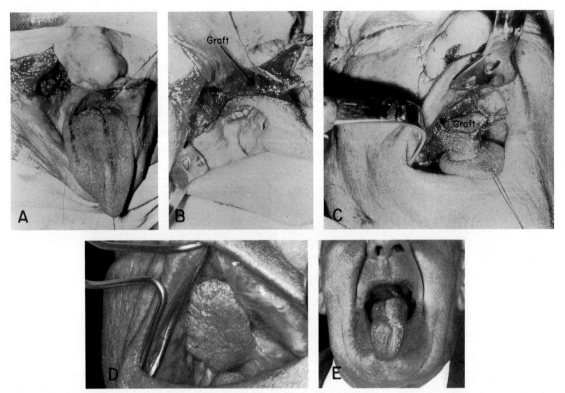

Figure 71–12. Repair of a partial maxillectomy defect of the palate, using the anteriorly based dorsal tongue flap. *A,* Excisional defect and tongue flap design. *B, C,* Tongue flap and skin graft. *D,* Healed recipient site. *E,* Healed donor site. (From Bakamjian, V. Y.: Tongue flaps in cancer surgery of the oral cavity. *In* Chretien, P. B., Johns, H. E., Shedd, D. P., Strong, E. W., and Ward, P. H. (Eds.): Head and Neck Cancer. Vol. 1. Proceedings of International Conference, Baltimore, MD, July 22-27, 1984. Toronto, B. C. Decker, 1985, p. 169.)

upward into the defect with a twist of 180 degrees at the base (Fig. 71–12*B*). It was sutured medially to the line of excision in the hard palate, posteriorly to that in the soft palate, and laterally to the cheek mucosa. A split-thickness skin graft was applied at the same time to the raw surface, leaving an anterior fistulous opening (Fig. 71–

12*C*). The latter was closed at three weeks, when it was time to divide the pedicle (Fig. 71–12*D*), leaving behind a slender but functionally unimpaired tongue (Fig. 71–12*E*).

Transverse Dorsal Tongue Flap. In bipedicle form, such a flap may be transferred

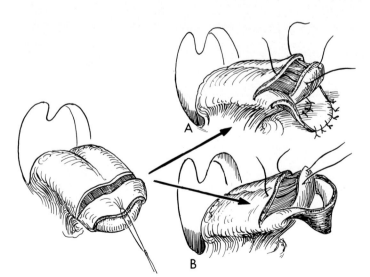

Figure 71–13. Bipedicle transverse tongue flap *(A)* to the anterior floor of the mouth and *(B)* to the lower lip. The donor defect is closed by primary approximation.

anteriorly from the tongue to the oral floor (Fig. 71–13*A*) or to the lip (Fig. 71–13*B*). As with the longitudinal flaps, the donor wound is easily closed by direct suture, but this maneuver considerably diminishes the length and blunts the free end of the tongue. Routine or indiscriminate use of the flap, therefore, is not recommended unless the tongue is extra long and larger than average in size.

Example 8. A 56 year old man presented with a recurrent squamous cell cancer that had destroyed the lower lip and infiltrated the chin after radiotherapy (Fig. 71–14*A*). A resection of the lip included the soft tissues of the chin, the outer table of the symphyseal bone, the alveolus, and the anterior lower teeth (Fig. 71–14*B*). A bipedicle transverse flap was outlined across the dorsum of the distal third of the tongue (Fig. 71–14*C*). After the donor wound was closed by direct suture, the flap was advanced forward (Fig. 71–14*D*). With a 90 degree twist at the pedicles to direct its raw face outward, and a little fold at one edge to simulate the vermilion, the flap was used to supply

the lining layer for a new lip (Fig. 71–14*E*). Bilateral, inferiorly based nasolabial skin flaps were medially rotated to meet in the midline and complete the first stage of the reconstruction (Fig. 71–14*F*). Although it was shortened and blunted, the end of the tongue was surprisingly functional, even before the pedicles were divided to release it from the reconstructed lip (Fig. 71–14*G,H*). The final appearance obtained with revision of the scars was satisfactory (Fig. 71–14*I,J*).

FLAPS FROM LINGUAL TIP

Intended for defects in which a reconstruction may prove difficult or not easily amenable to the more orthodox lip-switch and/or cheek advancement techniques, these flaps basically fall into two groups: perimeter flaps from the lingual margin for vermilion repairs and flaps dorsoventrally disposed on the lingual tip for lining and vermilion replacements.

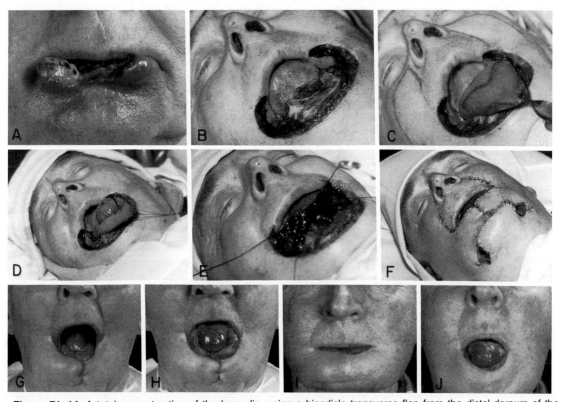

Figure 71–14. A total reconstruction of the lower lip, using a bipedicle transverse flap from the distal dorsum of the tongue and two inferiorly based flaps of nasolabial skin. *A,* Lesion. *B,* Excisional defect. *C, D, E,* Outline and transfer of tongue flap. *F,* Bilateral nasolabial and submental skin flap. *G, H,* Before division of pedicles. *I, J,* Final result. (From Bakamjian, V. Y.: Tongue flaps in cancer surgery of the oral cavity. *In* Chretien, P. B., Johns, H. E., Shedd, D. P., Strong, E. W., and Ward, P. H. (Eds.): Head and Neck Cancer. Vol. 1. Proceedings of International Conference, Baltimore, MD, July 22-27, 1984. Toronto, B. C. Decker, 1985, p. 169.)

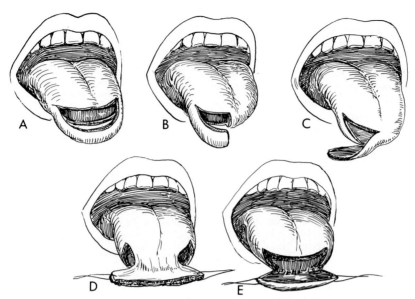

Figure 71–15. Perimeter flaps from the lingual tip for vermilion repairs.

Perimeter Flaps. Developed by a vertical incision a little inside and parallel to the border of the tongue, the perimeter flaps are narrow flaps that may be bipedicle or unipedicle. The bipedicle variety (Fig. 71–15A), usable for the vermilion border on either lip, may be likened to the transverse dorsal tongue flap. Because of the anastomotic ranine arch, however, it suffers no lack of vascular crosslinkages between its two limbs. Consequently, in a partial replacement of the vermilion border a unipedicle from a lateral base (Fig. 71–15B) may extend, if necessary, beyond the midline or one may extend laterally from a central base (Fig. 71–15C). Two of the latter kind, one from each side, may be joined to form a biwinged structure, with an appearance reminiscent of a hammerhead shark. With the incisions on its ventral side connected (Fig. 71–15D), the resultant flap, based centrally on the dorsal side of the lingual tip, may be used in reconstructions of the lower lip. With the incisions on the dorsal side connected (Fig. 71–15E), the ventrally based variant may be used in reconstructions of the upper lip.

Example 9. A 9 year old boy presented with an aggressively growing angioendothelioma that involved most of the upper lip, the floor of the right nasal vestibule, and the right paranasal and medial canthal areas of the cheek (Fig. 71–16A). His past history included radon seed implants at the age of 2 years, several attempts at excision between the ages of 4 and 8 years, and pronounced acceleration of the infiltrating tumor growth after the last excision. An abdominal tube flap was attached to the left wrist in preparation for immediate transport to the anticipated large defect on the face, at the time of the planned resection (Fig. 71–16B). Both the inner and outer layers of the missing lip portion were reconstituted by skin derived from division of the abdominal flap in subsequent stages (Fig. 71–16C). The patient returned in his teens, desiring a vermilion border for a more normal-looking lip. A single pedicle, centrally based perimeter flap from the right border of the tongue was mounted on to the edge of the reconstructed portion of the lip (Fig. 71–16D). When the pedicle was divided two weeks later, the old scars were revised with considerable improvement of the final appearance (Fig. 71–16E). There was no impairment in tongue function (Fig. 71–16F).

Example 10. A 59 year old man, with a previous history of a wedge resection, presented with a squamous cell cancer recurrent in the lower lip (Fig. 71–17A). A total vermilionectomy was performed, with a repeat wedge resection to encompass the involved scar from the previous operation (Fig. 71–17B). Closing the wedge defect in the usual manner, a biwinged, dorsocentrally based perimeter flap was elevated on the end of the tongue (Fig. 71–17C). This was inserted as vermilion border on the raw edge of the sutured lip (Fig. 71–17D). Speech and feeding were inconvenienced only minimally during an interim period of two weeks, and a satisfactory result was achieved upon release of the tongue from the repaired lip (Fig. 71–17E,F).

Example 11. A 58 year old man presented with a verrucous squamous cell cancer that involved the entire lower lip (Fig. 71–18A). A total resection

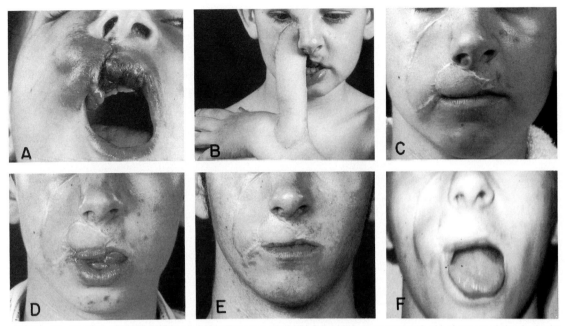

Figure 71–16. Vermilion border restoration of the upper lip (subtotally reconstructed with skin from an abdominal tube flap), using a centrally based perimeter flap from the lateral edge of the tongue. *A,* Lesion. *B,* Tube flap. *C,* After inset of the tube flap in the upper lip. *D,* Before division of the pedicle of the tongue flap. *E, F,* Final result.

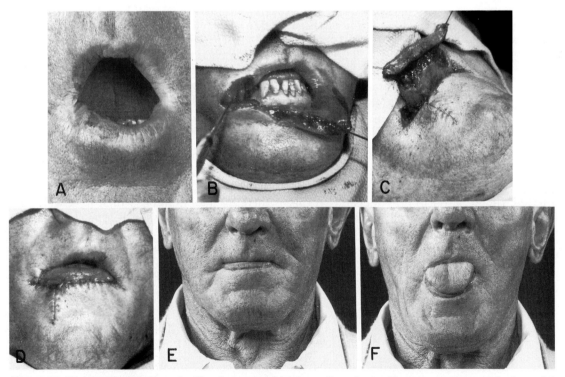

Figure 71–17. Vermilion border restoration (in a case of total vermilionectomy with wedge resection of the lower lip), using a biwinged, dorsocentrally based perimeter tongue flap. *A,* Lesion. *B,* Excisional defect. *C,* Elevation of the tongue flap. *D,* Tongue flap inserted into the lower lip. *E, F,* Final result. (From Bakamjian, V. Y.: Tongue flaps in cancer surgery of the oral cavity. *In* Chretien, P. B., Johns, H. E., Shedd, D. P., Strong, E. W., and Ward, P. H. (Eds.): Head and Neck Cancer. Vol. 1. Proceedings of International Conference, Baltimore, MD, July 22-27, 1984. Toronto, B. C. Decker, 1985, p. 169.)

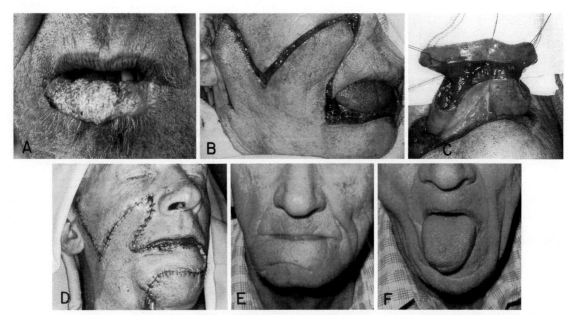

Figure 71–18. A total reconstruction of the lower lip, using a biwinged, dorsocentrally based perimeter tongue flap and a bilobed, inferiorly based skin flap from the face. *A,* Lesion. *B,* Cheek flap and excisional defect. *C,* Tongue flap. *D,* Inset of the cheek flap. *E, F,* Final result. (From Bakamjian, V. Y.: Tongue flaps in cancer surgery of the oral cavity. *In* Chretien, P. B., Johns, H. E., Shedd, D. P., Strong, E. W., and Ward, P. H. (Eds.): Head and Neck Cancer. Vol. 1. Proceedings of International Conference, Baltimore, MD, July 22-27, 1984. Toronto, B. C. Decker, 1985, p. 169.)

was performed. A bilobed, inferiorly based flap on the right face was developed to provide cutaneous coverage (Fig. 71–18*B*). A biwinged, dorsocentrally based perimeter tongue flap was developed (Fig. 71–18*C*). It was expanded open by spreading its layers apart, and the flap was apposed to the front limb of the rotated bilobar skin flap as lining and vermilion border for the reconstructed lip (Fig. 71–18*D*). In appearance and function the result was satisfactory upon division of the tongue from the reconstructed lip (Fig. 71–18*E,F*).

Dorsoventrally Disposed Flaps. This second group of flaps is derived from the lingual tip by a horizontal incision, rather than by a vertical incision inside and parallel to the edge. Equal in their breadth to the width of the tip of the tongue, these are short

flaps that are wider than they are long. A flap reflected dorsally on a posterior base (Fig. 71–19*A*) may supply lining for an upper lip reconstruction, while the smooth edge of the tongue itself provides the vermilion border. Another flap reflected ventrally on an anterior base (Fig. 71–19*B*) may do the same in a lower lip reconstruction. The vermilion in this instance is established at the second stage when, by division along the underside of the lingual tip, the smooth mucosa can be turned forward onto the edge of the reconstructed lip. Another possibility is that of forming double flaps, which may well be described as the fishmouth type (Fig. 71–19*C*). One component is reflected dorsally for vermilion and the other ventrally for lining, or

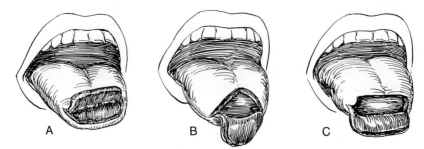

Figure 71–19. Flaps dorsoventrally disposed from the lingual tip for providing lining and vermilion reconstruction of the lip (see text).

vice versa, depending on the requirements of the particular reconstruction. Although these flaps are durable and safe to use, their main disadvantage is that they tend to shorten the tongue. Discretion is therefore warranted to avoid unwanted consequences.

Example 12. A 70 year old man presented with a large basal cell cancer in the upper lip, recurring several years after radiotherapy. An extensive resection to encompass the lesion included all except the right one-fifth of the upper lip, with the left commissure, the floor of both nasal vestibules, and the lower half of the columella (Fig. 71–20A). A broad and short flap on a posterior base was dorsally reflected on the lingual tip for lining (Fig. 71–20B). A flap of submental skin with a broad base on the left cheek provided the covering layer, and the smooth edge of the tongue formed the vermilion border (Fig. 71–20C). Feeding was by a nasogastric tube during the two weeks before the tongue was released (Fig. 71–20D). At a third stage, a satisfactory result was achieved by divid-

ing the skin pedicle and eliminating the dog-ear deformity on the cheek (Fig. 71–20E,F).

Example 13. A 71 year old man presented with an advanced squamous cell cancer of the lower lip, which persisted after radiotherapy. A commissure to commissure resection was performed to encompass the lesion (Fig. 71–21A). A bilobed, inferiorly based flap of skin on the left face was elevated and rotated forward (Fig. 71–21B), so that its anterior limb provided the covering layer for the new lip. An incision dorsally placed just inside the edge of the tongue was used to split the tip, forming a pair of flaps, a shorter one reflected dorsally for vermilion and a longer one reflected ventrally for lining (Fig. 71–21C,D). Healing occurred without complications (Fig. 71–21E). After discovery of a metastatic left cervical node a radical neck dissection was performed, postponing the final stage for release of the tongue another three weeks (Fig. 71–21F). Although satisfactory in appearance, the functional result was marred by noticeable impairment in speech and oral incontinence during eating.

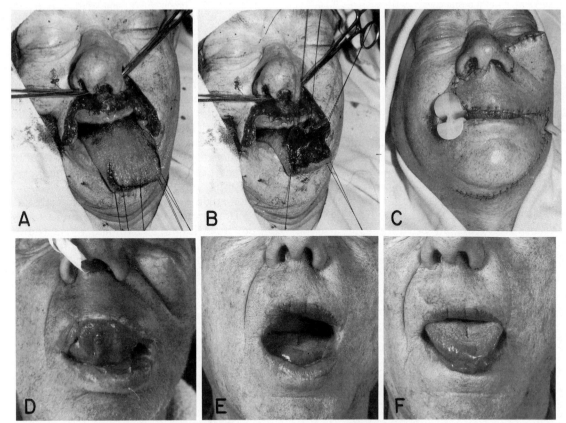

Figure 71–20. A near-total reconstruction of the upper lip, using a broad and short tongue flap, dorsally reflected on a posterior base on the lingual tip, and a flap of submental skin, superiorly based on the right face. *A, B,* Excisional defect and elevation of the tongue flap. *C,* After inset of the flaps. *D,* Before tongue flap division. *E, F,* Final result. (From Bakamjian, V. Y.: Tongue flaps in cancer surgery of the oral cavity. *In* Chretien, P. B., Johns, H. E., Shedd, D. P., Strong, E. W., and Ward, P. H. (Eds.): Head and Neck Cancer. Vol. 1. Proceedings of International Conference, Baltimore, MD, July 22-27, 1984. Toronto, B. C. Decker, 1985, p. 169.)

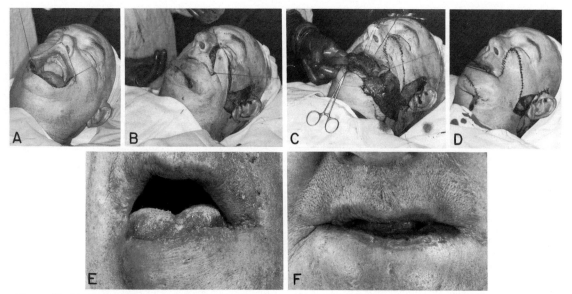

Figure 71–21. A total reconstruction of the lower lip, using a pair of dorsoventral flaps (fishmouth fashion) from the lingual tip and a bilobed, inferiorly based flap of facial skin. *A,* Excisional defect. *B,* Cheek skin flap. *C, D,* Tongue flap and inset of skin flaps. *E,* Before division of the tongue flap. *F,* Final result. (From Bakamjian, V. Y.: Tongue flaps in cancer surgery of the oral cavity. *In* Chretien, P. B., Johns, H. E., Shedd, D. P., Strong, E. W., and Ward, P. H. (Eds.): Head and Neck Cancer. Vol. 1. Proceedings of International Conference, Baltimore, MD, July 22-27, 1984. Toronto, B. C. Decker, 1985, p. 169.)

FLAPS FROM VENTRAL SURFACE OF TONGUE

The flaps so far described have been totally or largely from the dorsum of the tongue. The ventral aspect of the tongue may also find a limited usefulness in flap design. However, since the ventral mucosa is less extensive in area and since a deficiency in this area would inexcusably impair lingual function, the donor sites cannot be closed by direct approximation. However, an advantageous use of ventral tongue flaps is that in which a pair of posteriorly based flaps, one from each side, may be rotated medially and anteriorly to cover an anterior floor defect in the mouth, extending over a resected alveolar margin of the mandible to the inner aspect of the lip (Fig. 71–22). The combined donor wound is skin grafted. In this location the graft is much better tolerated than it would be if applied to the defect described, since the tongue provides a muscular, more substantial base and a convex surface. Thus, the problems of graft contraction and, paradoxically, limitation of tongue mobility are avoided by actually transferring tissue from the tongue to the defect in the oral floor.

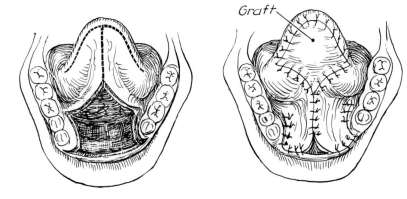

Figure 71–22. Two flaps from the ventral surface of the tongue used to close a defect of the anterior floor of the mouth.

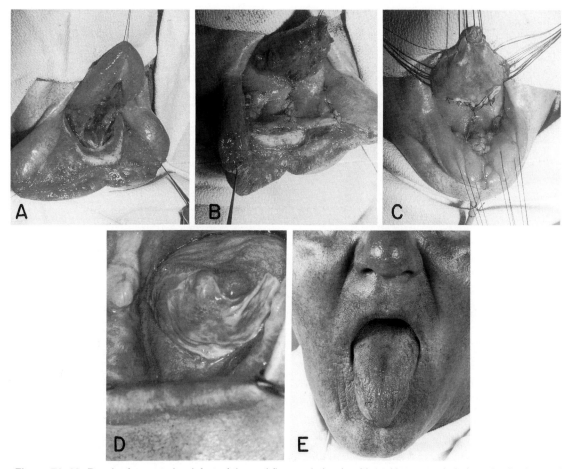

Figure 71–23. Repair of an anterior defect of the oral floor and alveolar ridge with a posteriorly based pair of ventral tongue flaps. *A,* Excisional defect. *B,* Transfer of tongue flaps. *C,* Inset of the tongue flaps and skin grafting of the tongue donor sites. *D,* Healed skin grafts. *E,* Tongue mobility. (From Bakamjian, V. Y.: Tongue flaps in cancer surgery of the oral cavity. *In* Chretien, P. B., Johns, H. E., Shedd, D. P., Strong, E. W., and Ward, P. H. (Eds.): Head and Neck Cancer. Vol. 1. Proceedings of International Conference, Baltimore, MD, July 22-27, 1984. Toronto, B. C. Decker, 1985, p. 169.)

Example 14. A 50 year old man presented with a squamous cell cancer in the anterior oral floor, extending over the alveolus into the gingivolabial sulcus. Through a midline lip-splitting approach, the resection circumvented the lesion and included the alveolar half of the mandibular height with the specimen (Fig. 71–23*A*). Two posteriorly based flaps, one from each half of the ventral side of the tongue, were elevated, and by medial rotation toward one another they were advanced to cover the large defect in the oral floor and over the mandibular resected margin (Fig. 71–23*B*). The remaining donor defect on the front ventral surface of the tongue was grafted with split-thickness skin (Fig. 71–23*C,D*). There was no impairment in tongue mobility (Fig. 71–23*E*).

REFERENCES

Bakamjian, V. Y.: Use of tongue flaps in lower-lip reconstruction. Br. J. Plast. Surg., *17:*76, 1964.

Bakamjian, V. Y.: Anteriorly and posteriorly based flaps from the dorsum of the tongue. *In* Conley, J., and Dickinson, J. T. (Eds.): Plastic and Reconstructive Surgery of the Face and Neck. Proceedings of the First International Symposium. Vol. 2. Stuttgart, Georg Thieme Verlag, 1972, p. 158.

Bakamjian, V. Y.: Tongue flaps in cancer surgery of the oral cavity. *In* Chretien, P. B., Johns, M. E., Shedd, D. P., Strong, E. W., and Ward, P. H. (Eds.): Head and Neck Cancer. Vol. 1. Proceedings of International Conference, Baltimore, MD, July 22–27, 1984. St. Louis, MO, B. C. Decker, 1985, p. 169.

Calamel, P. M.: The median transit tongue flap. Plast. Reconstr. Surg., *51*:315, 1973.

Fernandez-Villoria, J. M.: Tonsillar area reconstruction. Plast. Reconstr. Surg., *40*:220, 1967.

Guerrero-Santos, J.: Use of a tongue flap in secondary correction of cleft lips. Plast. Reconstr. Surg., *44*:368, 1969.

Guerrero-Santos, J., and Altamirano, J. T.: The use of lingual flaps in repair of fistulas of the hard palate. Plast. Reconstr. Surg., *38*:123, 1966.

Guerrero-Santos, J., Vazquez-Pallares, R., Vera-Strathmann, A., Machain, P., and Castaneda, A.: Tongue flap in reconstruction of the lip. *In* Transactions of the Third International Congress of Plastic Surgeons. Amsterdam, Excerpta Medica Foundation, 1964, p. 1055.

Jackson, I. T.: Use of tongue flaps to resurface lip defects and close palatal fistulae in children. Plast. Reconstr. Surg., *49*:537, 1972.

Klopp, C. T., and Schurter, M.: Reconstruction of palate with tongue flap and repair of tongue. Cancer, *9*:1, 1956.

Lexer, E.: Wangenplastik. Dtsch. Ztschr. Chir., *100*:206, 1909.

McGregor, I. A.: The tongue flap in lip surgery. Br. J. Plast. Surg., *19*:253, 1966.

72

Augustus J. Valauri

Maxillofacial Prosthetics

HISTORY

The origins of maxillofacial prosthetics are difficult to trace, but it may be assumed that the prosthetic restoration of missing parts of the face was practiced before surgical procedures became feasible. According to Popp (1939), artificial ears, noses, and eyes were found on Egyptian mummies. The ancient Chinese also reconstructed missing parts of the nose and ears, using wax and resins of various types.

The prosthetic restoration of missing parts of the face and jaws, as well as teeth, was performed by surgeons who also practiced dentistry. Paré (1575) was probably the first to use an obturator to close palatal clefts. In his writings, Paré illustrated a prosthetic nose fashioned of silver and attached to the face by means of a string; the prosthesis was probably painted to match the patient's complexion. He also illustrated a prosthetic ear made of paper or leather with an extension around the head for its retention.

In 1728, Fauchard utilized perforations of the palate to retain artificial dentures. Kingsley (1880) described the use of artificial appliances to restore both congenital and acquired defects of the palate, nose, and orbit. Martin (1889) described ingenious devices for the replacement of missing sections of the maxilla and mandible. Kingsley and Martin occupy preeminent positions as pioneers in the development of modern maxillofacial prosthetics.

Martin's technique consisted of a combination of intraoral and extraoral prosthetic restorations, in which the intraoral component was used to support and retain the extraoral component. At the Ninth International Congress in Washington in 1887, Martin presented a paper entitled "Artificial Nose Made in Ceramic and Retained Without the Aid of Spectacles."

In 1894, Tetamore illustrated a number of patients with loss of the nose and parts of the face that he had reconstructed prosthetically. The prostheses were fabricated of a light plastic material, which was nonirritating, and the color of the material approximated the patient's natural coloring. The prostheses were secured to the face by bow spectacles made especially for this purpose. Since the new plastics introduced at that period were made of cellulose nitrate, it is assumed that this is the material Tetamore used. In 1901, the use of vulcanite for the fabrication of prosthetic ears and noses was described by Upham.

Kazanjian's (1932) contributions during and after the First World War provided the impetus for dental surgeons, maxillofacial prosthodontists, and plastic surgeons to work together for the successful rehabilitation of the facially injured or deformed patient. Various types of maxillofacial appliances and extraoral prosthetic restorations were used, and basic principles were outlined.

To treat casualties of the wars of this century, prosthodontic and facial prostheses were constructed mainly to serve as temporary supports for the soft tissues of the face when these were deprived of their skeletal framework; such prostheses were indispensable for the rehabilitation of the patient. Although surgical progress in the last 60 years has eliminated the need for some types of artificial appliances, maxillofacial prostheses continue to play an important role in reconstructive surgery of the face and jaws.

INDICATIONS

Advances in head and neck tumor surgery and the dramatic improvement in survival statistics resulting from the modern concept of en bloc resection have produced another problem, namely, the surviving patient with facial disfigurement. A similar problem must be faced in patients with post-traumatic deformities. The loose remaining mandibular fragments and the loss of dental occlusal relationships make mastication impossible; soft tissue defects of the cheeks or lips result in constant drooling; retention of food in the oral cavity is difficult; and swallowing may be affected. The patient has a repulsive appearance to onlookers and even to himself. Outwardly alive, he is inwardly dead.

The cure of cancer requires the removal of a sufficient margin of uninvolved tissue, combined with the resection of the regional lymph nodes, to ensure eradication of the disease process. In the past, the disease-oriented surgeon proceeded with the necessary mutilating resection, following the philosophy that all means are necessary to preserve life, irrespective of the esthetic and functional consequences to the patient. This philosophy no longer prevails. The patient demands more than the preservation of life; he requires rehabilitation and restoration of function and form.

In the wide variety of maxillofacial deformities resulting from congenital malformation, trauma, or excision of malignant tissue, restoration of function and of facial form is achieved by the replacement of missing soft tissue, by repositioning of malpositioned bone, by bone grafting of osseous defects, and by restoration of adequate contour.

A facial prosthetic appliance may be fabricated of solid material or soft and flexible material. If it is made of hard acrylic resin, it should have solid, immobile margins not affected by the muscles of expression or mastication, because mobility of the margins directs attention to the prosthesis. It thus is often preferable to restore the mobile parts of the face by plastic surgical procedures as a preliminary to the insertion of a rigid type of appliance. Prosthetic restorations in the oral or nasal cavity must also rest on a base of healthy tissue. For example, when the soft tissues are expanded after resection of intranasal scar tissue and are to be supported by a prosthesis, they must be lined with a skin or mucosal graft before the appliance is inserted (Fig. 72–1).

Prosthetic and prosthodontic appliances are required in the following conditions:

1. For realignment and fixation of mandibular fragments in adequate dental occlusal relationship with the teeth of the opposing upper jaw after loss of a portion of the mandible, until continuity of the jaw can be re-established by bone grafting.

Following loss of a portion of the mandible, the remaining fragments are subjected to the inexorable traction of the attached muscles. After loss of the anterior half of the mandible, including the symphysis and the anterior portion of the body on each side, the remaining mandibular fragments are subjected to a lingual displacement from the contraction of the mylohyoid muscle, and an upward and backward displacement from the contraction of the musculature of mastication. When the mandible is destroyed between the symphysis and the ramus on one side, the remaining portion of the mandible is displaced medially by the traction exerted by the mylohyoid muscle; the ramus is usually subjected to the forward, medial, and upward pull of the masticatory muscles. Some method of fixation of the mandible is required to avoid osseous displacement by the constriction of the soft tissues. If this is not done, rehabilitation at a later date becomes extremely difficult and in many cases impossible.

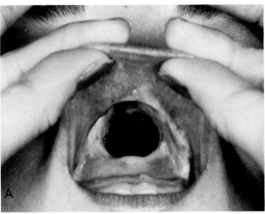
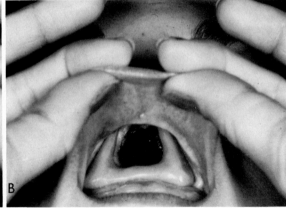

Figure 72–1. *A,* Intranasal cavity, deficient of lining, relined with a split-thickness skin graft. *B,* The prosthesis supports the skin grafted area and restores contour.

2. As obturators for the occlusion of defects of the palatal region after loss of the palatal and maxillary bone.

3. For the maintenance of facial form and contour and prevention of contraction during the healing period following the reconstruction of lips or cheeks. Prostheses are also used to secure intraoral skin or mucosal grafts, to support the grafts and prevent contraction in the nasal and orbital regions (Fig. 72–2), and to maintain a reconstructed alveolar buccal sulcus and retentive alveolar ridge.

Prostheses are often used as temporary or transitional modalities, before or during surgical treatment, to maintain the soft tissues during the healing period. The prosthesis, in such cases, is discarded after skeletal restoration.

4. For the restoration of facial features, such as the nose, auricle, or orbital region, when reconstructive surgery is not advisable, either because it is not indicated for fear of tumor recurrence or because the patient is too old or ill to undergo multiple-stage reconstructive procedures.

In post-traumatic deformities, prosthetic restoration of missing parts of the face is indicated when surgical procedures cannot be expected to produce satisfactory functional or esthetic results. For example, when teeth are lost, a prosthodontic restoration is the only means of rehabilitation. Similarly, when a section of the palate or alveolar ridge is destroyed, a prosthesis may often be preferable to surgery.

A large defect of the skull can be corrected by transplantation of bone (see Chap. 18), but when reconstruction by bone grafts is con-traindicated because the patient is too old to undergo reconstructive procedures or the cranial defect is too extensive, a metal or plastic cover for the defect is occasionally indicated (Fig. 72–3).

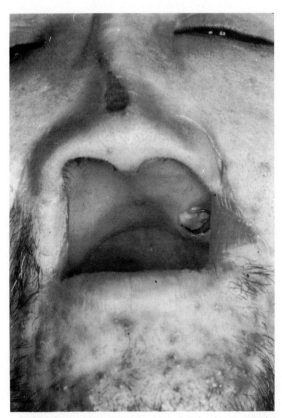

Figure 72–2. A patient who had sustained an extensive gunshot wound wearing an obturator prosthesis to prevent contraction of the nasal soft tissues and to aid in deglutition and speech.

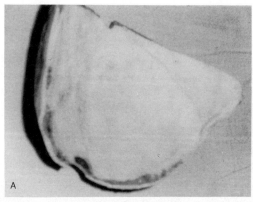 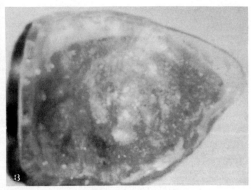

Figure 72–3. *A,* Section of the cranium that has been removed. *B,* A duplicate of the removed bone is made of clear methylmethacrylate (acrylic) reinforced with metal mesh to replace the cranial defect.

FIXATION OF MANDIBULAR FRAGMENTS

There are many techniques to implement the principles of prosthetic fixation. The method of choice should be the one that offers the simplest and most direct approach to successful and positive fixation.

The following types of appliances are employed in maintaining mandibular fragments: arch and band appliances, biteblocks or dentures maintained in position by circumferential wiring, biphase appliances, and buried appliances made of inert materials. When there is sufficient mandibular bone remaining, extraoral fixation may be employed (see Figs. 72–10 and 72–11).

Arch and Band Appliances, Splints, and Biteblocks. While bimaxillary fixation by interdental wiring is satisfactory, arch and band appliances and splints are to be preferred when facilities are available for their construction. They provide monomaxillary fixation, permit movement of the jaw, and are the appliances of choice when the fragments have teeth upon which bands may be placed. They can be maintained in position for a long time before the definitive reconstructive procedures. They also constitute the most stable means of maintaining fixation of the fragments after bone grafting.

When the fragments are edentulous, biteblocks or dentures may be maintained by circumferential wiring around the body of the mandible; the maxillary appliance may be fixed by internal wire suspension to the zygomatic process of the frontal bone, the zygomatic arch, or the piriform aperture. Circumferential wires placed at strategic

positions in order to maintain fixation are looped around the mandibular fragments and over the biteblock or denture (Fig. 72–4*A*). When the upper jaw is edentulous, the upper denture is maintained by internal wiring placed through the zygomatic fossa and looped through a hole drilled through the posterior margin of the frontal process of the zygoma. Additional reinforcing wires may be placed through the edge of the piriform aperture or looped around the anterior nasal spine (Fig. 72–4*B,C*). Such internal and circumferential wiring of maxillary and mandibular prostheses has been maintained for periods of six to 12 weeks after the transplantation of a large segment of bone graft to restore a major portion of the mandible.

When the teeth are in poor condition and are unable to support a fixation appliance, appliances such as those illustrated in Figure 72–5 can be maintained by means of circumferential wiring. In more recent years the author has used with more frequency the Morris (1949) biphase fixation appliance (see Figs. 72–6 to 72–10).

The Twin-Screw Morris Biphase Appliance. The twin-screw Morris biphase appliance (Morris, 1949; Fleming and Morris, 1969) is highly versatile. The Morris external fixation splint (Fig. 72–6) employs vitallium bone screws $\frac{1}{8}$ inch in diameter. The screws are threaded at both ends; one end is inserted into bone, and the other receives a washer-faced nut that secures an acrylic bar that joins the two units of parallel screws. A stab-like soft tissue incision is made over the proposed site of insertion of the screw, and a hole is drilled into the bone with a $\frac{3}{32}$ inch twist drill (Fig. 72–7). A drill of smaller dimension is preferred to place holes into the

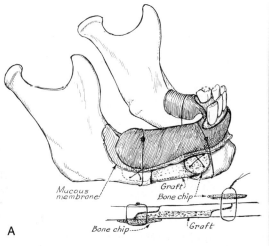

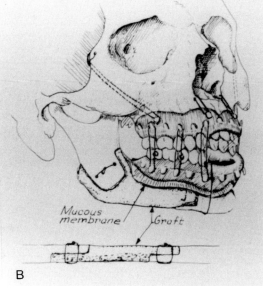

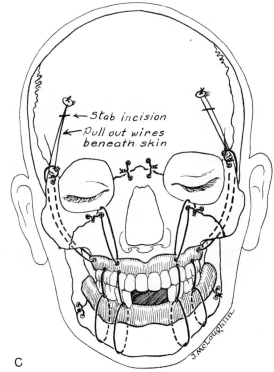

Figure 72–4. *A,* The loose ramus fragment. Control and fixation of the ramus by a prosthodontic appliance. The patient's denture was relined (in the operating room) and was maintained by circumferential wiring after placing of the bone graft. Excessive pressure over the mucoperiosteum should be avoided to prevent necrosis. *B,* Retention of the prosthesis with circum-mandibular and craniofacial suspension wires. *C,* Method of interosseous wire fixation and internal wire suspension utilizing the patient's own dentures in an edentulous patient with multiple facial fractures. The lower front teeth are removed from the denture to facilitate feeding.

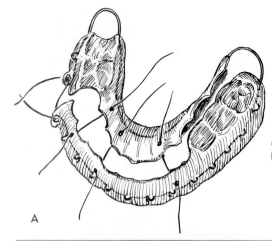

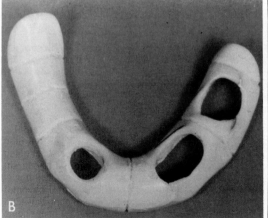

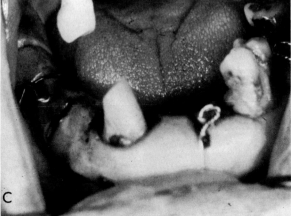

Figure 72–5. *A,* Split acrylic fixation appliance. *B,* Overlay acrylic splint. *C,* The overlay is secured with circumferential wires placed around the mandible.

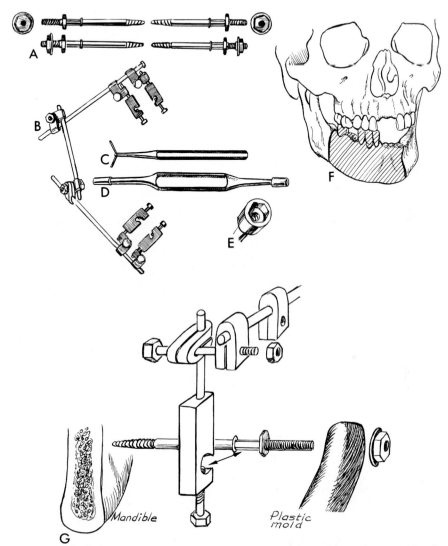

Figure 72–6. The biphase external skeletal fixation appliance. *A,* Vitallium bone screws with special heads and washer-faced lock nuts. *B,* Primary assembly of the splint fixation appliance with rods and screw clamps in position for adjustment. *C,* Antitorque wrench. *D,* The wrench. *E,* The end of the wrench that accepts hexagonal nuts. *F,* The shaded area represents the mandibular defect that is to be repaired. *G,* Details of the vitallium bone screw and clamp. The hexagonal surface of the screw facilitates positive no-skid fixation. Rod clamps are shown above as they maintain the primary splint rods in position. (From Kazanjian and Converse.)

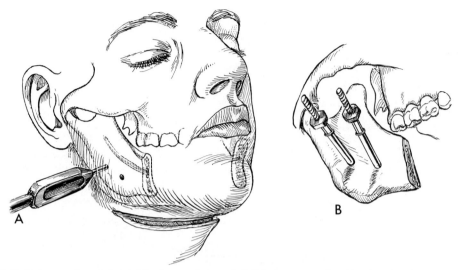

Figure 72–7. Biphase external skeletal fixation appliance. *A,* Drill holes are made with a hand drill to receive the bone screws. *B,* The bone screws are threaded into position. (From Kazanjian and Converse.)

ramus. The screws are inserted with a distance of at least 2 cm between each screw of the pair. After realignment of the fragments is achieved, the two units of parallel screws are joined by a connecting portion of the apparatus (the first phase), which is designed to maintain the position of the two units (Fig. 72–8) until an acrylic bar (the second phase) ensures permanent fixation (Fig. 72–9). The term "biphase" defines this double maneuver. Quick-curing acrylic resin, while in its rubber-like, pliable state (Fig. 72–9), is molded

and adapted over the ends of the screws of each unit (Fig. 72–10). Before the acrylic bar has hardened, a washer-faced nut is secured to the exposed thread of each screw. The temporary connecting splint is removed.

The Morris apparatus is strong, although light in weight. The vitallium screws are well tolerated and can be left in position for long periods (Fig. 72–11). The external splint controls the remaining mandibular fragments during the period of consolidation of the bone grafts. Before bone grafting, the external fix-

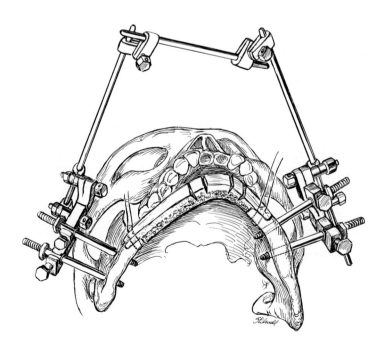

Figure 72–8. Biphase external skeletal fixation appliance. The primary splint appliance and the bone graft in position before the fixation wires are twisted. (From Kazanjian and Converse.)

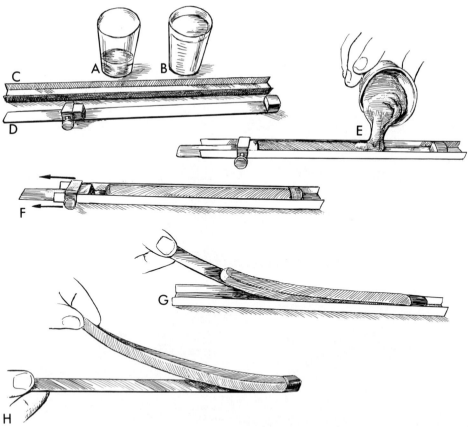

Figure 72–9. Fabrication of an acrylic resin bar. *A,* Acrylic liquid monomer. *B,* Acrylic resin polymer powder. The liquid monomer and powdered polymer are mixed in a 1 to 3 ratio. *C, D,* The metallic tray and rod that make up the take-apart mold. *E,* Acrylic mixture being poured into the take-apart mold. *F,* Mold being separated from the "room temperature curing" acrylic splint. *G, H,* The still pliable acrylic bar is carefully removed from the mold without deforming its shape. (From Kazanjian and Converse.)

ation appliance is used to retain the edentulous fragments in position. After the bone is transplanted and fastened with interosseous wires or miniplates to the remaining mandibular segments, additional fixation methods are not required.

If a portion of the mandible is to be excised with the tumor, it must be established whether mandibular reconstruction with a bone graft replacement should be the treatment of choice and whether replacement is to be done at the time of resection or within a reasonable time soon after. It is best to apply an external device such as the biphase apparatus *before the mandibular bone is removed* (Fig. 72–12).

The fixation may be simply applied with the screws at a distance well away from the surgical area. The acrylic frame is applied and allowed to set. After the acrylic has hardened, the frame near the mesial screws is keyed so that the center portion of the

acrylic frame may be cut away and replaced at the same predetermined position at any time during or after the excision of the tumor and mandibular section (Fig. 72–12). This method of fixation allows the surgeon to perform the surgery and still return the remaining fragments of the mandible to their presurgical position without any deviation of the remaining fragments. The resected fragment of the mandible can be duplicated, and a template of the exact size of the resected bone is fabricated in acrylic or metal and used as a guide in harvesting the appropriate size of bone graft needed to replace the missing bone.

If reconstruction of the mandible with a bone graft is immediately performed, the continuity of the mandibular fixation acrylic bar may be maintained with stainless steel wires. This can be assembled and disassembled until the appropriate bone graft is shaped to replace the bone removed. When the graft is fixed in position, all surgical procedures are

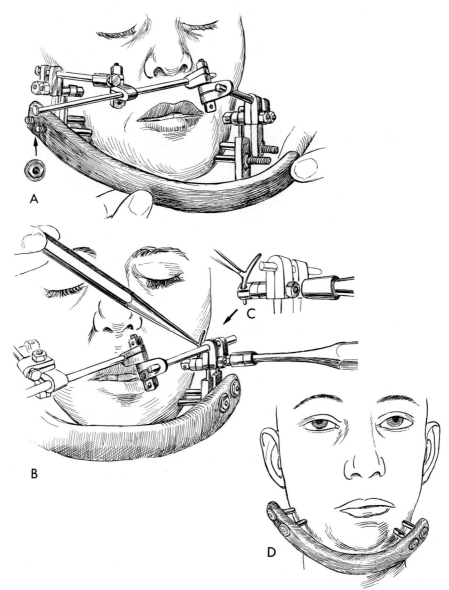

Figure 72–10. Adapting the acrylic resin splint. *A,* While still in a semiputty condition, the acrylic bar is gently pressed onto the machined threads of the bone screws. Washer-faced lock nuts are initially twisted to a position just short of being flush with the end of the screw. *B, C,* After the heat of polymerization has dissipated three to five minutes later and the acrylic bar has hardened, final tightening of the lock nuts is performed. To overtighten the lock nut while the acrylic is soft invites weakness in the splint owing to excessive thinning of the bar at this site. The primary mechanical splint is removed in the reverse order of its application. *D,* The secondary rigid, resilient, light acrylic bar (biphase splint) is relatively unobtrusive as the bone graft heals. When properly placed, the splint can be expected to maintain its mechanical stabilization for periods exceeding nine months. (From Kazanjian and Converse.)

to ten weeks or until there is clinical and radiographic evidence of sufficient strength in the graft area to release fixation support.

Immobilization of the graft segment is imperative to optimize the development of an intact graft and to avoid pseudarthrosis. The mandibular graft must intimately approximate the remaining mandibular segments. This can be accomplished only with proper fixations.

Inert Buried Appliances. These appliances find their major application when teeth are not available for fixation after the resection of the body of the mandible, and they serve to maintain the anatomic position of the mandibular angle and ramus. They include metallic plates and wires and appliances made of inorganic materials. They usually have a temporary function and are often well tolerated for a sufficient time before definitive bone graft reconstruction of the mandible. The author prefers a fenestrated tantalum tray that bridges the mandibular defect. The tray is wired to the mandibular fragments. Pieces of iliac bone are placed in

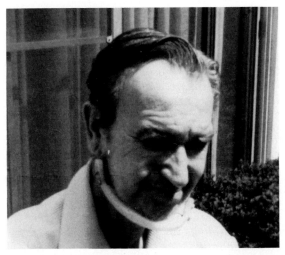

Figure 72–11. Morris appliance in position controlling the posterior fragments. A large portion of the body of the mandible had been reconstructed by a bone graft.

accomplished, and the incision is closed, the wire joints are reinforced with acrylic for a more permanent and stronger joint. The patient wears the extraoral prosthesis for nine

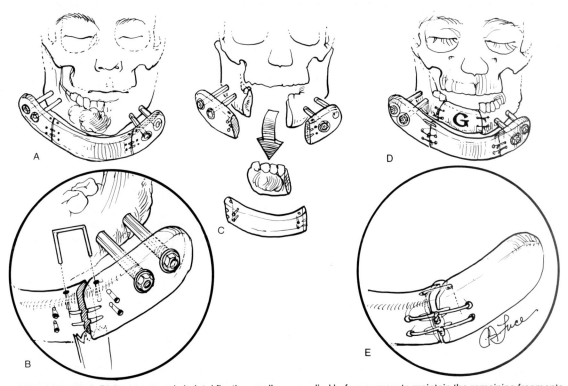

Figure 72–12. A, Biphase external skeletal fixation appliance applied before surgery to maintain the remaining fragments in proper relation after surgery. B, Acrylic frame is prepared with four holes and a U-shaped wire key before being cut and separated. C, Section of the acrylic frame has been cut and removed, allowing the surgeon to resect and remove the mandibular tumor. D, The resected mandibular segment has been replaced with a bone graft (G), and fixation accomplished with the acrylic frame reestablished in a predetermined position, placing the distal mandibular fragments in the same occlusal relationship as before surgical intervention. E, Final fixation of the acrylic frame with wires and acrylic.

the tray and joined with each other and with the ends of the mandibular fragments. The tray is subsequently removed prior to inlay skin grafting and reconstruction of the buccal sulcus. Boyne (1970) introduced the use of chrome-cobalt castings lined with a microporous filter filled with cancellous bone and marrow to restore bone contour and deficiencies. Telescopic metal sections were introduced and used by Hinds and associates (1963).

MANDIBULAR PROSTHESES

Mandibular deformities requiring special prosthetic reconstruction may be classified into two groups.

Group 1

Group 1 includes deformities of the mandible characterized by considerable loss of bone and teeth without disruption of the continuity of the mandible. These deformities result in a loss of the normal contour of the lower third of the face and an inability to masticate.

The primary aim of treatment is to prepare the oral structures for the successful retention of a denture of sufficient bulk to improve the contour of the face. The technique of the skin graft inlay for the restoration of a buccal sulcus and of the vertical increase of the alveolar ridge is described in Figure 72–16. The surgical preparation consists of incising the tissue on the buccal and labial aspects of the mandible, deepening the buccal sulcus, and applying a skin graft, which is maintained in position by a prosthetic appliance. A definitive prosthesis is constructed after final healing of the new retentive alveolar ridge has been achieved (Fig. 72–13).

Restoration of a Buccal Sulcus and a Functional Alveolar Ridge: Skin or Mucosal Graft Inlay Technique. Operative procedures that restore the external contour of the face and reestablish the bone continuity of the mandible should be supplemented by artificial dentures to restore masticatory function. Skin or mucosal grafting is often a necessary procedure to provide an adequate sulcus and a retentive alveolar ridge after bone graft reconstruction of the mandible.

The term "epithelial" inlay was first used by Esser (1917), who devised the technique of intraoral skin grafting. The term is a misnomer, since the graft, which includes both epidermis and dermis, is composed of more than epithelium alone, as the original term implies. It is preferable to use the term "skin graft" inlay. Esser conceived the technique for the purpose of establishing a buccal sulcus in patients in whom the mandible had been reconstructed by means of bone grafts. The purpose of restoring a vestibule was to increase the retention of a denture. Esser made an incision through the skin in the submandibular area, extending the incision to the lower border of the reconstructed mandible, then upward along the buccal aspect of the mandible as far as the mucosa of the floor of the mouth. Into this cavity he molded a piece of softened dental impression compound. Around the mold, a split-thickness skin graft, raw surface outward, was wrapped and the compound mold was placed into the cavity; the submandibular incision was sutured.

In a second-stage operation some weeks later, Esser incised through the mucosa of the floor of the mouth into the skin grafted cavity, removed the dental compound mold, and extended the buccal flange of the denture into the restored sulcus.

Waldron, an American surgeon during the First World War, modified the technique by placing the skin graft directly into the new sulcus through an intraoral incision (Waldron and Risdon, 1919). Since World War I, the skin graft inlay technique has been used extensively to restore an adequate lining in the oral cavity. The typical inlay technique consists of three parts: the incision, the prosthesis, and the graft (Fig. 72–14).

The Incision. The incision is made through the mucosa on the labiobuccal aspect of the alveolar ridge and extended to the periosteum. The reason for leaving the periosteum intact over the bone is that grafting is more successful over the vascular bed provided by the periosteum. The incision is extended downward along the buccal surface of the mandible, and the mucosal flap thus formed is reflected inferiorly and partially lines the labiobuccal aspects of the reconstructed sulcus (Fig. 72–14A,B). This type of incision has the advantage that the cut edges of the oral mucosa are not situated at the same level; thus, a constrictive scar band is not formed at the junction of the skin and the mucosa after the skin graft has healed. Careful hemostasis is obtained by fine forceps

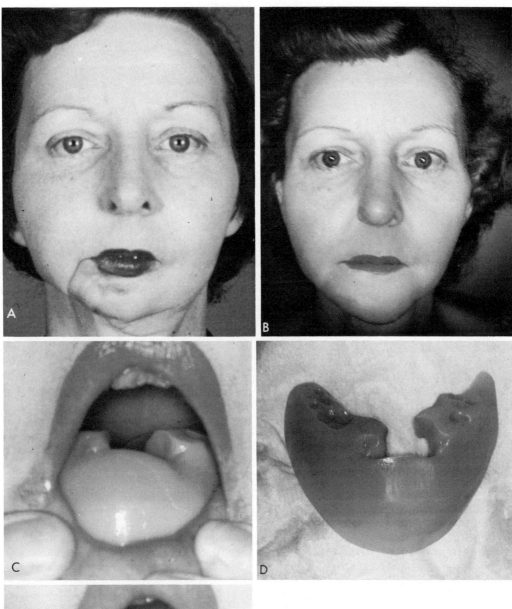

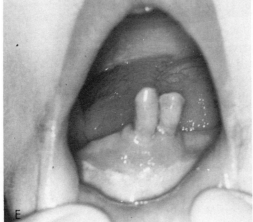

Figure 72–13. *A,* The patient had lost most of her dentition and a greater portion of the alveolar bone; the continuity of the mandible remained intact. *B,* The patient is shown wearing a large lower temporary prosthesis *(C, D).* The prosthesis, which has a downward extension into the skin grafted sulcus, will be gradually modified, and teeth will be added to achieve adequate dental contour. *E,* Photograph of the skin grafted sulcus.

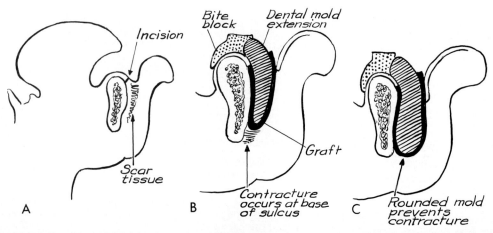

Figure 72–14. The skin graft inlay for restoration of the labiobuccal sulcus. *A,* The incision is made through the mucosa but does not extend through the periosteum. A flap is raised and reflected forward to line the lower lip (see *B*). *B,* The sulcus has been deepened; an impression has been taken with soft dental compound and hardened in situ with cold water. A split-thickness skin graft covers the dental compound mold. Note that the pointed shape of the tip of the mold will result in contracture of the grafted tissues postoperatively. *C,* Correct shape of the mold to maintain the depth of the sulcus. Fixation of the biteblock or denture that maintains the skin grafted mold is often best obtained by circumferential wiring around the mandible (see Fig. 72–15).

electrocoagulation. Complete hemostasis is essential to prevent hematoma, which would interfere with the vascularization of the skin graft.

In order that the revascularization of the graft may occur without interference, two conditions must be satisfied. First, the contact between the graft and host must be as intimate as possible, and there must be no interposition of blood or serum, which would act as a barrier to the ingrowth of host vessels. Second, satisfactory fixation and immobilization (Fig. 72–15) must be provided so that the vessels are not torn during the period of vessel penetration into the graft.

In large skin graft inlays, considerable distention of the soft tissues in the region of the symphysis is necessary to permit the introduction of a compound mold of sufficient size. In such cases, it may be necessary to sever the lower attachments of the musculature of the lower lip and the platysma to allow adequate stretching of the soft tissues.

The Prosthesis. Two features are essential in the construction of the dental compound mold: (1) it must provide an accurate impression of the new surgical cavity and (2) it must be considerably larger than the cavity in order to distend the tissues in every direction and be free of sharp edges that would cut into the tissues. One cannot overemphasize the need for considerable distention of the soft tissue and the construction of a grossly oversized mold, which can be reduced progressively during subsequent weeks. The construction of an oversized mold is important for two reasons. All skin grafts tend to contract during the healing period; if the skin graft is placed over a mold that is oversized, an excess of skin graft is implanted, thus counteracting the eventual contraction of the graft. Moreover, hematoma formation, which would interfere with the vascularization of the graft, is prevented.

Newly developed synthetic materials have made possible the fabrication of a definitive prosthesis while the patient is in the operating room. However, this procedure causes considerable delay despite the rapidity of curing of some of the new resins. In most complicated cases, it is more practical to prepare two appliances. The first is a temporary biteblock (occlusal wafer), which serves to anchor the compound mold for the primary skin grafting procedure; the second is a definitive denture with an oversized flange that fills the reconstructed sulcus. The flange is gradually reduced during the weeks subsequent to the operation. The shaping of the flange is important. It should fill the entire cavity and be of a shape that ensures retention (see Fig. 72–14C).

The Graft. Split-thickness skin grafts are the most frequently used tissue to reline the raw surface of the surgically prepared cavity. Their use is especially indicated in the inlay technique when large areas must be resurfaced.

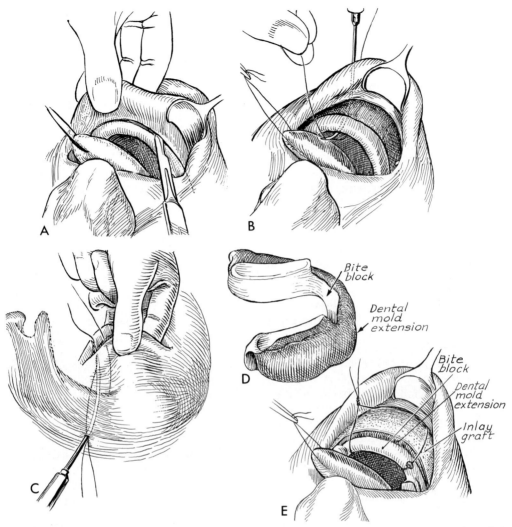

Figure 72–15. The skin graft inlay for the restoration of the labiobuccal sulcus in the edentulous patient. *A,* Incision through the mucosa. *B, C,* Passing a circumferential wire. *D,* The biteblock with the skin graft–carrying mold. *E,* Circumferential wires maintain the skin graft inlay in position.

Skin grafts have the disadvantage of lacking pliability, of having a keratin surface that is difficult to "wet," of being malodorous, and of occasionally transferring hair to the oral cavity. The "wetness" is an especially desirable feature when maxillary vestibuloplasties are performed (Steinhauser, 1971). To provide a more physiologic vestibular lining, a split-thickness graft of oral mucosa can be removed from the inner aspect of the lower lip by a Castroviejo mucotome (a small electric dermatome) (Converse, 1964; Steinhauser, 1969). The cheeks and the undersurface of the tongue can also serve as donor sites. The entire hard palatal mucoperiosteum has also been used (Hall and O'Steen, 1970). In an effort to increase the area of coverage,

Morgan, Gallegos, and Frileck (1973), using the mucoperiosteum of the hard palate, placed the graft through a skin mesher to expand the graft; thus, a greater surface area could be covered by the limited amount of graft. The denuded hard palate reepithelized spontaneously.

The skin graft inlay was originally made with very thin split-thickness grafts. The thin graft has the advantage of becoming vascularized rapidly and having what is referred to as an excellent "take." The inconvenience of the thin graft is its contraction during the postoperative healing period. For this reason, thicker split-thickness grafts are employed. The usual thickness is 0.014 inch, as calibrated on American dermatomes. The skin graft should be removed from a hairless area of the body to prevent subsequent growth of hair inside the oral cavity.

Fixation of the Skin Graft–Carrying Prosthesis. The fixation of the appliance that maintains the skin graft in the newly made sulcus varies according to the status of the dentition. When the patient has teeth, it is possible to provide fixation of the partial denture by fixed band and arch appliances. When the patient is edentulous, a complete denture or biteblock (occlusion rim) is maintained by circumferential wiring around the body of the mandible (Fig. 72–15*E*). A denture can be made in patients who have teeth on portions of the adjacent mandible. Clamps keep the denture stabilized to the teeth, and circumferential wires ensure completion of the fixation. Softened dental compound is added to the denture and extended into the deepened sulcus; a definitive appliance can be made immediately in the operating room with quick-curing methylmethacrylate.

Postoperative Care. The skin graft is immobilized for a period of seven to ten days, after which the compound mold is removed under sedation, regional anesthesia, or general anesthesia. Any excess skin graft overlapping the edges of the sulcus is trimmed and any points where granulation tissue is seen are cauterized with a silver nitrate stick. The appliance is immediately replaced to prevent contraction of the graft and diminution of the sulcus. At no time during the subsequent months should the prosthesis be left out of the skin grafted cavity, since contraction of the skin graft prevents replacement of the prosthesis. The duplicate acrylic resin mold is used to replace the primary mold. The prosthesis is left undisturbed for another four or five days, after which it is removed for cleansing. After this, it is removed every few days.

As emphasized above, the prosthetic mold should be grossly oversized for all large skin graft inlays. After a period varying between three and five weeks, the size of the acrylic resin prosthesis is reduced by progressively grinding it down to the desired size and shape. All skin grafts contract; the period of maximal contracture spans several weeks, and the reduction in size should be slow and progressive. The best results are obtained if a period of approximately eight to ten weeks is spent in developing the final size and shape of the prosthesis. The patient should be told to avoid removing the appliance for any length of time, in order to prevent contraction in the skin grafted area.

Increasing the Vertical Projection of the Edentulous Mandibular Arch. Exposure of the alveolar process is obtained preferably through an intraoral approach. A bone graft is fashioned and fitted over the bone and maintained by circumferential wires laid into grooves on the upper surface of the graft (Fig. 72–16). There is usually sufficient mucosa to redrape it over the bone graft and deepen the sulcus. There is considerable resorption of the grafted bone, but usually sufficient bone remains to protect the inferior alveolar nerve and furnish a retentive alveolar process. Although bone resected from the lower border of the mandible is less prone to resorption, the edentulous mandible is often so tenuous that little bone is available for this purpose. Autogenous cartilage grafts have also been successfully employed. Inorganic implants remain in position for a limited period before being extruded.

More recently there has been some success in increasing the vertical height of the mandibular and maxillary ridges with hydroxyapatite (Fig. 72–17).

Autogenous bone grafts appear to be the most satisfactory replacement material for mandibular reconstruction, as illustrated in the following case report with over 20 years of follow-up. The chief complaints of the 43 year old woman shown in Figure 72–18*A,B* were:

1. Difficulty in wearing the lower denture because of inadequate retention due to a severely diminished ridge (Fig. 72–18*C*), and pain due to exposure of the inferior alveolar nerve, which was inadequately protected by osseous covering.

2. Problems with facial esthetics owing to prognathic jaw relationships.

Treatment. The patient's jaw dysharmony was first corrected by means of a bilateral vertical osteotomy of the ramus, obtaining a more favorable arch relationship. The upper and lower dentures were modified and were used as surgical splints to maintain a predetermined fixed position while postoperative healing took place.

Approximately ten months later, the patient was prosthetically prepared for the second stage of surgical rehabilitation. Accurate impressions of the upper and lower jaws were obtained; centric and vertical relations were

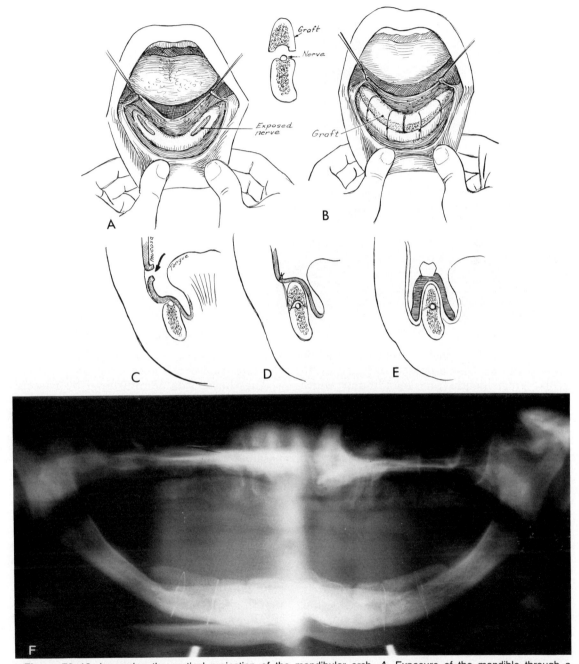

Figure 72–16. Increasing the vertical projection of the mandibular arch. *A,* Exposure of the mandible through a labiobuccal incision. The inferior alveolar nerves are exposed. *B,* The bone graft is shaped to fit over the nerves and is secured by circumferential wires. *C,* The labiobuccal incision is made. *D,* Suture completed. *E,* The denture now has better retention as a result of the increased height of the alveolar process. Often the labiobuccal sulcus must be reconstructed as a secondary procedure. *F,* Panoramic radiograph 16 years after the above procedure.

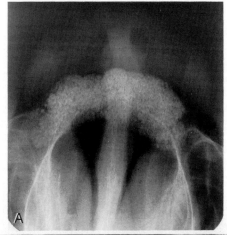

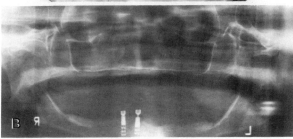

Figure 72–17. *A,* Augmentation of the anterior maxillary envelope with hydroxyapatite. *B,* Panoramic radiograph showing ridge augmentation with alveolar ridge graft and core vent implants one year postoperatively.

recorded and the models were articulated on an articulator. The proposed increase in alveolar ridge height and mandibular width was designed by means of wax. This was duplicated in stone and used for the construction of a surgical guide tray in clear acrylic. The tray was used as a guide for the height and width of bone needed to increase and protect the lower alveolar ridge.

The operation was carried out under general anesthesia. An incision was made along the buccal mucosa 1.5 cm anterior to the lower alveolar arch. The mucosal flap was elevated and the periosteum of the alveolar arch was raised with a periosteal elevator. The nerves were found through the foramen in the upper edge of the lower alveolar arch. A bone graft was taken from the right iliac crest. The bone graft, measuring 9 cm, was placed over the lower alveolar arch and held in position with circumferential wire (Fig. 72–18*D*). The mucosal flap was applied over the bone graft and sutured.

Seven months later the patient was prepared for the final surgical phase: the creation of a labial sulcus. The patient's upper denture was used and two accurate-fitting presurgical lower biteblocks were prepared with pliable stainless steel loops on the buccal phalanges to create a buccal extension and a sulcus for the retention of the lower denture.

Anesthesia was administered by nasotracheal intubation. An incision was made close to the buccal surface of the alveolar bone with care not to incise the periosteum. The incision was extended carefully, whenever possible with a blunt instrument, thus forming a sulcus or pocket freeing the tissues so that maximal extension could be attained. After a satisfactory pocket was formed, the preoperative splint was introduced into the mouth and the wire loops were bent into the area for maximal retention. Dental compound was softened in hot water and molded onto the wire loops, while the compound was still soft. This was once again introduced into the mouth and fitted into the freshly formed cavity. It was essential at this time to overbuild the contour and construct an oversized mold. With a Hanau hand torch, the sharp edges and dead spaces were eliminated and the compound seared and sealed to the acrylic splint.

After an acceptable prosthesis was prepared by the method described above, a split-thickness graft was taken from a hairless area, e.g., the inner aspect of the arm, and laid gently "raw surface out" over the dental

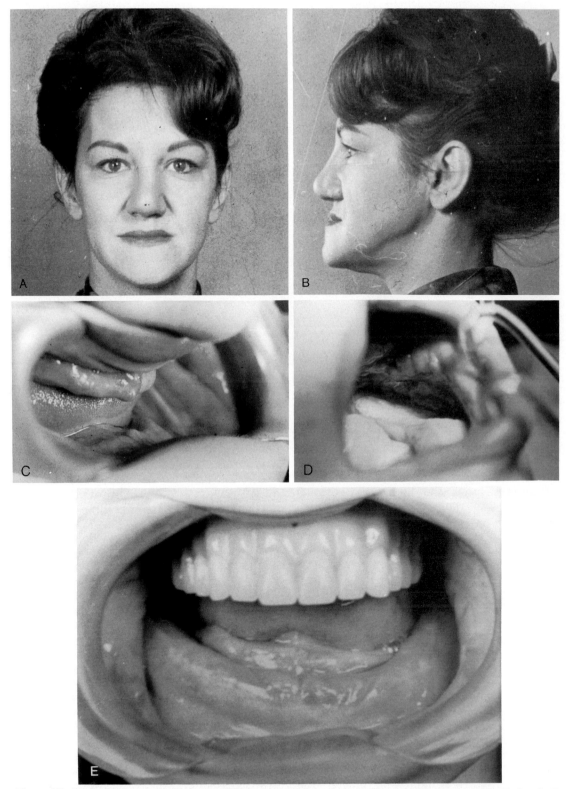

Figure 72–18. *A, B,* A patient showing mandibular prognathism. *C,* Severely resorbed alveolar ridge. *D,* Surgically created sulcus with skin graft. *E,* New alveolar ridge created with bone graft and skin graft inlay of the sulcus.

Illustration continued on following page

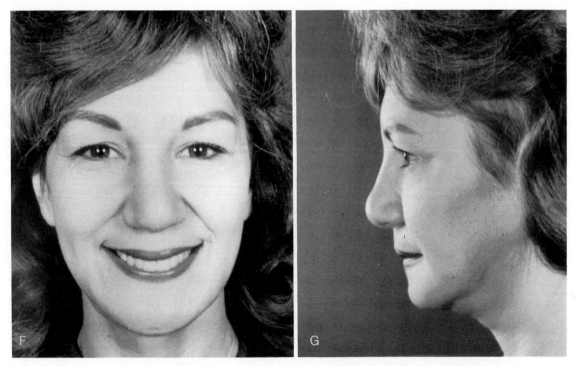

Figure 72–18 *Continued F, G,* The patient with dentures and her new profile.

compound impression that covered the raw area of the sulcus to be formed. Dabs of dermatome cement were used to maintain contact of the graft with the prosthesis. The prosthesis, with the skin graft in place, was introduced into the oral cavity, where it was immobilized by circumferential wires.

Ten days later, the temporary surgical prosthesis was replaced by a transitional acrylic prosthesis. It is important to emphasize to the patient that the prosthesis is not to be left out of its sulcus longer than a few minutes for the first four to six weeks after the operation (Fig. 72–18*D*).

When the alveolar skin graft had healed (Fig. 72–18*E*), the patient was treated almost as any individual requiring an upper and lower denture. The lower was first impressioned in alginate from which an acrylic tray was made, allowing room for a rubber base impression. The peripheral borders were trimmed in compound; the tray was partially cut over the ridge area and a rubber base impression was taken of the lower arch. The top of the tray was completely cut away and the tray was reinserted in place leaving the ridge area overlying the bone graft exposed. A creamy mixture of impression plaster was brushed over the ridge and on the acrylic tray for the final impression of the newly created

alveolus. This two-phase impression was boxed and poured. The upper was impressioned in the conventional manner. The patient was supplied with well-fitting, full upper and lower dentures (Fig. 72–18*F,G*).

Deformities caused by malunited fractures are also included in Group I. Repair of such deformities is usually achieved by surgical methods. Borderline cases, however, may be encountered in which one may hesitate to subject the patient to osteoplastic repair; a prosthetic appliance can be constructed, the mouth being prepared for its reception by less drastic surgical procedures. The technique illustrated in Figure 72–19 was employed for a patient who had suffered a compound comminuted fracture of the lower jaw, and in whom the fragments had been permitted to consolidate without considering the occlusion of the teeth. As a result, the remaining lower teeth slanted lingually, completely out of contact with the upper teeth. An osteoplastic procedure would have involved an osteotomy through the median section of the mandible, immobilization of the fragments to restore adequate occlusion, and transplantation of bone to fill the gap in the mandible. Less drastic prosthetic measures were employed. An upper partial ramp was placed lingual to the maxillary posterior teeth, and carved to

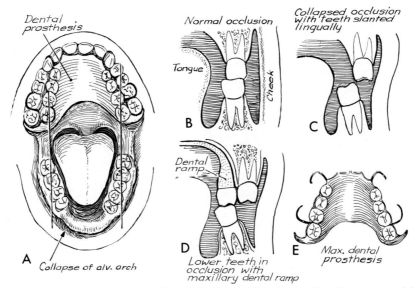

Figure 72–19. *A,* Occlusal view of a patient with mandibular alveolar collapse. Note the upper partial ramp. *B,* Normal occlusion. *C,* Mandibular teeth slanted lingually out of normal occlusion. *D,* A ramp is placed lingual to the posterior maxillary teeth and carved to restore occlusal interdigitation. *E,* Maxillary dental prosthesis.

proper occlusal interdigitation to allow for mastication and freedom of mandibular movements. A lower partial denture was made to restore the missing teeth and augment the soft tissues to the desired facial contour. It may be necessary in some cases to extend the labial sulcus for better denture retention and restoration of the facial contour. This type of occlusal ramp is also useful in improving masticatory function after hemimandibulectomy. In general, it is preferable to restore the occlusion by osteotomies.

In patients in whom the few remaining teeth have been fractured or badly destroyed by caries and only two or three remaining roots are present, it is advisable to retain the roots and treat them with endodontic therapy. The roots can then serve as strong and efficient anchors when joined together by means of endodontic gold posts and a connecting metal bar, which can be used to retain an overdenture (Fig. 72–20).

Group 2

The second group of mandibular deformities are those in which a full-thickness section of the mandible is missing. It should be emphasized that defects of the mandible, even though extensive, can be repaired by bone grafting; however, prosthetic surgical splints may be necessary. In this chapter the possibilities of prosthetic devices are outlined for patients in whom surgery is contraindicated.

In cases such as these in which the opportunity of mandibular junction is limited, the degree of function that can be restored is dependent on the size and anatomic position of the existing bone and on the presence or absence of teeth. The cases differ, depending on the degree of lateral and backward displacement and the resulting disturbance of occlusion and normal jaw function. In favorable cases the correction of the deformity may be achieved by mechanical manipulation and by orthodontic or orthopedic appliances; in others, the presence of cicatricial tissue necessitates surgical intervention.

Loss of Median Section of Major Portion of Body of Edentulous or Semiedentulous Mandible. It is difficult to secure the retention of a denture in an edentulous patient, but a degree of stability may be attained by the formation of a deep pocket lined with a skin graft, using the skin graft inlay technique. The pocket permits the wearing of a prosthesis, which restores the contour of the missing bone. The raw area resulting from the formation of the pocket is lined with a split-thickness skin graft or a skin flap (Fig. 72–21). Figure 72–22 illustrates a semiedentulous patient who has lost the median section of the mandible from molar to molar. He is wearing cast metal splints, which will subsequently be used as fixation appliances for a mandibular bone graft.

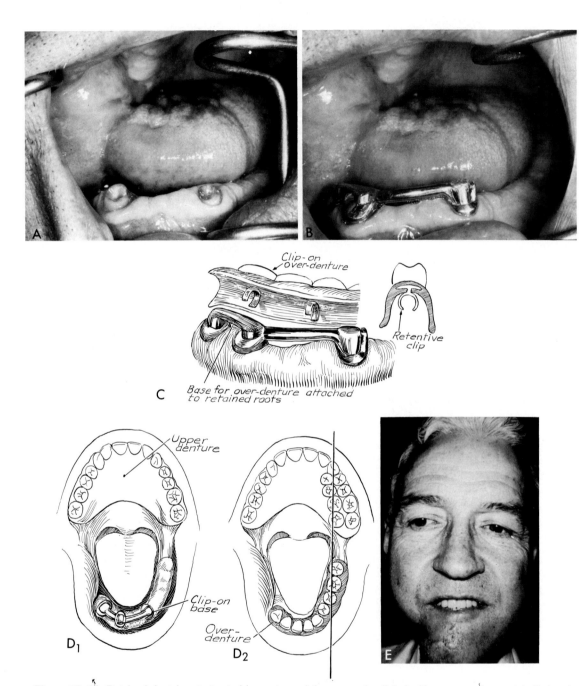

Figure 72–20. Retained dental roots treated by root canal therapy and splinted with a connecting metal clip bar for retention of a prosthesis. *A,* Intraoral view of the remaining roots prepared for gold posts. *B,* Retained roots splinted with clip-on gold bar. *C,* Retaining clips. *D,* The maxillary occlusal ramp accommodates the occlusion of the deviated mandibular fragment with the overdenture. *E,* Appearance of the patient in centric occlusion wearing the upper and lower prostheses.

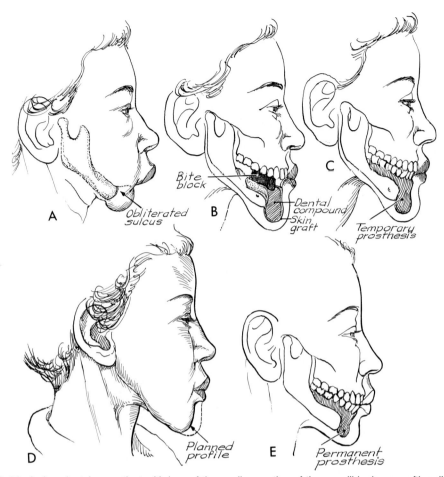

Figure 72–21. *A,* An edentulous patient with loss of the median section of the mandible; bone grafting did not restore the contour of the lower face. *B,* Surgical prosthesis fitted into a deep skin grafted pocket. *C,* The retentive mandibular prosthesis, which restores the mandibular contour. *D,* Planned profile of the mandibular contour. *E,* Contour of the patient wearing the permanent prosthesis.

When chin contour is being restored with a prosthesis or a combination of bone grafting, skin grafting, and prosthesis, the proportions of the entire face must be considered (Fig. 72–22*B*).

Loss of a Lateral Section of Mandible. Loss of bone in this group may be limited to the mandibular condyle and part of the ramus, may extend to the body of the mandible, and may be sufficiently extensive to involve the symphysis and a portion of the contralateral body, leaving only a small segment to act as a base for artificial restoration. The number of teeth in the remaining part of the mandible is an important factor, since the prosthesis is designed primarily to utilize these teeth for purposes of retention and also to assume the burden of mastication.

The loss of a part of the ramus may not necessarily interfere with mandibular func-

tion if the remaining portion of the mandible is free of trismus and distortion from adherent scar. Adhesions and scars require surgical treatment. Following surgery, an appliance is made employing the principle of the simple inclined plane or occlusal guide to attain correct occlusal relationships (Fig. 72–23).

When destruction of one side of the mandible includes the ramus and part of the body on the same side, the articulation of the remaining teeth is disturbed by a lateral and posterior displacement of the mandible. The primary object of a prosthesis in this situation is to retain the mandible in an anatomic position in order to maintain adequate occlusion of the remaining teeth. Various types of prosthetic appliances are used successfully in such cases. A practical type is a retention appliance, constructed to correct the facial contour and to facilitate functioning of the

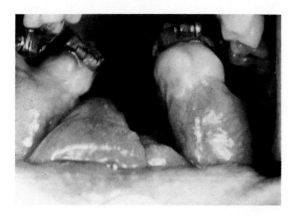

Figure 72–22. *A*, Appearance following loss of the median section of the body of a semiedentulous mandible. Note the medial collapse. The patient is wearing cast metal splints on the retained molars for intermaxillary fixation. *B*, Facial proportions according to Leonardo's square.

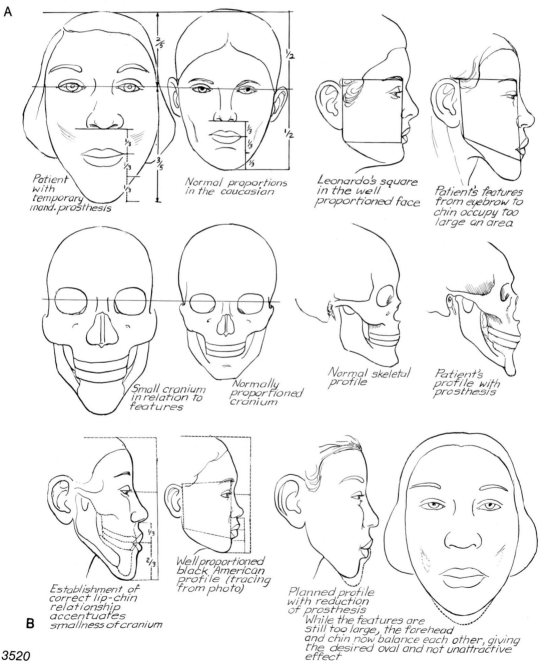

A

Patient with temporary mand. prosthesis

Normal proportions in the caucasian

Leonardo's square in the well proportioned face

Patient's features from eyebrow to chin occupy too large an area

Small cranium in relation to features

Normally proportioned cranium

Normal skeletal profile

Patient's profile with prosthesis

Establishment of correct lip-chin relationship accentuates smallness of cranium

B

Well proportioned black American profile (tracing from photo)

Planned profile with reduction of prosthesis

While the features are still too large, the forehead and chin now balance each other, giving the desired oval and not unattractive effect

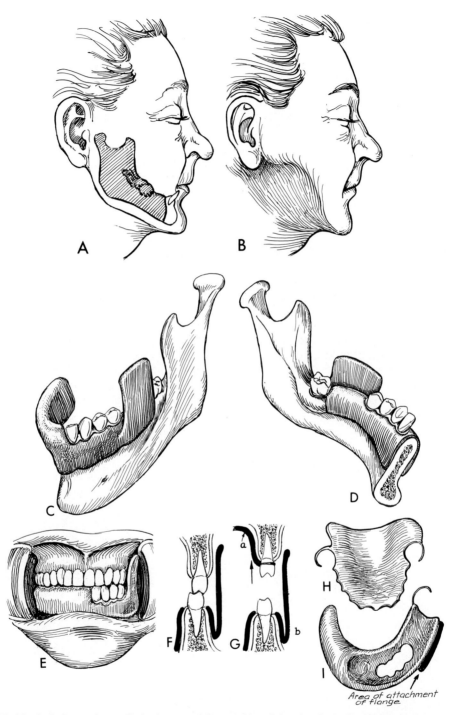

Figure 72–23. *A, B,* Loss of mandibular bone and the resulting deformity. *C, D,* Position and design of the flange appliance as it fits the remaining mandibular fragment. *E,* Flange appliance in position, extending into the labial sulcus and maintaining the mandible in adequate functional and occlusal relationships. *F, G,* Diagram illustrating the function of the maxillary and mandibular prostheses. The maxillary prosthesis (a) supports the lingual aspect of the upper teeth and minimizes trauma to them when the flange (b) is in function. *H, I,* The maxillary and mandibular prostheses, respectively.

remaining mandibular segment. Such an appliance may extend from the last tooth of the anterior segment on the side of the defect backward and upward toward the maxillary third molar, where a pseudotemporomandibular joint is established in the form of either a groove or a ball-and-socket joint (Fig. 72–24).

Successful treatment depends on the willingness of the surgeon and the prosthodontist to collaborate in the reconstruction of major defects. The surgeon and the prosthodontist should be aware of the limitations and the possibilities of the prosthesis in order that the surgical technique and prosthetic therapy may complement each other. The prosthodontist should plan for the patient's present and future by doing a thorough intraoral clinical examination, obtaining a full mouth series as well as a panoramic roentgenogram, making impressions and casts of the patient's dentoalveolar ridges, and registering a satisfactory maxillomandibular occlusal relationship for future use. Dental care should be given to all teeth to be retained and an oral prophylactic treatment should be undertaken before surgical intervention.

The prosthodontist in consultation with the surgeon should fabricate surgical prosthetic appliances to be used at the time of surgery. Temporary prosthetic appliances, such as an obturator, are perhaps one of the greatest services that modern dentistry can offer a patient with a palatal defect resulting from loss of a major portion of the maxilla (see Chap. 68). The temporary palatal surgical obturator can be fabricated quickly. It should be light and simple, and should lend itself to being adjusted and altered in the operating room. It should also be capable of being altered after the secondary tissue changes associated with healing. Contemporary materials such as rapid-setting acrylic resins and soft tissue conditioners are a boon to this type of patient care. The temporary surgical obturators are of importance in supporting packing and surgical scaffolding and in maintaining contour and form in the defective area. The patient is thus helped in recovering the functions of speech, mastication, and deglutition (Fig. 72–25).

In mandibular surgery, temporary splint appliances listed earlier in the chapter may be employed to maintain normal maxillomandibular jaw relationships. As surgical rehabilitation techniques advance, transitional prosthetic appliances may be necessary to assist surgical procedures (Fig. 72–26).

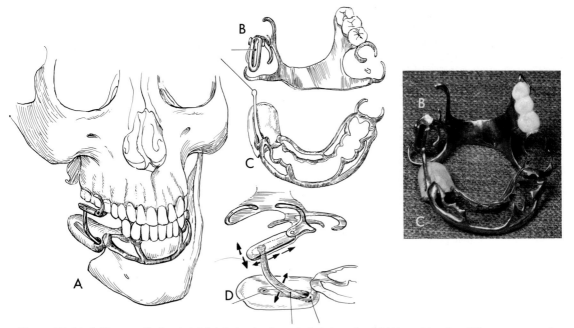

Figure 72–24. *A,* The mandibular skeletal defect extends posteriorly from the right bicuspid region. If the upper posterior teeth are missing, the patient is supplied with two partial dentures *(B, C).* A hinged bar extends from the last molar region of the upper denture to the bicuspid region of the lower jaw. When the patient occludes his teeth, the intermaxillary hinged bar forces the lower jaw into an adequate position. *B, C,* Upper and lower dentures. *D,* Mechanism of the forward displacement provided by the intermaxillary hinged bar.

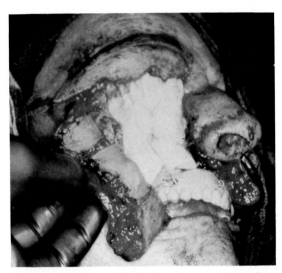

Figure 72–25. A surgical obturator supporting a large packing over a skin graft following maxillectomy.

Upon completion of all major reconstructive surgical procedures, the surgeon clears the patient for final prosthetic care.

MAXILLARY PROSTHESES

Defects of the palate, varying in size from small perforations to complete loss of the hard and soft palate, can be successfully closed by means of prosthetic appliances. The missing alveolar process and teeth are restored harmoniously; the appliance, when indicated, can be extended into the nasal cavity to support the soft tissues of the nose.

Preliminary surgical measures simplify the problems attending prosthetic design. The chief difficulty lies in finding a means of retention for the appliance. Remaining teeth and remnants of the hard palate and alveolar process are generally required for anchorage and to provide a base for stability during mastication. Figure 72–27 illustrates the retention obtained by using a resilient hollow bulb obturator. When a portion of the maxilla is missing and an insufficient number of teeth remain, however, it is necessary to find other support, such as that available in the nasal fossa (Fig. 72–28).

Temporary Dentures. Patients with large defects of the maxilla are usually referred to the prosthodontist long after the original traumatic or surgical destruction. Contraction of soft tissues may therefore offer an additional obstacle to the successful construction of the prosthesis. *Consequently, the use of dentures prepared preoperatively, to serve as temporary supports, has been advocated.* Such dentures can be utilized immediately

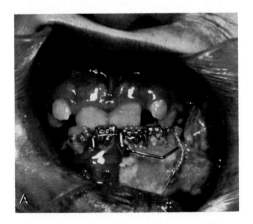

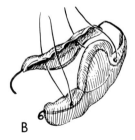

Figure 72–26. *A,* A patient wearing the surgical fixation prosthesis with a guide flange and orthodontic bands to aid in intermaxillary fixation. *B,* The fixation appliance with the labial flange. *C,* The prosthesis wired in the patient's mouth during the healing phase. *D, E,* Labial and cross-sectional view of the flange prosthesis.

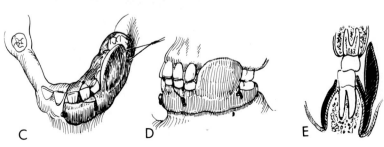

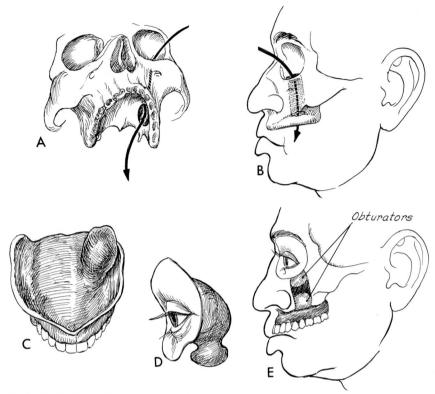

Figure 72–27. *A, B,* Orbitomaxillary defect. *C,* Full upper denture obturator with hollow flexible bulb. *D,* Orbital prosthesis with flexible extension for retention and obturation of the orbital cavity. *E,* Maxillary obturator and orbital prostheses in proper relationship.

after the resection in the operating room. The patient's denture can be modified for such a purpose, or a bite plate may be constructed even though the wound is as yet unhealed. Figure 72–29 shows a patient who had undergone hemimaxillectomy and orbital exenteration and in whom a temporary denture served to immobilize the parts after the surgical procedures. Such a temporary denture may be modified to serve as a permanent restoration at a later date.

A temporary denture that covers the defect adds to the patient's comfort. Difficulty experienced in speech and in eating is lessened, and secondary contraction and adhesions of the soft tissues are minimized (Fig. 72–30). The temporary denture, however, does not always prevent secondary contraction if the raw area is extensive; in such cases resurfacing by skin grafting is indicated.

Methods of Retention. Loss of part of the maxilla, coupled with loss of teeth, obviously creates an obstacle to stabilization. The remaining alveolar ridges, the palate, and the teeth should be utilized to retain artificial restorations by extending the denture through palatal spaces into the nasal cavity, and employing various spring attachments that extend from the lower jaw into the upper denture.

1. The purpose of using the maximal amount of the available portion of the palate and alveolar ridge surface is to retain the denture, afford stability, and increase masticating efficiency. Because the teeth are the most dependable means of anchorage, it is important to retain them whenever possible, employing light, resilient clasps (Fig. 72–31). Additional retention is obtained by means of a clip bar (Fig. 72–32).

2. Spaces leading to the nasal cavity are next in importance for retention. It is desirable, however, to survey the entire area and make the projections of the denture harmonize with the laws of leverage and with the existing conditions of the soft tissue. Projections of the denture may be extended above the posterior border of the palate, into the cavity of the movable portion of the nasal aspect. A denture may also be constructed in

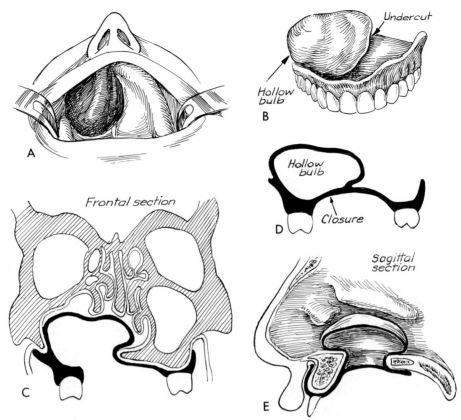

Figure 72–28. *A,* An edentulous patient with a maxillary defect after right hemimaxillectomy. *B,* Complete upper denture obturator. *C,* The tissue-bearing area of the hollow bulb extending into the anatomic undercut areas. *D,* The palatal closure obtained by the hollow bulb. *E,* Sagittal diagram demonstrating the nasal and distal extensions of the obturator used to aid in the retention and closure of the defect.

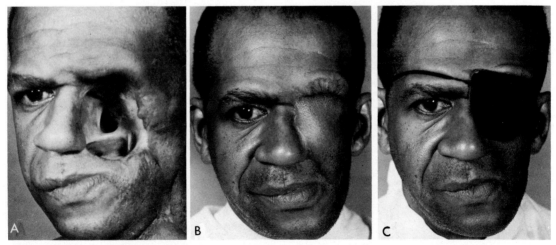

Figure 72–29. *A,* Appearance following a hemimaxillectomy and an orbital exenteration. *B, C,* The patient has undergone surgical reconstruction of the deformity. During the surgical phase, he wore a temporary obturator.

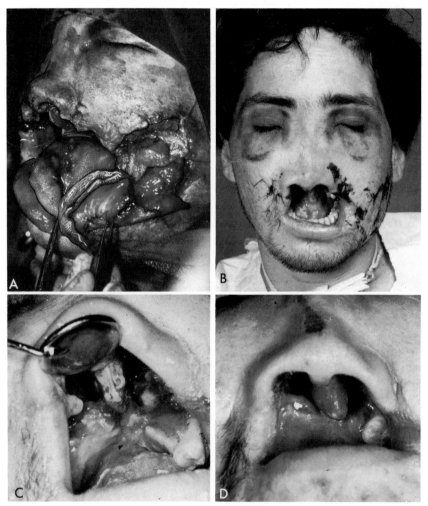

Figure 72–30. *A,* A patient with a gunshot wound of the face resulting in destruction of a major portion of the maxilla and upper lip. *B,* After emergency repair. *C,* Worm's eye view of the intraoral tissue loss. *D,* Intraoral view of the occlusal relationships.

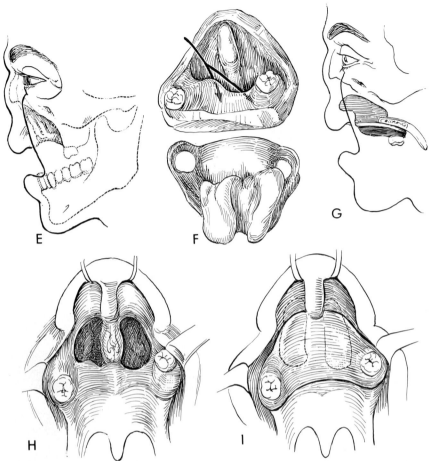

Figure 72–30 *Continued E,* Diagrammatic illustration of the deformity. *F,* The patient's dental model and the obturator fabricated from it. *G,* Position of the obturator extending into the nasal cavity to prevent further soft tissue contraction and to improve the functions of speech and deglutition. *H, I,* The deformity and its closure by the temporary obturator.

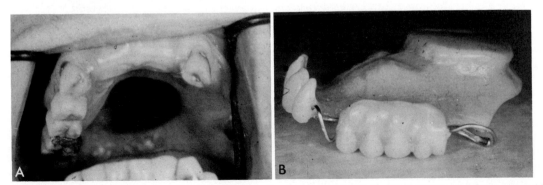

Figure 72–31. *A,* Large perforation of the hard palate with missing anterior teeth, left bicuspids, and first molar teeth. The second left molar has been retained. *B,* The denture with resilient gold wire clasps for the retention and extension of the obturator into the nasal surface. Note the replacement of the missing teeth.

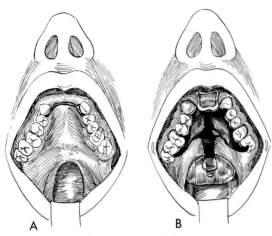

Figure 72–32. *A,* Palatal deformity extending into the nasopharynx. An anterior clip-bar splints the right and left canines. *B,* Upper partial prosthesis with an anterior frame resting on the clip-bar and resilient clasps provide adequate retention for the speech section of the obturator extending into the nasopharynx. Anterior teeth can also be placed on the frame.

two sections, introduced separately into the oral cavity and locked together with clasps or snap buttons after insertions (Fig. 72–33).

It is sometimes necessary to reoperate in order to establish a favorable space for the successful retention of a denture. In such cases, it is advisable to remove scarred mucous membrane and contracture bands and apply a skin graft within the oral cavity or nasal fossa, thus establishing a lining for a denture.

3. Spiral springs represent another means of denture retention and have been employed successfully in the past; the principles remain useful. The oldest and most generally used spiral spring is made of special gold wire about 0.5 mm in diameter and 5 cm in length. It is attached by means of suitable buttons on each side of the upper and lower dentures, at or about the first bicuspid region. The springs rest upon grooves on the buccal side of the denture; they assume a semicircular position (Fig. 72–34) when the teeth are in contact.

Another type, originally devised by Kazanjian (1915), consists of a horizontal spring connected with a lever. Two buttons are attached to the lower plate or bridge, one at the bicuspid region and the other in the third molar region. A horizontal spring is attached to the anterior button at one end and to the short arm of a lever at the other; the posterior button acts as a fulcrum to the lever. The long arm of the lever fits into a groove made

on the buccal aspect of the upper plate. The tension of the spring retains the denture as the patient opens and closes the mouth.

Spring devices employed for denture retention have some disadvantages. They do not serve a useful purpose unless they are accurately constructed and their strength is measured carefully. They require frequent repair, are not easy to keep clean, and at best afford a limited degree of stability for dentures. For these reasons, their use is limited to those cases in which other means have failed.

4. In deformities involving loss of part of the palate and nose, orbit, or side of the face, a facial prosthesis may be connected to an upper denture if there is no other means of support (Fig. 72–35).

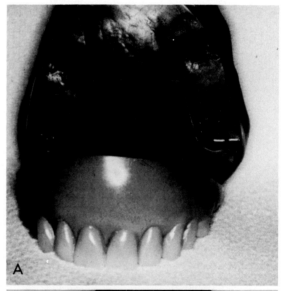

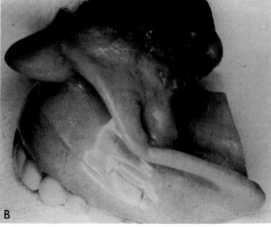

Figure 72–33. *A,* A two-piece full upper denture obturator illustrating plastic snap buttons. *B,* The two sections are joined and held together by three snap buttons.

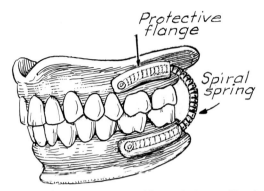

Figure 72–34. Full upper and lower dentures with spiral springs for retention. The spring rests on a groove made on the buccal side of the dentures.

Figure 72–36 illustrates a defect of the right side of the palate. Because teeth were present on the left side, a denture was made and retained with clasps. The right side of the denture extended into the defect to act as a seal, and a three-point contact for retention was achieved with an extension of the denture over the nasal surface of the defect.

Osseointegrated (Branemark) implant retention screws have revolutionized prosthetic retention for many types of maxillofacial patients. They have been used extensively for over 20 years by Branemark in Sweden, and more recently have been accepted in general by various specialists in the United States and Canada. They have been used experimentally in hemimandibulectomy patients for denture retention on successful mandibular bone grafts and atrophic mandibular alveolar bone (Fig. 72–37). Riediger (1988) recommended the use of enosseous implants in microsurgically revascularized bone transfers.

Bone and soft tissue reconstructive techniques have facilitated the closure of large maxillary defects and enabled a simpler type of denture to be employed. The necessary areas of resistance, however, have been ob-

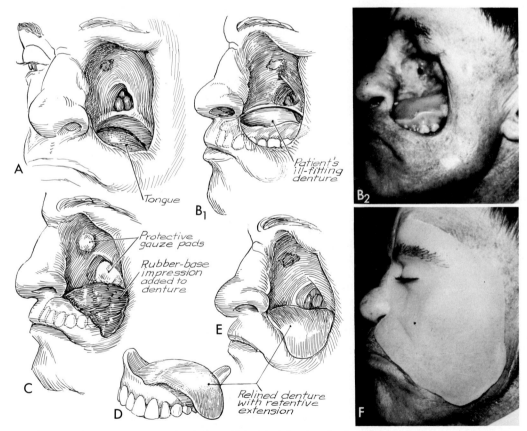

Figure 72–35. *A,* A patient with extensive maxillofacial deformity. *B₁,* Associated unstable, ill-fitting denture. *B₂,* Photograph of the denture. *C,* Denture impressioned with Thiokol rubber base for better retention and stability. *D, E,* The patient with a well-fitting and retentive acrylic prosthesis obturating the maxillectomy perforation and restoring physiologic functions. *F,* The patient wearing a noncosmetic facial prosthesis.

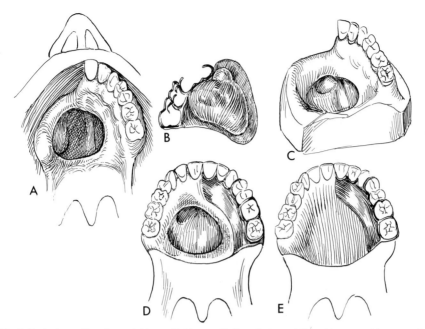

Figure 72–36. *A,* Defect resulting from right maxillectomy. *B,* Nasal view of the obturator with a nasal extension and multiple resilient-type cast clasps for retention on the remaining teeth. *C,* Study working cast of the maxilla. *D,* Maxillary obturator showing the hollow bulb. *E,* Finished obturator achieving palatal closure.

tained by means of an appliance that transfers the force to more distant structures, namely, the anterior surface of the frontal bone and the supraorbital ridges. A denture is made that also replaces the destroyed maxilla (Fig. 72–38).

It has been repeatedly emphasized in the preceding chapters that the contour of the soft tissues of the lower part of the face is dependent on the underlying framework. When the framework is lost, it should be replaced by transplanted bone plus an artificial denture. It has also been emphasized that when massive destruction of the maxilla and mandible occurs, the remaining parts should be preserved and retained in their anatomic positions by various devices outlined in the foregoing chapters. Subsequent reconstruction is aided by such procedures. Figure 72–39 illustrates a surgical prosthetic reconstructive procedure after massive destruction of the maxilla and mandible.

EXTRAORAL FACIAL PROSTHESES

Massive facial tissue destruction frequently leaves large defects that are most unsightly. Those that cannot be successfully repaired by reconstructive surgical procedures may be rehabilitated by a facial prosthesis. There are advantages to a facial prosthesis: the surgeon can remove the appliance whenever he wishes to examine the surgical areas; lengthy hospitalization is unnecessary; and the patient can be made presentable to the public soon after the facial deformity occurs.

The properties of the ideal material for external maxillofacial prostheses have been enumerated by various authors and were reconfirmed at the American Academy of Maxillofacial Prosthetics Workshop (Converse and Valauri, 1966):

1. Tissue compatibility. The material must not cause irritation or discomfort to the tissues on which it must rest.

2. Reproduction of true skin tones. The prosthesis should be soft and pliable, easily colored, and textured to simulate true skin tones.

3. Translucency. It should have the characteristic of translucency in order to give a lifelike appearance.

4. Flexibility. It must be flexible and resilient to simulate the feeling of soft tissue.

5. Durability. It must be durable to withstand sunlight, cold, and heat and not be affected by body fluids such as perspiration. It should be resistant to the effects of air

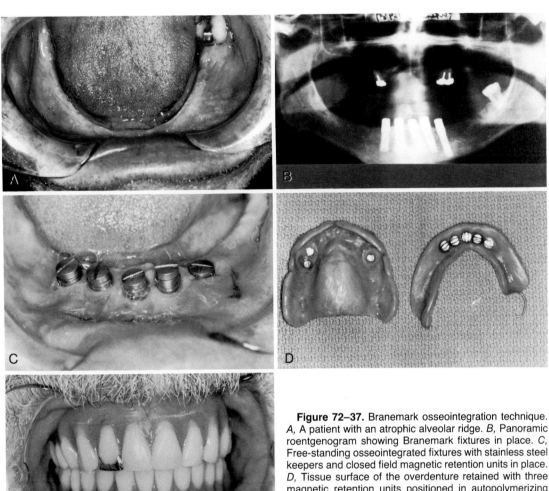

Figure 72–37. Branemark osseointegration technique. *A,* A patient with an atrophic alveolar ridge. *B,* Panoramic roentgenogram showing Branemark fixtures in place. *C,* Free-standing osseointegrated fixtures with stainless steel keepers and closed field magnetic retention units in place. *D,* Tissue surface of the overdenture retained with three magnetic retention units positioned in autopolymerizing methylmethacrylate. *E,* Intraoral view of the magnetically retained overdenture. (Courtesy of Dr. Bruce G. Valauri.)

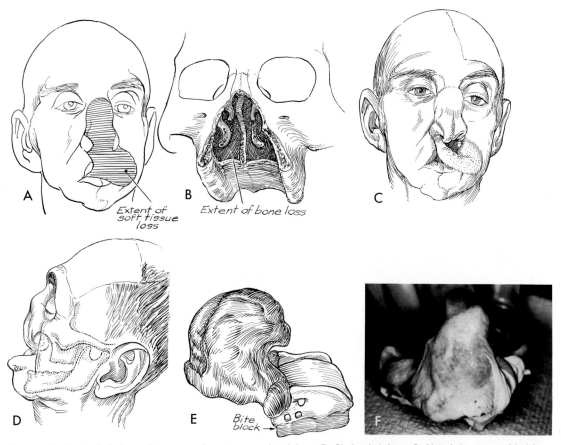

Figure 72–38. *A,* Soft tissue loss secondary to a gunshot injury. *B,* Skeletal defect. *C,* Nasal tissue provided by a forehead flap, and a tube flap to restore the upper lip. *D,* Lateral view of the patient. *E,* The upper surgical splint with an intranasal compound extension to carry a skin graft. *F,* The skin graft applied over the compound mold.

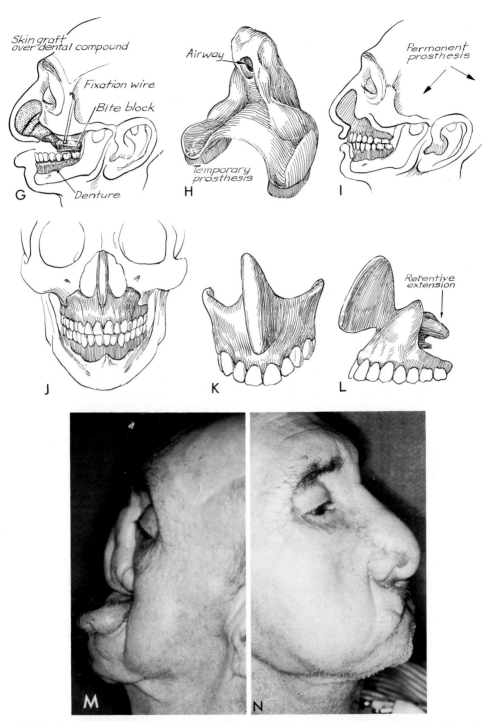

Figure 72–38 *Continued G,* Lateral view of the patient with the compound mold supporting the skin graft, which is maintained in position by wire suspension. *H,* The temporary acrylic prosthesis with a hole for breathing. *I,* Lateral view of the definitive denture, illustrating the nasal and paranasal extensions for the support of the nasal tissues and the retention of the prosthesis. *J,* Frontal view of the definitive full upper denture with the nasal extension allowing the passage of air. *K,* Frontal view of the definitive prosthesis. *L,* The maxillary denture with the intranasal extension supporting the nose. *M,* The patient before prosthetic reconstruction. *N,* The patient with prosthesis in place.

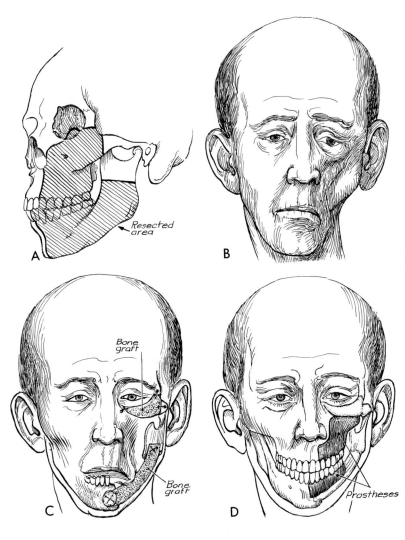

Figure 72–39. *A,* Skeletal defect including the maxilla and half of the mandible. *B,* Facial deformity resulting from loss of skeletal support. *C,* Bone grafts reestablishing the floor of the orbit, the contour of the zygoma, and mandibular continuity. *D,* Prosthodontic restoration to augment facial contour and restore masticatory function.

pollution and chemicals for a reasonable length of time.

6. Low thermal conductivity. It should be a poor or low conductor of heat or cold.

7. Lightness in weight. It should be light in weight so that it does not dislodge and fall easily. Adhesives should be able to retain it.

8. Moldability. It should be easy to mold into the desired anatomic shapes and forms of the ear, nose, and other facial features.

9. Ease of processing. It must be simple to process without the need for expensive equipment.

10. Ease of duplication. Duplication should be possible in order to produce identical or duplicate prostheses.

11. Easy cleaning. It should be easily cleanable without damage or deterioration.

12. Chemical and physical inertness and patient comfort. It should be comfortable to wear, and should not chemically or physically irritate the patient.

No material in use today fulfills all the criteria. Facial prosthetic materials such as polyvinylchloride (PVC), polyurethane, acrylic resin, and silicones are most commonly used today. Preparations of medical grade silicone have become the material of choice, and are used extensively for external prosthetic restorations (Fig. 72–40). These prosthetic restorations have a number of advantages over the hard acrylics in that they tend to produce a more natural skin tone. They are flexible, similar to soft tissue, and light in weight; they may be self-retentive, using undercut areas such as the orbit, and they provide patient comfort (Fig. 72–41).

Several methods have been developed for coloring and tinting; these may be intrinsic, extrinsic, or a combination of both in order

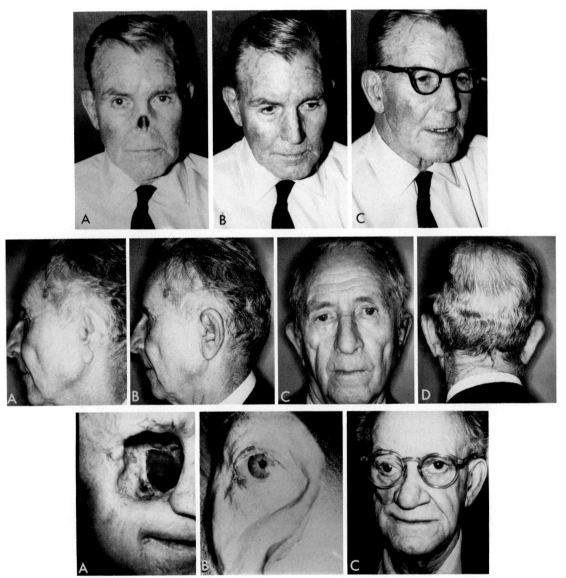

Figure 72–40. Examples of extraoral facial prostheses. *(Above) A,* A patient with partial loss of the nose. *B, C,* Same patient with a nasal prosthesis made of silicone. *(Center) A,* A patient with loss of a major portion of the auricle. *B to D,* Same patient with an auricular prosthesis made of flexible polyvinyl plastic. *(Below) A,* A patient with an orbital defect. *B,* Finished orbital prosthesis made of silicone and flexible polyvinyl plastic. *C,* The patient wearing glasses to camouflage the prosthetic margins.

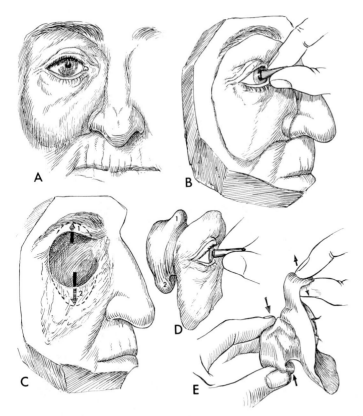

Figure 72–41. *A,* Orbital prosthesis in position. *B,* The prosthesis is removed with a suction cup applied to the ocular prosthesis. *C,* Recesses 1 and 2 behind the supraorbital and infraorbital rims are used for retention. *D,* Addition of a posterior extension, which fits into recesses 1 and 2. *E,* Demonstrating the resiliency of the prosthesis.

to obtain the more natural effect. The greatest disadvantage of the flexible materials is the deterioration of the prosthesis due to the perishable nature of the available materials and the consequent need for periodic replacement. This problem, however, can be easily rectified by retaining the mother mold used in the duplication of the prosthesis. Proper color records and charts should be maintained and adjusted at the final fitting of the prosthesis.

Fabrication of various flexible extraoral prosthetic restorations has been described by Bulbulian (1945) and in recent years by other clinicians who have used new flexible materials and slightly modified the basic technique according to the material employed. The first step in the fabrication of a prosthesis for facial restoration is to obtain an accurate impression of the defect. The next step is to make a cast from it. Many suitable impression materials are available, such as hydrocolloids, the alginates, and others of a similar nature. In most cases, it is advisable to use the elastic impression of undercut areas; they can be removed without being distorted, in contrast to rigid materials such as plaster, which are difficult to remove without breaking or injuring the tissues.

A combination of rigid and elastic impression materials gives the best results. An impression of the deformity, including the undercut areas, is first obtained by an elastic impression material, which in turn is reinforced by an outer jacket of plaster of Paris. The impression is the *negative* of the deformity; it is converted into an accurate cast (dental stone or metal), which is a *positive* reproduction of the deformity. Upon this cast the missing portion of the anatomy is sculptured with either clay or wax.

In many cases, if the maxillofacial prosthetist has been informed before the surgical intervention, he may be able to make an impression of the structure to be used as a model for the restorative prosthesis. Careful consideration should be given to the location of the *line of junction* between the restoration and the skin.

Since a dental stone cast is easier to make, it is preferred and used as a foundation; a preliminary pattern of the desired prosthesis is made of either wax or modeling clay. In some cases the form can be obtained from an individual with a similarly proportioned structure. Before duplicating the pattern in the final material, it is essential to try it on the patient and make any final adjustments.

When the desired criteria are satisfied, the pattern is fitted over the defect and used as the foundation for the final mold. The pattern must be fixed in proper position so that it does not move while the second or final parts of the mold are fabricated. In the case of a nose, a two-piece mold is usually necessary; however, in the fabrication of an ear or eye prosthesis, sectional three-piece molds are necessary to compensate for the undercuts. In some cases, a silicone mold may be used; this is more flexible and it may be possible to reproduce the undercuts in a two-piece mold. Employing the mold made for a particular pattern, one can proceed to construct a prosthesis in any of the flexible materials without destroying the mother mold. If a hard material is used, such as acrylic resin, part of the mold is usually destroyed. Following the manufacturer's instructions, the prosthetist may either pour, paint, or pack the material into the mother mold and fabricate the final prosthesis.

Retention of the flexible prosthetic restoration is usually obtained by means of various types of medical grade adhesives; in some cases mechanical aids, such as those described by Kazanjian (1932) (Fig. 72–42), may have to be employed. Figures 72–43 and 72–44 illustrate the use of resilient materials for purposes of mechanical retention.

Branemark Osseointegrated Implants. The application of osseointegrated fixtures to

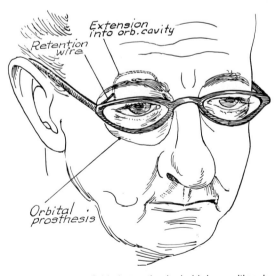

Figure 72–42. Orbital prosthesis held in position by spectacles, the frame of which fits into the groove on the nasal side, while a bar extends from the side of the spectacle frame to the outer border of the prosthesis. The dotted line indicates the extension into the orbital cavity.

the cranial skeleton for facial prosthesis retention made a revolutionary step in the search for a more perfect soft tissue replacement (see Figs. 72–53, 72–54). It is to be noted that not all patients with facial defects are candidates for this approach.

ORBITAL PROSTHESES

Ophthalmic Prostheses. When the ocular globe is destroyed or surgically removed, it can be replaced by an artificial eye when other orbital contents and the eyelids are present. Enucleation of the eye is commonly performed; the subsequent problem of fitting the patient with an ophthalmic prosthesis is in the province of the maxillofacial prosthodontist.

Ocular Prostheses. Anophthalmos is defined as a condition in which no eyeball, however small, can be found in the orbit (see Chap. 33). *Microphthalmos* has been described as a uniocular congenital deformity in which lack of development of an eye is in striking contrast to the development of the other. It is difficult to distinguish between a true anophthalmos and an extreme degree of microphthalmos in which there is a small ocular globe. Infants with these deformities should be treated within the first four weeks of life by placing a small ocular prosthesis (conformer) in the conjunctival socket. The conformer must be changed to one of larger size as conditions warrant so that shrinkage of the cul-de-sac is prevented and normal development is promoted. In some cases orbital expansion may be necessary; this is best determined by three-dimensional CT evaluation (see Chap. 33). When adequate expansion is obtained, an ocular prosthesis with an iris matching the normal eye should be made (Fig. 72–45).

UNUSUALLY LARGE EYE SOCKETS. In larger defects, the greater part of the orbital contents is often missing, although the eyelids remain intact. Surgery can reduce the size of the orbital space to accommodate an artificial eye. If surgery is not advisable, a silicone mold can be fitted to replace the missing part of a large orbit, and an artificial eye inserted anterior to the mold. To obtain the desired shape of the silicone prosthesis, softened dental compound or wax is inserted into the socket, and the artificial eye is set into a position that harmonizes with the contour and color of the unaffected eye.

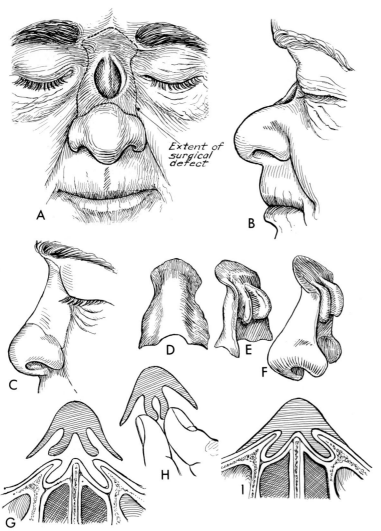

Figure 72–43. *A, B,* Extent of the nasal defect. *C, D,* Views of the partial nasal prosthesis. *E,* Side view of a complete nasal prosthesis. *F* to *H,* Illustration of the retention obtained with a flexible plastic material, which is easily adapted to the remaining anatomic areas. *I,* Partial flexible nasal prosthesis in position.

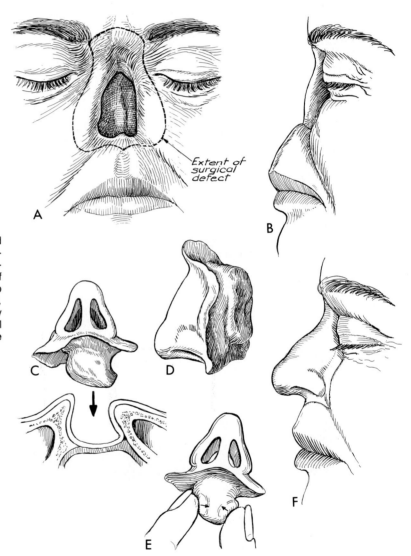

Figure 72–44. Flexibility and adaptability of a vinyl-plastic prosthesis. *A, B,* Deformity after ablation of the nose. *C,* Advantage of fitting flexible plastic material into the existing undercut areas. *D,* The nasal prosthesis. *E,* Flexibility of the prosthesis. *F,* The nasal prosthesis in position. Note the well-fitting flexible margins.

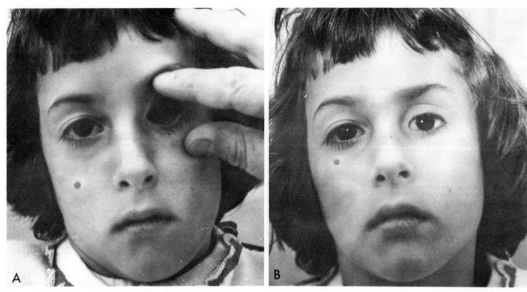

Figure 72–45. A patient with congenital microphthalmos. *A,* Dimensions of the expanded socket. *B,* The patient wearing the ocular prosthesis, which matches the contralateral eye.

A defect associated with destruction of the orbital contents, eyelids, and surrounding tissue leaves a large exposed cavity (Fig. 72–46 and see Fig. 72–40). Although surgical reconstruction may be considered, such a step is not always advisable, as total surgical reconstruction of the orbital contents has not always proved satisfactory. An esthetically modeled artificial restoration, however, is acceptable.

The first step in preparing an orbital prosthesis is to take an impression of the patient's face or the deformity, including the surrounding unaffected structures. This is done with a reversible hydrocolloid impression material, which is first heated in a double boiler until it is completely melted and boils. It is then allowed to cool to about 110°F before it is painted on the patient's face, starting from the deformity and extending outward until all the desired areas are covered without causing the patient discomfort. The patient is in a semireclining position, with an apron and towel draped around him. The procedure, including what to expect and what sensation he is going to feel with each step, is explained

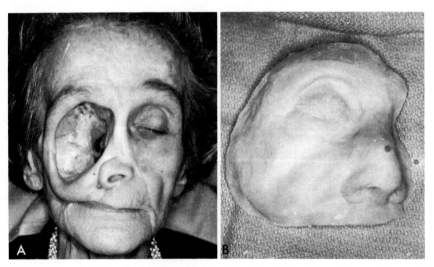

Figure 72–46. *A,* Postoperative deformity resulting from exenteration of the orbit and surrounding soft tissue. *B,* The facial anatomy has been restored by a combination (vinyl chloride) prosthesis of the orbit and surrounding soft tissue.

to the patient. The face is prepared by coating the eyelashes and eyebrows with Vaseline; a tube is inserted if the mouth is to be closed and impressioned. To prevent squinting, the patient is asked to relax and close the eyes, and adhesive tape is placed across the eyebrow and supraorbital tissues of the deformity. Using a camel's hair brush, after the impression material has been tested for heat, the prosthetist paints the impression material from the greatest depth of the deformity to the desired area to be impressioned. The brushing is continued until a thickness of approximately 3 mm is obtained, at which level strips of gauze impregnated with warm impression material are used to reinforce the impression and to act as partial anchors. Open paper clips or dry gauze are also used to reinforce and attach the plaster of Paris, which is employed to act as a backing for the impression material. When the plaster of Paris is set, the patient is asked to wrinkle his face, and the edges are gently freed. The impression is carefully removed and examined for accuracy and air bubbles. If the impression is acceptable, a positive cast in dental stone is made by carefully vibrating the stone into the impression until a desired thickness, sufficiently strong to be used as a working model, is obtained.

The next step is to match the patient's eye with an ocular prosthesis. This may be made by the maxillofacial prosthodontist, or a customized stock acrylic vision eye may be modified. The eye is chosen to match the contralateral eye in all details such as color, shape, size, and even blood vessels. When the criteria for the ocular prosthesis are obtained, a clay pattern is carved to match the eyelids and characteristics of the normal eye, such as wrinkles and folds. The ocular portion of the prosthesis should be placed so that the center of the pupil is the same distance from the dorsum of the nose as is that of the normal eye when the patient is looking straight ahead from an upright position. The depth of the eyeball in the socket should be the same as that of the normal eye when one looks down over the patient's forehead. The lids should be partially opened as if the patient were looking in the primary gaze; they should be correctly aligned in all proportions like the natural lids. Skin folds and texture should be made on the surface of the clay pattern.

Some maxillofacial prosthetists prefer at this stage to construct a metallic mold of the clay pattern. From this mold, the final prosthesis can be fabricated. The author prefers the stone mold, unless the prosthesis is to be refabricated three times or more, in which case a metal mold is desirable. After either type of mold is used and the desired material is selected, the final prosthesis should be made to match the patient's skin tones.

NASAL PROSTHESES

Post-traumatic deformities of the nose are treated surgically and rarely warrant artificial restoration. In the exceptional case, the stages in the construction of a prosthetic nose are best described under the following headings: (1) modeling the nose, (2) materials used for reproduction, (3) methods of retention, (4) coloring and camouflage, and (5) preliminary surgical procedures.

Modeling the Artificial Nose. A plaster or dental stone reproduction of the face serves as a working model. The procedure in making the stone working model is similar to that described for the orbital prosthesis. The nose is modeled on the cast with clay or wax. A knowledge of sculpturing is essential for shaping a nose to harmonize with the facial contour and individual type. For these reasons, the services of a sculptor are indicated. If sculpturing is difficult, an impression of a donor nose may be made and the nose duplicated and modified in wax to fit the patient's characteristics.

Materials Used for Reproduction. Material such as porcelain, celluloid, copper, silver, aluminum, gelatin compositions, vulcanite, and latex have been used in the past in the fabrication of a prosthetic nose. Some of these have been discarded in favor of acrylics, silicone, and vinyl plastics, depending on the laboratory facilities and the abilities of the prosthodontist.

The flexible types require adhesives for retention, and latex is not durable. Patients have also complained that they are unable to use handkerchiefs or control nasal secretions.

Hard acrylic resins are advantageous for several reasons. They are translucent and easily processed into the desired shape; modification of the shape is also possible after the work is completed. Furthermore, color may be incorporated into the material so that the artificial nose matches the color of the face. In most cases the author prefers polyvinyl resin or a combination of hard and soft plastics because they meet most of the desired properties previously listed in this chapter.

Methods of Retention. A rigid type of prosthetic nose may be retained by spectacles, by contact adhesion with the nasal cavities, and by various devices extending from the oral cavity to the nose. Figure 72–47 illustrates a typical prosthesis utilizing all available methods of retention. The inner surface of the prosthesis (A) fits over the boundaries of the nasal opening and covers an area consistent with the shape of the nose. Extensions of the restoration rest on the floor of the nose (B) to prevent it from slipping down on the lip. Lateral grooves (C) and also a metal clasp over the artificial bridge (D) fit the bridge and rim of the spectacles accurately. Even pressure is thus exerted by the spectacles on the upper half of the nose when the prosthesis is in place.

Successful retention of such a prosthesis is essential for the comfort of the patient and for a satisfactory appearance. Slight dislodgement invariably disturbs the fit of the appliance, and spaces between the prosthesis and the nose become conspicuous. All available means of anchorage must be utilized in each case; the undersurface of the appliance must fit the tissues accurately and must be in contact with the available tissue under its base to achieve stability.

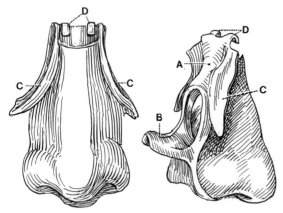

Figure 72–47. Nasal prosthesis. Main features of the prosthesis: (1) inner surface *(A)* base fits accurately and covers as much space as is consistent with the shape of the nose; (2) prolongation of restoration *(B)* rests on the floor of the nose, its purpose being to prevent the artificial nose from sliding down upon the lip; (3) lateral grooves as well as metal clasps over the bridge *(C, D)*, fitted accurately to the bridge and rims of spectacles so that when the nose is worn, there is even pressure from the spectacles against the face. (From Kazanjian, V. H.: Modern accomplishments in dental and facial prostheses. J. Dent. Res., *12:*651, 1932.)

The use of spectacles is one of the oldest and most common methods of retention, the spectacles being fastened to the bridge of the nose so that the entire weight of the appliance is supported by the auricles through the lateral arms of the spectacles. This method, however, has mechanical weakness unless other means of support are included. The spectacles cannot be secured sufficiently to achieve the desired degree of retention; when the spectacles are attached to the bridge of the nose, the pressure tends to dislodge the lower border. The pressure is therefore focused at the lateral aspects of the middle of the prosthesis to remedy the condition. Glasses with wide frames are used. The lower curvature on each rim and also the bridge are thus fitted accurately, the greatest amount of pressure being exerted at the lowest point. The glasses are not fixed to the prosthesis, the two appliances being maintained in their correct relationship when the spectacles are adjusted.

Spectacles, although accurately adjusted, do not prevent the prosthetic nose from sliding forward. To prevent this annoying feature, extensions of the appliance into the nasal cavity are necessary. An appliance that does not fit accurately and does not cover a considerable area is not tolerated by the delicate nasal mucosa; the floor of the nasal fossa is therefore the most practical location for the extensions.

According to Kazanjian (1932), whenever possible a nasal prosthesis should be anchored to an artificial denture because the combined prosthetic restoration results in a greater degree of stability. While this is true in terms of stability, the technique suffers the disadvantage that the nose may possibly move to the degree that the upper denture moves during mastication.

In recent years, better materials that approach the qualities desired for facial prostheses have been developed. The choice of materials has moved toward the vinyl resins and the silicones, which have various advantages over the acrylics, the most important being their resemblance to the normal tissues and their lightness of weight.

In the use of vinyl resins or silicones to fabricate a nasal prosthesis, an impression of the nasal defect is first made. A clay or wax pattern is made to fit the patient's face with the aid of a preoperative photograph; whenever possible, a model of the patient's own nose is taken before surgical removal. The pattern should be characterized to fit the face, reproducing the natural skin texture and wrinkles. Using the pattern, one can make a two-piece silicone or metal mold, which is used to fabricate a vinyl resin or silicone prosthesis.

Coloring and Camouflage. As described above, coloring and tinting may be intrinsic, extrinsic, or a combination of both methods in order to produce the desired effect and camouflage (Clarke, 1965).

Preliminary Surgical Procedures. A preliminary surgical procedure is often necessary to lessen the prominent demarcation lines; excision of a section of the lower end of the septum may also be required to stabilize the appliance. The prosthesis is less conspicuous if it does not extend to the mobile parts of the face and if the lines of demarcation are hidden by spectacles, by the natural folds of the face, or by the alar fold and base of the nose. Surgical procedures are also undertaken to reduce the size of the opening into the nasal cavity to conform to these boundaries.

Intranasal Prostheses

Prostheses have been employed to form a skeleton for the bridge of the nose when the nasal soft tissues are intact; this method is used only in selected cases. The most suitable patients are those in whom the anterior part of the palate and cartilaginous support of the nose are missing.

Secondary nasal deformities include the pinched tip deformity (see Chap. 36). If the treatment of this latter is not accomplished by surgery, it may be necessary to treat with *intranasal molds*, which may be combined with intranasal skin grafting.

Skin Grafting Within the Nose. Stenosis of the nasal airway, caused by lacerations, surgery, loss of nasal lining through destruction or avulsion may be corrected by the use of a dental mold carrier with mucosa or a split-thickness skin graft. The nasal vestibule is reconstituted by excising the scars, and the lateral wall is freed from the septum. Dental compound sticks are softened, molded into an oval core, and inserted into the nasal cavity. They are molded to adapt to the cavity and slightly overexpand for closer adaptation of the graft to the host area. This maneuver also allows for shrinkage during the healing

period. Usually two impressions are taken and two dental compound molds are made. The first compound mold is used immediately to serve as a graft carrier and to maintain the stenotic area in a state of dilation. The second mold is duplicated in acrylic, with an opening for the air to flow. The mold is retained for seven or ten days. When the temporary compound mold is removed, the thin, hollowed acrylic mold is introduced into the nostril. Shrinkage and constriction of the graft are thus minimized. The postoperative mold is retained for several months until the tendency for contraction of the skin graft has been overcome. When stenosis is the result of excessive removal of upper lateral and alar cartilage as well as nasal lining, the prosthesis supports the deficient cartilaginous structures and may be retained permanently to ensure patency of the airway and to support the alae (Fig. 72–48).

Nasomaxillary Skin Graft Inlay. A severe deformity results when the nasal bones and the middle portion of the maxilla have been destroyed or are underdeveloped. The condition has been referred to as a "dish-face" deformity. Gillies (1923) developed a technique that liberates the nose and the adjacent soft tissues from the atrophied or underde-

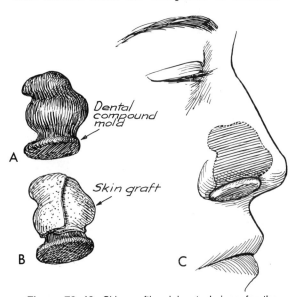

Figure 72–48. Skin grafting inlay technique for the correction of intranasal (vestibular) stenosis. *A,* A dental compound mold has been made from an impression of the nasal airway after resection of the scar tissue causing the intranasal contracture. A skin graft is wrapped around the mold. A duplicate mold is also made and sent to the laboratory for preparation of the definitive acrylic mold. *B,* The mold covered by the skin graft. *C,* The position of the mold inside the nasal cavity is outlined.

veloped skeletal structures, and lines the cavity with a skin graft and a prosthetic appliance. The nasomaxillary area thus freed from its constricted state is supported by a prosthesis. This technique has the inconvenience that the patient must continuously wear, cleanse, and replace the appliance. The nasal

skin graft inlay technique is illustrated in Figure 72–49.

A typical example of a patient requiring such reconstruction is shown in Figure 72–50. This technique has also been employed in a patient who was treated with radiation in the nasal area early in life and whose nose

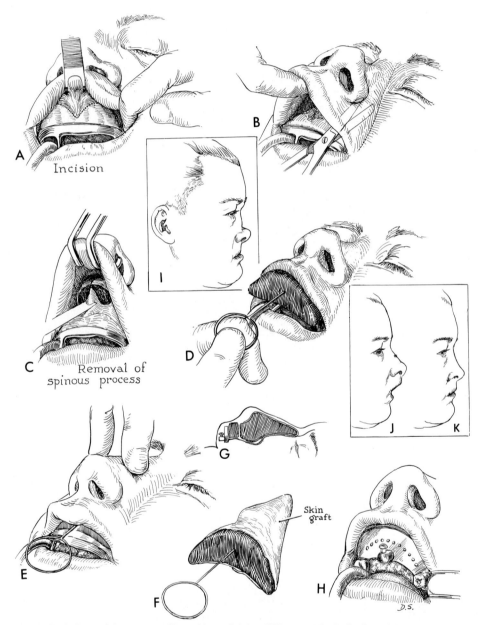

Figure 72–49. Technique of the nasomaxillary skin graft inlay (Gillies, 1923). *A,* Outline of the intraoral incision. *B,* The nasal cavity is entered through the mouth. *C,* The nasal spine is resected. *D,* A dental compound mold is fitted to the nasomaxillary cavity. *E,* The softened dental compound is molded to the nasomaxillary cavity by external digital pressure. *F,* The mold is covered with a split-thickness skin graft, dermal surface outward. *G,* The mold carrying the skin graft is placed inside the maxillary cavity. It is held in position by a splint anchored to the upper molar teeth. In this patient, the remainder of the maxillary teeth are absent. *H,* The dental appliance maintaining the mold in the nasomaxillary cavity. *I* to *K,* Appearance of the patient before, during, and after the skin graft inlay procedure.

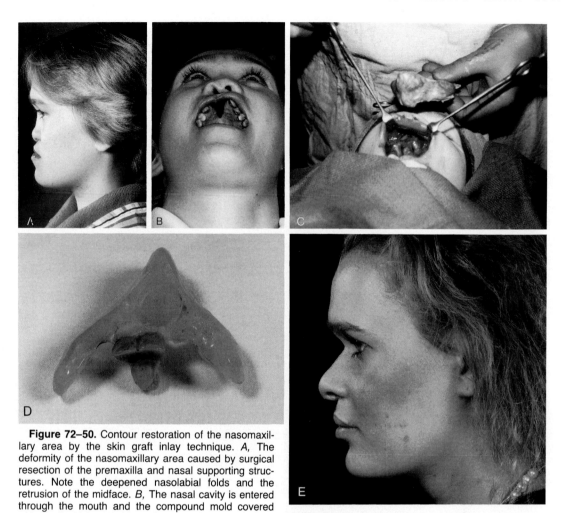

Figure 72–50. Contour restoration of the nasomaxillary area by the skin graft inlay technique. *A,* The deformity of the nasomaxillary area caused by surgical resection of the premaxilla and nasal supporting structures. Note the deepened nasolabial folds and the retrusion of the midface. *B,* The nasal cavity is entered through the mouth and the compound mold covered with a split-thickness skin graft, raw surface outward (see Fig. 72–49). *C,* The mold carrying the skin graft is placed inside the maxillary cavity. *D,* The transitional nasomaxillary prosthesis made of clear acrylic. *E,* Profile view of the patient wearing a transitional prosthesis. Note the change in contour of the midface and upper lip.

failed to develop (Fig. 72–51*A*). A description of the operative procedure follows.

Under *oroendotracheal* anesthesia, an incision is made in the upper buccal sulcus (Fig. 72–51*B*). The nasal fossa is entered from within the sulcus (Fig. 72–51*B*), and the nasal structures are freed of adhesions; an extensive raw area results. The nasal spine is removed and all sharp *bony* protuberances are filed smooth. A dental compound mold is constructed to fit the pyramidal cavity (Fig. 72–51*C*) with the apex pointing upward so that the mold can be inserted and removed easily. The mold is duplicated to construct a permanent acrylic resin prosthesis. A split-thickness skin graft from a nonhairy donor area is spread over the mold, raw surface outward, and is inserted into the nasal cavity (Fig. 72–51*D*). The skin graft carrier mold is maintained by a splint and, whenever necessary, is supported by the patient's teeth. The tissue should be distended by the compound mold in order to ensure close coaptation of the graft with the soft tissues and to counteract subsequent contraction of the graft (Fig. 72–51*E*).

The mold is removed after two weeks and the cavity is examined and cleansed. At intervals during subsequent weeks, the size of the mold is diminished. After a period of many weeks, a permanent acrylic resin prosthesis maintains the final contour of the nose (Fig. 72–51*F–I*). When the patient is edentulous, the nasal prosthesis is made as an upper extension of the denture (Fig. 72–52).

The application of osseointegrated fixtures to the craniofacial skeleton represents the latest step in nasal prosthesis retention (Fig.

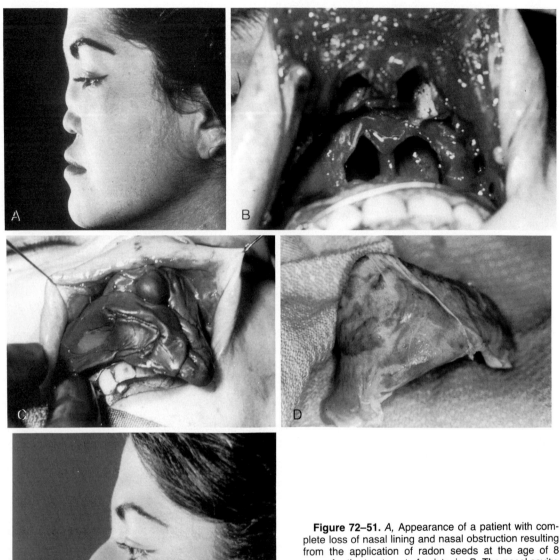

Figure 72–51. *A,* Appearance of a patient with complete loss of nasal lining and nasal obstruction resulting from the application of radon seeds at the age of 8 years for the treatment of epistaxis. *B,* The nasal cavity, which has been entered through the mouth. Note the metal arch attached to the teeth to support the compound stent. *C,* Dental compound impression of the nasal cavity. *D,* The compound mold covered with skin graft to be placed in the nasal cavity. *E,* Appearance of the patient wearing the oversize compound mold and skin graft.

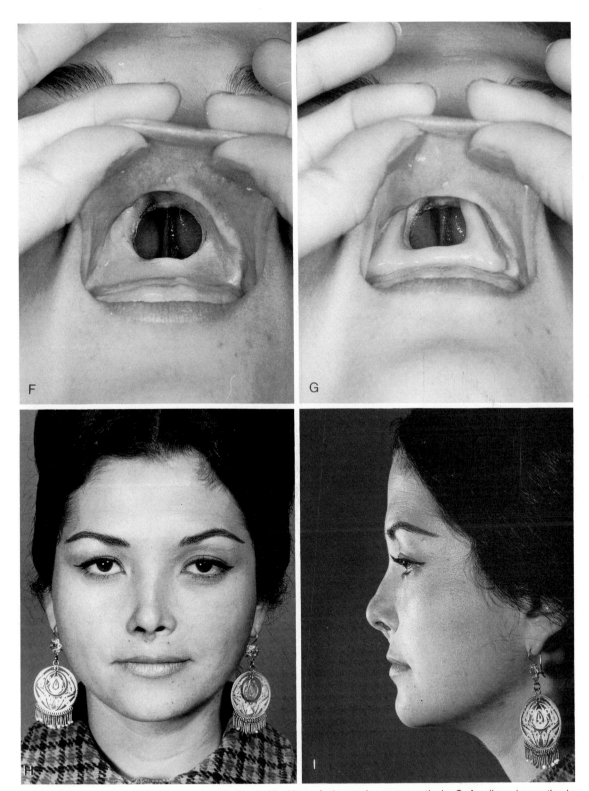

Figure 72–51 *Continued F,* The nasal cavity lined with skin graft six months postoperatively. *G,* Acrylic resin prosthesis with opening to allow unimpeded breathing in the nasal cavity. *H, I,* Postoperative views of the patient wearing the acrylic resin intranasal prosthesis.

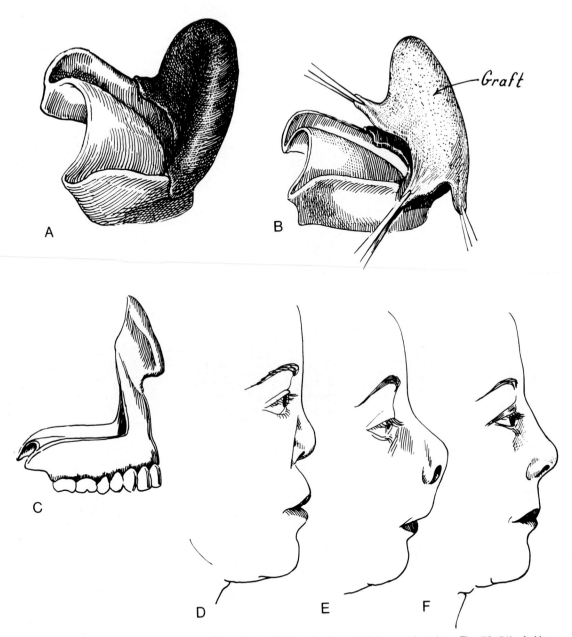

Figure 72–52. Technique of the nasomaxillary skin graft inlay for the edentulous patient (see Fig. 72–51). *A,* Upper denture with biteblock with compound stent that has an impression of the nasal cavity. *B,* Compound mold covered with skin graft. *C,* Definitive appliance. The denture is prolonged upward by an extension forming the nasal support and allowing an opening for the patient to breathe. *D to F,* Appearance of the patient before, during, and after the skin graft procedure.

72–53) (Parel, 1986; Parel and associates, 1986a,b).

AURICULAR PROSTHESES

Deformities of the ear may result from trauma or surgical ablation or may be congenital in nature; they may represent partial or complete defects.

When plans are made to restore a missing ear, it is first necessary to orient correctly the position of the ear so that it is a mirror image of the contralateral ear. The long axis, the adaptation, and the extension of the ear from the front or back of the head should be similar to those of the patient's existing ear (see Chap. 40). When a partial defect is to be replaced, it is imperative to observe the contralateral unaffected ear.

Modeling of the Artificial Ear. In most cases, it is best to make a plaster or stone reproduction of the patient's face, including the normal ear and the deformed side. The master cast is used to match that of the normal ear.

The detailed sculpting is completed with the patient seated in front of a mirror to facilitate matching the lines of contour of the normal ear as much as possible.

A three-piece stone or metal mold is constructed. This is used to reproduce a prosthetic ear in the desired material and color as described above for the orbital prosthesis.

Retention. It can be difficult to find ways of attaching and retaining the ear in proper position, and ingenious methods have been devised. When the prosthesis is light and flexible, the primary form of retention is by adhesives, several types of which are available. It is occasionally necessary to create surgical undercuts for retention; overhead bands and springs have been employed, and natural anatomic undercuts or auditory openings may be of great value. Glasses and hearing aid appliances have been effectively employed in many cases. Branemark osseointegrated implants (Branemark, Zarb, and Albrektsson, 1985) have demonstrated success in selected patients (Fig. 72–54).

POSTOPERATIVE INSTRUCTIONS

Patients should be instructed to keep the deformed area hygienically clean and healthy. If discomfort or pressure points are evident, they should not wear the prosthesis but should return to the prosthodontist for examination and adjustments.

Counsel should be given to patients on methods of retention, along with instructions on the care and cleansing of the prosthesis and the removal of adhesives. Patients should be warned about preventing destructive effects on the prosthesis, such as avoiding organic solvents that distort the color and dry the prosthesis. Smoking may produce nicotine stains and dry the prosthesis. Excessive sunlight and air pollutants affect the prosthetic material and cause it to deteriorate more rapidly.

Use of make-up may be of some help to patients in camouflaging the margins and making the prosthesis blend in with surrounding tissues.

LIMITATIONS OF FACIAL PROSTHESES

Prosthodontic appliances as adjuvants to surgery have a long life span once they are adequately adjusted. External facial prostheses, such as a prosthetic nose, orbit, or auricle, have a number of disadvantages. First, they are expensive to construct. Second, they tend to deteriorate with the passage of time; the color of the prosthesis changes, as does the color of the patient's skin with emotional changes or sun exposure. Therefore, the prostheses must be replaced at regular intervals. A third disadvantage, although a relatively minor one when adequate retention is achieved and a good quality adhesive is employed, is the possibility of detachment of the prosthesis. This is particularly a danger in auricular prostheses, which are maintained only by adhesive. More recently new techniques have been developed such as osseointegrated screws placed on bone and supported by magnets for the retention of facial prostheses. Surgical reconstruction, when possible and when esthetically acceptable, is preferable to replace extensive defects of the nose and ear.

CLEFT PALATE PROSTHESES

A cleft palate obturator can be an essential component in the rehabilitation of the cleft palate patient. Its fundamental objectives are

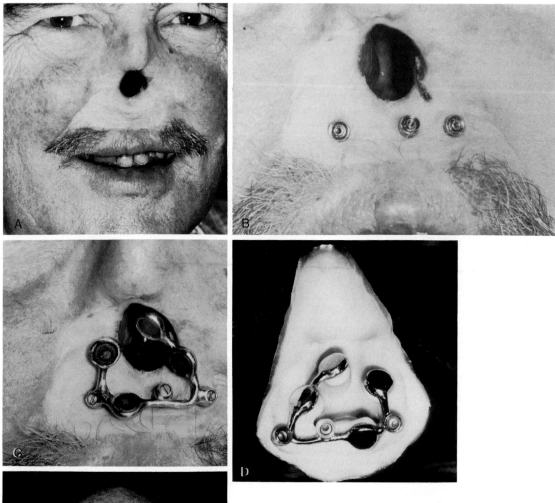

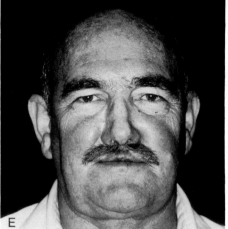

Figure 72–53. Application of osseointegrated fixtures for retention of a nasal prosthesis. *A,* A patient with a nasal deformity. *B,* Three osseointegrated implants placed in the superior maxilla immediately inferior to the piriform aperture, penetrating the healed skin graft. *C,* Design of the magnetic retention superstructure. All units are several millimeters above skin surface for hygiene and access. *D,* Tissue surface of the nasal prosthesis showing the distribution of an embedded magnetic retainer. *E,* Completed prosthesis. (Courtesy of Dr. Stephen M. Parel, D.D.S., Division of Maxillofacial Prosthetics, The University of Texas Health Science Center at San Antonio.)

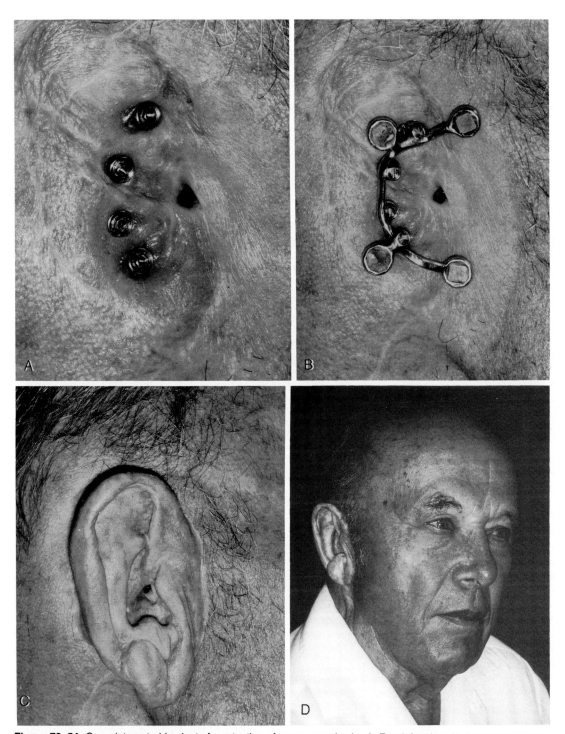

Figure 72–54. Osseointegrated implants for retention of an ear prosthesis. *A,* Ear deformity with four osseointegrated implants placed in the temporal bone posterior to the external auditory canal. *B,* Bar splint with cantilevered magnet retainers anchored to the four osseointegrated fixtures over the area where the prosthesis will be located. *C, D,* Prosthetic ear in place without adhesive.

to aid in developing normal speech, deglutition, and mastication by separating the oral cavity from the nasal cavity in the area of the hard or soft palate, or both. Intraoral prostheses are also required to improve esthetics, replace missing teeth, and provide functional dental occlusion (see Chap. 57).

The first recorded prosthesis designed to improve the speech of a cleft palate patient was constructed by Lusitanus in 1511. The improvement in prosthesis design is due to contributions from many prosthodontists dating from Paré, who in 1531 outlined the general principles of treatment for patients with cleft palate. Fauchard, in 1728, designed five different types of prostheses and recommended an extension to a dental base in order to improve speech. Others were Delabarre (1820) and Snell (1828), who first advocated and demonstrated the use of prostheses for patients with cleft palate. Kingsley (1880), Martin (1889), and Delabarre constructed mobile or movable prostheses. McGrath (1860) introduced an immobile prosthesis for acquired palatal deformities, but it was Suersen (1869) who explained the principle of the immobile prosthesis. Fitzgibbon (1929) advocated a rigid type of obturator constructed of gold. His theories are accepted today, but different materials are used. Most contemporary prostheses are of the immobile type made of a combination acrylic resin and supported by gold or cast chrome cobalt alloys (Harkins, 1960; Adisman, 1971).

A cleft palate prosthesis is indicated (1) as a feeding aid in infants, (2) as a palatal obturator in patients with the Pierre Robin sequence and cleft palate, (3) in children in poor physical health for whom surgery is contraindicated, (4) in wide clefts of the hard and soft palate that lack adequate tissue for surgical closure, (5) in patients with a neuromuscular deficit of the soft palate and pharynx, (6) in patients in whom surgery will interfere with growth and development of orofacial structures, (7) as an expansion prosthesis to improve arch relations, (8) in patients in whom surgical procedures have failed with resultant insufficient velopharyngeal closure or large fistulas, (9) in patients who are to have intermaxillary fixation for jaw surgery and need to be anesthetized through the nasal airways, and (10) in patients for whom the prosthesis is to be used as a surgical splint.

The maxillofacial prosthodontist is in-volved with care of a cleft palate patient almost from birth. The prosthodontist is called on to provide the child with a feeding aid obturator, which in a Pierre Robin-cleft palate infant (see Chap. 63) may also act as a life-saving device. The primary neonatal problem in these patients is often that of maintaining an airway, because, owing to defective mandibular development, there is inadequate anterior support of the tongue, which falls posteriorly and obstructs the pharynx. The inability to protrude the tongue also makes feeding difficult, apart from the problems associated with the cleft palate, if present (Cookson and Hall, 1968). The obturator separates the oral cavity from the nasal cavity and allows the food to be directed downward rather than to escape through the nasal cavity. In the Pierre Robin sequence, the obturator acts to prevent the tongue from occluding the nasopharynx and suffocating the patient.

The preparation of an obturator for an infant is in many cases difficult. The prosthesis is processed in clear or pink acrylic resin; it is finished and polished, reducing and contouring all edges. A hole is made in the anterior labial flange of the feeding aid obturator, and dental tape (Fig. 72–55) is passed through it and tied securely. A long section of the tape is left free to be secured on the child's face or garments; this acts as a handle for removal of the prosthesis from the mouth and prevention of choking.

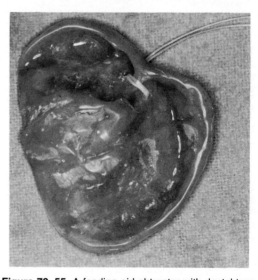

Figure 72–55. A feeding aid obturator with dental tape.

If the prosthesis is not self-retentive, the parents are advised to use denture powder or cream to aid in its retention. The child should wear the obturator as much as possible even when not feeding in order to become accustomed to it. In using the obturator as a feeding aid, the infant is able to take liquid by mouth and liquid is prevented from entering the nasal cavity with the unpleasant effects of choking, gagging, and regurgitating.

Types of Obturators

In general there are four types of prosthetic obturators: (1) the fixed or immobile prosthesis (Fig. 72–56); (2) the mobile or hinge prosthesis (Fig. 72–57); (3) the meatus type that extends into the nasopharynx (Fig. 72–58); and (4) the surgical splint prosthesis (Fig. 72–59).

At the present time the most popular obturator is the immobile fixed prosthesis, usually made of a combination of acrylic resin supported by a gold or chrome cobalt alloy metal frame and clasps. Provisional or temporary obturators are usually made of acrylic

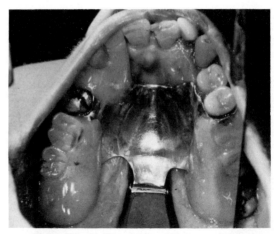

Figure 72–57. The mobile or hinge prosthesis.

resin and flexible metal arms for retention of the teeth.

Sections of the speech aid obturator are identified below with the anatomic oral structures to which they are adapted.

The Palatomaxillary or Maxillary Section. This portion covers the maxilla and any cleft present on the hard palate. It is the retentive part of the frame, and contains clasps and rests to provide adequate retention and to aid in the stability of the prosthesis. This section carries the necessary dental replacements, establishes functional occlusion, improves esthetics, and may aid in plumping out the facial contour if necessary (Fig. 72–60C). It is advisable that the patient wear

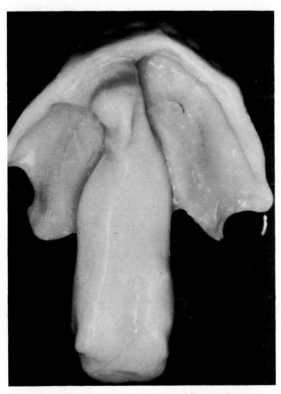

Figure 72–56. The fixed or immobile prosthesis.

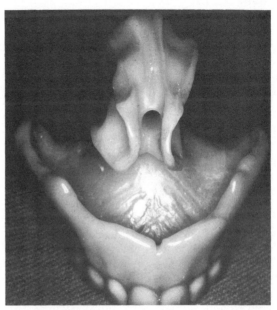

Figure 72–58. The meatus type of prosthesis.

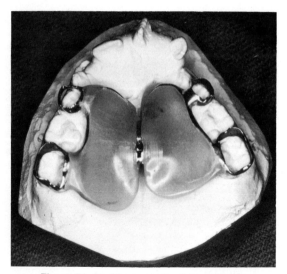

Figure 72–59. The surgical splint prosthesis.

this section and make sure it is stable and comfortable before advancing to the next stage (Fig. 72–60).

The Palatovelar Section or Palatal Extension. This section supplements the palatal cleft and must remain in constant lateral contact with the palatal muscle in repose or in activity, to increase deglutition efficiency and to subserve oral speech purposes. This section, which connects the maxillary portion to the nasopharyngeal section, is usually made of metal or acrylic resin reinforced by metal. It should extend beyond the posterior limits of the soft palate upward into the nasopharynx. In patients in whom an uvula is present but incompetent, a ring may be constructed around the uvula and extended superiorly (Fig. 72–61).

The Pharyngeal or Nasopharyngeal Section. This is the most important section to obtain physiologic velopharyngeal closure to subserve speech and deglutition. It extends posteriorly into the nasopharyngeal cavity near or above Passavant's ridge, where it is surrounded by the sphincteric action of the pharyngeal muscles during oral speech and deglutition. The retention loop at the end of the palatal extension section should extend into the nasopharynx, but it must be free of any contact with the soft tissues in any activity or muscular function. The patient should be allowed to wear the prosthesis with this section attached until it is comfortable before an impression is taken of the palatonaso-pharyngeal section. The impression of this

area is first taken in a combination of low-fusing wax (Fig. 72–62), which is relieved and covered with a thermolabile nasopharyngeal paste (Fig. 72–63) that flows at body temperatures when functional movements of the head, neck, and palatopharyngeal musculature are made.

When the prosthodontist and speech therapist are satisfied that the latter section is of the best form and shape for optimal speech, deglutition, and mastication, the prosthesis is removed from the patient and the nasopharyngeal section is immersed in cold water to harden and prevent distortion. This section of the prosthesis is reproduced in clear acrylic resin. The final fitting and adjustment on the patient should be made with the speech therapist present. In cases in which the speech bulb is of a large bulk, it may be made hollow to lighten its weight (Fig. 72–64).

The patient's age may influence the type of obturator to be constructed. In children during the period of deciduous teeth or mixed dentition and in their formative years, the obturator is usually made of acrylic resin reinforced with a metal rod and wrought wire clasps for retention. Abutment teeth may require orthodontic bands with buccal tubes for clasp retention. The construction of this appliance should usually be accomplished in sections, each section being tried for a period before the final nasopharyngeal bulb is constructed. The prosthesis will have to be adjusted and modified or replaced as growth and development proceed. In many cases orthodontic intervention is necessary; therefore, it is imperative that the orthodontist and prosthodontist work together and construct an ortho-speech prosthesis or a speech appliance in conjunction with the orthodontic appliance.

Speech appliances for the adult are of a more permanent nature. Orthodontic therapy and oral surgical revisions should be completed. If there are missing teeth, especially anterior teeth, they should be replaced with fixed bridge appliances. All selected abutment teeth may have to be protected and redesigned with full crown coverage. All teeth to be superimposed should be periodontally free of disease and protected with cast gold thimbles, or crowns that could be used for secondary retention. When the mouth and teeth are properly prepared, a preliminary impression is taken extending into the nasopharyngeal area. From this impression, a self-curing acrylic resin tray is made for the

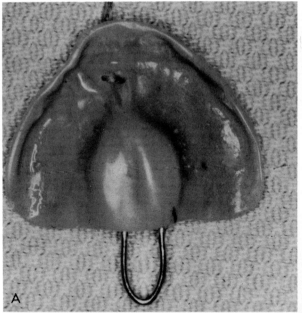

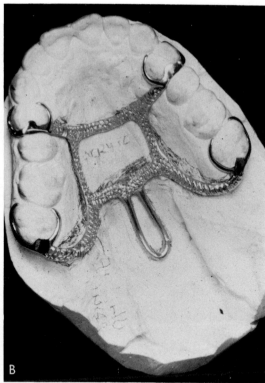

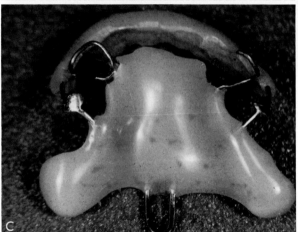

Figure 72–60. Section of the prosthesis before the addition of wax material to the impression of the palatovelar component. *A,* Acrylic base supported with a metal extension. *B,* Cast metal frame to carry the acrylic palatal section. *C,* With a labial plumper added.

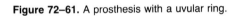

Figure 72–61. A prosthesis with a uvular ring.

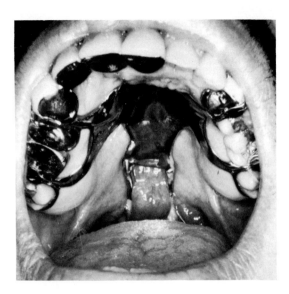

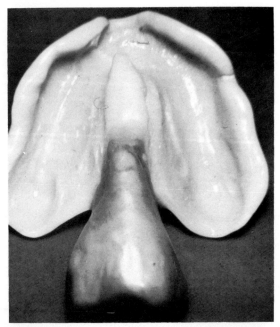

Figure 72–62. Full upper denture obturator prosthesis with low fusing wax extension into the palatonasopharyngeal area before the final impression.

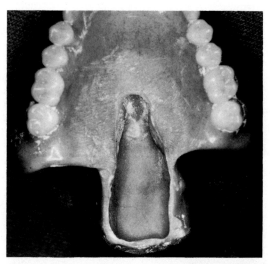

Figure 72–64. A speech bulb made hollow to lighten its weight.

final alginate or rubber base impression, which is made into a dental stone working model. Since growth and development are no longer a problem, the prosthesis is constructed of a supporting cast metal (Fig. 72–65) material for the frame and clasps and palatal extension, and completed in form and shape by processed acrylic resin. The main abutment teeth are usually covered with protective cast crowns designed for maximal retention without causing periodontal breakdown. The prosthesis is generally constructed in three stages or sections as described previously (Fig. 72–66).

In general, the design of a palatal lift prosthesis employs the principle of elevation of the soft palate as a means of decreasing the lumen of the velopharyngeal valve and producing obturation of the residual lumen. The most popular type is the strap and bulb prosthesis, which has a wide lateral expansion. A similar type of appliance can be used

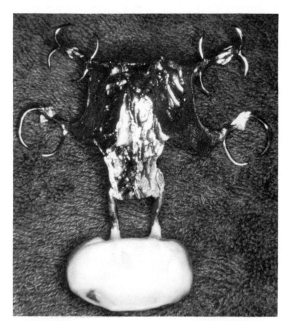

Figure 72–63. Impression with thermolabile (nasopharyngeal) paste.

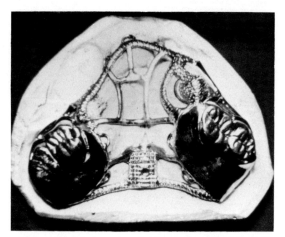

Figure 72–65. A cast metal frame to support the prosthesis.

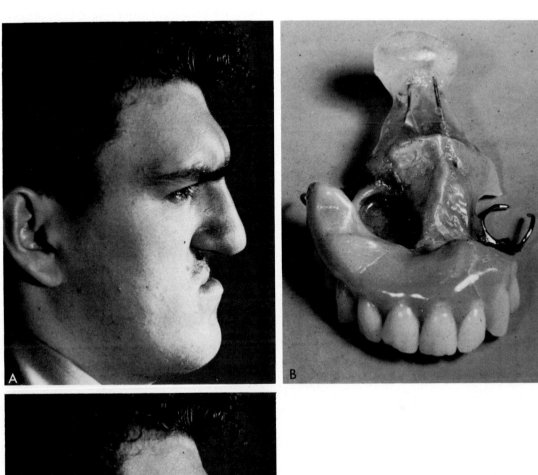

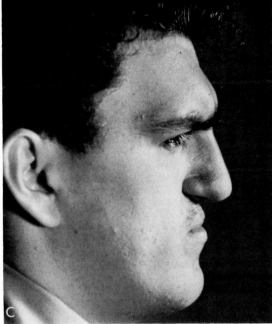

Figure 72–66. *A,* A cleft palate patient without an obturator prosthesis. *B,* A superimposed partial obturator prosthesis with a speech bulb and labial plumper to augment the facial contour. *C,* Profile view of the patient wearing the prosthesis.

for some palates that demonstrate insufficiency or paralysis. In these cases, the extension part of the prosthesis can be made narrower and in the shape of a lollipop, adjusted periodically to increase palatal elevation.

The palatal stimulating appliance (Adisman, 1971) has also proved successful in some cases.

REFERENCES

Adisman, I. K.: Cleft palate prosthetics. *In* Grabb, W., Rosenstein, S., and Bzoch, K. (Eds.): Cleft Lip and Palate; Surgical Dental and Speech Aspects. Boston, Little, Brown & Company, 1971, p. 617.

Antia, N. H.: The scope of plastic surgery in leprosy: A ten year progress report. Clin. Plast. Surg., *1*:69. 1974.

Bloomer, H., and Lang, B.: Principles and procedures in construction of the palatal lift appliance for patients with velopharyngeal insufficiency or incompetence. Presented at the meeting of the American Cleft Palate Association, April 26, 1968.

Boyne, P. S.: New concepts of bone grafting. *In* Goldman, H. M. (Ed.): Current Therapy in Dentistry. Vol. IV. St. Louis, C. V. Mosby Company, 1970, p. 320.

Branemark, P. -I., Breine, U., Lindstrom, J., Adell, R., Hansson, B. O., and Ohlsson, A.: Intra-osseous anchorage of dental prostheses. I. Experimental studies. Scand. J. Plast. Reconstr. Surg., *3*:81, 1969.

Branemark, P. -I., Zarb, G. A., and Albrektsson, T.: Tissue-Integrated Prostheses—Osseointegration in Clinical Dentistry. Chicago, Quintessence Publishing Company, 1985.

Bulbulian, A. H.: Facial Prosthesis. Philadelphia, W. B. Saunders Company, 1945.

Burston, W. R.: The early orthodontic treatment of cleft palate conditions. Dent. Pract. (Bristol), *9*:41, 1958.

Clarke, C. D.: Prosthetics. Butler, MD, Standard Arts Press, 1965.

Coccaro, P. J., and Valauri, A. J.: Orthodontics in cleft lip and palate children. *In* Converse, J. M. (Ed.): Reconstructive Plastic Surgery. 2nd Ed. Philadelphia, W. B. Saunders Company, 1977, p. 2213.

Converse, J. M.: Restoration of vestibular sulcus. In Converse, J. M. (Ed.): Reconstructive Plastic Surgery. 1st Ed. Philadelphia & London, W. B. Saunders Company, 1964, p. 941.

Converse, J. M., and Valauri, A. J.: The role of maxillofacial prosthetics in reconstructive surgery for defects of the head and neck. *In* Robinson, J. E., and Niiranen, V. J. (Eds.): Maxillofacial Prosthetics—Proceedings of an Interprofessional Conference, September, 1966, Washington, DC. Sponsored by the American Academy of Maxillofacial Prosthetics. U.S. Department of Health, Education and Welfare, Public Health Service Pub. No. 1950, 1966, p. 40.

Cookson, A., and Hall, B. D.: Use of obturators in the early management of a case of Pierre Robin syndrome (Pielou's method). Dent. Pract. Dent. Rec., *18*:264, 1968.

Cronin, T. D.: An overall plan of treatment of complete cleft lips and palate. *In* Hotz, R. (Ed.): Early Treatment of Cleft Lip and Palate. Berne, Huber, 1964.

Delabarre, F. A.: Cited by Harkins, C. S. (Ed.): *In* Principles of Cleft Palate Prosthesis: Aspects in the Rehabilitation of the Cleft Palate Individual. Published for Temple University Publications, Philadelphia, by Columbia University Press, New York, 1960, p. 5.

Esser, J. F.: Studies in plastic surgery of the face. Ann. Surg., *65*:297, 1917.

Fauchard, P.: Quoted by Kingsley, N. W.: *In* A Treatise on Oral Deformities. New York, D. Appleton & Company, 1880, p. 218.

Fitzgibbon, J. J.: The correction of congenital palate speech by the Fitzgibbon appliance. Apollonia, *4*:260, 1929.

Fleming, I. D., and Morris, J. H.: Use of acrylic external splint after mandibular resection. Am. J. Surg., *118*:708, 1969.

Gillies, H. D.: Deformities of the syphilitic nose. Br. Med. J., *29*:977, 1923.

Hall, H. D., and O'Steen, A. N.: Free grafts of palatal mucosa in mandibular vestibuloplasty. J. Oral Surg., *28*:565, 1970.

Harkins, C. S.: Principles of Cleft Palate Prosthesis: Aspects in the Rehabilitation of the Cleft Palate Individual. Published for Temple University Publications, Philadelphia, by Columbia University Press, New York, 1960.

Hinds, E. C., Spira, M., Sills, H. A., Jr., and Galbreath, J. C.: Use of tantalum trays in mandibular surgery. Plast. Reconstr. Surg., *32*:439, 1963.

Kazanjian, V. H.: Prosthetic restoration of acquired deformities of the superior maxilla. J. Allied Dent. Soc., *10*:1423, 1915.

Kazanjian, V. H.: Modern accomplishments in dental and facial prostheses. J. Dent. Res., *12*:651, 1932.

Kazanjian, V. H., and Converse, J. M.: Principles of maxillofacial prosthetics. *In* The Surgical Treatment of Facial Injuries. 3rd Ed. Vol. 2. Baltimore, Williams & Wilkins Company, 1974, Chap. 30.

Kent, J.: Reconstruction of the atrophic alveolar ridge with hydroxylapatite: a five year report. Study presented at the Second World Congress on Biomaterials. Washington, DC, April 27–May 1, 1984.

Kingsley, N. W.: A Treatise on Oral Deformities. New York, D. Appleton & Company, 1880.

Lew, D.: A method for augmenting the severely atrophic maxilla using hydroxylapatite. J. Oral Maxillofac. Surg., *43*:47, 1985.

Lindquist, A. F.: Prosthetic and orthodontic procedures for the cleft palate infants. Int. Dent. J., *13*:688, 1963.

Lusitanus, A.: Cited by Weinberger, H. W.: *In* An Introduction to the History of Dentistry. St. Louis, C. V. Mosby Company, 1948.

Martin, C.: De la Prosthèse Immediate. Paris, Masson, 1889.

McGrath: Cited by Harkins, C. S. (Ed.): *In* Principles of Cleft Palate Prosthesis: Aspects in the Rehabilitation of the Cleft Palate Individual. Published for Temple University Publications, Philadelphia, by Columbia University Press, New York, 1960.

McMahon, E. M.: Speech patterns with special reference to cleft palates. Aust. Dent. J., *6*:101, 1961.

McNeil, C. K.: Oral and Facial Deformity. London, Sir Isaac Pitman & Sons, 1954.

McNeil, C. K.: Orthopedic principles in the treatment of lip and palate clefts. *In* Hotz, R. (Ed.): Early Treatment of Cleft Lip and Palate. Berne, Huber, 1964.

Morgan, L. R., Gallegos, L. T., and Frileck, S. P.: Mandibular vestibuloplasty with a free graft of the mucoperiosteal layer from the hard palate. Plast. Reconstr. Surg., *51*:359, 1973.

Morgan, L. R., and Thompson, C. W.: Mandibular reconstruction. Current state of the art. Clin. Plast. Surg., 2:561, 1975.

Morris, J. H.: Biphase connector, external skeletal splint for reduction and fixation of mandibular fractures. Oral Surg., 2:1382, 1949.

Olin, W. H., and Schweiger, J. W.: Dental rehabilitation of the cleft lip and cleft palate patient. In Converse, J. M. (Ed.): Reconstructive Plastic Surgery. 1st Ed. Philadelphia & London, 1964, pp. 1489–1503.

Paré, A.: Les oeuvres de M. Ambroise Paré conseiller et premier chirurgien du roy. Avec les figures et portraits tout de l'anatomic que des instruments des chirurgie, et de plusieurs monstres, le tout divisé en vingt-six livres, comme il est contenue en la page suyvente. Paris, G. Buone, 1575.

Parel, S. M.: Implants and overdentures: the osseointegrated approach with conventional and compromised applications. Int. J. Oral Maxillofac. Implants, 1:93, 1986.

Parel, S. M., Branemark, P. -I., Tjellstrom, A., and Gion, G.: Osseointegration in maxillofacial prosthetics. Part II: Extraoral applications. Prosthet. Dent., 55:600, 1986a.

Parel, S. M., Holt, R., Branemark, P. -I., and Tjellstrom, A.: Osseointegration and facial prosthetics. Int. J. Oral Maxillofac. Implants, 1:27, 1986b.

Pielou, W. D., and Allen, A.: Pierre Robin syndrome. Dent. Pract. Dent. Rec., 18:169, 1968.

Popp, H.: Zur Geschichte der Prosthesen. Med. Welt., 13:961, 1939.

Riediger, D.: Restoration of masticatory function by microsurgically revascularized iliac crest bone grafts using enosseous implants. Plast. Reconstr. Surg., 81:861, 1988.

Rogers, B. O., and Valauri, A. J.: Harelip–cleft palate repair: postoperative dental problems. Dent. Pract. Dent. Rec., 4:7, 1966.

Schaff, N.: Maxillofacial prosthetics. In Carol, W., and Sako, K. (Eds.): Cancer and the Oral Cavity. Chicago, Quintessence Publishing Company, 1986.

Schweiger, J. W.: Prosthetic rehabilitation of the mandibulectomy patient. In Chretien, P. B., et al. (Eds.): Head and Neck Cancer. Vol. I. Philadelphia, B. C. Decker, 1984.

Smith, B., and Valauri, A. J.: The orbit. In Converse, J. M. (Ed.): Reconstructive Plastic Surgery. 1st Ed. Philadelphia, W. B. Saunders Company, 1964, p. 624.

Snell, J.: Cited by Harkins, C. S. (Ed.): In Principles of Cleft Palate Prosthesis: Aspects in the Rehabilitation of the Cleft Palate Individual. Published for Temple University Publications, Philadelphia, by Columbia University Press, New York, 1960.

Steinhauser, E. W.: Free transportation of oral mucosa for improvement of denture retention. J. Oral Surg., 27:955, 1969.

Steinhauser, E. W.: Vestibuloplasty—skin grafts. J. Oral Surg., 29:777, 1971.

Suersen, W.: Ueber die Herstellung einer dentlichen Aussprache durch ein neues System kunstlicher Gaumen bei angeborenen und erworbenen Gaumendefekten. Klin. Wochenschr., 6:110, 1869.

Tetamore, F. D. R.: Deformities of the face and orthopedics. Brooklyn, NY, Adams Printing Company, 1894.

Trauner, R.: Alveoloplasty with ridge extensions on the lingual side of the lower jaw to solve the problem of a lower dental prosthesis. J. Oral Surg., 5:340, 1952.

Udagama, A.: Dental oncology and maxillofacial rehabilitation. In Gunn, A. E. (Ed.): Cancer Rehabilitation. New York, Raven Press, 1984, p. 47.

Upham, R. H.: Artificial noses and ears. Boston Med. Surg. J., 145:522, 1901.

Valauri, A. J.: Correcting maxillofacial deformities. Use of surgical prosthesis and split-thickness skin graft. New York J. Dent., 33:2, 1963.

Valauri, A. J.: Prosthetic aids in the treatment of facial fractures and mandibular resection. In Robbett, W. (Ed.): Proceedings of the Centennial Symposium, Manhattan Eye, Ear, and Throat Hospital. Vol. II. Otolaryngology. St. Louis, C. V. Mosby Company, 1969.

Valauri, A. J.: Principles of maxillofacial prosthetics. In Kazanjian, V. H., and Converse, J. M.: The Surgical Treatment of Facial Injuries. 3rd Ed. Baltimore, Williams & Wilkins Company, 1974, p. 1408.

Valauri, A. J.: Maxillofacial prosthetics: in theory and practice. Dermatol. Surg., 1:52, 1975.

Valauri, A. J.: Maxillofacial prosthetics. In Epstein, E. (Ed.): Skin Surgery. Springfield, IL, Charles C Thomas, 1977a.

Valauri, A. J.: The orbit. In Converse, J. M. (Ed.): Reconstructive Plastic Surgery. 2nd Ed. Philadelphia, W. B. Saunders Company, 1977b, p. 962.

Valauri, A. J.: Cleft palate prosthetics. In Converse, J. M. (Ed.): Reconstructive Plastic Surgery. 2nd Ed. Philadelphia, W. B. Saunders Company, 1977c, p. 2283.

Valauri, A. J.: Maxillofacial prosthetics. In Converse, J. M. (Ed.): Reconstructive Plastic Surgery. 2nd Ed. Philadelphia, W. B. Saunders Company, 1977d, p. 2917.

Valauri, A. J.: Diagnostico e tratamento das lesoes adquiridas da face. In I Simposio Latino Americano De Reabilitacao Da Face E De Prostese Buco-Maxilo-Facial. (Proceedings of the First Latin American Symposium on Maxillofacial Prosthetics Rehabilitation of the Face.) Sao Paolo, Brazil, Published by Government of Brazil, 1979a, p. 5.

Valauri, A. J.: Resseccoes mandibulares. In I Simposio Latino Americano De Reabilitacao Da Face E De Prostese Buco-Maxilo-Facial. (Proceedings of the First Latin American Symposium on Maxillofacial Prosthetics Rehabilitation of the Face.) Sao Paolo, Brazil, Published by Government of Brazil, 1979b, p. 46.

Valauri, A. J.: Reconstrucao mandibular. In I Simposio Latino Americano De Reabilitacao Da Face E De Prostese Buco-Maxilo-Facial. (Proceedings of the First Latin American Symposium on Maxillofacial Prosthetics Rehabilitation of the Face.) Sao Paolo, Brazil, Published by Government of Brazil, 1979c, p. 197.

Valauri, A. J.: Maxillofacial prosthetics. Aesth. Plast. Surg., 6:159, 1982.

Valauri, A. J. (Ed.): Maxillofacial prosthetics. In McCoy, F. J., et al. (Eds.): The Yearbook of Plastic and Reconstructive Surgery, 1984. Chicago, Year Book Medical Publishers, 1984, p. 82.

Waldron, C. W., and Risdon, R.: Mandibular bone grafts. Proc. R. Soc. Med., 12:11, 1919.

Walsh, T. S., Jr.: Buried metallic prosthesis for mandibular defects. Cancer, 7:1002, 1954.

73

George L. Popkin

Tumors of the Skin: A Dermatologist's Viewpoint

Most skin tumors seen in dermatologic practice are benign lesions: verrucae, nevi, keratoses, cysts, and skin tags. However, a significant number are either premalignant or malignant. Proper management is therefore based on an understanding of the microscopic and gross pathology of the lesion. This should be coupled with an appreciation of the natural history and usual clinical course of the lesion to be treated.

The discussion will begin with the benign lesions and proceed to the premalignant and malignant lesions. Surgical excisional techniques will not be discussed except in a few instances; emphasis is placed on other dermatologic approaches to management.

VIRAL TUMORS

Verruca Vulgaris

The common wart (verruca vulgaris) is a benign, infectious skin tumor caused by a member of the papovavirus group (Rook, 1968). It is found on the surface of the skin, in the vagina and rectum, and infrequently on the oral mucous membrane.

Etiology. The papovavirus infects not only man but also other mammals, in which it causes papillomatosis of the skin and mucous membranes (Rook, 1968). Steward, Mack, and Foy (1968) and Lutzner (1963) observed that the virus is spherical and about 50 nm in diameter, and that it replicates in the nucleus of the epidermal stratum spinosum. Eventually it fills the nucleus and can be found in the cytoplasm as well. Virus particles may be found in the stratum corneum.

Incidence. Patients with warts account for 4 to 10 per cent of annual clinic and private

Table 73–1. Human Papillomavirus Types: Association With Particular Histologic Patterns and Potential Oncogenicity

HPV* Type	Associated Clinical Lesion	Histologic Pattern and Cytopathic Effect	Suspected Oncogenicity
1	Deep, solitary, painful, plantar warts	Endophytic, giant keratohyaline-like granules	None
2	Common warts; filiform warts; mosaic plantar warts; palatal warts	Exophytic, composite keratohyaline-like granules	None
3, 10	Flat warts (especially in children), also in some patients with EV†	Flat lesions; perinuclear vacuolization of cytoplasm; keratohyaline and tonofilaments pushed to periphery of cell	3 related sequences in EV cancers and some genital cancers
4	Dome-shaped, keratosis punctata–like warts, usually on hands (palms)	Clear cytoplasm compressing nuclei into crescents	None
5, 8, 9, 12, 14, 15	Macular lesions in patients with EV or renal allograft recipients (scaly, red, or pityriasis versicolor–like); flat, wartlike lesions on back of hands	Pale-staining cytoplasm; vacuolated nuclei; rounded keratohyaline granules	5 and 8 genomes found in Bowen's disease and squamous cell cancers
6	Anogenital condylomas, laryngeal papillomas	Exophytic fibropapillomas; outer cells may be binucleated; perinuclear halo	6 genome found in Buschke-Löwenstein tumors (giant condylomas)
7	Hand warts in butchers	Verrucous; nuclei are centrally located	None
11	Laryngeal papillomas; flat cervical "condylomas"	Koilocytes; some binucleated cells with perinuclear halos	11 genome found in cervical cancers
13	Focal epithelial hyperplasia of oral mucosa, especially frequently occurring in Greenland Eskimos and American Indians	"Bronze-age ax" rete ridge pattern; "mitosoid" nuclei; binucleated cells	None

*HPV indicates human papillomaviruses.
†EV indicates epidermodysplasia verruciformis.
From Lutzner, M. A.: The human papillomaviruses: a review. Arch. Dermatol., *119*:631, 1983. Copyright 1983, American Medical Association. Reproduced by permission.

dermatologic visits in the United States, and Rook (1968) noted an increase during a 20 to 30 year period from 3 or 4 per cent up to 10 to 15 per cent of new patients at some clinics in Great Britain. Blank and Rake (1955) found that warts appeared most commonly in patients between 10 and 20 years of age.

Epidemiology. The development of warts appears to be influenced by skin trauma. Warts may be found at sites of nail biting, picking of the skin, or plantar pressure caused by poorly fitting shoes or faulty weight bearing. The virus may be transmitted by direct or indirect contact. Individual susceptibility varies, and little is known about immunity. Experimental inoculation of human volunteers demonstrated an average incubation period of four months, with a range of one to 20 months (Goldschmidt and Kligman, 1958). Because of the great variability in the life cycle of individual warts and their known

response to suggestion therapy (Bloch, 1927; Allington, 1952), all forms of treatment must be evaluated against these factors.

Clinical Description. There are several clinical types of warts. Verruca vulgaris is the most frequently seen, and the fingers are the most common location for these tumors, which are firm and elevated and have a roughened surface (see Fig. 73–6). They are gray or brownish, and they may have small subsurface black specks that represent the tips of superficial capillary loops. At times, several warts aggregate into larger, plaque-type lesions. Common warts found around or under nails are designated periungual or subungual warts; in these locations they may cause considerable pain upon pressure.

Flat or plane warts (Fig. 73–1) occur on the face, hands, or legs. They are flat to slightly elevated lesions, ordinarily a few millimeters in diameter, although they can

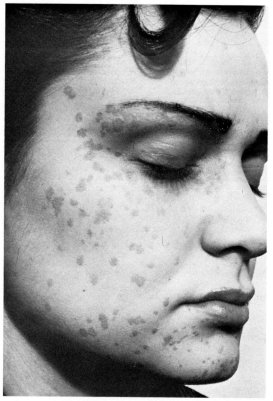

Figure 73–1. Plane warts. [Used by permission of New York University School of Medicine (Skin and Cancer Unit).]

(Fig. 73–3) but may also be around the anus, in the web spaces (Rook, 1968), in the angles of the mouth, and occasionally on the conjunctiva (Blank and Rake, 1955). Although often called venereal warts, they may or may not be transmitted by sexual intercourse, depending on individual host factors.

Pathology. Almeida, Hawatson, and Williams (1962) noted that the virus infects the nuclei of the epidermal cells, becoming detectable first in the upper portion of the stratum spinosum. Common warts are characterized by acanthosis, papillomatosis, and hyperkeratosis, with areas of parakeratosis. According to Lever (1967), verruca vulgaris is distinguished from other papillomas by the presence of large vacuolated cells in the upper portions of the stratum spinosum. This feature pertains only to young lesions. The rete ridges slant downward from the periphery toward the center. In plantar warts the picture is similar except for a thicker horn layer.

Plane warts show a loose, lamellar type of hyperkeratosis, acanthosis, and thickening of the granular layer; there is no papillomatosis. More extensive vacuolation of the cells is seen in the upper stratum spinosum and granular layer (Lever, 1967).

Acuminate warts have pronounced acanthosis and papillomatosis. The sharply defined lower border of the epidermal-dermal

become considerably larger, the color varying from pink or skin colored to a darker hue. The lesions may be seen in scratch marks.

Digitate and filiform warts are found on the face, neck, and scalp.

Plantar warts (Fig. 73–2) are characterized by slightly elevated lesions usually surrounded and covered by callus. After removal of the callus, the wart is visible. Palmar warts may resemble plantar warts. Occasionally, plantar corns may appear like warts. Both may be quite painful when squeezed between the thumb and index finger. However, scalpel paring of the callus overlying the corn reveals a yellowish shiny core. When a similar procedure is performed on a plantar wart, small bleeding points are usually encountered. Mosaic wart is the designation for plantar warts that are packed so closely together as to suggest a mosaic arrangement.

Acuminate warts are found on moist parts of the body. In contrast to the horny hard coverings of other types of warts, these lesions are soft and pink and white in color. They are most often found on the external genitals

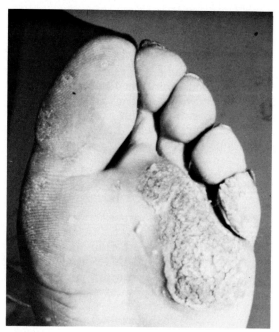

Figure 73–2. Plantar warts [Used by permission of New York University School of Medicine (Skin and Cancer Unit).]

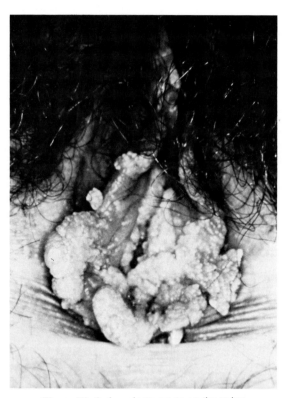

Figure 73–3. Acuminate warts on the vulva.

junction and cellular orderly arrangement distinguishes this lesion from carcinoma (Lever, 1967). The vacuolation of the cells helps to confirm the diagnosis. Lever (1967) emphasized that such vacuolation is found in the upper portions of the normal mucosa, so that it must be found in the deeper portions of the epithelial ridges to substantiate the diagnosis of a virus-induced lesion.

Malignant Transformation of Warts. Epidermodysplasia verruciformis (EV) is a type of skin eruption resembling plane warts distributed in a generalized pattern. Typical common warts are often noted also in the patient with EV. In some cases of EV, the lesions are pink, pigmented, or of violet hue. Histologic findings in EV are similar to those of plane warts.

According to Nagington and Rook (1979), the lesions of EV may remain unchanged for a long time. However, squamous cell carcinoma has developed in about 20 per cent of cases reported. These authors note that malignant change occurs most often in lesions on sun-exposed skin.

Human papillomaviruses (HPV)-5 and -8 and the -3 related genome are found in cancers of EV (Lutzner, 1983). In Buschke-

Löwenstein tumor (squamous cell carcinoma), HPV-6 genome copies have been noted (Lutzner, 1983). HPV-11 may be found in cervical cancers.

Treatment. "The treatment of warts is an art" (Blank and Rake, 1955). Since warts are benign lesions, one should strive for minimal destruction of normal tissue, thereby reducing healing time and scarring.

Verruca Plana. Suggestion therapy should be tried first if the lesions are at all extensive. This can take the form of sterile saline intradermal injections at weekly intervals for two to three weeks, combined with applications of a bland cream "carefully" rubbed into the warts twice a day with a small cotton-tipped applicator. Liquid nitrogen or carbon dioxide slush lightly applied for three to five seconds exerts a psychotherapeutic and a physical effect. On the face, other surgical methods, such as light electrodesiccation or mild curettage, carry the risk of scarring. Should the latter methods of treatment be necessary, it is wise to try treatment of a few inconspicuous areas, if possible, to determine the degree of residual scarring.

Common warts may be approached by several techniques. One of the simplest, if the warts are not extensive, is the use of sharp curettage followed by light electrodesiccation or the application of a styptic for hemostasis. After local anesthesia has been secured, the curved pointed scissors are used to sever the entire periphery of the wart at its junction with normal skin (Figs. 73–4, 73–5). Following this, a sharp dermal curette is used with a firm scraping motion to remove the wart from its bed. Inspection of the wart base with a good light will show whether the removal is complete. When curettage is finished, electrodesiccation with monopolar spark gap current (of low intensity) may be used for hemostasis, or a styptic, such as a 35 per cent solution of aluminum chloride in 50 per cent isopropyl rubbing alcohol compound, can be employed to stop capillary bleeding (Heinlein 1970). Some physicians prefer to electrodesiccate the entire wart as the first maneuver after local anesthesia has been secured. This softens the hyperkeratotic mass and renders curettage quite simple. The patient is instructed to keep the treated area as dry as possible and to use nonadherent dressings during the healing period.

By keeping normal tissue destruction to a minimum, more rapid healing is ensured and

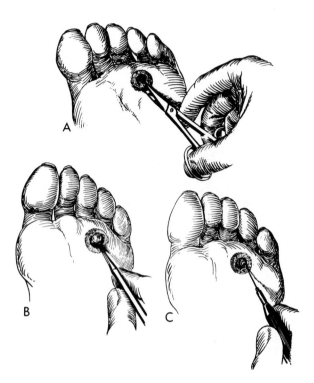

Figure 73–4. Curettage of a plantar wart. *A,* Incising the wart—normal skin junction. *B,* Curettage of wart. *C,* Light electrodesiccation of the curetted bed for hemostasis.

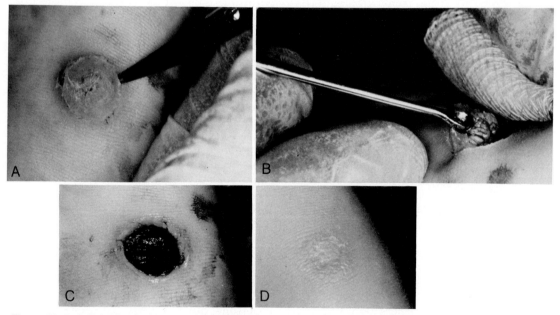

Figure 73–5. *A,* Painful plantar wart. Junction of skin at the edge of the wart incised with pointed scissors. *B,* Curettage of plantar wart. *C,* Defect following removal of the plantar wart. Hemostasis secured by application of 35% aluminum chloride in 50% isopropyl alcohol and pressure. *D,* Nonpainful scar several months after treatment.

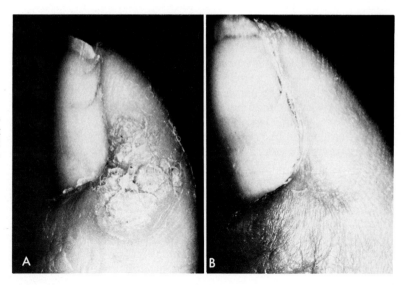

Figure 73–6. Treatment of a periungual wart by curettage and light electrodesiccation. *A,* Periungual wart. *B,* Several weeks after treatment.

there is less likelihood of scarring. Warts so treated ordinarily leave little or no scar (Fig. 73–6). Exceptions are large warts that have been present for a long time. The skin of some individuals reacts to minor trauma with scarring. In anticipation of the latter, as mentioned before, it is wise to treat one or two warts and observe the course of healing before removing multiple lesions.

When warts are quite extensive, other methods of treatment are desirable. Liquid nitrogen (−195.8°C) is applied to the warts with a cotton-tipped applicator. Liquid nitrogen may be stored in the office in insulated containers of 5, 10, 25, or 31 liters. The 31 liter container appears to retain its liquid nitrogen for the longest time. By means of a small dipper, the liquid nitrogen is ladled out into a Styrofoam drinking cup. This provides sufficient insulation to treat one patient with the liquid nitrogen. A cotton-tipped applicator is dipped into the liquid nitrogen and held against the wart with light pressure until freezing of the wart, as well as a rim of 1 to 2 mm of normal skin, occurs. This usually requires 10 to 20 seconds. Heavier treatment for a longer period is required if the wart is extremely thick or hyperkeratotic. At times, a blister is produced, but this is not necessary in order to achieve the desired end result. Liquid nitrogen treatments may be repeated at intervals of two weeks until the wart disappears. Heavier treatments induce greater inflammatory response, hemorrhagic blisters, and considerable pain.

Other methods of therapy include the local application of various acids, such as mono-, bi-, and trichloroacetic acids.

Plantar warts in young children may be treated by the application of 40 per cent salicylic acid plaster cut to the size of the lesions. This is left in place for five days. Frequently in young children the entire wart comes away when the dressing is changed in one week. For older children or adults with one or more plantar warts, under local infiltration anesthesia, the same technique of sharp curettage is used as for warts on the finger (see Fig. 73–4). If hyperhidrosis occurs or if faulty weight bearing is noted, attempts should be made to correct both of these conditions in an effort to lessen recurrence of plantar warts.

Other methods of treating the warts include the use of flexible collodion with lactic acid and salicylic acid in concentrations of 5 to 10 per cent each (Lerner and Lerner, 1960). This preparation may be applied to the wart daily, discontinuing treatment if erythema and pain develop. Cantharidin, 0.7 per cent, in equal parts of collodion and acetone may be effective when applied to warts under adhesive tape dressings kept in place for nine to ten days, unless excessive pain supervenes (Epstein and Kligman, 1958).

Acuminate warts of the anogenital area may respond dramatically to applications of 25 per cent podophyllum resin in compound tincture of benzoin. It is suggested to patients that they wash the application off after three hours. A small circumscribed area should be tested prior to wider application. If excessive irritation does not occur, the next time the patient is treated the medication may be left in place for a longer period until it is finally left on overnight and washed off the following day. The treatment may be done at intervals of one to two weeks, depending on the inflammatory response. In treating resistant acuminate warts, it may be necessary to use local or general anesthesia to remove the warts by electrodesiccation and curettage.

Podophyllum resin should not be applied to large areas at one time because of the possibility of systemic absorption and toxicity.

Control or elimination of associated vaginal discharge is helpful in the management of vulval and vaginal acuminate warts, and proctologic examination may be indicated in persistent anal-perianal warts to rule out the presence of warts of the anal canal and rectum.

Molluscum Contagiosum

This disease is caused by a virus that morphologically resembles the pox viruses and is usually classified as a member of this group of viruses despite the absence of antigenic cross reaction (Rook, 1968). The lesion clinically consists of skin-colored papules (Fig. 73–7) varying in size up to 1 cm, although most of the lesions are a few millimeters in size. One important clinical characteristic is the central, often porelike depression, which becomes more noticeable upon light freezing of the skin surface with Freon-ethyl chloride mixtures.

The incidence is not known, but in private practice it is seen infrequently in comparison with the common wart; it may be seen in wrestlers, and it is presumed to be transmitted by direct contact. Some individuals may acquire immunity through previous subclinical infection.

Etiology. The viral agent is 300 × 200 × 100 nm in size (Lutzner, 1963). It affects the cells of the deeper layer of the epidermis, forming cytoplasmic oval hyaline bodies. Multiplication of the virus results in the formation of molluscum bodies in the dermis. These bodies destroy the fibrous matrix of the superficial layers of the skin (Lever, 1967), and thus the central pore is formed.

The diagnosis of the lesions ordinarily offers no difficulty when they are seen in crops

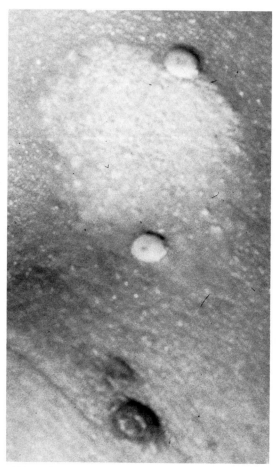

Figure 73–7. Molluscum contagiosum. Note the central depression after light freezing with ethyl chloride–Freon spray.

on young adults or children. Occasionally, a single lesion occurs on the face and may be clinically confused with a basal cell epithelioma or other lesions. However, biopsy readily confirms the characteristic histopathology.

Therapy. The spontaneous disappearance of lesions is known. Simple sharp curettage under local spray anesthesia is curative, but the patient must be followed for several months, since clinically inapparent lesions may gradually become manifest. Other methods of treatment consist of touching the lesion with trichloroacetic acid or expressing the contents of each lesion with a comedo extractor. Liquid nitrogen therapy as described for common warts is also effective.

SEBORRHEIC KERATOSIS

Seborrheic keratosis (seborrheic wart, senile wart, basal cell papilloma) is a light to

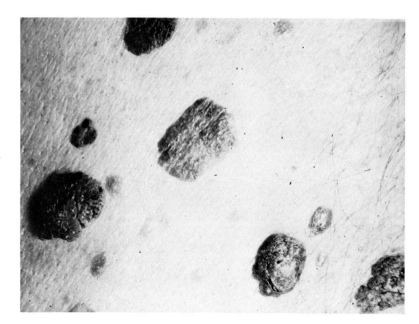

Figure 73–8. Multiple seborrheic keratoses.

very dark brown raised papular lesion. The surface of the lesion varies from smooth to wartlike, with pitting visible on the surface of some lesions (Fig. 73–8). The lesions may be sessile or pedunculated and may occur singly, but more often are seen in clusters. They tend to exist more frequently in the middle to older age group and are benign growths.

Smooth, slightly elevated, small pigmented papules on the malar and forehead areas of blacks are termed dermatosis papulosa nigra. These occur earlier in life than seborrheic keratoses, but under the microscope they show resemblance to lesions of seborrheic keratosis (Hairston, Reed, and Derbes, 1964).

Etiology. The etiology is unknown, but it is believed that there is a familial predisposition with an autosomal mode of inheritance (Sanderson, 1968a).

Lesions may be seen following an inflammatory dermatosis or uncommonly as a manifestation of internal malignancy. The Leser-Trélat sign is the sudden eruption of seborrheic keratoses with pruritus as a manifestation of internal malignancy (Ronchese, 1965).

Seborrheic keratoses are usually seen on the face, neck, and thorax and may be seen at times on the hands and arms. Ordinarily, the diagnosis of seborrheic keratosis is reasonably simple for the experienced physician. In the differential diagnosis, pigmented basal

cell epithelioma, melanoma, and pigmented nevus must be considered. In the relatively flat type of seborrheic keratosis, senile lentigo and malignant melanoma in situ must also be ruled out. When the lesion shows no play of colors, is not translucent, and does not have telangiectasis on the surface, basal cell epithelioma and malignant melanoma are less likely diagnoses. Surface pits and skin line markings, as well as a verrucous surface, favor the diagnosis of seborrheic keratosis. The differentiation of flat seborrheic keratosis from senile lentigo may be difficult. At times only a small biopsy provides the answer. Deeply pigmented seborrheic keratoses have been widely excised erroneously because the clinical diagnosis of malignant melanoma had been made.

Pathology. Acanthosis, papillomatosis, and hyperkeratosis are common to all types of seborrheic keratoses. The base of the lesion does not dip below the epidermal line of the adjacent skin (Lever, 1967). The keratosis itself is made up of basal-like cells with a relatively large nucleus. Sanderson (1968a) believed that seborrheic keratoses develop because of local arrest in maturation of keratinocytes. Melanocytes are found in the epidermal-dermal line and also in the upper layers. Melanin is discharged into the tumor (Sanderson, 1968a).

Occasionally a seborrheic keratosis that has been irritated produces a histopathologic

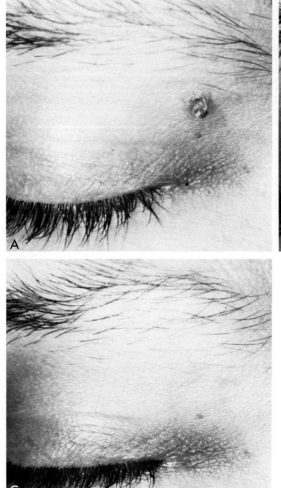

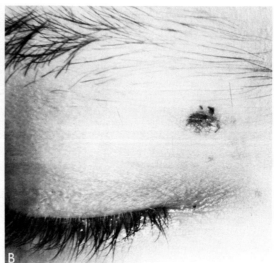

Figure 73–9. Seborrheic keratosis. *A,* Before treatment by curettage and light electrodesiccation. *B,* Immediately after treatment. *C,* Appearance several months later.

picture that may suggest a squamous cell carcinoma. However, the presence of pseudo–horn cysts, the general structure, and the history aid in the differentiation of an irritated seborrheic keratosis from squamous cell carcinoma (Lever, 1967).

Therapy. Seborrheic keratosis may be scalpel shaved to the base for biopsy, when indicated, followed by sharp curettage and light electrodesiccation (Figs. 73–9, 73–10). Simple currettage also suffices for most lesions. When multiple elevated small lesions are present, 50 per cent trichloroacetic acid may be applied at intervals of three weeks until the lesions have disappeared. Cryotherapy is also effective (Zacarian, 1969).

RHINOPHYMA

Rhinophyma is seen relatively infrequently in dermatologic practice (see also Chap. 37). The cause of this gradual enlargement of the nose, and at times the adjacent cheek tissues, often associated with acne rosacea, is not known. However, the disorder may result in considerable hypertrophy of the nasal skin, causing emotional distress to the patient. There may be an increase in the number and size of sebaceous glands, accompanied by an increase in the amount of dermal collagen. Dilatation of blood vessels and an inflammatory infiltrate may also be seen (Lever, 1967; Rook, 1968).

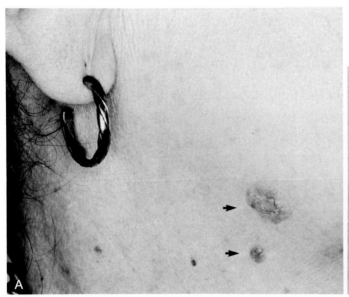

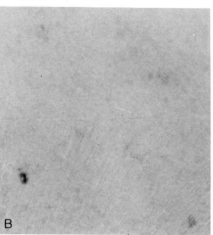

Figure 73–10. *A*, Two seborrheic keratoses. *B*, Five months after treatment by curettage alone. Note the absence of scarring (close-up view).

Biterminal electrocutting spark gap currents provide a simple and relatively bloodless method of electroshaving and electrocutting the excess tissue down to a reasonably acceptable and cosmetically agreeable contour. This can be done in the office under a combination of local infiltration and nerve block anesthesia.

The beginner is advised to proceed slowly with this type of sculpting. He should pause frequently in the course of treatment to have the patient sit up so that both sides of the

nose can be observed as tissue removal proceeds (Figs. 73–11 to 73–13).

The author prefers to use a small wire loop electrode and the biterminal current generated by a spark gap apparatus. This technique provides some degree of tissue coagulation and hemostasis, the degree dependent on the speed at which the wire loop (or other active electrode) is drawn through or over the skin (the more slowly, the greater is the electrocoagulation and hemostatic effect).

EPIDERMAL AND PILAR CYSTS (SEBACEOUS CYST, WEN, ATHEROMA, STEATOMA)

These common benign tumors are found on the scalp, ears, retroauricular areas, scrotum, face, and thorax. Epidermal cysts of the inclusion type are occasionally found on the hands and feet. Varying from a few millimeters to several centimeters in size, these lesions are subcutaneous in location, are sometimes marked by a dilated pore with or without a comedo, and are usually attached at some point to the overlying skin. They usually are freely movable unless episodes of inflammation, infection, or leakage have caused development of a surrounding fibrous tissue reaction.

Etiology. Beyond a familial tendency toward the development of scalp pilar cysts and a history of trauma in epidermal inclusion

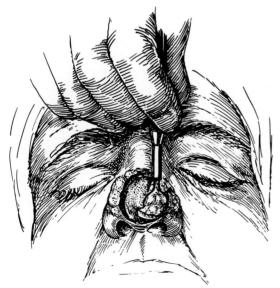

Figure 73–11. Biterminal electrocutting current for removal of rhinophymatous tissue.

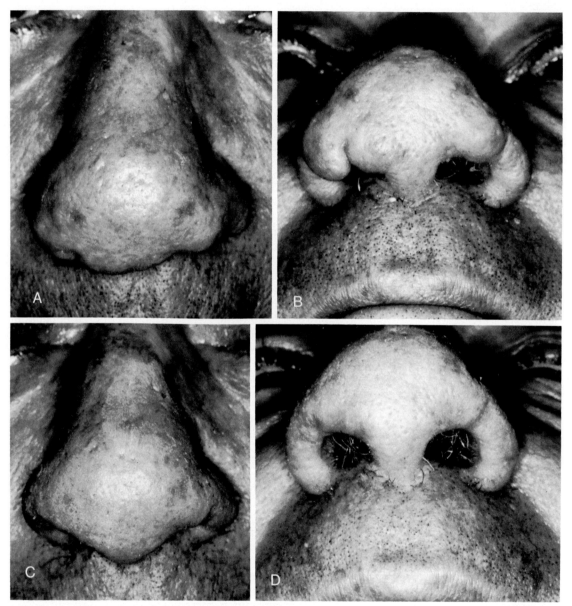

Figure 73–12. *A,* Rhinophyma involvement of the ala and tip of the nose and the nares. *B,* Basilar view. *C,* Appearance five weeks after treatment by biterminal electrocutting current. *D,* Postoperative basilar view.

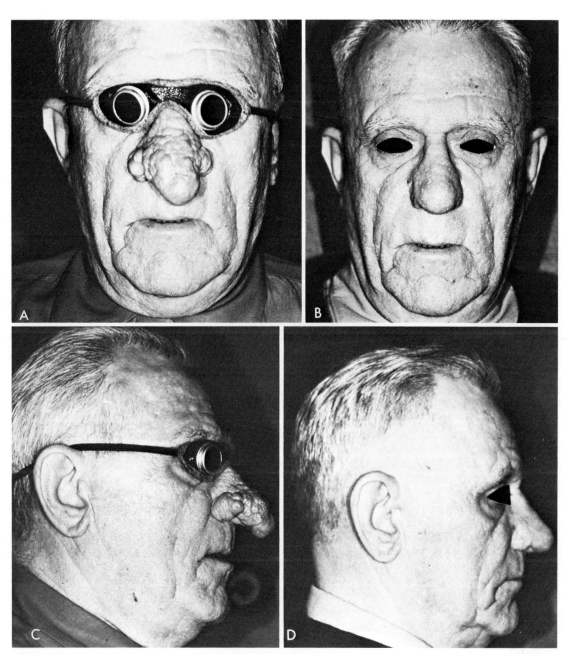

Figure 73–13. Patient with rhinophyma. *A, C,* Appearance before electrocutting current treatment. *B, D,* Posttreatment appearance. (From Niedelman, M. L.: Rhinophyma—treatment by electroshaving. Arch. Dermatol., *70*:91, 1954. Copyright 1954, American Medical Association.)

cysts of the palms and soles, little is known about the cause of these lesions. Sanderson (1968a) suggested that "sebaceous cyst" be used as a generic term until the histologic diagnosis is known. Lever (1967) noted that differentiation in a pilar cyst is "toward" hair keratin and not toward sebaceous material.

The cysts are found chiefly in adults, but children are not infrequently seen with epidermal cysts of the face. Elderly individuals may come for treatment of large scalp cysts of many years' duration.

Pathology. Epidermal cysts show the cellular layers of the epidermis with formation of keratinous material arranged in layers. Young cysts show the characteristic epidermal layers. Old cysts become thinned out, reducing the number of visible layers (Lever, 1967). When rupture of the wall takes place, a foreign body reaction with foreign body giant cells is noted. Occasionally a pseudocarcinomatous picture develops that, as emphasized by Raab and Steigleder (1961), simulates a squamous cell carcinoma. Possibly this phenomenon accounts for some of the earlier reports of malignant degeneration in the epidermal cysts. In the author's experience, it must be an exceedingly rare occurrence. Pilar, tricholemmal, and sebaceous cysts have neither a granular layer nor intercellular bridges in the epithelium that lines them (Lever, 1967; Rook, 1968). The contents of the cysts are amorphous, often showing calcium. The cysts also rupture, with ensuing foreign body reaction. According to Sanderson (1968a), the cells of the cyst walls resemble the root sheath cells of anagen or telogen hairs.

Treatment. There are several therapeutic methods employed by dermatologists. When the cyst is inflamed, it is best to incise and drain the lesion. Following this, a small cotton-tipped applicator made with a toothpick or the broken fine end of a wooden applicator stick is dipped in liquefied phenol, and the excess phenol is removed on the mouth of the bottle. The interior of the cyst cavity is swabbed with the phenol-dipped applicator. An alcohol swab neutralizes the phenol on the skin surface. This often constitutes sufficient treatment. If any sac remnants remain, the residuum is excised at a later date when the inflammation has subsided.

If the cyst is on the face and has not been previously inflamed, a No. 11 blade is used to make a 2 to 3 mm incision in the skin line over the thinnest portion of the skin overlying the cyst. A 2 mm biopsy punch (Lieblich, Geronemus, and Gibbs, 1982) may also be used (Fig. 73–14). Manual expression of the contents frequently results in the extrusion of the sac wall in the opening. If this does not occur, the curettes (Fig. 73–14C) may be used to engage the interior surface of the wall of the cyst and bring it to the surface. After grasping the wall with a small hemostat, the physician can roll it back on its long axis; the entire cyst wall may be teased out through the small incision, leaving little if any scarring (Fig. 73–14G).

If this technique is not possible, conventional excision may be performed at a later date. Depending on the amount of redundant skin, the fusiform excision, including the central pore when present, is extended to a few millimeters beyond the largest diameter of the cyst. The previously marked excision line is scored lightly with the scalpel. Beyond the cyst the excision is carried down to the subcutaneous fat. At this point the skin hook retracts the skin margin away from the cyst wall, and small curved scissors are used to find the cleavage plane and sever the overlying scored skin without rupturing the sac wall. The skin hook is used as a retractor holding the lateral skin surface away from the cyst while dissection continues. Following the removal of the cysts, the wound is closed with appropriate sutures.

MILIA

These lesions are seen not uncommonly after dermabrasion of the face and also occur without known antecedent trauma. They are observed on the face, below the eyes, and elsewhere on the body after certain blistering diseases such as pemphigus and epidermolysis bullosa. They are firm, white, papular lesions 1 to 2 mm in diameter. Their diagnosis ordinarily poses no problem.

According to Sanderson (1968b) and Love and Montgomery (1943), these lesions may arise following trauma to sweat or pilosebaceous ductal structures. Epstein and Kligman (1956) viewed some milia as benign keratinizing tumors.

Treatment of these lesions is by simple incision using the point of a No. 11 blade. A comedo extractor is used to extrude the milium contents.

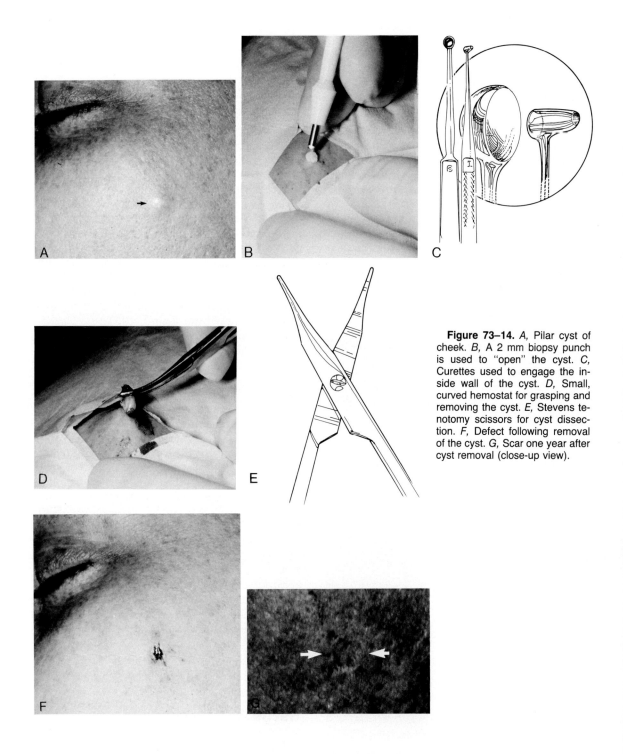

Figure 73–14. *A,* Pilar cyst of cheek. *B,* A 2 mm biopsy punch is used to "open" the cyst. *C,* Curettes used to engage the inside wall of the cyst. *D,* Small, curved hemostat for grasping and removing the cyst. *E,* Stevens tenotomy scissors for cyst dissection. *F,* Defect following removal of the cyst. *G,* Scar one year after cyst removal (close-up view).

EPIDERMAL APPENDAGE TUMORS

Sebaceous Hyperplasia

Sebaceous hyperplasia (senile sebaceous nevi) consists of a white to skin-colored tumor, 2 to 10 mm in size and slightly elevated above the skin with a noticeable central depression. The lesions are located on the face, especially on the forehead, in middle-aged or older individuals. When multiple lesions are seen, little difficulty is encountered in making the diagnosis. Single lesions, unless studied carefully, may at times be confused with basal cell epitheliomas (Fig. 73–15).

According to Lever (1967), these lesions consist of mature sebaceous glands grouped around one central duct or multiple ducts in larger lesions.

Treatment consists of eradication by electrosurgery and curettage, cryosurgery, or simple excision. Superficial treatment by light electrosurgery or chemical application results in persistence of the lesion.

Nevus Verrucosus (Nevus Unius Lateris)

This lesion, seen at birth or shortly after birth, consists of skin-colored to brownish, slightly elevated, wartlike patches on the face, scalp, neck, thorax, and extremities (Fig. 73–16). It occurs with equal frequency in both sexes (Haber, 1955). The lesions vary in magnitude from a small plaque on the scalp or a linear arrangement of wartlike papules to a generalized systematized nevus affecting much of the body surface. In the latter case, lesions consisting of whorls and swirls may be seen. Rook (1968) noted that developmental defects may be seen in association with these lesions. Basal cell epithelioma may arise in the localized variety, possibly with increased frequency in lesions arching over the ear (Litzow and Engel, 1961).

Pathology. The localized variety shows hyperkeratosis, papillomatosis, and elongation of the rete ridges (Lever, 1967). At times, apocrine glands and sebaceous glands may be found in this lesion (Lever, 1967). The presence of sebaceous and apocrine glands may account for the enlargement of these lesions at puberty.

The systematized form of nevus verrucosus shows hyperkeratosis, increase in the granular layer of the epidermis, and a vacuolization or ballooning of cells in the midepidermis (Lever, 1967). At times, coalescing of the vacuoles forms small, cavity-like structures.

The isolated verrucous nevi occasionally cause difficulty by pubertal enlargement and symptomatology of an irritative nature, depending on the location of the nevus.

Treatment. Total excision remains the best method of treatment. When small lesions are treated by thorough curettage and electrosurgery, recurrence of the lesions is not infrequent. Cryosurgery may also prove useful for some lesions (Zacarian, 1969).

Nevus Sebaceus

This is a benign epidermal appendage tumor tending toward sebaceous differentiation (Lever, 1967). Seen most frequently on the

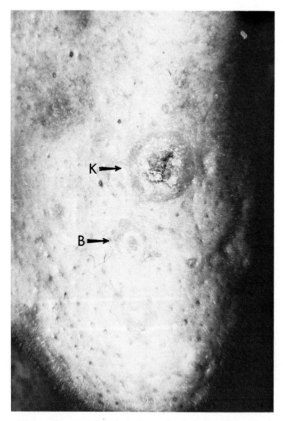

Figure 73–15. Multiple lesions of sebaceous hyperplasia of the nasal skin showing clinical resemblance to basal cell epithelioma *(B)* and keratoacanthoma *(K)*.

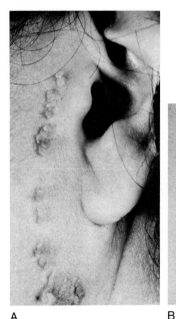

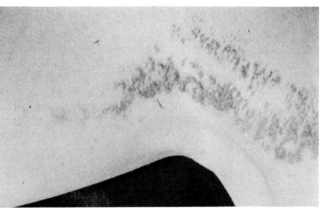

Figure 73–16. Nevus verrucosus. *A,* Of the preauricular area. *B,* Of the extremity. [Photographs *A* and *B* used by permission of New York University School of Medicine (Department of Dermatology).]

A   B

scalp, it also appears on the face (Fig. 73–17) and around the nose and mouth (Rook, 1968).

Developing at birth or shortly thereafter, it is skin colored to yellowish orange, with closely set papules making up a plaque that is slightly elevated, and in the scalp it may be partially or completely devoid of hair. Lacking the orange-yellow color, it is often confused in early life with nevus verrucosus.

Mehregan and Pinkus (1965) noted small, underdeveloped sebaceous glands and hair follicles without hair in the nevus sebaceus lesions of younger individuals, sometimes with a rapid increase in size at puberty because of endocrine effects. The sebaceous glands become more well developed; the hair follicles show hairs occasionally, and the apocrine glands become active. The same authors noted increased vascularity and proliferation of the fibrous tissue in the dermis. They also pointed out that a number of associated tumors may be seen with this lesion, including syringocystadenoma papilliferum, sebaceous epithelioma, apocrine cystoadenomas, infundibulomas, and basal cell epitheliomas. According to Rook (1968), published statistics range from a 10 to a 50 per cent incidence of basal cell epithelioma development, but Lever (1967), citing several authors, reported a 15 to 20 per cent incidence. Wilson, Jones,

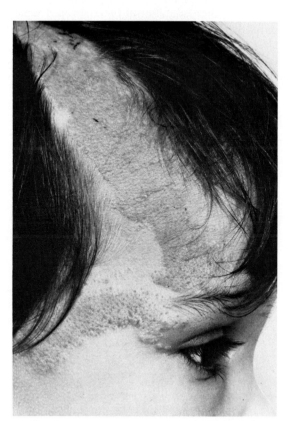

Figure 73–17. Nevus sebaceus. [Used by permission of New York University School of Medicine (Skin and Cancer Unit).]

and Heyl (1970) showed a 6.5 per cent incidence in 140 nevi. They also noted that squamous cell epithelioma may develop from nevus sebaceus but that this is a rare occurrence. The clinical picture changes from the slightly elevated plaque to a more papillomatous, verrucous, enlarged, and thickened lesion that may later undergo ulceration and crusting, depending on whether any of the associated tumors develop within it.

Surgical excision is the treatment of choice.

Pilomatrixoma (Benign Calcifying Epithelioma of Malherbe)

Pilomatrixoma should be considered in the differential diagnosis of an epidermal cyst and is a relatively uncommon tumor. Located chiefly on the head, neck, and upper extremities and occasionally on the lower extremities, it occurs usually as a solitary subcutaneous tumor attached to the skin surface with occasional episodes of tenderness and inflammation. Diagnosis should be suspected when palpation of an apparent epidermal cyst discloses an angular, firm lesion in the dermis.

Pathology. The tumor consists of cells that stain intensely basophilic at the periphery and eosinophilic nearer the center (Sanderson, 1968b). Lever (1967) noted that the basophilic cells show little cytoplasm and have indistinct cell boundaries. In older lesions there are fewer basophilic cells, and shadow cells predominate, these being cells with eosinophilic cytoplasm and absent or "shadow" areas in which the nuclei were formerly located. On the basis of histochemical and electron microscopic studies, evidence indicates that these lesions probably represent tumors differentiating toward hair (Hashimoto, Nelson, and Lever, 1966).

Treatment is by surgical excision. During dissection of the lesion, a friable, capsule-like structure is noted surrounding the tumor material. Cornification and calcification may be encountered.

SWEAT GLAND TUMORS

These are divided into two categories: those arising from eccrine glands and those arising from apocrine glands. While the entire group of lesions is uncommon in clinical practice, these lesions are sometimes seen, and some familiarity with them helps the physician in making a diagnosis.

Syringoma

One type of sweat gland tumor that may be seen is a syringoma (Fig. 73–18). The papular or cystlike lesions are found commonly on the lower eyelids, face, neck, and chest and may be white, yellowish, or skin colored. The lesions may have an abrupt onset at puberty or later, women being affected more than men.

By light and electron microscopy, the tumors show cystic duct structure with microvilli. Biochemical reactions indicate similarities to eccrine rather than apocrine structures (Mustalko, 1959; Winkelmann and Mueller, 1964; Hashimoto, Gross, and Lever, 1966). Colloidal material is present in the lumina of the ducts. "Comma-like" configurations of the ducts suggest a "tadpole"-like appearance to histopathologists. Frequently there is a dense stromal reaction.

Treatment is by electrosurgical destruction or excision.

Eccrine Poroma

Occurring chiefly on the palms and soles as a pink pedunculated tumor with a hyperkeratotic periphery, the tumor is about 1 cm in size or smaller and may resemble a pyogenic granuloma without an eroded surface (Fig. 73–19). Pyogenic granuloma usually has a

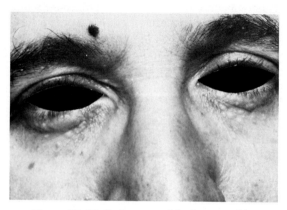

Figure 73–18. Syringomas of the lower eyelids.

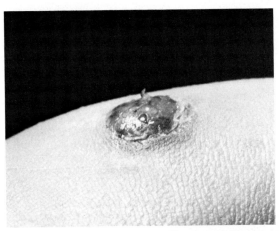

Figure 73–19. Eccrine poroma. (Courtesy of Dermatology in Practice, *3*, No. 7, 1970, and Dr. Arthur Hyman.)

history of a much shorter growth period and frequently is crusted, with episodes of bleeding and ulceration.

On histologic study, cuboidal cells may be seen occupying the epidermis, sometimes showing ductlike structures. Histochemical reactions and electron microscopy relate these cells to eccrine structures and embryonic intraepidermal sweat ducts (Hashimoto and Lever, 1964). This benign tumor is best treated by surgical excision.

Hidradenoma Papilliferum

Hidradenoma papilliferum is an uncommon benign tumor of the anogenital area of adult females and occurs most frequently on the labia majora, varying in size to 4 cm. Mobile and rounded to palpation, it may be cystlike in consistency.

According to Lever (1967), it is an adenoma with apocrine characteristics. Surgical excision is indicated.

Cylindroma (Turban Tumor)

This relatively uncommon tumor (Fig. 73–20) occurs in solitary and multiple forms. It is of sweat gland origin, and despite conflicting studies it is believed to be of the apocrine type and most often involves the scalp. Females are affected more than males, and it has its onset in adult life. The multiple type, according to Sanderson (1968b), is inherited as an autosomal dominant trait. The involvement over the scalp may rarely be so extensive as to suggest a turban.

The histopathology is distinctive, with islands of epithelial cells in a hyalin sheath. Two cell types are noted: undifferentiated cells with dark nuclei, and cells with large pale nuclei showing a tendency to differentiate toward ductal or secretory cells (Lever, 1967). There have been rare reports of malignancy arising from cylindromas.

Extensive surgical excision may be necessary for patients who show widespread involvement with this type of tumor.

Trichoepithelioma

This is an uncommon benign tumor, pinkish to flesh colored, differentiating toward

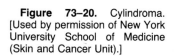

Figure 73–20. Cylindroma. [Used by permission of New York University School of Medicine (Skin and Cancer Unit).]

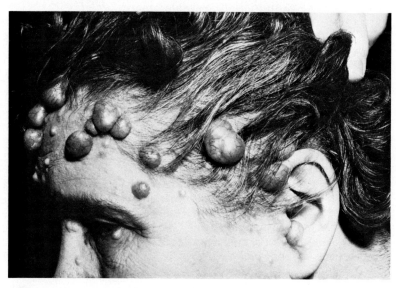

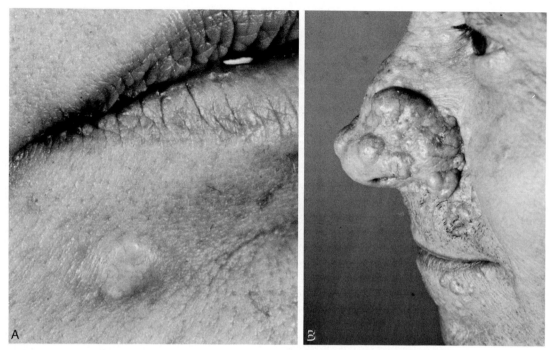

Figure 73–21. *A,* Solitary trichoepithelioma of the lower lip. *B,* Multiple trichoepitheliomas of the face. [Photographs *A* and *B* used by permission of New York University School of Medicine (Department of Dermatology).]

hair structures (Lever, 1967; Rook, 1968) and occurring as multiple symmetric lesions on the midareas of the face, particularly the nasolabial folds, eyelids, and forehead (Fig. 73–21). Occasional lesions show a bluish discoloration and appear cystic. It tends to be familial in incidence. Solitary lesions occasionally occur. The lesions tend to be under 1 cm in size, and occasionally one sees a transition of the lesions into basal cell epithelioma.

Microscopic examination reveals many horn cysts, occasional calcification, and melanin granules in and around the cysts. The cells resemble those of basal cell epithelioma in a fibrous stroma with peripheral palisading in evidence; incompletely developed hair shafts and papillae may also be seen. Occasionally, when horn cysts are few, clinical information is necessary to differentiate this lesion from basal cell epithelioma (Lever, 1967).

On occasion, ulceration and increase in size of a trichoepitheliomatous lesion may herald the presence of basal cell epithelioma (Rook, 1968). However, in their series of 109 lesions in 50 patients, Gray and Helwig (1963) did not note this type of transformation despite the presence of spontaneous ulceration.

Treatment of multiple lesions with extensive involvement is difficult and requires palliative, locally destructive measures, such as liquid nitrogen therapy, dermabrasion, or application of full strength trichloroacetic acid to individual lesions. With any treatment short of complete surgical removal, one can expect the lesions to persist and enlarge.

DERMATOFIBROMA, (HISTIOCYTOMA, NODULUS CUTANEUS, SCLEROSING ANGIOMA, LIPOIDAL HISTIOCYTOMA, FIBROMA SIMPLEX, FIBROMA DURUM)

Dermatofibroma is a benign dermal tumor that occurs in solitary or multiple fashion, chiefly on the legs but also on the thorax and upper extremities. It varies in appearance from a depressed pigmented area to a fairly large (1.5 to 2.0 cm) lesion that may be firm, pink, skin colored, or purplish brown (Fig. 73–22). The lesion is slightly elevated to almost sessile in contour.

Beare (1968) believed that these lesions

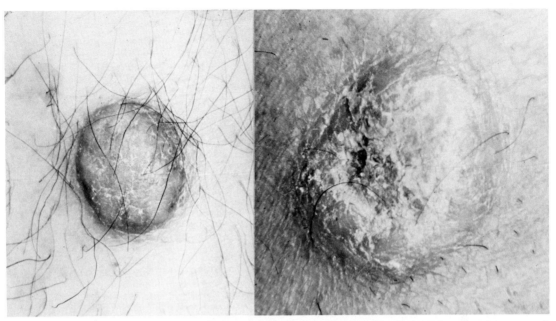

Figure 73–22. Two examples of dermatofibroma; the right lesion shows hyperkeratotic and scaling changes on the surface.

represent a reactive overgrowth of reticulo-endothelial, vascular, and fibrocytic cells.

The histologic picture varies according to the age of the lesion; younger lesions may show more vascularity, older lesions more fibrosis. Spindle-shaped cells abound, while some lesions show more fibroblasts and others more histiocytic reaction. In the latter, Lever (1967) noted that the histiocytes may contain lipid or hemosiderin. The overlying epidermis is acanthotic in most cases. Although overlying basal cell epithelioma has been reported (Yannowitz and Goldstein, 1964), Lever (1967) felt that the epidermis is stimulated to produce immature hair structures or "even primary epithelial germ formations" resembling basal cell epithelioma without having the biologic potential of epitheliomas.

Differential clinical diagnosis depends to a certain extent on the clinical experience of the observer and the number of variants of the lesion he has seen. Other diagnoses that must be considered are nevus cell nevus, dermatofibrosarcoma, and xanthoma.

Treatment is by simple surgical excision. Horizontal shave-type biopsies ordinarily fail to leave a scar more cosmetically acceptable than the original lesion. The use of liquid nitrogen to treat these lesions has been evaluated (Torre, 1970). Zacarian (1969) reported the eradication of the lesion with minimal residual scarring in several patients treated with liquid nitrogen.

SKIN TAGS (ACROCHORDON, SOFT FIBROMA, CUTANEOUS TAGS)

Skin tags are small, benign skin tumors (Fig. 73–23) that are seen most often on the sides of the neck, axillae, and groin and occasionally on the thorax. They vary in diameter from 1 to 6 mm and are pedunculated, soft in consistency, and usually skin colored although occasionally brownish.

The differential diagnosis includes nevus cell nevus and early seborrheic keratosis. The lesions are also found in women during pregnancy and later in life.

Histopathologic examination shows a connective tissue core with a thinned out overlying epidermis. Increased pigmentation may be seen.

Treatment is by several modalities. Larger lesions are easily grasped with a fine-toothed forceps and excised with a pair of scissors at the base. Light electrodesiccation (Fig. 73–24) using an epilating needle and epilat-

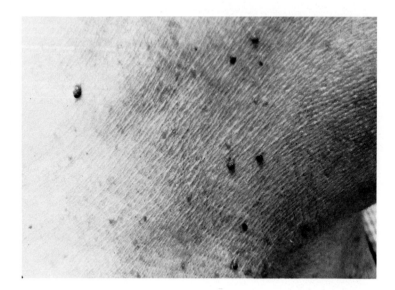

Figure 73–23. Skin tags.

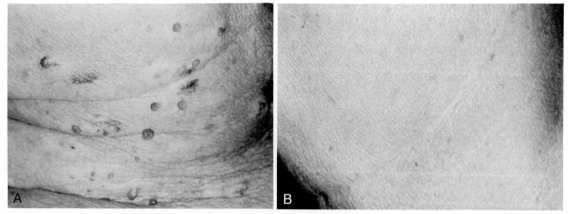

Figure 73–24. *A,* Skin tags (fibroepithelial polyps) of the neck. *B,* Appearance three months after treatment by electrodesiccation with a current of low intensity.

ing current of the monopolar electrodesiccating spark is effective, but patients should be cautioned that they may develop new lesions. A minor complication may be the replacement of skin tags with a "white spot" in individuals with a dark complexion.

MUCOUS CYSTS

A mucous cyst is a benign tumor (Fig. 73–25) formed by the extravasation of saliva or mucous following rupture of the salivary duct (Lattanand, Johnson, and Graham, 1970). It is located chiefly on the lower lip or occasionally on the tongue. The size varies from a few millimeters to 2 cm.

Pathology. The cysts are lined not by epithelium but rather by granulation tissue with histiocytes and fibroblasts (Lever, 1967). Those cysts present for a longer time show fibrous tissue in their walls.

Treatment. Simple surgical excision usually suffices. Electrodesiccation of the cysts and their contents is usually also curative.

MYXOID CYSTS (MUCOUS CYST OF FINGERS OR TOES)

A myxoid cyst is a small lesion usually located in or about the distal phalanx of the finger or the toe, which may, when involving the cuticle or proximal nail fold area, cause a canal-like dystrophy of the adjacent nail. It is often located near the joint, and when punctured exudes a heavy, clear, viscous fluid.

Etiology. Johnson, Graham, and Helwig (1965) found no correlation between the cystic

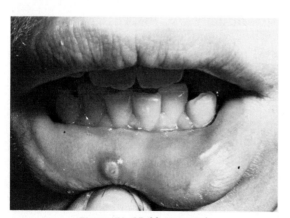

Figure 73–25. Mucous cyst.

areas and any underlying structures. On the other hand, Eliassow and Frank (1942) demonstrated that contrast media injected into such a cyst made its way into the adjacent joint cavity. Lever (1967) postulated that cysts are formed from fibroblastic production of hyaluronic acid associated with deficiency of local collagen formation. A high incidence of osteoarthritis was demonstrated in these patients by roentgenograhpic study of the affected distal phalanx (Constant and coworkers, 1969).

Pathology. Mucous material with an increase in the number of fibroblasts is seen. The mucin is made up chiefly of hyaluronic acid. Early cleftlike structures give way to typical cyst formation in a sub- or intraepidermal location (Lever, 1967).

Treatment. Despite presumably adequate excision, recurrences are well known unless some of the underlying bony exostosis is removed. Injection of triamcinolone acetonide solution, carefully done once or twice, merits a trial.

VASCULAR TUMORS (LESIONS)

During childhood, the more common vascular tumors are the hemangiomas and the pyogenic granulomas. Later in life the angioma (venous lakes) is seen, a thin-walled lesion occurring on the scrotum, lips, face, and ears. On the thorax of some individuals of both sexes, small red capillary ectasias called senile angiomas are often seen (Fig. 73–26). However, these ruby spots or cherry angiomas are seen in a significant number of young people (Keller, 1957; Bean, 1958), and the term "senile angioma" should be discarded.

The hemangiomas of infancy consist of nevus flammeus and the superficial and cavernous hemangiomas.

These lesions are also discussed in Chapter 66.

Nevus Flammeus (Port-Wine Stain)

The nevus flammeus (port-wine stain) may be found over the occiput or on the face, thorax, and extremities (Fig. 73–27). Occasionally, the lesions may be associated with other anomalous blood vessels in the Sturge-

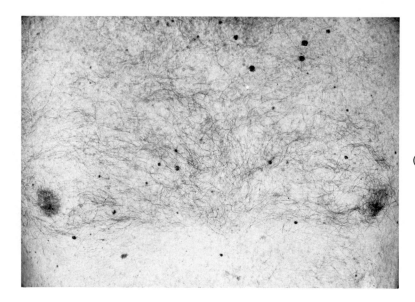

Figure 73–26. Cherry angioma ("senile" angioma) of the thorax.

Weber and Klippel-Trenaunay-Weber syndromes. The former is a port-wine stain in the distribution of the trigeminal innervation of the face. However, the vascular lesion may also involve additional areas of the head, neck, and torso. There may be associated contralateral hemiplegia and focal and jacksonian epilepsy due to angioma of the leptomeninges. Upon radiographic examination, calcification in the meningeal angioma may be seen in older children. Mental retardation is often seen. Various degrees of ophthalmic involvement include buphthalmos, megalocornea, and hydrophthalmos. Angiomatosis may be present in the various tissues of the eye.

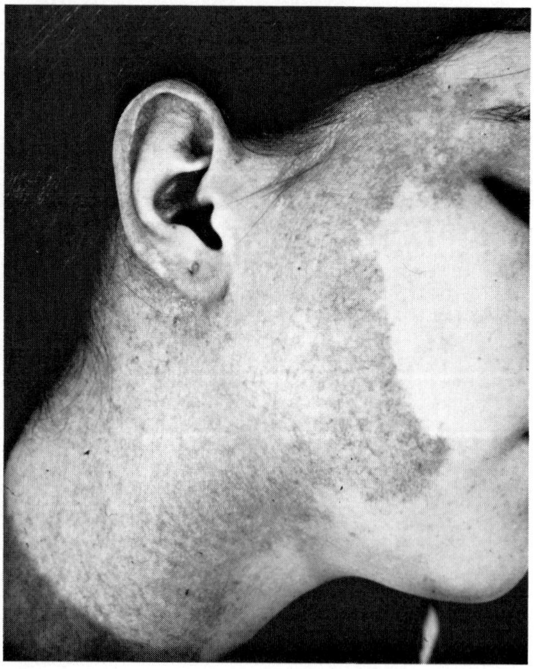

Bean (1958) summarized the history of these syndromes and suggested that various eponyms be discarded in favor of the term "congenital dysplastic angiopathies of the skin and underlying tissues."

The Klippel-Trenaunay-Weber syndrome (hemangiectatic hypertrophy) may show capillary hemangiomas and cavernous hemangiomas and is associated with deeper venous varicosities, arteriovenous fistulas, increased skin temperature, and perspiration of the affected extremity. Osteohypertrophy may result in gross deformity of the affected extremity (Van der Harst, 1951).

The histopathology of nevus flammeus consists of dilatation of the capillaries in the dermis. These changes and the capillary ectasias are usually seen later in the child's life (Lever, 1967).

Capillary Hemangiomas (Strawberry Marks or Superficial Hemangiomas)

Figure 73–27. Nevus flammeus (port-wine stain) of the face.

These may be found on any part of the thorax, neck, head, or extremities. The le-

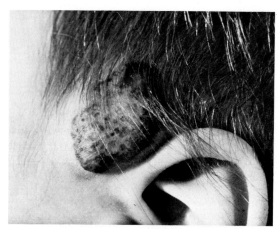

Figure 73–28. Strawberry hemangioma of the temporal area.

sions consist of a bright red or bluish red, elevated, soft, compressible tumor in a plaque type of configuration (Fig. 73–28). Later in life, cutaneous angiomas may be seen in association with spinal cord arteriovenous anomalies (Doppman and associates, 1969). The childhood lesion arises shortly after birth and may increase in size for six to 12 months (Bowers, Graham, and Tomlinson, 1960) or for a longer period in a lesser number of cases. Most of the lesions gradually undergo spontaneous involution over the next two to seven years, ordinarily leaving little or no scarring. In a pediatric practice survey of 1735 children, Jacobs (1957) found a hemangioma incidence of 10.1 per cent up to year 1, dropping to 1.5 per cent in children over 5 years of age. Extensive cases may show persistent telangiectasis and superficial atrophic scarring.

Exceptions to spontaneous resolution are lesions involving the mucous membranes. These lesions may persist into adult life.

Complications include ulceration, tissue necrosis, secondary infection, early hemorrhage, and scarring.

Ulceration is more common around the mouth and in the anogenital area, with problems secondary to the increase in hemangioma bulk occurring in these locations. Obstruction of vision, if sufficiently severe during the first six months, may result in permanent visual defects of the affected eye (Norden and Maumenee, 1968), and it is wise to have ophthalmologic consultation for hemangiomas that may be sufficiently large to infringe on the field of vision.

Selected lesions require excisional surgery. These include bulky and persistent, painful, ulcerated lesions of the periorificial or other areas that do not respond to conservative treatment. Later, plastic surgical correction for deformity secondary to involuted and/or previously ulcerated hemangiomas may be indicated.

Cavernous Hemangioma

These deeper hemangiomas may occur with or without overlying capillary lesions, being circumscribed masses located in the subcutaneous tissue (Fig. 73–29). They may be seen by themselves in children but may also be associated with two syndromes: Maffucci's syndrome and the blue rubber bleb nevus syndrome.

Maffucci's syndrome, or dyschondroplasia with cavernous hemangioma, shows gross defects in ossification resulting in severe deformities. Chondrosarcoma and other neoplasms have been observed and death is believed to be the result of multiple genetic defects (Bean, 1958).

In the blue rubber bleb nevus syndrome, soft compressible hemangiomas may be found on the trunk and extremities. In addition, similar lesions may be found in a submucous

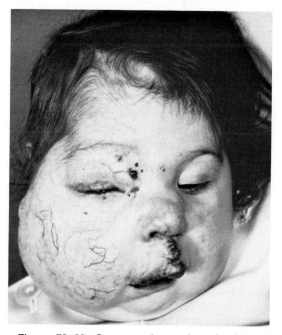

Figure 73–29. Cavernous hemangioma involving the right side of the face.

location in the gastrointestinal tract (Bean, 1958). The number of lesions varies from a few to many, and the size of the individual lesions may reach 4 cm. Their presence in other organs has also been noted. Bleeding may be a problem.

Therapy must be individualized for each case. Recent ideas sharply contrast with the older aggressive therapeutic approach involving cryotherapy, radiation, and injection of sclerosing solutions. At present, the recommendation is that watchful waiting is most desirable if the physician can secure the cooperation of the family of the affected individual (see Chap. 66).

Kasabach-Merritt Syndrome (Hemangioma with Thrombocytopenia)

This is an uncommon type of hemangioma of the skin associated with thrombocytopenia, purpura, anemia, bleeding, and coagulation defects. According to Bureau and associates (1967), it occurs in infants from birth to 4 months of age, and undergoes rapid evolution to a large subcutaneous hemangioma of the involved area. The lesion frequently appears to be inflammatory and is associated with hemorrhage both within the hemangioma and at distant sites. Sequestration of platelets within the lesion has been demonstrated. Radiation therapy or the administration of systemic corticosteroids may be required, and involution of the hemangioma is associated with elevation of the platelet count.

PATHOLOGY OF HEMANGIOMAS

In cavernous hemangiomas, there are varying numbers of blood-filled spaces in the lower dermis and subcutaneous tissues. Endothelial cells line the spaces, and depending on the age of the lesions, increasing connective tissue stroma develops with fibrosis (Lever, 1967). The strawberry mark type of hemangioma shows endothelial cell proliferation during the period of active growth (Lever, 1967). Later during the period of regression, fibrosis takes place.

As evidenced by the scarcity of hemangiomas in the adult population, spontaneous resolution is the rule for most hemangiomas. Whether resolution is complete depends on the type and location. Hemangiomas involv-

ing the mucous membranes may persist into adult life. Fibrofatty remnants of fibrosed cavernous hemangiomas may be seen in older children, and telangiectatic vessels may be seen at the sites of strawberry hemangiomas. Capillary hemangiomas of the port-wine type persist into adult life.

A variant of hemangiomas is the so-called hyperkeratotic hemangioma (Imperial and Helwig, 1967). This entity is distinguished from angiokeratoma corporis circumscriptum and termed "verrucous hemangioma." The lesion persists into adult life and is often found in a linear arrangement on the extremities, interfering with the wearing of shoes. Excision, when feasible, is the treatment of choice.

Pyogenic Granuloma (Granuloma Telangiectaticum)

This is a rapidly developing vascular papular lesion that tends to bleed freely on slight trauma (Fig. 73–30).

The lesion appears as a rounded, red, often sessile papule with intact epidermis or with a crust. The tumor is variable in size, most lesions being under 1 cm in diameter. They are located commonly on the face, the thorax and the fingers. They grow to a certain size and tend to remain stationary. Occasionally, the lesion is seen on the mucosal surfaces. Histologic confirmation avoids the rare clinical confusion of this lesion with a malignant melanoma (Fig. 73–31).

Pathology. Microscopic examination shows many newly formed dilated capillaries. Endothelial proliferation with prominent endothelial cells is noted. The stroma is loose and rich in mucin. In older lesions, fibrosis is more prominent. The overall configuration is that of a pedunculated lesion covered by a flattened epidermis and surrounded at its base by a collarette of epidermis (Lever, 1967; Sanderson, 1968b).

Treatment. After a biopsy of the lesion is taken, the commonest dermatologic therapy involves sharp curettage and electrodesiccation; surgical excision is also an acceptable modality.

Complications. At times, hypertrophic scarring is seen following therapy on the upper portion of the chest. Sanderson (1968b) reported that after injudicious therapy, benign satellite lesions may develop with the

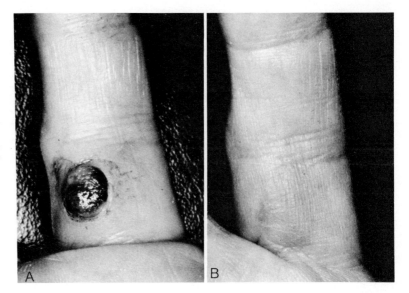

Figure 73–30. *A,* Pyogenic granuloma of the finger. *B,* One month after biopsy; treatment by curettage and electrodesiccation. Note the absence of scarring.

same histopathologic picture as in the original lesion. Recurrence of the lesion may also be seen after apparently adequate therapy.

Nevus Araneus (Spider Nevus or Spider Telangiectasis)

This is a lesion having a central blood vessel that is slightly elevated and from which fine dilated vessels radiate. It is found in children and adults, most frequently on the face; it may also be seen on the thorax and upper extremities. The lesion may be pulsatile. Such lesions may arise during pregnancy and in cirrhosis of the liver, suggesting a relationship to elevated estrogen levels. Following termination of pregnancy, all or some of the lesions may disappear, but they may recur with future pregnancies.

On microscopic examination a central arteriole is seen opening into a subepidermal-level ampulla. From this structure the vessels resembling venules radiate and divide into capillaries. Occasionally a glomus type of lesion is noted with a Sucquet-Hoyer–like structure, located just below the ampulla portion (Bean, 1958; Lever, 1967; Champion and Wilkinson, 1968).

Treatment. Fine electrodesiccation or an epilating current applied to the central vessel may be curative, but the recurrence rate is high. There is also a calculated risk of skin pitting. At times, excisional surgery may be required. Cryotherapy with liquid nitrogen, using a fine applicator for 15 seconds with moderate pressure, has also been useful in selected instances. Figure 73–32 illustrates treatment of telangiectasia by biterminal electrocoagulating current of low intensity. Laser therapy (see Chap. 75) is also effective.

Lymphangioma

Lymphangiomas are tumors consisting of dilated lymph channels lined with a single layer of endothelium. The size and clinical type vary according to the depth of involve-

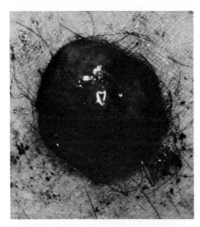

Figure 73–31. Eroded nodular malignant melanoma. Note the resemblance to pyogenic granuloma.

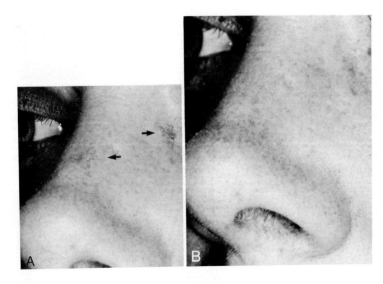

Figure 73–32. *A,* Telangiectasia of the nose. *B,* One month after treatment with biterminal electrocoagulating current of low intensity.

ment, vessel size, location, and so on. Therapy of such lesions warrants a surgical approach.

Glomus Tumor

These are single or multiple, pink to purple tumors, 0.1 to 2.0 cm in size (Fig. 73–33), consisting of glomus cells, vascular channels,

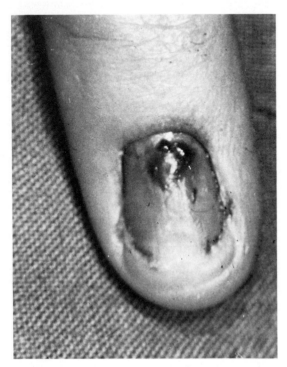

Figure 73–33. Glomus tumor in the nail bed. The fingernail has been removed.

and nonmyelinated nerve fibers. The multiple type of tumor appears to have an autosomal dominant inheritance and is more common in children (Rook, 1968). Single lesions are likely to be quite painful with the application of pressure or temperature change, and occur on the fingers, penis, ears, head, and neck. Multiple tumors are not ordinarily painful and clinically resemble hemangiomas. They may be located in any of the above locations or may be widely scattered over the integument. Neither type of lesion is particularly common.

Pathology. The solitary type is believed to be derived from the Sucquet-Hoyer canal of the skin glomus body. Smaller, more painful tumors are quite cellular with numerous glomus cells (Sanderson, 1968b). Vascular lumina lined by endothelium and surrounded by glomus cells are also present (Lever, 1967); multiple lesions show more dilated vascular channels surrounded by endothelial cells and fewer glomus cells than the solitary type. In both types nonmyelinated fibers traverse the tumor. The lesions are benign, and surgical excision is the treatment of choice. Recurrences may follow incomplete excision.

TUMORS OF NEURAL TISSUE

Granular Cell Myoblastoma

This is a tumor composed of cells with a granular cytoplasm. The lesions seen on the tongue and elsewhere appear as a firm tumor, sometimes without sharp borders. At times the tumor may be raised, papular, or sessile. It occurs most commonly in the tongue (Fig. 73–34) and has been reported in various internal organs. The tumor is uncommon, usually solitary, but may be found occasionally as multiple lesions (Cave, Kopf, and Kerdel-Vegas, 1955). It occurs in both children and adults.

Pathology. Originally this tumor was believed to be derived from striated muscle cells because of its close relation to such cells when found in the tongue. Histochemical studies by Alkek, Johnson, and Graham (1968) led these authors and others to believe that the tumor is derived from nerve sheath Schwann cells or fibrocytic or fibrohistiocytic cells. The histologic picture shows cells with pale cytoplasm and eosinophilic granules (Lever, 1967); small round and vesicular nuclei are noted (Sanderson, 1968b). Shear (1960) suggested that the lesion is reactive rather than neoplastic. Lever (1967) noted that pseudocarcinomatous hyperplasia seen overlying the lesions, particularly in the oral mucosa, may be confusing unless a sufficiently deep biopsy has included some of the tissue showing the typical granular cells.

Therapy. Excision, when complete, is curative. A rare metastasizing type of granular cell myoblastoma has been reported. It is called a malignant granular cell schwannoma and has two histopathologic patterns (Gamboa, 1955): in one type, a benign histopathologic appearance is noted in the primary and metastatic tissues, whereas in the second type, both primary and metastatic tissues are malignant in appearance. These variations are seen despite clinically malignant behavior in both types.

NEVOCELLULAR NEVI AND SELECTED PIGMENTED LESIONS

Freckles (Ephelides)

These pigmented lesions, which are commonly found on light-exposed surfaces, make their appearance early in life. They are believed to be due to an autosomal dominant gene (Brues, 1950). They darken in the summer and fade in the winter, and tend to be seen more often in blue-eyed individuals with fair skin and red or blond hair. Within the freckles, the melanosomes may be decreased in number but appear to resemble those melanosomes found in darker-skinned individuals (Breathnach and Wyllie, 1964). The melanosomes form melanin more rapidly upon stimulation by sunlight than do those of the surrounding skin. On light microscopy, an increase in the epidermal pigment is seen.

Treatment. Superficial chemical destructive methods, such as application of a 30 to 50 per cent solution of trichloroacetic acid, may be used. Cryodestructive techniques utilizing liquid nitrogen or carbon dioxide slush in a quantity sufficient to produce superficial desquamation may also be used as treatment. In a similar fashion, light dermabrasion may be employed. Results vary and may be compromised by subsequent sunlight exposure. It is wise to treat a small test area before undertaking the treatment of widespread lesions.

Lentigines

These are flat, pigmented lesions that are divided into two types—solar and simple. The solar lentigo is seen following sunlight damage on exposed areas of skin. The lesions may fuse with adjacent lentigines to form pigmented patches of several centimeters.

The simple lentigo is brown to black and occurs on any part of the body, including the mucous membranes. Usually it is less than 5 mm in size (Rook, 1979).

Both types retain their dark color during all the year. Freckles are lighter, often show

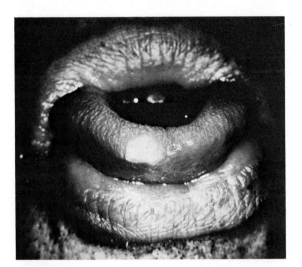

Figure 73–34. Granular cell myoblastoma of the tip of the tongue.

a mottled appearance (Maize and Ackerman, 1987) and tend to darken in the summer.

Simple lentigines may be seen as part of certain syndromes, e.g., Peutz-Jeghers (gastrointestinal polyposis). Microscopic examination of solar lentigines shows epidermal proliferation with different patterns in rete ridges; increased melanin, particularly in the basal layer; and solar damage in the underlying dermis (Maize and Ackerman, 1987).

Simple lentigines show hyperpigmentation, epidermal hyperplasia with increase in the numbers of melanocytes (benign), elongated rete ridges, and an increased number of melanocytes in the basal layer (Maize and Ackerman, 1987).

In the differential diagnosis, solar lentigines may resemble the superficial flat types of seborrheic keratosis. The latter tend to be more irregular in outline and to show slight hyperkeratosis on their surface. Hutchinson's melanotic freckle (malignant melanoma in situ) is usually more irregular in outline, shows a play of shades of brown and black, and tends to increase in size gradually over the years.

Solar lentigines may be treated by application of liquid nitrogen with a cotton-tipped applicator for periods of 10 to 15 seconds, with light pressure. Electrodesiccation with a fine epilating type of monopolar spark gap current may also be used.

Nevus Cell Nevus

Pigmented lesions of the skin cause much concern and are responsible for sharp differences of opinion between the various specialties. Despite much up-to-date work, old ideas persist regarding biopsy and treatment. Patients have different reasons for wanting treatment of nevi. Some are concerned about possible malignancy; other wish to have nevi removed for cosmetic reasons.

Since Masson's hypothesis (1926), there is fairly general acceptance of his idea that the cells from the neural crest of the embryo migrate to the skin surface and produce a number of different types of pigmented nevus cell nevi.

There are three major categories of nevus cell nevus: *junction, compound,* and *intradermal.* They take their names from the microscopic position that most nevus cells occupy in the skin.

While it is not always possible to distinguish clinically one type from another, some guidelines may be helpful. Lesions that are flat are likely to be a lentigo or a junctional nevus. Shaffer (1955) suggested certain clinical histopathologic correlations. Those that are slightly raised are likely to be compound nevi. Nevi with a central elevation and a peripherally pigmented base are likely to be junction nevi. Verrucoid pigmented nevi are junction nevi in about 75 per cent of cases, and sessile and dome-shaped lesions are intradermal nevi in the vast majority of cases. Pigmented papillomas are probably intradermal nevi.

Pathology. The junction nevus shows a preponderance of nevus cells singly and in nests occupying the lower portion of the epidermis. Some nevus cells extend downward into the dermis, and some are found in the upper adjacent portion of the dermis. Melanocytes are also found in the epidermis (Lever, 1967).

In the compound nevus, in addition to junctional activity, a considerable number of nevus cells are noted in the dermis.

In the intradermal type, most nevus cells are found within the cutis. However, Kopf and Andrade (1963) found that careful serial sectioning of intradermal nevi showed that in nearly all there was histologic evidence of junctional activity.

According to Lever (1967), although there is some potential for malignant transformation in junction nevi, it is small when only well-circumscribed nevus cells are found.

If malignant transformation is suspected, i.e., if there has been a recent change in pigmentation or size, inflammation, or bleeding, a conservative total excision biopsy should be performed if possible. If the lesion is too large for simple total excisional biopsy, a partial (incisional) biopsy is indicated, especially if definitive therapy will result in extensive surgery as for malignant melanoma.

Occasionally, hairy pigmented nevi show a sudden increase in size with erythema and the development of a pustule or abscess within or under the nevus. Patients complain of tenderness at the site of the nevus, and voice understandable fears about malignancy. This situation is usually due to a folliculitis of one of the hairs or inflammation in an underlying epidermal cyst (Duperrat, 1954; Haber, 1962; Freeman and Knox, 1962).

Treatment is conservative, consisting of warm compresses and topical and/or systemic antibiotics, but incision and drainage may be required. At a later date, conservative excision of the nevus and the underlying area of fibrotic reaction is desirable, although the author has treated such lesions by biopsy and electrodesiccation. The latter technique will be further discussed.

Therapy. Although fusiform surgical excision carefully performed with observation of the lines of minimal skin tension is an excellent method, dermatologists tend to reserve this treatment for selected lesions, making use of simpler methods for most pigmented papular nevi, particularly those on the face.

For suspicious lesions, those with a large amount of hair, and flat junction nevi, surgical excision appears best suited. For those lesions with a few hairs, epilation may be performed first. At a later date, with a No. 15 scalpel blade, the nevus is excised to a level slightly above the skin. The removed tissue is submitted for histopathologic examination. Following excision, an electrodesiccating spark of low intensity is applied to the remainder of the nevus until the base is leveled to the skin surface (Figs. 73–35 to 73–37). On occasion it is necessary to curette the electrodesiccated tissue for greater visibility and control of the level of removal of tissue.

Complications of this simple technique are few. Ordinarily, little or no visible scar is noted. In a small percentage of cases, pigment persists or returns to the site at a later date (Cox and Walton, 1965). Liquid nitrogen applied with a cotton-tipped applicator for 10 to 15 seconds with moderate pressure is helpful in blanching much if not all of this pigment; in rare instances, benign regrowth of the nevus will take place over a period of years, requiring further therapy.

This method of treatment is particularly suited to the management of multiple intradermal nevi of the face and nose.

Giant Pigmented Nevus or Bathing Trunk Nevus

This term is applied to a congenital pigmented nevus that may cover large areas of the skin surface. Later in childhood, these lesions become thickened, verrucous, and

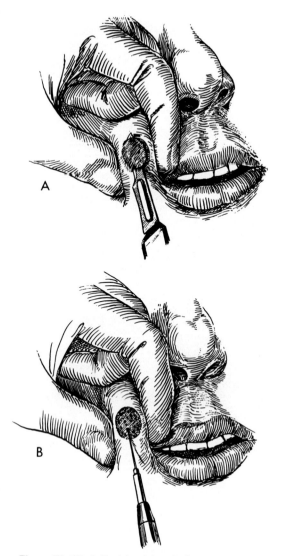

Figure 73–35. *A,* Excision (shave) of a nevus at its base. *B,* Electrodesiccation of the base of the nevus.

hairy. A small percentage may give rise to malignant melanoma (10 per cent in one series: Greeley, Middleton, and Curtin, 1965). Giant pigmented nevi may be associated with intracranial melanocytosis and other abnormalities such as spina bifida, meningocele (if the skin lesion is located over the vertebral column), other nevi, lipomas, and neurofibromatosis (Rook, 1968).

Pathology. According to Lever (1967), three components may be found in the giant pigmented nevus: nevocellular nevus cells, neuroid nevus cells, and blue nevus cells. Parts of the lesion may show a histopathology suggesting benign juvenile melanoma. When it occurs, melanoma may arise from a position

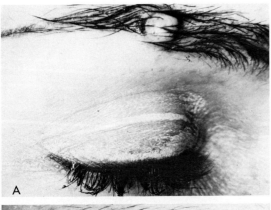
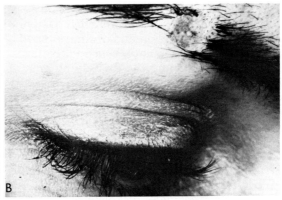
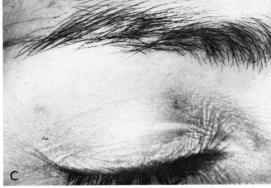

Figure 73–36. *A,* Intradermal nevus of the eyebrow. *B,* After "shave" type of biopsy and electrodesiccation. *C,* Site of the intradermal nevus several months after treatment.

Figure 73–37. *A,* Intradermal nevus. *B,* Several months following treatment by "shave" type of biopsy and electrodesiccation.

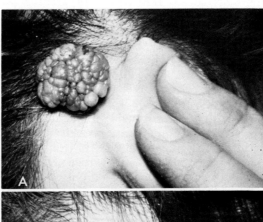
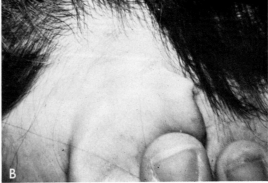

deep within the lesion and not at the junction of the dermis and epidermis. With leptomeningeal involvement, melanocytes are found coating blood vessels and may infiltrate the brain substance. Melanomas may also arise in the leptomeninges.

Treatment remains an especially difficult problem because of the extent of involvement in some cases and the potential threat of melanoma developing at some time. Plastic surgical excision with skin graft coverage is the current method of treatment.

Blue Nevus

Blue nevi are slate blue to dark blue-black or brown papular lesions with a smooth surface. These occur in two forms, the common and the cellular types. Cellular blue nevi may show either a smooth or an irregular surface and are usually larger than the common type (Fig. 73–38). Blue nevi are located most often on the dorsum of the hands and feet; the buttocks and the face may also show involvement. However, Rodriquez and Ackerman (1968) noted cellular blue nevi to be more common in females and to be present on the buttocks and sacrococcygeal regions in over half of their cases.

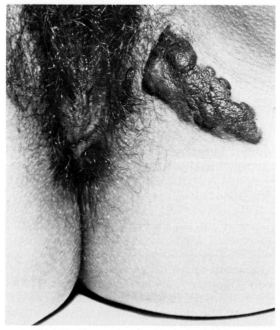

Figure 73–38. Blue nevus adjacent to the labia. [Photograph used by permission of New York University School of Medicine (Skin and Cancer Unit).]

These lesions may arise early in life but can develop in adults (Dorsey and Montgomery, 1954), and ordinarily do not change in size or appearance.

Pathology. In the common type, elongated, flattened, spindle-shaped melanocytes and melanophages are found in the mid- or lower portions of the dermis (Lever, 1967). The cellular type, in addition to the above pathology, shows islands of larger cells, rounded or spindle shaped, with nuclei of different shapes. The cellular type of lesion may extend deeply into the subcutaneous fat (Lever, 1967). A very small percentage of the cellular-type lesions may undergo malignant transformation. Confusion with malignant melanoma may occur, but the absence of mitotic activity and the absence of other criteria of malignancy help to distinguish these lesions.

Sanderson (1968b) regarded blue nevi as a defect in the development of melanocytes that were to migrate to the epidermal junction.

Treatment. Treatment is by simple excision but must be adequate in the deeper lesions.

When malignant degeneration takes place in a cellular blue nevus (a rare occurrence), metastases may result (Kwittken and Negri, 1966). An important histopathologic feature, in addition to the usual criteria of neoplasia, is the presence of areas of necrosis within the lesion.

Halo Nevus (Leukoderma Acquisitum Centrifigum)

This term is applied to a nevus cell nevus that develops an area of surrounding leukoderma (Figs. 73–39, 73–40), which may be followed by the gradual depigmentation and ultimate disappearance of the nevus. The area of depigmentation may persist and may even be associated with true vitiligo elsewhere on the body (Frank and Cohen, 1964). The lesion commonly appears on the posterior aspect of the trunk, but is seen elsewhere on the body (Kopf and Andrade, 1965-66). Its clinical importance lies in its possible confusion by clinicians with malignant melanoma.

While the central lesion is commonly a nevus, other halo lesions may rarely be one of several neuroectodermally derived tumors, i.e., a blue nevus, a neurofibroma, or a malig-

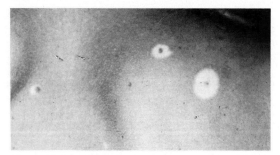

Figure 73–39. Multiple halo nevi on the back of a child.

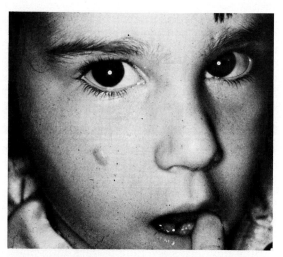

Figure 73–41. Spitz nevus. [Photograph used by permission of New York University School of Medicine (Skin and Cancer Unit).]

nant melanoma (Kopf, Morrill, and Silverberg, 1965).

Histopathology. Lever (1967) noted that an early lesion shows multiple nests of nevus cells at the epidermal-dermal junction and in the dermis. Around and beneath the nevus cells, there are cells resembling lymphocytes and histiocytes. A reduction in the number of or the absence of melanocytes is noted in the hypopigmented halo zone (Kopf, Morrill, and Silverberg, 1965). Later in the histogenesis of the lesion, the infiltrate and melanin disappear. Electron microscopy of the halo shows that the dopa-negative epidermal clear cells are Langerhans' cells (Wayte and Helwig, 1968).

Therapy. Ordinarily no therapy is required unless clinical doubt exists as to the nature of the lesion. If excision is performed, inclusion of the hypopigmented area is warranted for cosmetic reasons, in view of the persistence of leukoderma in some lesions.

Spitz Nevus (Epithelioid Cell–Spindle Cell Nevus)

This is a benign skin tumor seen chiefly in children but also occurring in adult life (Kopf and Andrade, 1965–66). Lever (1967) was of the opinion that the lesion represents a compound nevus. Its clinical importance lies in the fact that it has a histologic picture that may be confused with malignant melanoma. Spitz (1948) was the first to point out that certain histopathologic findings would distinguish this entity from malignant melanoma. Clinically, the typical lesion is a firm pink to red to reddish purple nodule that has a smooth or occasionally scaly surface (Fig. 73–41). It is firm to palpation, is often seen on the face, and varies from 1 to 2 cm in diameter, unusual lesions being even larger (Kopf and Andrade, 1965–66; Sanderson, 1968b). Most lesions are pink and smooth, but occasionally brown to black lesions are seen, and a verrucous surface may be evident (Fig. 73–42).

Spitz nevus cells may be junctional, compound, or intradermal in location (Maize and Ackerman, 1987; Rhodes, 1987). They are composed of spindle-shaped and epithelioid cells; giant and multinucleated cells are also seen. Telangiectasis and edema of the stroma are noted with increasing maturation of the cells in the deeper portions of the tumor (Lever, 1967). Melanin is usually diminished or absent. Mitoses are seen, but anaplasia is lacking (Sanderson, 1968b).

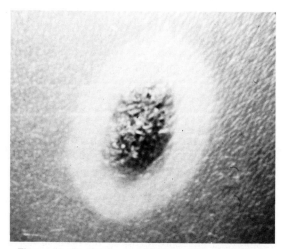

Figure 73–40. Halo nevus. (Courtesy of Dr. Sam Frank.)

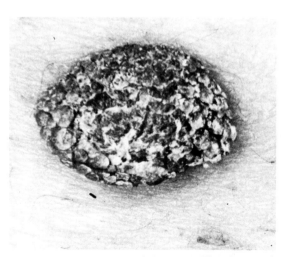

Figure 73–42. Verrucous Spitz nevus. The photograph does not show the reddish hue present in this pigmented lesion.

Therapy. Conservative surgical excision with submission of material for histopathologic examination should suffice.

Dysplastic Nevus

This term is used to describe a heterogeneous group of unusual melanocytic nevi that show a histologically distinctive picture (Friedman and associates, 1985). These nevi occur in a sporadic and a familial form. Their importance lies in the fact that dysplastic nevi may be precursors and/or clinical markers of malignant melanoma (Greene, 1982; Dixon, 1983; Fitzpatrick and associates, 1984).

In 1952 Cawley described cases of familial malignant melanoma. Other authors noted larger numbers of nevi in patients with familial malignant melanoma. Clark and associates (1978) described atypical moles occurring in patients with familial malignant melanoma in the families B and K, and designated the syndrome the B-K mole syndrome. In one-third of the patients with nonfamilial melanoma, morphologically and histologically similar precursor lesions were noted (Greene, 1982). In a study of 234 primary cutaneous melanomas, dysplastic nevi were reported in histologic association with melanomas in 21.8 per cent of patients (Rhodes and associates, 1983).

In the familial form of malignant melanoma, patients with dysplastic nevi are at a much higher risk of developing melanoma than are the general population. It was estimated in 1985 that one of 150 individuals in the United States will develop melanoma during his lifetime (Friedman, Rigel, and Kopf, 1985). In patients with dysplastic nevi, the risk of developing melanoma with a background of familial malignant melanoma is several hundred times higher (Greene, 1982). The risk of melanoma developing in patients with the sporadic form of dysplastic nevi is not yet known. Melanoma has been known to arise directly from dysplastic nevi in the familial malignant melanoma syndrome (National Institutes of Health, 1984).

Greene and associates (1985) proposed a classification of dysplastic nevi either associated with a personal or family history of melanoma or without such a history. The four types, in order of increasing risk of melanoma, are: (1) Type A (so-called sporadic type), dysplastic nevi with no familial history of dysplastic nevi or melanoma and no personal history of melanoma; (2) Type B, similar to Type A except that other family members have dysplastic nevi; (3) Type C, patients with both dysplastic nevi and melanoma but a negative family history for both; and (4) Type D, patients who have either one (type D_1) or two or more (type D_2) members of their family with melanoma and dysplastic nevi. Type D_2 patients are at the highest risk of development of melanoma.

Clinical Picture. Dysplastic nevi typically measure 5 to 12 mm in diameter, although some may actually be smaller (Fig. 73–43). They may have both flat and elevated components. The color ranges from light tan to dark brown and may show a pink background. The borders of the dysplastic nevus, in contrast to common nevi, are often indented and poorly defined. The lesions are found anywhere in the body, but frequently are noted on sun-exposed areas and also in covered areas such as the female breasts, buttocks, pubic area, and scalp. Lesions begin to appear in adolescence and continue to appear after the age of 35, their numbers ranging from a few to more than 100 (Greene, 1982; National Institutes of Health, 1984; Friedman and associates, 1985).

The microscopic picture of "dysplastic nevi" may be that of a junctional or compound type of melanocytic nevus with unusual features:

1. The presence of an increased number of melanocytes arranged both singly and in nests along elongated rete ridges on the basal layer of the epidermis and extending

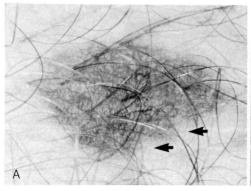
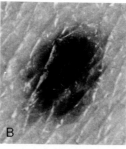

Figure 73–43. Dysplastic nevus. Note the irregular borders and lack of sharp definition of the edges of the nevus. *B,* Note the lack of sharp definition between the edge of the nevus and the surrounding skin. [Photographs *A* and *B* used by permission of New York University School of Medicine (Department of Dermatology).]

to the side of the bulk of the lesion (so-called "shoulder" of the nevus).

2. Cytologically atypical melanocytes (Clark and associates, 1978) in a random and variable fashion in the "shoulder" component. These cells may also be seen along the remainder of the junctional component and, at times, within the dermis.

3. Two patterns of epidermal growth of melanocytes have been described: lentiginous melanocytic hyperplasia (common) and epithelioid cell melanocytic dysplasia (less common).

4. Other histologic features commonly associated with the melanocytic changes include:
   a. Lamellar fibroplasia.
   b. Concentric eosinophilic fibroplasia.
   c. A patchy lymphocytic infiltrate in the dermis (National Institutes of Health, 1984; Friedman and associates, 1985).

Management. The entire integument must be examined, including the scalp and the periorbital region. A typical lesion should be excised to establish the diagnosis. When dysplastic nevi show changes in the margins or color or the lesions become inflamed, they should be excised for histologic evaluation. Lesions suggestive of malignant melanoma should be excised. Dysplastic nevi should be removed from areas, such as the scalp, which are difficult to examine. The importance of periodic self-examination by the patient for change in preexisting lesions should be emphasized. Patients with dysplastic nevi should minimize exposure to ultraviolet light (Dixon, 1983).

Careful attention should be given to nevi during periods of hormonal changes such as during puberty and pregnancy (Fitzpatrick and associates, 1984). In familial cases and in patients with large numbers of dysplastic

nevi, referral to a dermatologist is advisable for periodic follow-up examinations at three to six month intervals. Photographic documentation is important in the management and follow-up of patients with the dysplastic nevus syndrome.

BOWENOID PAPULOSIS

This disease (Hoyt, 1970; Kopf and Bart, 1977; Wade, Kopf, and Ackerman, 1979) is characterized by red-brown to violaceous papules ranging in size from 2 to 10 mm. The papules may show scaling on the surface, and have been noted to appear on the genitalia of both sexes as well as in extragenital locations (Bart, 1984) (Fig. 73–44).

Guillet and associates (1984) noted differences from Bowen's disease. Bowenoid papulosis occurs in a younger age group (21 to 38 years), and the location tends to be multicentric (in the inguinal and crural areas and genitalia). One of these authors' patients developed condylomata acuminata following spontaneous improvement of bowenoid papulosis.

At the present time, this disease entity is of interest because of the apparently non-aggressive course (Bart, 1984) despite the histologic appearance of Bowen's disease (intraepidermic squamous cell carcinoma). Spontaneous disappearance of some lesions can occur.

Of interest is the finding in bowenoid papulosis of human papillomavirus, Type 16 (Zachow and associates, 1982; Oriel, 1984), which has been associated with cervical carcinoma (Crum and associates, 1984). Bart (1984) noted that bowenoid papulosis of the penis is frequently associated with a history of viral conditions such as recurrent herpes

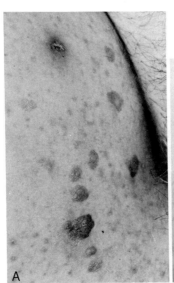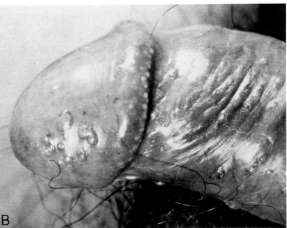

Figure 73–44. *A, B,* Bowenoid papulosis. [Photographs used by permission of New York University School of Medicine (Department of Dermatology).]

simplex and condylomata acuminata. Using immunoperoxidase techniques, Penneys and associates (1984) demonstrated papillomavirus common antigen in both verruca and bowenoid papulosis.

In view of the histologic appearance and the lack of knowledge about the ultimate fate of untreated lesions of bowenoid papulosis, it is recommended that the lesion should be conservatively destroyed. Liquid nitrogen therapy may be employed (a cotton-tipped applicator dipped into liquid nitrogen and held against the lesion for 10 to 15 seconds) or the lesion may be removed by electrodesiccation and curettage.

ACTINIC (SOLAR, SENILE) KERATOSIS

This lesion is a roughened, keratotic, flat to elevated patch found chiefly on the light-exposed skin of individuals who may show other skin manifestations of actinic damage. The color varies and may be skin colored, reddish, grayish, or light yellow-brown. These lesions are often palpated as a roughened patch by the patient before they become particularly visible.

The lesions are seen chiefly on the face, ears, neck, dorsum of the hand and arm, and exposed portions of the legs. If the occupation has resulted in actinic exposure of the thorax, they will also be seen in this location.

Histologic changes may occur in the epidermis that resemble Bowen's disease or early squamous cell carcinoma. The pathologic picture may reflect the clinical appearance. Pinkus (1966–67) and Lever (1967) observed that the dermis shows the effects of actinic damage in the collagen, together with an abundant lymphocytic infiltrate with plasma cells and eosinophils in some cases. A small percentage of actinic keratoses may transform into squamous cell carcinoma (Fig. 73–45). Actinic keratoses must be considered precancerous (Andrade, 1964). Bendel and Graham (1970) reported no evidence of metastases in 156 patients with squamous cell carcinoma arising from actinic keratoses. On the other hand, Lund (1965) noted that an estimated 0.1 per cent of such squamous cell carcinomas metastasize.

Traditional dermatologic therapy has involved sharp curettage and electrodesiccation, but newer methods may yield superior cosmetic end results. Perhaps the most important of these are topical 5-fluorouracil and cryodestructive methods. For the isolated few lesions of actinic keratosis, liquid nitrogen applied with a cotton-tipped applicator for 10 to 15 seconds with light to moderate pressure results in removal of the keratosis with satisfactory cosmetic results (Fig. 73–46). Shortly after the treatment, a local edematous response is noted. This is replaced in a few days with a crust that falls off, leaving a pink surface that gradually returns to normal

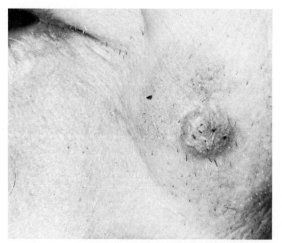

Figure 73–45. Squamous cell carcinoma arising in an area of actinic keratosis on the face adjacent to the mouth.

skin color. In some individuals, the treated site may remain "whiter" than the surrounding untreated skin; carbon dioxide snow "pencils" are used in a similar fashion.

Dillaha and associates (1963) described the use of 5-fluorouracil (5-FU) for the treatment of actinic keratoses. In individuals with a severe degree of actinic skin damage, the use of a 1 to 5 per cent preparation of 5-FU yields the best cosmetic result. The treatment consists of twice daily application of the 5-FU preparation. Care must be exercised to avoid getting the medication into the eyes. Handwashing should follow finger application of this medication. Sunlight may accentuate the inflammatory response, which becomes quite severe. Topical steroid creams may be pre-scribed for use after 5-FU therapy is finished, to allay some of the inflammatory response. Treatment of the face is continued up to two to six weeks, depending on the intensity of the inflammatory response. On the dorsum of the hand, arm, and back the results are less predictable, and therapy may need to be continued for at least six to eight weeks.

The chemical is also able to destroy actinic keratoses that are not clinically visible (Fig. 73–47). While this method of therapy cannot prevent the appearance of new actinic keratoses, it may be repeated at a later date when new crops of lesions appear.

As far as the mode of action is concerned, Eaglestein, Weinstein, and Frost (1970) showed that 5-FU appears to inhibit the synthesis of deoxyribonucleic acid and ribonucleic acid, an action that in turn leads to interference with cellular functions and alterations in the mitotic rate.

LEUKOPLAKIA

Leukoplakia is a condition of the vermilion border of the lips, the mucosa of the mouth, and the vulva, characterized by white patches displaying a distinctive histopathology.

Etiology. The lesion is believed to be a response to external noxious agents (such as sunlight, tobacco, snuff, poorly fitting dentures, and carious teeth) and intrinsic disease (such as involutional atrophic changes in the vulva, the atrophic glossitis of syphilis, and lichen sclerosus et atrophicus) (Lever, 1967;

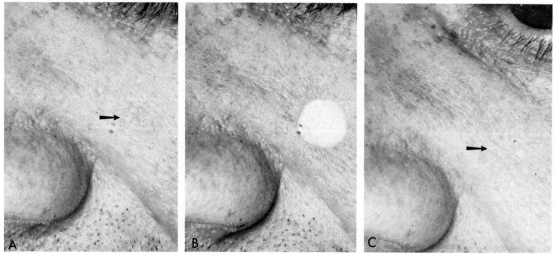

Figure 73–46. *A,* Actinic keratosis *(arrow). B,* During treatment with liquid nitrogen. *C,* Healed result after treatment.

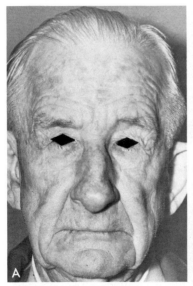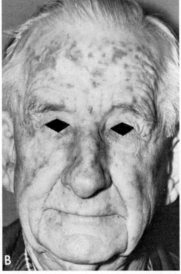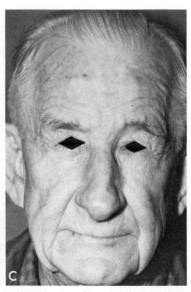

Figure 73–47. Actinic keratoses. *A,* Before treatment. *B,* During treatment with 5-fluorouracil. Note the many clinically inapparent lesions "picked out" by the chemical. *C,* Appearance after subsidence of the inflammatory response associated with 5-fluorouracil therapy. (Courtesy of Dr. G. T. Jansen and Arch. Dermatol., Vol. 88, 1963. Copyright 1963, American Medical Association.)

Pindborg, 1972; Wilkinson, 1972). According to Wallace and Whimster (1951), leukoplakia is found coexistent with lichen sclerosus et atrophicus in about 25 per cent of cases.

Clinical Picture. Whitish patches resulting from a disturbance in keratinization characterize the disorder. The patches may be glistening, shiny, or dull. On the lower lip the lesions may be dry and fissured and may complicate actinic cheilosis. On the oral mucosa the lesions often are flat but may become verrucous, suggesting a change from benign to malignant status (Fig. 73–48). Leukoplakia of the vulva is seen in the form of gray or whitish patches, and the clinical picture is likened to hardened, cracked white paint (Wallace, 1962). On the vulva, the condition is often preceded by chronic itching.

Authorities do not agree on the incidence of malignant transformation of leukoplakia into squamous cell carcinoma, but there is a consensus that it is lower than previously believed. Silverman (1970) noted that in 800 patients with oral carcinoma, 15 per cent of the cancers were directly associated with leukoplakia. The same authors found that in 117 patients with leukoplakia followed for an average of five years, 6 per cent developed malignancies at the site of the leukoplakia.

Pathology. White lesions of the vulva or oral mucosa do not necessarily represent leukoplakia, and histopathologic examination is

required before such a clinical impression can be verified.

Lever (1967) noted that the oral and vulval histologic findings are similar. In some cases, the atrophic epithelium shows a picture of anaplastic bowenoid changes (King, 1964). In other lesions of leukoplakia, hyperkeratosis and a granular layer (usually absent on the oral and vulvar mucosa) are seen. Atypical cells must be present to substantiate the diagnosis.

Therapy. Oral lesions may regress upon removal of the causal irritants. Localized

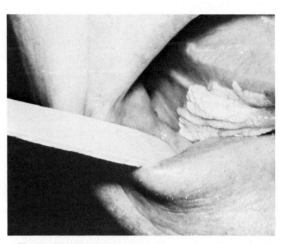

Figure 73–48. Leukoplakia of the oral cavity. Note the verrucous changes.

patches may be selectively destroyed by electrodesiccation and curettage. Suspicious patches that are indurated or verrucous should be biopsied, and the patient should be followed closely when simple eradication or excision is not feasible. Since carcinoma of the tongue and the floor of the mouth has a poor prognosis, any change of leukoplakia toward malignancy requires surgical attention.

A technique for biopsy and excision of suspected vulval lesions, as well as for follow-up procedures after surgery of the vulva for carcinoma, has been described by Collins, Hausen, and Theriot (1966). Making use of Richart's technique for cervical staining, they paint the vulva with 1 per cent toluidine blue, leaving it on for three minutes and then washing the stain off with 1 per cent acetic acid solution. Areas retaining the stain should be biopsied. False-positive staining does occur with some benign and superficial vulval ulcerations.

MALIGNANT MELANOMA IN SITU (MELANOTIC FRECKLE OF HUTCHINSON, LENTIGO MALIGNA, PRECANCEROUS MELANOSIS OF DUBREUILH)

This a dark macular lesion occurring chiefly on the face and characterized by a gradual increase in size, eventually giving rise in a percentage of patients to malignant melanoma. Miescher (1928) thought that about one-third of the lesions develop into malignant melanoma.

While the etiology is unknown, the large preponderance of the lesions in older individuals on exposed areas leads one to postulate that actinic exposure probably plays a major contributory role.

The clinical picture is that of a flat, pigmented lesion showing several shades of black and brown coloration (Figs. 73–49, 73–50). Jackson, Williamson, and Beattie (1966) noted that when the lesion is examined with a hand lens one may see pigmented points and lines in the lesion that merge with apparently normal skin. After a variable length of time, induration may occur, with formation of the nodules of malignant melanoma. It is generally agreed that even when a malignant melanoma supervenes, it represents a less

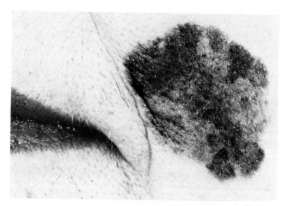

Figure 73–49. Melanotic freckle of Hutchinson involving the cheek. [Used by permission of New York University School of Medicine (Skin and Cancer Unit).]

malignant process than the variety arising de novo or from junctional nevi (Pinkus, 1966–67; Lever, 1967; Sanderson, 1968b). A better prognosis exists even after metastases to regional nodes (Lever, 1967).

Mishima (1966) also believed that these melanomas differ biologically in behavior. Melanomas arising from melanocytes of junctional nevi have a more serious prognosis. Lever (1967) felt that another explanation of this phenomenon may lie in the fact that melanomas arising in the melanocytes of melanotic freckle develop on skin chronically damaged by sunlight. This factor may modify their biologic behavior. As emphasized by Pinkus (1966–67), the transformation of this lesion from hyperplasia of junctional epidermal melanocytes to frank melanoma proceeds slowly. No nevus cells are involved, the melanocytes being changed into melanoma cells.

Treatment. The treatment varies, depending on whether there is coexistent malignant

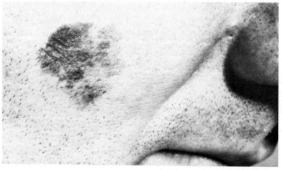

Figure 73–50. Melanotic freckle of Hutchinson. [Used by permission of New York University School of Medicine (Skin and Cancer Unit).]

melanoma or not. It is also important to be aware that the diseased melanocyte may extend downward into the pilosebaceous unit in the eccrine duct.

In the freckle stage alone or malignant melanoma in situ (Maize and Ackerman, 1987), surgical excision and Mohs microscopically controlled excision are useful treatment modalities. Care must be taken to include some of the normal skin at the periphery of the lesion because of the tendency of a melanotic freckle to spread peripherally.

The treatment method of Miescher and Storck (Petratos and associates, 1972), utilizing irradiation by means of a special low voltage aparatus, has found favor in some European clinics. This method was abandoned at the Skin and Cancer Unit of the New York University Medical Center because of recurrences and problems connected with its use (Kopf, Bart, and Gladstein, 1976; Pitman and associates, 1979).

BASAL CELL EPITHELIOMA (CARCINOMA)

From the dermatologist's point of view, many if not most of the basal cell epitheliomas seen in the office and clinic practice at the present time are handled successfully by dermatologic techniques. For the management of difficult or unusual skin tumors, including basal cell epitheliomas, a combined specialty tumor conference represents an important advance. At such conferences, the services of a dermatologist, plastic surgeon, pathologist, radiologist, and Mohs chemosurgeon are essential in deciding the optimal therapeutic approach for a particular tumor (see Chap. 74).

One method of therapy for basal cell carcinoma by the dermatologist is curettage and electrodesiccation. Other methods of dermatologic treatment include superficial x-ray therapy, cryodestructive measures with liquid nitrogen, excisional therapy, and Mohs chemosurgery (see p. 3652). The choice of therapy depends on several factors relevant to the particular patient and the individual lesion: the patient's age, occupation, and physical and emotional status; the location of the lesion; the general condition of the skin; and the clinical and histopathologic type.

The technique of curettage and electrodesiccation depends on the fact that the average basal cell epithelioma is mushy in consistency, and yields readily to separation from the surrounding normal skin and dermis by means of curettage. This is partly the result of the fact that the fibroblastic stroma underlying the basal cell epithelioma is rich in mucopolysaccharides (Sweet, 1963; Freeman, Knox, and Heaton, 1964.)

Local infiltration anesthesia is satisfactory for this technique. Following vigorous curettage and careful inspection of the bed of the treated area, an electrodesiccating spark of medium intensity is directed carefully point by point into and onto the curetted bed, including a rim of normal surrounding skin. Curettage and electrodesiccation is repeated carefully two or more times, depending on the operator's sense of feel with the curette and the amount of mushy material that he encounters in the course of subsequent curettage (Fig. 73–51).

Five to seven days later, the treated site begins to ooze and show an inflammatory response. The exudation and separation of the necrotic cutis and epithelium proceed for a period of two or more weeks, depending on the extent and depth of the initial involvement and treatment. A simple ointment such as bacitracin may be applied for a few weeks, together with nonadherent dressings. Approximately two to four weeks after therapy, a firm crust forms under which epithelization occurs (Figs. 73–52 to 73–54).

Because this technique requires that the tissue be soft and easily separable from surrounding normal tissue, certain types of basal cell epitheliomas are not suitable for this treatment. Morphea or fibrosing types of lesions, as well as lesions recurring in heavily scarred areas where fibrotic stromal reaction makes such separation with the curette unlikely, are better treated by other techniques. Similarly, basal cell lesions invading bone or cartilage or excessively large lesions, except those of superficial basal cell epithelioma, should be treated by other methods.

The management by curettage and electrodesiccation of large lesions involving the nasal tip and ala, the canthi and eyelids, and the lip vermilion–skin junction may result in a functional or anatomic deficit. Such lesions may be more amenable to x-ray therapy, with better maintenance of anatomic and functional integrity. However, Knox (1968) did not hesitate to treat selected small eyelid margin lesions by curettage and electrodesiccation. This technique may be used on le-

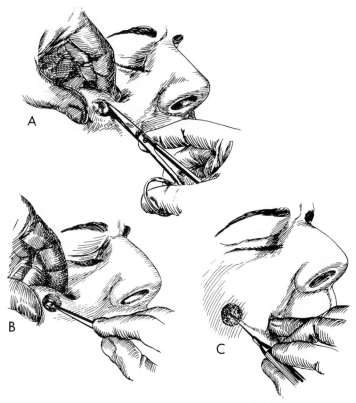

Figure 73–51. Technique of curettage and electrodesiccation. *A,* Biopsy of a basal cell epithelioma. *B,* Vigorous curettage of a basal cell epithelioma. *C,* Monopolar spark gap electrodesiccation for treatment of a basal cell epithelioma.

sions of superficial basal cell epithelioma on the trunk and elsewhere. In some instances, for treatment of large superficial basal cell epitheliomas the author prefers the use of liquid nitrogen. By means of application or spray, the tumor and 3 to 5 mm of the surrounding normal skin are frozen for a period of 30 seconds or for one to two freeze–thaw cycles. This results in edema, exudation, and possible blistering within one to two days. The area later becomes dry and scaly, leaving a scar that is smooth and quite acceptable, with the exception of some degree of mild hypopigmentation.

Grenz radiation therapy of superficial basal cell epitheliomas is another useful modality in selected instances (Gladstein, 1970). It may be used when electrosurgery is likely to result in hypertrophic or keloidal scarring. Lesions in areas such as the midchest and deltoid region may be treated by grenz radiation. Superficial basal cell epitheliomas of the eyelids may also be treated by this modality.

Grenz ray therapy, with 10 to 12 kilovolts at 10 to 15 milliamps with a half value layer of 0.035 mm of aluminum, generates x-rays of low penetration, most radiation energy being absorbed in the upper portions of the skin surface consistent with the location of

the pathology. The half value layer should be adjusted to reflect the thickness of the lesion.

These treatments are given in doses of 500 R three times a week for a total dose of 5000 R.

The technique of curettage and electrodesiccation is well suited for the many lesions found in the basal cell nevus syndrome (Gorlin's syndrome), which is a genetically determined condition characterized by the presence of a few to many tumors on the face and other parts of the body indistinguishable histopathologically from basal cell epithelioma. Other features of the syndrome are dentigerous cysts, bifid ribs, characteristic dyskeratotic pits of the palms and soles, vertebral abnormalities, increased interpupillary distance, broad nasal root, and other anomalies (Howell and Caro, 1959; Gorlin, Yunis, and Tuna, 1963; Zackheim, Howell, and Loud, 1966). The skin lesions may develop into invasive and destructive basal cell epitheliomas.

Complications and Disadvantages of Curettage and Electrodesiccation. Postoperative bleeding is rarely encountered five to seven days later. This is easily controlled by pressure or a suture. Hypertrophic scarring may occur in certain anatomic sites such

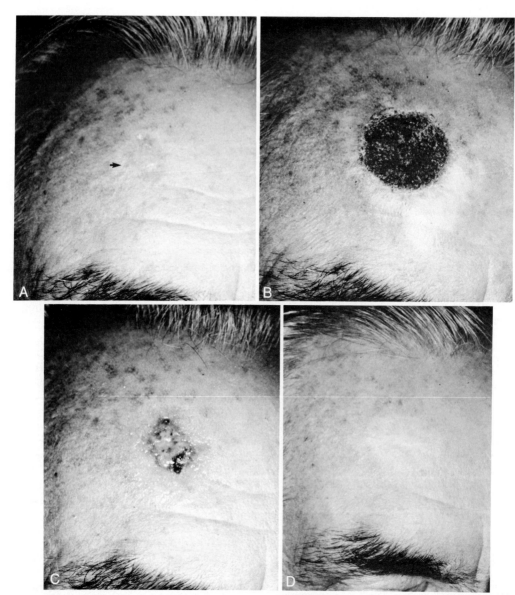

Figure 73–52. *A,* Basal cell carcinoma after incisional biopsy *(arrow). B,* Extent of the defect after treatment by curettage and electrodesiccation. *C,* Two weeks after treatment by curettage and electrodesiccation. *D,* Over one year after treatment. Note the hypopigmentation, a typical appearance after treatment of a lesion of this size.

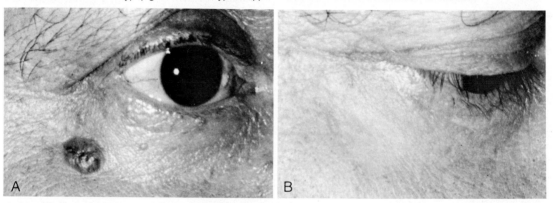

Figure 73–53. *A,* Basal cell carcinoma of medium size. *B,* One year after treatment by curettage and electrodesiccation.

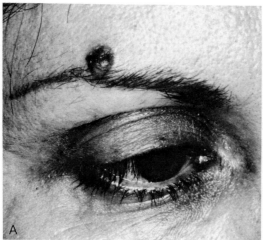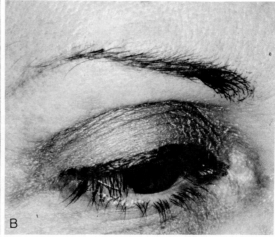

Figure 73–54. *A,* Basal cell carcinoma, small lesion. *B,* Seven years after treatment by curettage and electrodesiccation.

as the upper chest, the neck, the deltoid area, the vermilion junction, or the oral commissures. In the latter two areas, other methods of treatment are suggested. Usually, hypertrophic scarring subsides spontaneously over a period of several months (Fig. 73–55), but

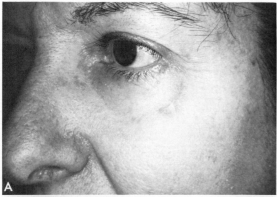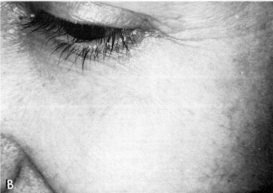

Figure 73–55. *A,* Basal cell carcinoma site six weeks after curettage and electrodesiccation. Note the hypertrophic scar of the zygomatic area. *B,* Nine months later, the scar has become inconspicuous.

this may be hastened by the intralesional injection of a few drops of triamcinolone acetonide suspension (3 to 5 mg per ml) at monthly intervals. True keloids rarely develop in individuals who are susceptible. A persistent fold of skin may result from the use of the technique on lesions of the nose medial to the inner canthus (Fig. 73–56). Persistent hypopigmentation is also seen following sharp curettage and electrodesiccation on actinically damaged skin (Fig. 73–57).

A surgical specimen for histopathologic examination of the margins is not provided by the technique of sharp curettage and electrodesiccation, but the sense of feel that the operator experiences with the curette determines how widely and deeply he proceeds in the eradication of a particular lesion.

Despite some drawbacks, this technique provides a simple and rapid outpatient treatment for many cases of basal cell epithelioma. The cure rate (96 per cent or better in selected cases) in patients treated by experienced dermatologists (Popkin, 1968) compares favorably with that obtained by irradiation or excisional surgery. It is exceeded only by the exacting, time-consuming, microscopically controlled chemosurgery technique of Mohs (Popkin, 1968).

Superficial Radiation Therapy. Superficial x-ray therapy as practiced by dermatologists also yields a high rate of cure. In a series of 500 basal cell epithelioma lesions treated at the New York University Skin and Cancer Unit, the cure rate was 92.7 per cent at five years and 88.9 per cent at ten years. This method of treatment is outpatient or office oriented and is especially useful for

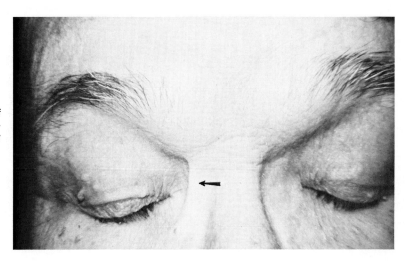

Figure 73–56. Development of an epicanthal fold following curettage and electrodesiccation therapy in the medial canthus region.

lesions in the face, neck, and ears of individuals beyond middle age (Bart, 1970). For lesions involving the canthus and eyelid margins, the nasal tip and ala, and the lip vermilion–skin junction, the author feels that radiation therapy offers the best functional and cosmetic end result. In addition, the treatment borders of clinically noninvolved tissue can be more easily extended (in contrast to surgery) to prevent persistence of disease due to failure to eradicate peripheral extensions.

The technique of radiation therapy also suffers from the absence of histopathologic verification of the tumor margins. Another drawback is that, whereas surgical scars generally improve with age, radiation therapy scars do not. Atrophy and telangiectasis be-

come more apparent over the years, especially in individuals with fair skin.

Despite these drawbacks, dermatologic x-ray therapy is an important and useful modality for the treatment of basal and squamous cell carcinoma.

In the technique used at the New York University Skin and Cancer Unit, the surrounding area is shielded to within 5 to 10 mm of the visible and palpable border of the lesion (the width of the margin depending on the lesion size and clinical and histopathologic type). The patient receives 680 R per treatment three times a week, for a total of 3400 R for basal cell epithelioma and 5400 R for squamous cell carcinoma. The factors are 0.8 to 1.0 mm half value layer of aluminum, 65 to 100 kvp at a target skin distance of 15

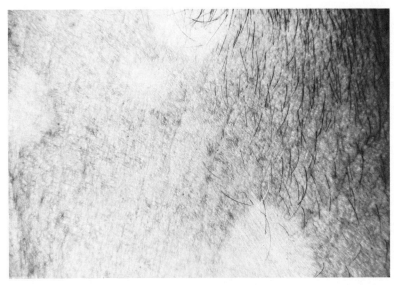

Figure 73–57. Persistent hypopigmentation after curettage and electrodessication for a basal cell carcinoma.

to 20 cm. The surrounding uninvolved skin, as well as the eyes, thyroid, and gonadal areas, are lead-shielded. When eyelid canthi and margins are treated, brass eye or lead "tongue"-type shields are inserted into the conjunctival sac to protect the eye.

Following x-ray therapy, a reaction develops with considerable inflammatory and exudative response. It gradually subsides, leaving a hairless scar.

BOWEN'S DISEASE

This is a skin condition characterized by chronic scaling and, at times, a crusted, elevated lesion with an erythematous or purplish base (Fig. 73–58). It is found on both exposed and nonexposed surfaces of the body. On the vulva, the lesions may be smooth and velvety or wartlike, brownish, and polycylic (Fig. 73–59). The labia majora are involved more often than the labia minora. According to Sanderson (1968b), itching is a prominent symptom in vulval lesions. Considered a carcinoma in situ that has not broken through the epidermal-dermal junction, it may after a variable period of time become frankly invasive squamous cell carcinoma.

Work by Graham and Helwig (1959, 1964) and others has demonstrated a higher than average association of Bowen's disease with other primary skin and internal malignancies. Lever (1967) and others felt that these findings posed some difficulties in interpretation, since both visceral cancer and Bowen's

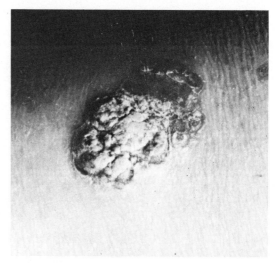

Figure 73–58. Bowen's disease. [Used by permission of New York University School of Medicine (Skin and Cancer Unit).]

disease are likely to occur in patients of the cancer prone age groups.

The pathology of Bowen's disease shows a disordered epidermis with multinucleated giant cells, dyskeratotic cells, and mitotic figures. Despite acanthosis, the dermoepidermal border is intact in Bowen's disease.

However, when invasion does occur, Graham and Helwig (1964) reported that the likelihood of metastases is high. In one series, eight of 155 patients with Bowen's disease showed invasion as carcinoma. Of those eight patients, three had metastases to internal organs.

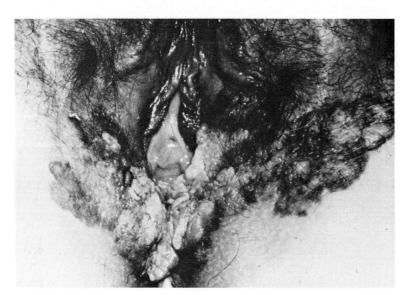

Figure 73–59. Bowen's disease (intraepithelial squamous cell carcinoma) of the vulva. (Courtesy of Dr. Earle Brauer and Dr. Stephen Gumport.)

Treatment. Dermatologists have successfully treated small lesions by thorough curettage and electrodesiccation. However, Graham and Helwig (1964) noted that 72 per cent of the lesions recurred following such treatment, and 87 per cent recurred after x-ray therapy. They recommended surgical excision.

Zacarian (1969) successfully used liquid nitrogen in a small series of patients with Bowen's disease. Gladstein (1970) reported that selected cases of Bowen's disease may be successfully eradicated using the grenz ray irradiation technique previously outlined for the treatment of superficial basal cell epithelioma.

ERYTHROPLASIA OF QUEYRAT

This lesion is characterized as a red patch involving predominantly the glans penis but also affecting the shaft of the penis, the vulva, and the oral mucosa (Fig. 73–60). Blau and Hyman (1955) considered this lesion a variant of Bowen's disease. Graham and Helwig (1964) noted the lower rate of associated cancer of patients with erythroplasia of Queyrat as compared with those with Bowen's disease. They also felt that there was a greater likelihood of local invasion occurring in the form of squamous cell carcinoma. Accordingly, despite the histologic similarity of Bowen's disease and erythroplasia of Queyrat, Graham and Helwig considered them to be two distinct entities. Hyman (1970) was of the opinion that the greater likelihood of local invasion can be explained by the location of the lesion

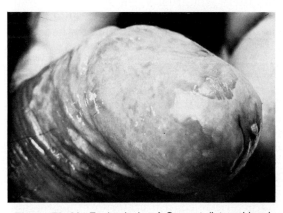

Figure 73–60. Erythoplasia of Queyrat (intraepidermic squamous cell carcinoma). [Courtesy of Dr. Arthur Hyman. Used by permission of New York University School of Medicine (Skin and Cancer Unit).]

on the penis (semimucous membrane), and further believed that the so-called associated cancer proneness noted by Graham and Helwig may be explained by the age group of patients with Bowen's disease.

Grenz ray therapy and 5-fluorouracil (5-FU) have been used for treatment of erythroplasia of Queyrat, microscopically controlled Mohs chemosurgery being reserved for difficult or complicated cases.

PAGET'S DISEASE OF NIPPLE AND EXTRAMAMMARY PAGET'S DISEASE

Paget's disease of the nipple is usually manifest as a crusted, oozing type of dermatitis and may be accompanied by a serosanguineous discharge from the nipple. It is, however, the surface manifestation of ductal breast carcinoma, and dermatologists are aware that persistent eczema-like lesions of the nipple may represent Paget's disease. Early and deep biopsy is recommended in these eczema-like lesions of the nipple that are unresponsive to topical therapy (Baer and Witten, 1959–60).

The treatment for Paget's disease of the nipple is the same as that for carcinoma of the breast.

Extramammary Paget's disease (Fig. 73–61) is usually an erythematous patch or plaque on or about the genitalia, but the lesion may also be found in the axilla and occasionally on other portions of the thorax. Itching and burning are prominent symptoms, and the condition may masquerade as a chronic and persistent eczema with surface scaling and crusting. Graham and Helwig (1964) reported that this condition is seen chiefly in older patients, the median age of onset being 59 years. They also noted that subjacent adnexal apocrine carcinoma was present in slightly less than one-third of their patients. Primary carcinoma of other organs was noted by Graham and Helwig (1959) in about 20 per cent of their cases.

Surgery is the treatment of choice and must be wide and deep because of possible recurrence. Multiple biopsies must be taken to ensure that the periphery is tumor free (Pitman and associates, 1982). The lesion is capable of spreading by direct contiguity into the vagina, anus, urethra, and bladder.

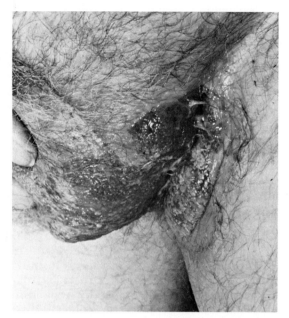

Figure 73–61. Extramammary Paget's disease of the genital region. [Used by permission of New York University School of Medicine (Skin and Cancer Unit).]

SQUAMOUS CELL CARCINOMA (EPIDERMOID CARCINOMA, PRICKLE CELL EPITHELIOMA)

Squamous cell carcinoma is a malignancy of epidermis arising de novo or following damage or injury to the skin. It is composed of both mature squamous cells in varying degrees and anaplastic or immature squamous cells and horn cells. The differentiation in the direction of horn cells is expressed by pearl formation. The invasion of the dermis and other elements of the distinctive histopathology characterize the lesion.

Etiology. The lesion may arise de novo but most commonly arises in an area with preexisting damage to the skin, such as sites of previous irradiation or actinic damage (see Fig. 73–45), chronic burn ulcers, sinuses of osteomyelitis, long-standing granulomas due to syphilis, lupus vulgaris, and leprosy (Sanderson, 1968b). It has also been observed in chronic discoid lupus erythematus scars (Sutton and Sutton, 1949). The role of previous irradiation in certain lesions as a carcinogen or co-carcinogen must be given serious consideration (see Chap. 25). Chronic arsenic ingestion predisposes to the development of a wide variety of skin malignancies, including basal cell epithelioma, Bowen's disease, and squamous cell carcinoma.

Chronic ulcers of the lower legs with heaped-up, rolled borders not found in locations usually associated with varicose ulcerations, vasculitis, and arteriosclerosis should arouse suspicion. A small incisional biopsy should be performed if any doubt exists about the nature of the lesion.

Patients with xeroderma pigmentosum may develop squamous cell carcinoma when exposed to sunlight. Cleaver and Trosko (1969) and Cleaver (1970), working with fibroblasts cultured from actinically damaged xeroderma pigmentosum skin, demonstrated deficiency of an enzyme (absence of endonuclease) needed for the repair of sunlight-damaged DNA strands. This work may point the way to a better understanding of the relationship of sunlight and carcinogenesis.

Actinic keratoses may give rise to squamous cell carcinoma (see Fig. 73–45). An estimated 0.1 per cent of such carcinomas metastasize, according to Lund (1965). However, Bendel and Graham (1970) found no examples of metastases in their series of 156 patients with squamous cell carcinomas arising from actinic keratoses.

Sanderson (1968b) noted that squamous cell carcinoma is chiefly a disease of older individuals, the age incidence rising sharply after ages 55 to 59. Males are affected twice as frequently as females.

Pathology. Broders (1920) classified squamous cell carcinoma according to the proportion of differentiated to undifferentiated and atypical cells, but Lever (1967) emphasized that the depth of penetration of the tumors is also important in establishing the degree of malignancy. On histopathologic examination there is a great variation, ranging from the low grade malignancy and well-differentiated squamous cell carcinoma to the highly anaplastic squamous cell carcinoma. The low grade lesions show horn pearls, an inflammatory dermal infiltrate, invasion to sweat gland depth or less, and maintenance of the basement membranes in some areas. In the anaplastic variety, most tumor cells are atypical and lacking in intercellular bridges (Lever, 1967).

Clinical Picture. The de novo form shows an erythematous papule on normal skin, which grows relatively slowly and lacks the characteristic central crateriform depression filled with keratinous material seen in keratoacanthoma. The de novo form must be distinguished from the relatively rare amelanotic melanoma—a firm pink nodule that may show scaling.

According to Sanderson (1968b), induration is the first evidence of malignancy. In palpating a hyperkeratotic lesion on damaged skin, one notes a thickening that extends beyond the lesion, a finding that should arouse suspicion that malignant changes have supervened (Fig. 73–62). The same author noted that the findings of persistent fissures or ulcers are indicative of malignant change in mobile structures, such as the lip or penis. In rare instances, giant condylomata may show malignant low grade changes. The incidence of associated metastases varies.

Treatment. Treatment of the lesions, as in other forms of skin cancer, depends on the anatomic location, the degree of malignancy and invasiveness, the presence or absence of metastatic lymph nodes, the age of the patient, and the training and specialty of the treating physician.

Early noninvasive lesions may be treated very satisfactorily by sharp curettage and electrodesiccation, surgical excision, Mohs chemosurgery, and cryodestructive methods. On the face and ears, x-ray therapy is useful. A fractionated dose of 600 R per treatment is used at 65 to 120 kvp, 3 to 5 ma (half value layer of 0.9 mm of aluminum), given every two days for a total dose of 5400 R. The

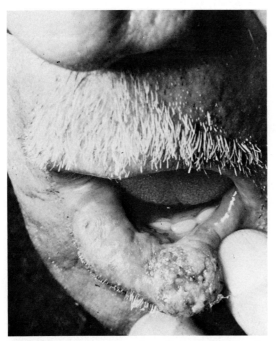

Figure 73–62. Squamous cell carcinoma of the lower lip.

therapeutic and cosmetic results are excellent, particularly in the older age group and in lesions involving the eyelid margins, canthi, nose, lips, and ears. If cartilaginous or bony invasion has occurred, surgery is preferred. Inoperable advanced lesions may be ameliorated by appropriate chemotherapy.

Cryodestruction is useful in small and large noninvasive lesions and larger inoperable masses. In the latter, cryosurgery is undertaken for palliation and removal of foul-smelling, fungating portions of the tumor. Mohs chemosurgery is a painstaking, at times painful, but excellent method of microscopically controlled excision of selected lesions (see p. 3652).

KERATOACANTHOMA (MOLLUSCUM SEBACEUM)

This is a benign, self-healing skin tumor composed of keratin and squamous cells, the more common variety showing a characteristic crateriform clinical picture.

While the etiology of the lesion is unknown, it is believed to originate in the hair follicle (Kalkoff and Macher, 1961; Baer and Kopf, 1962–63), However, Bart (1971) noted that keratoacanthoma may occur on the palms and soles, where hair follicles ordinarily are absent.

Etiology. The cause of the lesions is not known, but the fact that most of the common solitary-type keratoacanthomas occur on exposed surfaces suggests that sunlight may play some role (Baer and Kopf, 1962–63). Infection has also been suggested but not proved as a cause, and the role of mineral oil and tar products may have some importance (Baer and Kopf, 1962–63). The rare multiple type of keratoacanthoma appears to have a familial predisposition (Baer and Kopf, 1962–63).

Andrade (1971) observed that Hutchinson's melanotic freckle, benign juvenile melanoma, and keratoacanthoma are all clinicopathologic entities. As such, the diagnosis must be based on the clinical appearance, history, and histopathologic picture. The keratoacanthoma begins as an erythematous papule that appears most often on the cheeks, nose, hands, or fingers (Baer and Kopf, 1962–63). It progresses rapidly to form a central crateriform depression filled with keratinous material. The lesion is not fixed to underlying deeper tissues. If left untreated, the lesion expels the horny plug, and the sides of the crater are resorbed, leaving a characteristic, slightly atrophic hairless scar with a crenelated border (Fig. 73–63). The entire process requires an average of two to eight months (Baer and Kopf, 1962–63). The same authors noted that most lesions measure under 2 cm in diameter. Sanderson (1968b) reported that the lesion affects males three times more frequently than females, and in many series there is a 1:3 ratio of keratoacanthoma to squamous cell carcinoma. The lesion is most common in fair-skinned individuals.

The histopathology is distinctive when a central fusiform biopsy segment is available for microscopic examination (Popkin and associates, 1966). This shows the typical central keratinous plug with overhanging lips at the edge. Other features are pseudoepitheliomatous hyperplasia and a lymphocytic and histiocytic cellular infiltrate in the dermis. If the lesion lacks the central fusiform segment with normal skin at each edge and some of the underlying cutis, and the clinical history is not characteristic, the pathologist may have difficulty in distinguishing this lesion from squamous cell carcinoma. Indeed, the pathologist often requires a satisfactory biopsy specimen, the clinical history, and the physical appearance to make this diagnosis with some assurance (Andrade, 1971).

Therapy. Because the end result of spontaneous involution is not always cosmetically pleasing, curettage and electrodesiccation or surgical excision is suggested after the diagnosis has been established. The advantage of surgical excision for small lesions is, of course, that it removes the tumor and secures a pathology specimen in one maneuver.

TATTOOS OF SKIN

Although tattoos are not skin tumors, recent developments in the treatment of tattoos are of interest to both plastic surgeons and dermatologists.

The problem of removal of tattoos applied by professional tattoo artists as well as by amateurs is a vexing one. Treatment techniques such as overtattooing, multiple excisions, and excision with skin grafting all have drawbacks. In the past, one-stage deep dermabrasion achieved removal of much of the tattoo but resulted in unacceptable scarring.

Boo-Chai (1963) and Clabaugh (1968) made important contributions to the cosmetic removal of tattoos. Clabaugh (1968) demonstrated by skin window techniques that mac-

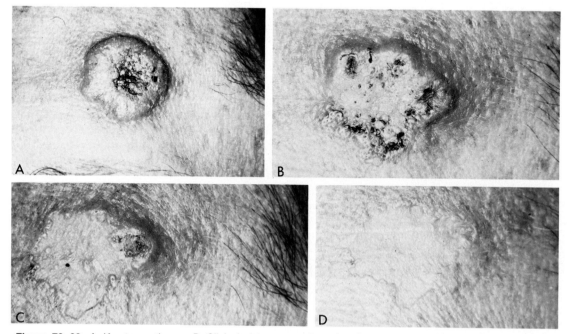

Figure 73–63. *A,* Keratoacanthoma. *B,* Clinical picture several weeks after incisional biopsy. *C,* Two months after biopsy. *D,* Healed scar.

rophages mobilized the pigment of tattoos, bringing it to the surface following superficial dermabrasion.

Utilizing fine diamond fraises with local refrigerant spray anesthesia, Clabaugh (1968) achieved excellent cosmetic removal of tattoos by means of very superficial dermabrasion (Fig. 73–64). For several days after dermabrasion, the gauze dressings placed on the dermabraded surface show the pigment of the tattoo. Whether daily change of gauze dressings allows greater mobilization of pigment than immediate air drying and crust formation remains to be determined.

Crittenden (1971) achieved tattoo removal by means of "salabrasion." Rubbing table salt crystals over the unanesthetized skin by means of lightly moistened gauze sponges wrapped around the finger, he produced sat-

isfactory results. The tattoo was abraded by this method until a uniform red color was noted on the abraded surface. The "salabrasion" was repeated at intervals of four to six weeks and it was noted that the epidermis was easily removed by subsequent "salabrasions."

Both Clabaugh (1968) and Crittenden (1971) noted that tattoos applied by tattoo artists responded better than those put on by amateurs. They postulated that tattoo pigments were probably deposited at more uniform depths when applied by tattoo artists.

Robinson (1985) used superficial dermabrasion followed by scissor excision for small tattoos in fingers, hands, arms, and legs. Bailin, Ratz, and Levine (1980) found CO_2 laser useful in treating decorative tattoos. Landthaler and associates (1984) found that

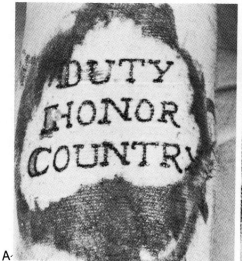

A

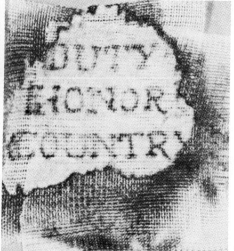

B

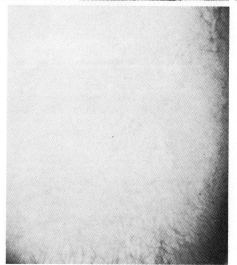

C

Figure 73–64. *A,* Tattoo site 48 hours after dermabrasion. Note that the dermabrasion is very superficial and that the pigment remains. *B,* Tattoo site dressing 48 hours after dermabrasion showing the amount of pigment deposited. *C,* Tattoo site two months after one full dermabrasion with a second touch-up dermabrasion. (Courtesy of Dr. W. Clabaugh. From Epstein, E.: Skin Surgery, 4th Ed., 1970. Courtesy of Charles C Thomas, Publisher, Springfield, IL.)

the argon laser could be used for decorative tattoo removal. They noted scar formation, including keloids, and their experience demonstrated that dermabrasion remained the treatment of choice for removal of decorative tattoos. Laser treatment of tattoos is also discussed in Chapter 75.

REFERENCES

Alkek, D. S., Johnson, W. C., and Graham, J. H.: Granular cell myoblastoma. Arch. Dermatol., 98:543, 1968.

Allington, H. V.: Review of psychotherapy of warts. Arch. Dermatol. Syph., 66:316, 1952.

Almeida, J. D., Hawatson, A. F., and Williams, M. G.: Electron microscope study of human warts. J. Invest. Dermatol., 38:337, 1962.

Andrade, R.: Precancerous and cancerous lesions of the epidermis and its appendages. Handbuch Haut Geschlechts Krankheiten, 1:344, 1964.

Andrade, R.: Personal communication, 1971.

Baer, R. L., and Kopf, A. W.: Keratoacanthoma. Year Book of Dermatology. Chicago, IL, Year Book Medical Publishers, 1962–63, p. 7.

Baer, R. L., and Witten, V. H.: Year Book of Dermatology and Syphilology (editorial comment on article, Strawberry Hemangiomas: Natural History of Untreated Lesion by A. H. Jacobs). Chicago, IL, Year Book Medical Publishers, 1957–58, p. 325.

Baer, R. L., and Witten, V. H.: Editorial comment on extramammary Paget's disease with metastasis to lymph nodes, by Prose, P. H., and Hyman, A. B. (Arch. Dermatol., 80:398, 1959). In Year Book of Dermatology, Chicago, IL, Year Book Medical Publishers, 1959–60, p. 164.

Bailin, P. L., Ratz, J. L., and Levine, H. L.: Removal of tattoos by CO_2 laser. J. Dermatol. Surg. Oncol., 6:997, 1980.

Bart, R. S.: X-Ray Therapy of Skin Cancer. Sixth National Cancer Conference Proceedings. Philadelphia, J. B. Lippincott Company, 1970, pp. 559–569.

Bart, R. S.: Personal communication, 1971.

Bart, R. S.: Bowenoid papulosis of the chin. J. Dermatol. Surg. Oncol., 10:821, 1984.

Bean, W. B.: A note on the development of cutaneous arterial "spiders" and palmar erythema in persons with liver disease and their development following the administration of estrogens. Am. J. Med. Sci., 204:251, 1942.

Bean, W. B.: Vascular Spiders and Related Lesions of the Skin. Springfield, IL, Charles C Thomas, 1958.

Beare, J. M.: Histiocytic proliferative disorders. In Rook, A., Wilkinson, D. S., and Ehling, F. J. G. (Eds.): Textbook of Dermatology. Vol. 2. Oxford, Blackwell Scientific Publications, 1968.

Bendel, B. J., and Graham, J. H.: Solar keratosis with squamous cell carcinoma—a clinico-pathologic, histochemical study. Sixth National Cancer Conference Proceedings. Philadelphia, J. B. Lippincott Company, 1970, pp. 471–488.

Blank, H., and Rake, G.: Viral and Rickettsial Diseases. Boston, Little, Brown & Company, 1955, pp. 160, 163, 171.

Blau, S., and Hyman, A. B.: Erythroplasia of Queyrat. Acta Derm. Venereol., 35:341, 1955.

Bloch, B.: Über die Heilung der Warzen durch Suggestion. Klin. Wochenschr., 6:2271, 1927.

Boo-Chai, K.: The decorative tattoo: its removal by dermabrasion. Plast. Reconstr. Surg., 32:559, 1963.

Bowers, R. E., Graham, E. A., and Tomlinson, K. M.: Natural history of strawberry nevus. Arch. Dermatol., 82:667, 1960.

Breathnach, A. S., and Wyllie, L. M.: Electron microscopy of melanocytes and melanosomes in freckled human epidermis. J. Invest. Dermatol., 42:389, 1964.

Broders, A. C.: Squamous cell epithelioma of the lip; a study of 537 cases. J.A.M.A., 74:656, 1920.

Brues, A. M.: Linkage of body build with sex, eye color, and freckling. Am. J. Hum. Genet., 2:215, 1950.

Bureau, Y., Barriere, H., Litoux, P., and Bureau, R.: L'angiome geant thrombopeniant (syndrome de Kasabachet Merritt). Ann. Dermatol. Syphiligr. (Paris), 94:5, 1967.

Cave, V. G., Kopf, A. W., and Kerdel-Vegas, F.: Multiple myoblastomas in children. Arch. Dermatol., 71:579, 1955.

Cawley, E. P.: Genetic aspects of malignant melanoma. Arch. Dermatol., 65:440, 1952.

Champion, R. H., and Wilkinson, D. S.: Disorders affecting blood vessels. In Rook, A., Wilkinson, D. S., and Ebling, F. J. G. (Eds.): Textbook of Dermatology. Vol. 1. Oxford, Blackwell Scientific Publications, 1968.

Clabaugh, W.: Removal of tattoos by superficial dermabrasion. Arch. Dermatol., 98:515, 1968.

Clark, W. H., Jr., Reimer, R. R., Greene, M. H., et al.: Origin of familial malignant melanoma from heritable melanocytic lesions. "The B-K mole syndrome." Arch. Dermatol., 114:732, 1978.

Cleaver, J. E.: DNA, damage and repair in light sensitive human skin disease. J. Invest. Dermatol., 54:181, 1970.

Cleaver, J. E., and Trosko, J. E.: Xeroderma pigmentosum: a human disease defective in an initial stage of DNA repair. Proceed. Natl. Acad. Sci. Cited in editorial in J.A.M.A., 210:2390, 1969.

Collins, C. G., Hausen, L. H., and Theriot, E.: A clinical stain for use in selecting biopsy site in patients with vulvar disease. Obstet. Gynecol., 28:158, 1966.

Constant, E., Royer, J. R., Pollard, R. J., Larsen, R. D., and Posch, J. L.: Mucous cysts of the fingers. Plast. Reconstr. Surg., 43:241, 1969.

Cox, A. J., and Walton, R. A.: The induction of junctional changes in pigmented nevi. Arch. Pathol., 79:429, 1965.

Crittenden, F. M.: Salabrasion removal of tattoos by superficial abrasion with table salt. Cutis, 7:295, 1971.

Crum, C. P., Ikenberg, H., Richart, R. M., and Gissman, L.: Human papillomavirus type 16 and early cervical neoplasia. N. Engl. J. Med., 310:880, 1984.

Dillaha, C. J., Jansen, G. T., Honeycutt, W. M., and Bradford, A. C.: Selective cytotoxic effect of topical 5-fluorouracil. Arch. Dermatol., 88:247, 1963.

Dixon, S. L.: The dysplastic nevus syndrome. A review. J. Assoc. Milit. Dermatol., 10:3, 1983.

Doppman, J. L., Wirth, F. P., Jr., DiChiro, G., and Ommaya, A. K.: Value of cutaneous angiomas in the arteriographic localization of spinal cord arteriovenous malformations. N. Engl. J. Med., 281:1440, 1969.

Dorsey, C. S., and Montgomery, H.: Blue nevus and its distinction from mongolian spots and the nevus of ota. J. Invest. Dermatol., 22:225, 1954.

Duperrat, B.: Suppurations folliculaires torpides sous les nevi mélaniques. Ann. Dermatol. Syphiligr. (Paris), 81:251, 1954.

Eaglestein, W. H., Weinstein, G. D., and Frost, P.:

Fluorouracil: mechanism of action in human skin and actinic keratoses. Arch. Dermatol., *101*:132, 1970.

Eliassow, A., and Frank, S. B.: Pathogenesis of synovial lesions of the skin. Arch. Dermatol. Syph., *46*:691, 1942.

Epstein, W. L., and Kligman, A. M.: The pathogenesis of milia and benign tumors of the skin. J. Invest. Dermatol., *26*:1, 1956.

Epstein, W. L., and Kligman, A. M.: Treatment of warts with cantharidin. Arch. Dermatol., 77:508, 1958.

Fitzpatrick, T. B., Parrish, J. A., Haynes, H. A., and Gonzalez, E. (Eds.): Identification of precusors to malignant melanoma. Dermatologic Capsule and Comment, 6·1, 1984.

Frank, S. B., and Cohen, H. J.: The halo nevus. Arch. Dermatol., *89*:367, 1964.

Freeman, R. G., and Knox, J. M.: Epidermal cysts associated with pigmented nevi. Arch. Dermatol., *85*:590, 1962.

Freeman, R. G., Knox, J. M., and Heaton, C. L.: The treatment of skin cancer. Cancer, *17*:535, 1964.

Friedman, R. J., Heilman, E. R., Rigel, D. S., and Kopf, A. W.: The dysplastic nevus: clinical and pathologic features. Dermatol. Clin., *3*:239, 1985.

Friedman, R. J., Rigel, D. S., and Kopf, A. W.: Early detection of malignant melanoma: the role of physician examination and self-examination of the skin. CA, *35*:130, 1985.

Gamboa, L. G.: Malignant granular cell myoblastoma. A.M.A. Arch. Pathol., *60*:663, 1955.

Gladstein, A.: Personal communication, 1970.

Goldschmidt, H., and Kligman, A. M.: Experimental inoculation of humans with ectodermotropic viruses. J. Invest. Dermatol., *31*:175, 1958.

Gorlin, R. J., Yunis, J. J., and Tuna, N.: Multiple nevoid basal cell carcinoma, odontogenic keratocysts and skeletal anomalies: a syndrome. Acta Derm. Venereol., *93*:39, 1963.

Graham, J. H., and Helwig, E. B.: Bowen's disease and its relationship to systemic cancer. Arch. Dermatol., *80*:133, 1959.

Graham, J. H., and Helwig, E. B.: Precancerous skin lesions and systemic cancer. *In* Tumors of the Skin. Chicago, Year Book Medical Publishers, 1964, p. 209.

Gray, H. R., and Helwig, E. B.: Epithelioma adenoides cysticum and solitary trichoepithelioma. Arch. Dermatol., *87*:102, 1963.

Greeley, P. W., Middleton, A. G., and Curtin, J. W.: Incidence of malignancy in giant pigmented nevi. Plast. Reconstr. Surg., *36*:26, 1965.

Greene, M. H.: The dysplastic nevus syndrome. The Melanoma Letter. Skin Cancer Foundation, *1*(1):2, 1982.

Greene, M. H., Clark, W. H., Jr., Tucker, M. A., Elder, D. E., Kraemer, K. H., et al.: Acquired precursors of cutaneous malignant melanoma. The familial dysplastic nevus syndrome. N. Engl. J. Med., *312*:91, 1985.

Guillet, G. Y., Braun, L., Massé, R., Aftimos, J., Geniaux, M., and Texier, L.: Bowenoid papulosis. Demonstration of human papillomavirus (HPV) with anti-HPV immune serum. Arch. Dermatol., *120*:514, 1984.

Haber, H.: Verrucous nevi. Trans. St. John's Hosp. Dermatol. Soc., *34*:20, 1955.

Haber, H.: Some observations in common moles. Br. J. Dermatol., *79*:224, 1962.

Hairston, M. A., Jr., Reed, R. J., and Derbes, V. J.: Dermatosis papulosa nigra. Arch. Dermatol., *89*:655, 1964.

Hashimoto, K., Gross, B. G., and Lever, W. F.: Syrin-goma: histochemical and electron microscope studies. J. Invest. Dermatol., *46*:150, 1966.

Hashimoto, K., and Lever, W. F.: Eccrine poroma: histochemical and electron microscopic studies. J. Invest. Dermatol., *43*:237, 1964.

Hashimoto, K., Nelson, R. G., and Lever, W. F.: Calcifying epithelioma of Malherbe. J. Invest. Dermatol., *46*:391, 1966.

Heinlein, J. A.: Personal communication, 1970.

Howell, J. B., and Caro, M. R.: Basal cell nevus: its relationship to multiple cutaneous cancers and associated anomalies of development. Arch. Dermatol., *79*:67, 1959.

Huyt, K. M.: Multicentric pigmented Bowen's disease. Arch. Dermatol., *101*:48, 1970.

Hyman, A.: Personal communication, 1970.

Imperial, R., and Helwig, E. B.: Verrucous hemangioma. Arch. Dermatol., *96*:247, 1967.

Jackson, R., Williamson, G. S., and Beattie, W. G.: Lentigo maligna and malignant melanoma. Can. Med. Assoc. J., *195*:346, 1966.

Jacobs, A. H.: Strawberry hemangiomas: natural history of untreated lesions. Calif. Med., *86*:8, 1957.

Johnson, W. C., Graham, J. H., and Helwig, E. B.: Cutaneous myxoid cyst: clinicopathologic and histochemical study. J.A.M.A., *191*:15, 1965.

Kalkoff, K., and Macher, E.: Zur Histogenese des Keratoalkanthoms. Hautarzt, *12*:8, 1961.

Keller, R.: Clinical and histologic features of senile angioma. Dermatologica, *114*:345, 1957.

King, O. H., Jr.: Intraoral leukoplakia. Cancer, *17*:131, 1964.

Klein, E., and Holtermann, D. A.: Immunotherapeutic approaches to the management of neoplasms. Natl. Cancer Inst. Monogr., *35*:379, 1972.

Knox, J. M.: Comments made during Cutaneous Tumor Panel Discussion at Academy of Dermatology Meeting, Chicago, 1968.

Kopf, A. W., and Andrade, R. A.: A histologic study of the dermoepidermal junction in clinically "intradermal" nevi employing serial sections. Ann. N.Y. Acad. Sci., *100*:200, 1963.

Kopf, A. W., and Andrade, R.: Benign juvenile melanoma. *In* Year Book of Dermatology. Chicago, Year Book Medical Publishers, 1965–66, p. 7.

Kopf, A. W., and Bart, R. S.: Multiple bowenoid papules of the penis: a new entity? Tumor Conference 11. J. Dermatol. Surg. Oncol., *3*:265, 1977.

Kopf, A. W., Bart, R. S., and Gladstein, A. H.: Treatment of melanotic freckle with x-rays. Arch. Dermatol., *112*:801, 1976.

Kopf, A. W., Morrill, S. D., and Silverberg, I.: Broad spectrum of leukoderma acquisitum centrifugum. Arch. Dermatol., *92*:14, 1965.

Kwittken, J., and Negri, L.: Malignant blue nevus. Arch. Dermatol., *94*:64, 1966.

Landthaler, M., Haina, D., Waidelich, W., and Braun-Falco, O.: A three year experience with the argon laser in dermatotherapy. J. Dermatol. Surg. Oncol., *10*:456, 1984.

Lattanand, A., Johnson, W. C., and Graham, J. H.: Mucous cyst (mucocele): a clinicopathologic and histochemical study. Arch. Dermatol., *101*:637, 1970.

Lerner, M. R., and Lerner, A. B.: Dermatologic Medications. Chicago, Year Book Medical Publishers, 1960, p. 181.

Lever, W. F.: Histopathology of the Skin. 3rd Ed. Philadelphia, J. B. Lippincott Company, 1961; 4th Ed., 1967; 5th Ed., 1975.

Lieblich, L., M., Geronemus, R. A., and Gibbs, R. C.: Use of a biopsy punch for removal of epithelial cysts. J. Dermatol. Surg. Oncol., 8:1059, 1982.

Litzow, T. J., and Engel, S.: Multiple basal cell epitheliomas arising in linear nevus. Am. J. Surg., 101:378, 1961.

Love, W. R., and Montgomery, H.: Epithelial cysts. Arch. Dermatol. Syph., 47:85, 1943.

Lund, H. Z.: How often does squamous cell carcinoma of the skin metastasize? Arch. Dermatol., 92:635, 1965.

Lund, R. H., and Ihnen, M.: Malignant melanoma: clinical and pathologic analysis of 93 cases. Surgery, 38:652, 1965.

Lutzner, M. A.: Molluscum contagiosum verruca and zoster viruses. Arch. Dermatol., 87:436, 1963.

Lutzner, M. A.: The human papillomaviruses: a review (editorial). Arch. Dermatol., 119:631, 1983.

Maize, J. C., and Ackerman, A. B.: Pigmented Lesions of the Skin. Clinicopathologic Correlations. Philadelphia, Lea & Febiger, 1987.

Masson, P.: Les naevi pigmentaires tumerus nerveuses. Ann. Anat. Pathol., 3:417, 657, 1926.

Mehregan, A. H., and Pinkus, H.: Life history of organoid nevi. Arch. Dermatol., 91:574, 1965.

Miescher, G.: Präcanceröses Vorstadium des Melanoms, präcanceröse Melanose. In Jadassohn, J. (Ed.): Handbuch der Haut und Geschlechts Krankheiten. Vol. 12, Part 3, Geschwulste der Haut II. Berlin, Springer-Verlag, 1928.

Mishima, Y.: Cellular and subcellular differentiation of melanin phagocytosis and synthesis by lysosomal and melanosomal activity. J. Invest. Dermatol., 46:70, 1966.

Mustalko, K. K.: Succinic dehydrogenase activities of syringomas. Acta Derm. Venereol., 39:318, 1959.

Nagington, J., and Rook, A.: Virus and related infection. In Rook, A., Wilkinson, R. S., and Ebling, J. (Eds.): Textbook of Dermatology. 3rd Ed. Oxford, Blackwell Scientific Publications, 1979, pp. 626–627.

National Institutes of Health: Precursors to Malignant Melanomas, Consensus Development Conference Summary. U.S. Dept. of Health and Human Services, Public Health Service, Bethesda, MD. Vol. 4, No. 9, 1984, U.S. Govt. Printing Office.

Norden, G. von., and Maumenee, A. E.: Stimulus-deprivation amblyopia. Am. J. Ophthalmol., 165:220, 1968.

Oriel, J. P.: Genital warts, what kind of association with cervical cancer? Sex. Transm. Dis. (Bull.), 4:2, 1984.

Penneys, N. S., Mogallon, R. J., Madji, M., and Gault, E.: Papillomavirus common antigens. Arch. Dermatol., 120:859, 1984.

Petratos, M. D., Kopf, A. W., Bart, R. S., Grieswood, E. N., and Gladstein, A. H.: Treatment of melanotic freckle with x-rays. Arch. Dermatol., 106:189, 1972.

Pindborg, J. J.: Disease of the oral cavity and lips. In Rook, A., Wilkinson, S. D., and Ehling, F. J. G. (Eds.): Textbook of Dermatology. 2nd Ed. Oxford, Blackwell Scientific Publications, 1972.

Pinkus, H.: The borderline between cancer and non-cancer. In Year Book of Dermatology. Chicago, Year Book Medical Publishers, 1966–67, p. 5.

Pitman, G. H., Kopf, A. W., Bart, R. S., and Casson, P. R.: Treatment of lentigo maligna and lentigo maligna melanoma. J. Dermatol. Surg. Oncol., 5:727, 1979.

Pitman, G. H., McCarthy, J. G., Perzin, K. H., and Herter, F. P.: Extramammary Paget's disease. Plast. Reconstr. Surg., 69:238, 1982.

Popkin, G. L.: Curettage and electrodesiccation. N.Y. Stage J. Med., 68:866, 1968.

Popkin, G. L., Brodie, S. J., Hyman, A.B., Andrade, R., and Kopf, A. W.: Technique of biopsy recommended for keroacanthoma. Arch. Dermatol., 94:191, 1966.

Raab, W., and Steigleder, G. K.: Fehldiagnosen bei Horngsten. Arch. Klin. Exp. Derm., 212:606, 1961.

Rhodes, A.: Neoplasms: benign neoplasias, hyperplasias, and dysplasias of melanocytes. In Fitzpatrick, T. B., Eisen, A. Z., Wolf, K., Freedberg, I. M., and Austin, K. F. (Eds.): Dermatology in General Medicine. New York, McGraw-Hill Book Company, 1987.

Rhodes, A. F., Harrist, T. J., Day, C. L., Mihm, M. C., Fitzpatrick, T. B., and Sober, A. J.: Dysplastic melanocytic nevi in histologic association with 234 primary cutaneous melanomas. J. Am. Acad. Dermatol., 9:563, 1983.

Robinson, J. K.: Tattoo removal. J. Dermatol. Surg. Oncol., 11:14, 1985.

Rodriquez, H. A., and Ackerman, L. U.: Cellular blue nevus. Cancer, 21:393, 1968.

Ronchese, R.: Keratoses, cancer and "the sign of lesser Trélat." Cancer, 18:1003, 1965.

Rook, A.: Naevi and other developmental defects and virus infections. In Rook, A. J., Wilkinson, D. S., and Ebling, F. J. G. (Eds.): Textbook of Dermatology. Vol. I. Oxford, Blackwell Scientific Publications, 1968, Chaps. 6, 24.

Rook, A.: Naevi and other developmental defects. In Rook, A., Wilkinson, D. S., and Ebling, F. J. A. (Eds.): Textbook of Dermatology. Vol. 1. Oxford, Blackwell Scientific Publications, 1979.

Sanderson, K. V.: The structure of seborrhoeic keratoses. Br. J. Dermatol., 80:588, 1968a.

Sanderson, K. V.: Malignant and premalignant lesions in diseases of the perianal and genital region; and Tumors of the skin. In Rook, A. J., Wilkinson, D. S., and Ebling, F. J. G. (Eds.): Textbook of Dermatology. Vol. 2. Oxford, Blackwell Scientific Publications, 1968b, Chaps. 52, 57.

Shaffer, B.: A clinical appraisal of pigmented nevi in the light of present day histopathologic concepts. Arch. Dermatol., 72:120, 1955.

Shear, M.: The histogenesis of the so-called "granular cell myoblastoma." J. Pathol. Bacteriol., 80:225, 1960.

Silverman, S.: Dialogues in dermatology. Excepts quoted in Dermatol. Pract., 3:2, 1970.

Spitz, S.: Melanomas of chilldhood. Am. J. Pathol., 24:591, 1948.

Steward, E. E., Mack, W. N., and Foy, R. B.: Demonstration of human papoviruses in wart tissue by electrophoresis. Lab. Invest., 19:40, 1968.

Sutton, R. L., and Sutton, R. L., Jr.: Handbook of Diseases of the Skin. St. Louis, MO, C. V. Mosby Company, 1949, p. 627.

Sweet, R. D.: The treatment of basal cell carcinoma by curettage. Br. J. Dermatol., 75:137, 1963.

Torre, D.: Personal communications, 1970.

Van der Harst, L. C. A.: Three cases of Klippel-Trenaunay osteohypertrophic varicose nevus. Ann. Dermatol. Syphiligr., 78:315, 1951.

Wade, T. R., Kopf, A. W., and Ackerman, A. B.: Bowenoid papulosis of the genitalia. Arch. Dermatol., 115:306, 1979.

Wallace, H. J.: Vulvar leukoplakia. Br. J. Obstet. Gynaecol. 69:865, 1962.

Wallace, H. J., and Whimster, I. W.: Vulvar atrophy and leukoplakia. Br. J. Dermatol., 63:241, 1951.

Wayte, D. M., and Helwig, E. B.: Halo nevi. Cancer, 22:69, 1968.

Wilkinson, D. S.: Disease of the perianal and genital

regions. *In* Rook, A., Wilkinson, D. S., and Ehling, F. J. G. (Eds.): Textbook of Dermatology. Vol. 2. 2nd Ed. Oxford, Blackwell Scientific Publishers, 1972.

Wilson, C. W., Jones, E. W., and Heyl, T.: Nevus sebaceous: a report of 140 cases with special regard to the development of secondary malignant tumours. Br. J. Dermatol., *82*:99, 1970.

Winkelmann, R. K., and Mueller, S. A.: Sweat gland tumors. Arch. Dermatol., *89*:827, 1964.

Yannowitz, M., and Goldstein, M.: Basal cell epithelioma overlying a dermatofibroma. Arch. Dermatol., *87*:709, 1964.

Zacarian, S. A.: Cryosurgery of Skin Cancer. Springfield, IL, Charles C Thomas, 1969.

Zachow, K. R., Ostrow, R. S., Bender, M., et al.: Detection of human papillomavirus DNA in anogenital neoplasms. Nature, *300*:771, 1982.

Zackheim, H. S., Howell, J. B., and Loud, A. U.: Nevoid basal cell carcinoma syndrome: some histologic observations in cutaneous lesions. Arch. Dermatol., *93*:317, 1966.

74

Phillip R. Casson
Perry Robins

Malignant Tumors of the Skin

The common malignant tumors of the skin, basal cell and squamous cell carcinoma, are, for practical purposes, diseases of Caucasoid populations and, when seen in pigmented races, are associated with unusual etiologic factors and anatomic sites. Basal cell carcinoma is more frequently seen, with a preponderance in the 3:1 or 4:1 range, depending on the latitude. These tumors share many features and have a similar cause, distribution, and age incidence. Melanoma is also a skin tumor of Caucasoids, and, when it affects dark-skinned people, is located predominantly on the foot.

The less common malignant skin tumors have neither specific etiologic factors nor a demonstrable racial predilection; they include adnexal skin tumors, hemangioendotheliosarcoma, leiomyosarcoma, dermatofibrosarcoma, Merkel's cell tumor, and atypical fibroxanthoma. These rare tumors are not easily diagnosed on clinical grounds, and they have an unpredictable prognosis. Their management is based on precise clinical findings and the pathologic features of representative biopsy specimens.

BASAL CELL CARCINOMA

This skin cancer is considered to arise from pluripotential cells of the epidermis (Kint, 1976). The typical cells have a deep-staining nucleus and are ovoid in shape, resembling the cells of the basal layer of the epidermis (hence the name).

It is the most common skin cancer and occurs almost exclusively in people of European descent; when seen in members of the pigmented races, it is associated with predisposing conditions such as nevus sebaceus, albinism, or xeroderma pigmentosum.

In subtropical countries that have received several waves of immigrants from Europe in the past 200 years, the incidence of basal cell carcinoma is extremely high. For example, in Queensland, Australia, an incidence of 265 cases per 100,000 population per year has been recorded, a rate ten times the incidence in South-West England where a similar ethnic population exists (Gordon and Silverstone, 1976).

Etiologic Factors

The primary cause of basal cell carcinoma is exposure to ultraviolet (UV) radiation derived from sunlight, although the evidence remains circumstantial. It also occurs in association with specific disease entities such as the basal cell nevus syndrome, xeroderma pigmentosum, and nevus sebaceus. It may be observed in epidermodysplasia verruciformis and Gardner's syndrome.

Ultraviolet Radiation. Ultraviolet radiation is arbitrarily divided into three wave bands: (1) UVA, from 320 to 400 nm; (2) UVB, from 290 to 320 nm; and (3) UVC, from 200 to 290 nm. UVC is filtered out by the ozone layer of the atmosphere, but it may become a factor if ozone depletion continues; it may also be encountered from artificial sources. The UVB band is involved in sunburn, chronic sun damage, and skin cancer carcinogenesis (Kelner and Taft, 1956). UVA is less obvious in its effects but is thought to be additive to the adverse effects of UVB on the skin (Pathak, Fitzpatrick, and Parrish, 1982). It is the principal wavelength generated by tanning salon sunlamps, the use of which is controversial and should certainly be avoided by people with a known sensitivity to the sun.

The skin of Caucasians, in particular those of Celtic origin, is sensitive to the long-term effects of ultraviolet radiation. Those with fair skin, blue eyes, and blond to red hair may respond to such exposure by the development of hyperkeratoses and solar keratoses at an early age; they may also develop basal cell carcinoma and squamous cell carcinoma despite minimal sun exposure. It should be emphasized that the Mediterranean races are not immune to the effects of the sun, and they also develop these forms of skin cancer.

The changes induced in the epidermal cells that stimulate the onset of tumor metamorphosis are the result of a direct effect on cellular DNA, as determined in cell cultures (Cleaver, 1968). Adjacent pyrimidines in DNA link together to form dimers; these in turn block the normal DNA resynthesis process, the extent of the interference being dependent on the UV wavelength and exposure time (Carrier, Snyder, and Regan, 1982). It appears that the combination of cell damage and imperfect repair leads to cell mutation and ultimately carcinomatous changes.

Ultraviolet radiation also serves as an additive factor in the production of basal cell carcinoma when it is a sequel to radiation dermatitis, xeroderma pigmentosum, or posttransplant immunosuppression.

Exposure to Radiation. Before the longterm effects of x-ray therapy were recognized, various forms of radiation therapy were used for a variety of benign conditions, from hemangioma in all its variants to female hirsutism, acne, and fungus infections. Only years later was it noted that radiation dermatitis could progress to the development of basal cell carcinoma and squamous cell carcinoma in some people (Fig. 74–1).

Experience with 361 patients with skin cancer after radiation therapy, which was administered mainly for benign conditions, was reported. Sixty-three per cent of the tumors observed were basal cell cancer, most of the remainder being squamous cell lesions. A relatively low cure rate of basal cell carcinoma (only 60 per cent) was achieved (Martin, Strong, and Spiro, 1970). This condition is rarely seen now. However, these patients required careful observation for the remainder of their lives, and they were advised to avoid sun exposure, as this further insult aggravated their problem. Benefit was obtained from the excision and grafting of unstable areas of radiation-induced dermatitis as a preventive measure. It was also noted that neoplasms developed at the site of radiation therapy for other forms of cancer.

Another group exposed to repeated small doses of x-rays were medical personnel unaware of the dangers; they also developed radiation dermatitis, which frequently progressed to a neoplasm after a latent period of many years (Conway and Hugo, 1966). The most frequent site for this type of skin tumor was the hands (Hartwell, Huger, and Pickrell, 1964).

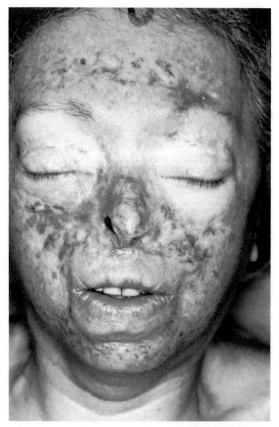

Figure 74–1. A 58 year old woman with radiation dermatitis of the face after being given superficial x-ray treatments for acne as a teenager. Several basal cell carcinomas had been excised previously.

Basal Cell Nevus Syndrome. This disease was first described as a clinical entity by Howell and Caro in 1959. It has three essential components: (1) multiple basal cell nevi of the skin (Fig. 74–2), (2) jaw cysts, and (3) small pits in the skin of the palms and soles (the pink palmar pits). Other anomalies observed are pseudohypertelorism, frontal bossing, syndactyly, spina bifida, and neurologic disorders.

It is a hereditary disease, transmitted as an autosomal dominant trait without sex linkage, and most individuals who inherit the gene show evidence of the syndrome to some degree (Anderson and associates, 1967). Spontaneous mutation may occur. The skin tumors that are observed in children are clinically benign until the onset of puberty, and they vary in number from a few to hundreds. After the disease is diagnosed, careful and frequent observation is essential. The age of onset of demonstrable malignancy is variable, and, when malignancy develops, the clinical behavior is similar to that of basal cell carcinoma in the normal person. Each lesion must be treated as it develops or control of the disease will be lost (Howell, Anderson, and McClendon, 1964). Metastatic disease has been described in lymph nodes and lungs in individuals with the syndrome (Taylor and associates, 1968; Winkler and Guyuron, 1987). The jaw cysts, which are odontogenic keratocycts, may required treatment if they become symptomatic.

Xeroderma Pigmentosum. This is a systemic disease that occurs primarily as a skin condition. It was first recognized by Kaposi (1872), who emphasized the poor prognosis and reported a death from metastasis. It is a rare genetic disease transmitted via an incomplete sex-linked recessive gene (El-Hefnawi, El-Nabawi, and Rasheed, 1962). Individuals with the gene exhibit extreme sensitivity to sunlight from an early age. In addition, there are a number of associated metabolic abnormalities, which include elevation of serum copper and gamma globulin levels (El-Hefnawi, El-Nebawi, and El-Ha-

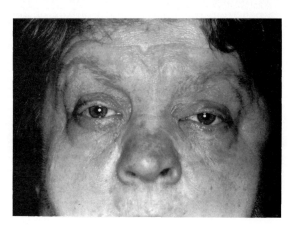

Figure 74–2. The facial appearance of a patient with basal cell nevus syndrome with pseudohypertelorism and the typical nevi. The patient also has palmar skin pits. The disease in this patient was relatively nonaggressive.

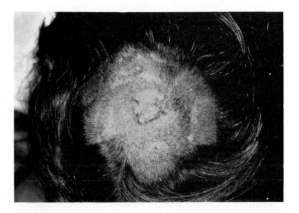

Figure 74–3. Nevus sebaceus of the scalp. It is yellowish, non-hair bearing, and elevated above the surrounding skin.

wary, 1962). There is an increased excretion of urinary amino acids and a decreased excretion of 17-ketosteroids and 17-hydroxycorticosteroids (El-Hefnawi and associates, 1963). The disease commences in early childhood; clinical signs include an unusual sensitivity to sun exposure with diffuse freckling initially, followed by progressive drying and thinning of the skin. Keratoses subsequently develop, and, by early adult life, malignant changes in the skin occur: basal cell carcinoma, squamous cell carcinoma, or melanoma. The disease is unpredictable, the commonest form exhibiting multiple tumors on the exposed surfaces of the body and ocular symptoms. Death eventually occurs as a result of metastatic disease, although a few long-term survivors have been observed. Management consists of absolute protection from sun exposure, constant observation, and early, aggressive treatment of skin tumors as they occur. Prolongation of life has been reported with this regime (Woolf and associates, 1959; Pickrell, 1972). Laboratory research using fibroblast tissue cultures from affected individuals has demonstrated the defective DNA repair considered to occur with ultraviolet light exposure (Cleaver, 1968).

Albinism. The various forms of albinism are inherited disorders. The most common, oculocutaneous albinism, is characterized by hypomelanosis of the skin, the hair, and the eyes; it is a predisposing factor in the occurrence of the skin cancer in affected individuals. Albinos of European origin are able to keep the incidence of skin cancer relatively low with avoidance of sun exposure and the use of protective sun creams. However, the occurrence of albinism in the pigmented races is of more serious import. In the Bantu with the condition, a high incidence of squamous cell carcinoma is noted on exposed surfaces, basal cell carcinoma being less common (Oettlé, 1964). In areas where inbreeding occurs the incidence of albinism may be extremely high, as observed in the Cuna Indians on the San Blas islands of Panama (Bleehen and Ebling, 1986).

Nevus Sebaceus. Nevus sebaceus (nevus of Jadassohn) is a superficial skin lesion present either at birth or in early childhood. Its extent varies, with most lesions being 2 to 3 cm in size; the shape is irregular. It is most common in the head and neck area. The appearance is diagnostic, the lesion being elevated above the surrounding skin by 1 to 2 mm with an irregular verrucoid surface, which is yellow to pinkish in color; it is non-hair bearing in the scalp and beard area (Fig. 74–3). Basal cell carcinoma may develop in the skin lesion (Fig. 74–4), a 6.4 per cent incidence being reported in an unselected series of 140 cases in England (Jones and Heyl, 1970) and 15 per cent by Mehregan and Pinkus (1965). Excision is recommended both for aesthetic reasons and for the prevention of basal cell carcinoma.

Immunosuppression. Organ transplant recipients managed by conventional immunosuppressive therapy (azathioprine, prednisone, and antilymphocytic globulin) have an increased risk of developing a variety of malignant tumors (Marshall, 1973; Penn, 1975). Skin and lip cancer composed 40 per cent of the tumors recorded at the Cincinnati Transplant Tumor Registry; squamous cell carcinoma predominated, constituting more than 50 per cent of the total, followed in frequency by basal carcinoma and melanoma (Penn, 1987). Multiple tumors are often observed, and sun exposure and the duration of therapy are factors that appear to increase the inci-

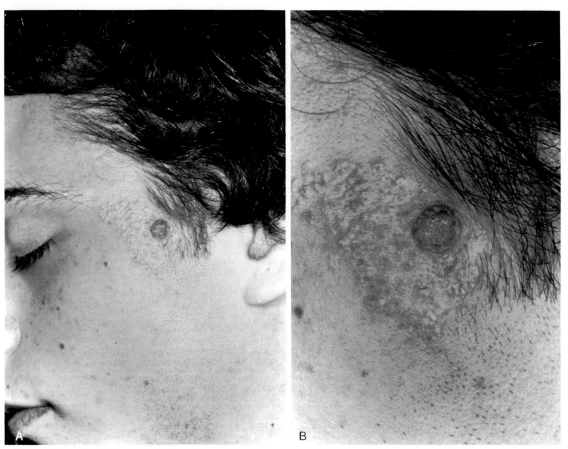

Figure 74–4. *A, B,* Nevus sebaceus of the temporal skin in a 17 year old male patient. A nodule had appeared four months prior to presentation, which was determined to be basal cell carcinoma.

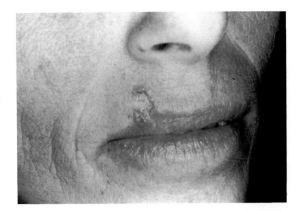

Figure 74–5. Superficial basal cell carcinoma of the upper lip.

dence (Sheil, 1977; Boyle and associates, 1984). The use of cyclosporin as the primary immunosuppressive drug is changing this aspect of organ transplantation; the incidence of skin tumors is more recently reported as 16 per cent (Penn, 1988).

The exact cause of the substantially increased tumor incidence with immunosuppression, up to ten times that in the normal population, may be postulated as a depression of the cellular immune system or perhaps a direct effect on DNA itself. The organ transplant recipient must be under close observation. Biopsy of any suspicious lesion is performed, as many other skin lesions such as warts and keratoacanthoma are also seen in this group of patients (Penn, 1979).

Trauma. The occurrence of basal cell carcinoma in scar tissue is rare but well documented and suggests that previous injury may be a predisposing factor. It has been described in chronic leg ulcers (Burns and Calnan, 1978), vaccination scars (Hazelrigg, 1978), and even tattoos (Earley, 1983).

Clinical Features

The typical basal cell carcinoma is a palpable tumor that is elevated above the level of the skin. It has pearly, translucent edges; telangiectasia is noted on close examination. It may vary from erythematous to violaceous and is occasionally pigmented. It may occur anywhere on the body but is most common on the exposed skin surfaces of the face (Fig. 74–5) and the anterior chest.

This skin tumor may mimic any lesion from psoriasis to a sebaceous cyst. Biopsy of virtually all skin lesions is advisable for identification before treatment. An exception may be the small superficial lesion (less than 3 mm in diameter), which may be excised with direct primary closure or removed by a scalpel shave excision without a preliminary biopsy.

Lever (1975) listed seven clinical types of basal cell carcinoma, based on gross appearance:

1. *Noduloulcerative basal cell carcinoma.* It begins as a small waxy nodule that often

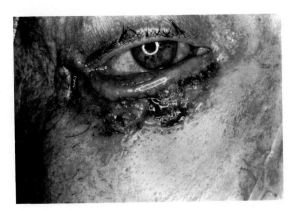

Figure 74–6. Example of a localized invasive basal cell carcinoma of the lower eyelid with a four year history. There is minimal peripheral extension.

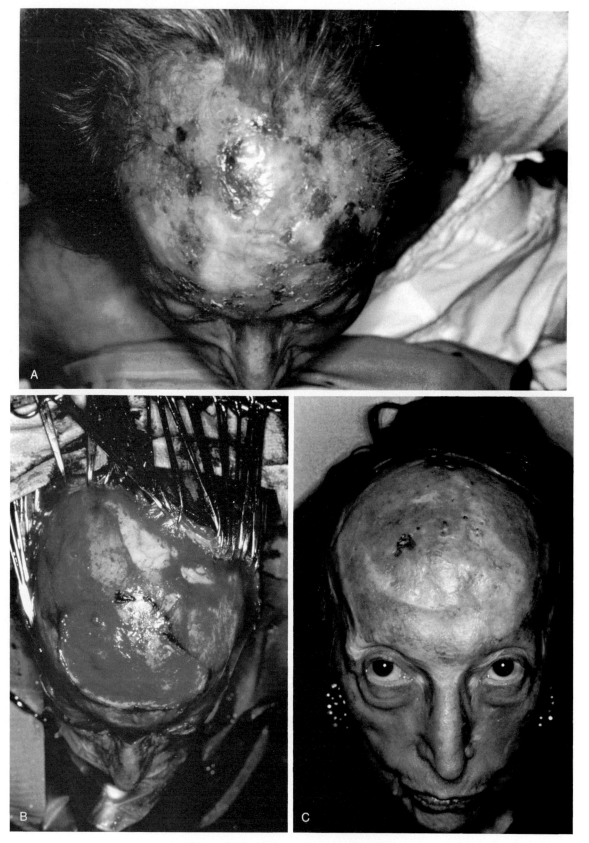

Figure 74–7. *See legend on opposite page*

shows on its surface a few small telangiectatic vessels. The nodule usually increases slowly in size and undergoes central ulceration. A typical lesion consists of a slowly enlarging ulcer surrounded by a pearly, rolled border. This category is by far the most common type and includes the "rodent ulcer."

2. *Pigmented basal cell carcinoma.* This lesion differs from the noduloulcerative type only by its irregular brown pigmentation.

3. *Morphea-like or fibrosing basal cell carcinoma.* It is manifest as a slightly elevated, firm, yellowish plaque with an ill-defined border, over which the skin remains intact for a long time before ulceration occurs.

4. *Superficial basal cell carcinoma.* This lesion consists of one or several erythematous, scaling, only slightly infiltrated patches surrounded by a fine, threadlike, pearly border. The patches usually show small areas of superficial ulceration and crusting. In addition, their centers may show smooth, atrophic scarring. Whereas the three types of basal cell carcinoma described above are commonly situated on the face, superficial basal cell carcinoma occurs predominantly on the trunk.

5. *Premalignant fibroepithelioma.* This lesion consists of one or several raised, moderately firm, often pedunculated nodules, covered by smooth, slightly reddened skin. They clinically resemble fibromas. Ulceration occurs only rarely. The most common lesion is usually located on the back.

6. *Nevoid basal cell epithelioma syndrome.* This entity, in which the cutaneous lesions are often referred to as basal cell nevi, is dominantly inherited. Lesions begin to appear in childhood or adolescence and continue to accumulate throughout life. The lesions consist of elevated, firm, smooth nodules that either have the color of normal skin or are slightly pigmented. Some gradually increase in size and eventually may ulcerate. Aside from the cutaneous lesions, mandibular or maxillary cysts are regularly present, and other anomalies of the skeletal and nervous systems may occur.

7. *Linear basal cell nevus.* This lesion consists of several bands composed of brownish nodules. It is not inherited, is not associated with other anomalies, and is the rarest of the basal cell epitheliomas.

Basosquamous cell epithelioma is a term frequently found in the literature. Lever (1975) believed that this lesion does not actually represent transition of a basal cell epithelioma into a squamous cell carcinoma but rather is actually a basal cell epithelioma with keratinizing differentiation. Nodular basal cell carcinoma may differentiate into several subtypes (i.e., solid, cystic, adenoid, keratotic).

The growth of basal cell carcinoma is characteristically slow. With the passage of time ulceration is seen in most patients. Two groups may be clinically differentiated according to mode of spread, the first remaining localized and eventually invading underlying tissues (Fig. 74–6) and the second group tending to spread in a superficial plane (Fig. 74–7). Several variations have been described: the nodular type (Fig. 74–8), the sclerosing or morphea type, the superficial basal cell carcinoma, and the pigmented basal cell carcinoma (Fig. 74–9). There is some correlation between the clinical appearance and the pathologic findings; for example, the architectural pattern of the nodular type is solid masses and that of the morphea type shows thin strands of tumor cells surrounded by dense fibrosis.

A person with a basal cell carcinoma may live for years without treatment of the disease. Death from it alone is rare and is the result of long-standing, untreated or uncontrolled disease that invades the periorbital bone and eventually the brain by direct extension.

Metastases from basal cell carcinoma occur only rarely, with less than 200 examples recorded in the world literature up to 1984 (von Domarus and Stevens, 1984), although some cases are not reported (Casson, 1980). A history of long neglect or treatment failure with multiple recurrences is usually obtained. The characteristic clinical finding in patients with lymph node involvement is a stony hard, roughened sensation on palpation. The metastases should be managed by regional node dissection, and cures are obtainable (Conway and Hugo, 1965). Metas-

---

Figure 74–7. Extensive superficial basal cell carcinoma of the forehead and scalp in a 90 year old woman with a 30 year history of the lesion without treatment. *A*, Preoperative appearance. *B*, Treatment by excision of the entire lesion, including the underlying periosteum. The outer table of the cranium was removed, and a split-thickness skin graft was applied. *C*, Result six months postoperatively.

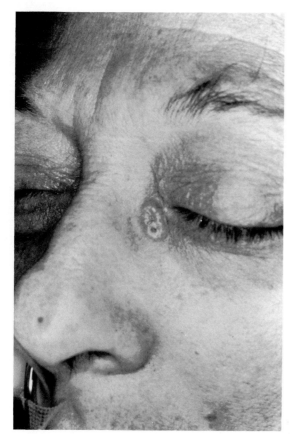

Figure 74–8. Nodular basal cell carcinoma of the medial canthus.

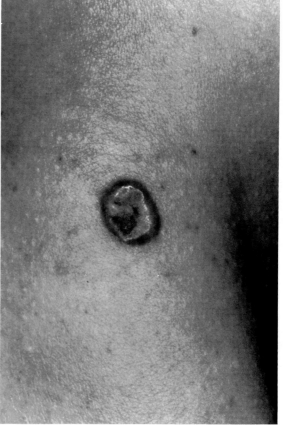

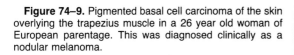

Figure 74–9. Pigmented basal cell carcinoma of the skin overlying the trapezius muscle in a 26 year old woman of European parentage. This was diagnosed clinically as a nodular melanoma.

tases to the lung and bone are also observed (Farmer and Helwig, 1980).

All patients with a history of previous treatment of a basal cell cancer are at an increased risk for development of new skin tumors. Approximately one-third of patients have a new lesion within five years (Robinson, 1987). These individuals should be counseled to avoid the sun, use sunscreen creams, and be evaluated at a maximum of six month intervals.

Treatment

Because of the extreme rarity of metastases in this disease, control of the local disease is synonymous with cure. The majority of previously untreated basal cell carcinomas are seen as small lesions; they are readily managed by a variety of methods, which have comparable cure rates in experienced hands. These include: (1) curettage and electrodesiccation; (2) radiation therapy; (3) surgery, either conventional procedures or Mohs excision; and (4) cryotherapy.

CURETTAGE AND ELECTRODESICCATION

This is the primary method used by dermatologists who undoubtedly treat the vast majority of basal cell carcinomas in the United States; in the hands of the experienced practitioner cure rates in the 95 per cent range are obtained (Popkin, 1968; Kopf and associates, 1977).

The technique entails removal of the lesion with a skin curette under local anesthesia, followed by electrodesiccation of the treated area. This defect is covered and allowed to heal over a period of days, or weeks, depending on its size. It is the most suitable therapy for superficial or previously untreated lesions less than 1 cm in extent. Apart from an occasional hypertrophic scar and residual depigmentation, it produces an acceptable cosmetic result. It should not be used for tumors overlying the alar cartilages or tumors of the eyelids, where contraction of the scar may occur; it is also contraindicated in the treatment of any recurrent lesion. Its obvious disadvantage is the lack of a specimen for histopathologic determination of the adequacy of treatment.

RADIATION THERAPY

Most basal cell carcinomas are controlled by radiation therapy in one of its various forms, and the reported cure rates (approximately 95 per cent) are comparable with those of conventional surgery and curettage and desiccation (von Essen, 1960). A margin of normal tissue is included in the treatment field, as with surgical excision; the cure rate tends to drop as the field of treatment increases in size (von Essen, 1960).

This modality provides a comparably effective therapeutic choice, particularly in areas where tissue preservation is important, for example, the periorbital skin (Fitzpatrick and associates, 1984), the nose, and the lip. The cosmetic result is at first acceptable but tends to deteriorate as depigmentation and skin atrophy occur over a period of years; use of radiation therapy should be restricted to older patients (i.e., those over the age of 60 years). Skill and experience are required to avoid the effects of overtreatment; these include late ulceration (Fig. 74–10) and injury to adjacent structures such as the eye (Fig. 74–11). Treatment by radiation therapy is also indicated for palliation in old patients in whom a major resection would otherwise be indicated. Remarkable control of the disease process is obtainable in such individuals by the use of carefully administered radiation therapy. Recurrence after radiation therapy does not respond to secondary radiation treatment and should be managed only by surgical excision.

SURGICAL TREATMENT

The diagnosis of basal cell carcinoma should be established and documented by biopsy before any surgical excision is performed, except for the smallest lesions, which may be excised with a small margin for both histopathologic examination and treatment.

Visual examination in adequate light with magnification combined with palpation enables the clinician to determine the extent of skin involvement and the degree of invasion of the underlying soft tissues and bone, when present. Computed tomographic (CT) scans are important aids in the evaluation of larger tumors to determine the extent of the cancer and the amount of bone involvement. In the patient previously treated by whatever modality, clinical examination is rendered less

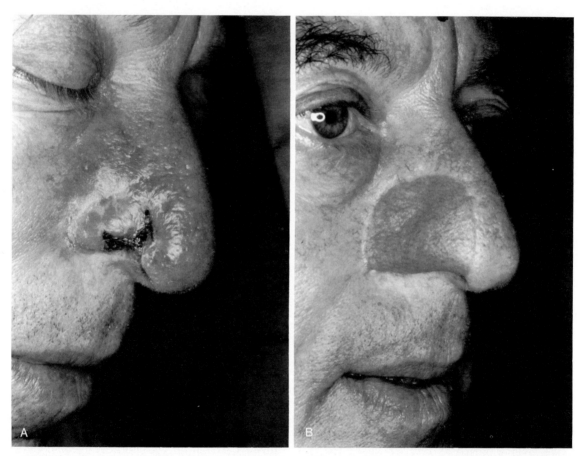

Figure 74–10. A 55 year old man with a basal cell carcinoma of the nasal ala treated by radiation therapy. *A,* Ulceration occurred within 18 months after radiation. Histologic examination of the entire area of ulceration failed to show any residual carcinoma. *B,* Alar reconstruction by a forehead flap.

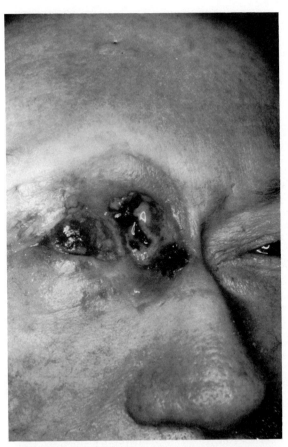

Figure 74–11. Appearance after radiation therapy for a basal cell carcinoma in an 80 year man with ulceration, bone necrosis, and destruction of the globe. Severe pain necessitated surgical resection. No basal cell carcinoma was found on histologic examination of the specimen.

accurate by the presence of post-treatment scarring, skin grafts, and flaps (Fig. 74–12). Prior radiation therapy may also cause radiographic changes in the underlying bone in the absence of true tumor invasion.

In the previously untreated lesion, margins of 2 to 5 mm may be adequate; in larger tumors with a longer clinical history the possibility of extension beyond detectable borders is more likely and a wider margin (in the 1 cm range) is advisable. In recurrent basal cell carcinoma even larger margins should be part of the treatment plan, depending on the size and location of the tumor (Burg and associates, 1975). The known clinical behavior of the more diffuse morphea type of basal cell carcinoma also dictates an additional margin if the primary treatment

is to be successful. The ability to obtain an immediate skin closure should also be determined during treatment planning, and reconstructive alternatives should be discussed with the patient. A three-dimensional concept is required, as well as an evaluation to include the possibility of the invasion of deeper structures, such as the parotid gland, the ear canal, the facial musculature, or the cartilages of the nose. It is only with such an approach that an en bloc resection with uninvolved margins on pathologic examination is obtainable.

After a clinically adequate resection in the larger cancers, frozen section examination may be necessary to determine if the tumor has been eradicated; this examination is mandatory if reconstruction by a flap technique is contemplated. If the involvement of bone margins is suspected, frozen section examination may not be technically possible; under these circumstances a delayed closure or a temporary split-thickness skin graft is permissible.

If delay of closure for two, three, or four days is chosen, it is safe to apply an occlusive dressing until an examination of the suspect margins is completed. The author has not experienced any problem with infection when this method has been used. Cooperation between the surgeon and the pathologist is assumed, and the surgeon should personally orient the specimen for the pathologist who will be examining it. If the tumor remains incompletely resected, additional excision must be performed until it is determined that all tumor is eradicated. The concern with the presence of residual tumor is most important if the need to use a flap for coverage exists, as is the usual situation in the more advanced, often recurrent lesions.

The presence of flaps makes the detection of deep recurrence more difficult; a delay in the treatment of the recurrent disease then occurs, with all its implications. An alternative is the application of a split-thickness skin graft as a temporary measure, after which the patient may undergo a period of observation before definitive reconstruction. A sufficient duration of follow-up is difficult to determine, as the author has witnessed several recurrences in advanced tumors six and eight years after excision.

Surgeons are sometimes confronted with a pathology report indicating that tumor cells

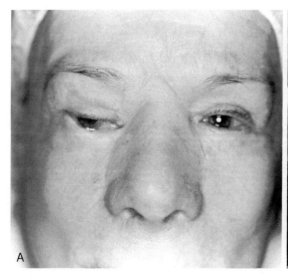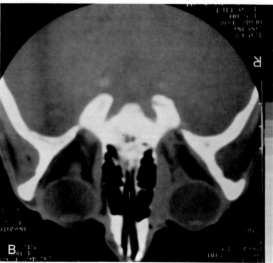

Figure 74–12. *A,* Recurrent basal cell carcinoma of the medial canthus under a local skin flap with a fixed medial rectus muscle, necessitating resection of the orbital contents, part of the frontal bone, and the ethmoid sinuses. *B,* CT scan showing recurrent tumor extending along the entire medial wall of the orbit. (Patient of Dr. Glenn Jelks.)

are present at the margin of the resection, several days after surgery has been completed. Approximately one-third of basal cell carcinomas eventually recur (Gooding, White, and Yatsuhashi, 1965), with most of the recurrences being detected within 24 months (Pascall and associates, 1968). On the basis of these findings there has been a tendency to employ observation only with follow-up at short intervals. In the author's opinion virtually all patients in this group should have excision as soon as the wound is healed, a recurrence rate of 30 per cent being unacceptable, particularly in the current litigious climate. In a series of 12 such patients who underwent immediate reexcision, 58 per cent had residual tumor present and no recurrences were reported (Koplin and Zarem, 1980).

The cure rate obtained by trained surgeons treating previously untreated basal cell carcinoma can be greater than 95 per cent, depending on its size at the initial examination (Rank and Wakefield, 1959; Hayes, 1962; Shanoff, Spira, and Hardy, 1967; Binns and Sherriff, 1975).

The overall cure rate in previously untreated basal cell carcinoma obtained by Mohs (1978), using microscopically controlled excision technique, is a remarkable 99.9 per cent. Analysis of these figures shows that the cure rate for basal cell tumors greater than 3 cm falls to 90.5 per cent (Mohs, 1978). The prognosis for cure of the larger lesions is

substantially less than that for the small superficial lesions included in most of the statistical series reported from dermatology units. It is the larger tumors that the plastic surgeon is most often asked to treat.

TREATMENT OF RECURRENT LESIONS

A history of prior treatment of basal cell carcinoma, by whatever modality, indicates that the physician is no longer dealing with a simple basal cell carcinoma. The postsurgical recurrence rate in previously treated lesions is much higher than that obtained after surgery for a primary lesion. It was reported as 15 per cent by Rank and Wakefield (1959) and 24 per cent by Hayes (1962), who reported only a 3 per cent recurrence rate after surgery for previously untreated lesions, a substantial difference.

The surgical margins considered adequate for a primary tumor are not satisfactory for recurrent lesions and should be extended if possible to 1.5 to 3 cm. If a recurrence is situated in one part of the scar, skin graft, or flap, resection of the entire scar, graft, or flap should be considered; it has been the author's experience that control of recurrence in one area may be followed by reappearance of the tumor in another (e.g., around the periphery of a skin graft or radiation field). The presence of post-treatment scarring renders the treatment of the large recurrent lesions technically more difficult, and hypotensive anesthesia is of benefit, permitting the operator to perform the dissection in a relatively blood-free field, an aid in detecting tumor extensions beyond the plane of the dissection.

If possible, the tissue planes should be used as margins, and there should be no hesitation in planning a full-thickness resection of the cheek, the nose, or the calvarium if this is considered necessary. It is most difficult to manage patients in whom the recurrence is present in the periorbital area; direct invasion into the anterior cranial fossa is possible because of the thinness of the bones of the orbit and the proximity of the cranial fossa and cribriform plate. Frequently treatment by both surgery and radiation fails, and the eye has already been destroyed or resected (Fig. 74–13). Treatment planning is guided by CT findings and the clinical examination results, with emphasis on the need to operate beyond the tumor using uninvolved anatomic structures as margins.

The microscopically controlled excision of Mohs has a special role in the management of the recurrent lesion and is invaluable in tracing tumor extensions beyond clinically detectable disease (see below under Mohs Micrographic Surgery). The cure rate reported by Mohs (1978) in the management of recurrent basal cell carcinoma is 96.8 per cent, substantially higher than that usually obtainable by conventional surgery.

CRYOTHERAPY

The use of various freezing techniques for the treatment of skin tumors, both benign and malignant, has been reported for many years (Cahan, 1965). There has been a resurgence in the popularity of this method coinciding with commercial production of more sophisticated equipment. This technique provides the physician with consistent temperature control and a freeze-thaw cycle that is the basis for satisfactory tumor destruction. In a series of more than 3000 patients a cure rate of 96.4 per cent was obtained (Zacarian, 1983), and for smaller noninvasive lesions cryotherapy seems to be a suitable nonsurgical alternative.

After treatment, edema, blistering, and skin necrosis may be observed as tissue destruction progresses; late sequelae are hypopigmentation, skin atrophy, and scarring. It is not suitable for the management of tumors larger than 2 cm and for lesions that recur after any treatment modality. As with radiation therapy and desiccation with curettage, no tissue specimens are available for pathologic examination.

5-FLUOROURACIL

5-Fluorouracil (5-FU) in the management of basal cell carcinoma has been evaluated since 1962. The original enthusiasm (Snyderman and Starzynski, 1968) has abated, and it has no place in the management of invasive basal cell carcinoma (Mohs, Jones, and Bloom, 1978). It may be useful for the patient with extensive sun damage and multiple solar keratoses in whom significant resolution of these lesions will occur. Any lesion that persists after treatment with 5-fluorouracil

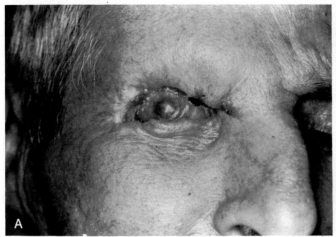
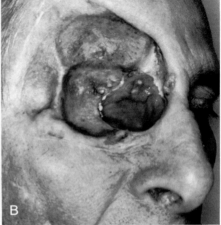

Figure 74–13. Recurrent basal cell carcinoma of the orbit after radiation therapy and surgery. *A,* Appearance of the patient. *B,* Result after periorbital resection and closure with a skin graft. Reconstruction of the defect was not recommended because of the poor prognosis in this 77 year old man.

should undergo biopsy and be treated accordingly.

Reconstruction

The high cure rate obtained in the surgical management of smaller basal cell carcinomas of the head and neck area and the extremities is compatible with immediate reconstruction in virtually every patient.

Direct primary closure after undermining is applicable in small lesions; for larger tumors other reconstructive methods will of necessity be employed. These may be either a full-thickness skin graft or a local flap from the periphery of the defect. Larger resections require transposition flaps, either random or myocutaneous. Microvascular free flaps may also be used.

The timing of the reconstruction depends on the location of the defect, its interference with function, and the adequacy of the resection as determined by the surgeon. Although the author does not accept the concept of delaying reconstruction until the possibilities of recurrence are minimal, there are clinical situations (e.g., large multirecurrent tumors) in which simple closure either with a skin graft or with a relatively limited reconstruction should be considered, at least until the surgical specimen has been adequately examined. The use of tissue expansion methods then becomes feasible; excision of the skin graft and replacement with expanded tissue is a preferable method of reconstruction in selected patients (see Chap. 13).

Perioral defects are reconstructed immediately to restore function; similarly treatment of the periorbital tumor for which eyelid resection is planned must include protection of the globe as part of the surgical procedure.

SQUAMOUS CELL CARCINOMA

This pathologic entity has many clinical features in common with basal cell carcinoma; they share similar causes, anatomic sites, and age incidence. It is less common than basal cell carcinoma by a ratio in the range of 1:4, varying with the latitude. It may develop de novo in previously undamaged skin or be preceded by one of several premalignant lesions, actinic keratosis, Bowen's disease, or, if located on the penis, erythroplasia of Queyrat.

It is more aggressive than the basal cell carcinoma; it tends to ulcerate earlier, grow more rapidly, and invade underlying structures sooner. It does metastasize in a small but significant number of patients.

Etiologic Factors

The primary cause of squamous cell carcinoma is exposure to ultraviolet radiation in the UVB range (290 to 320 nm) (Fig. 74–14). The evidence is only circumstantial at this time as indicated by the following findings: (1) occurence of the lesions on exposed portions of the body, usually the head and neck area; (2) an increased incidence in outdoor workers; (3) an increased incidence as the equator is approached; and (4) rarity in the pigmented races.

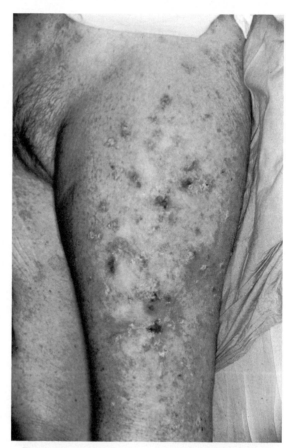

Figure 74–14. Chronically sun-damaged skin with actinic keratoses and squamous cell carcinomas on the thighs of a 50 year old woman with psoriasis. The areas had been treated for years by natural sun exposure and sun lamps. Metastatic lymph node disease developed from one of the many lesions.

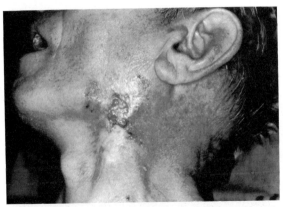

Figure 74–15. Radiation-induced squamous cell carcinoma of the neck in a 68 year old man treated by irradiation for carcinoma of the larynx 16 years previously.

Radiation Therapy. The incidence of squamous cell carcinoma at the site of previously administered radiation therapy is now rare; this is the result of improved equipment and skin-sparing techniques, in association with increased precautions by medical personnel with potential exposure risk. The indications for radiation treatment are also now more precise, and the use of radiation therapy to treat benign conditions is virtually nonexistent.

The onset of squamous cell carcinoma in a previously radiated field is preceded by many years of radiation dermatitis, characterized by skin atrophy, telangiectasia, alopecia, loss of skin pigmentation, and keratosis (Fig. 74–15).

Xeroderma Pigmentosum. As described above, this hereditary disease is a precursor to squamous cell carcinoma of the skin in affected individuals. The complete avoidance of sun exposure and the aggressive treatment of all tumors as they occur may prolong life.

Immunosuppression. Shortly after the acceptance of renal transplantation as a practical form of management of renal failure, it was recognized that some surviving patients developed a variety of tumors (Penn and associates, 1969). The Transplant Tumor Registry (as of September 1987) contained data on 3427 tumors in 3203 patients (Penn, 1988); 40 per cent of the tumors are skin cancers, with squamous cell carcinoma exceeding basal cell carcinoma in immunosuppressed patients by a ratio of 1.9:1, a departure from the ratio encountered in normal individuals.

The exact cause of this phenomenon is not clear; it may be a direct oncogenic effect on the involved tissue or the result of a depressed immune system and a reduction therefore in immune surveillance (loss of immune competence).

This effect is even more pronounced in transplant recipients exposed to sunlight; long-term transplant survivors in Queensland, Australia, have an incidence 20 times that of the general population (Hardie and associates, 1980); a similar but less pronounced incidence in a comparable population group has been noted in England (Boyle and associates, 1984). The effect of the immunosuppressive drugs seems to be compounded by sun exposure, which itself may impair cellular immune responses (Fisher and Kripke, 1977; Parrish, 1983).

Chemical Carcinogenesis. Exposure to a variety of chemicals contained in coal tar (Fig. 74–16), pitch, soot, and petroleum products has been recognized as a cause of skin cancer for many years (Pott, 1775; Bell, 1876) and the identification and investigation of these chemicals was an exciting chapter in carcinogenesis research (Kennaway, 1955; Miller, 1970). Exposure occurs in the workplace in most instances, as it did in Pott's day; the enforcement of industrial regulations and preventive measures for those at risk has reduced the incidence of new cases to a minimum, and exposure to chemicals has little significance in the present day epidemiology of skin cancer in most countries.

Chronic exposure to arsenic by ingestion as a medication or as a vapor in agricultural sprays has also been recognized as a cause of skin cancer (Hutchinson, 1888). Of particular interest was the report of both basal cell and

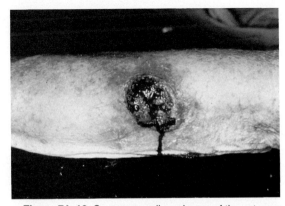

Figure 74–16. Squamous cell carcinoma of the extensor aspect of the forearm in a person exposed to coal tar products at work. There were associated axillary metastases.

squamous cell carcinoma in an otherwise nonsusceptible population in Taiwan as the result of arsenic in the drinking water (Yeh, 1973). With the recognition of arsenic as an etiologic agent, new examples of such skin cancers have become increasingly rare.

Viral Carcinogenesis. Epidermodysplasia verruciformis is a rare autosomal recessive disease, characterized by multiple warts on exposed surfaces of the body. Approximately 35 per cent of individuals with the disease develop squamous cell carcinoma on sun-exposed surfaces (Lutzner, 1978). The human papillomavirus may be found in the warts before the development of cancer, thus confirming a link between this virus and the development of squamous cell carcinoma of the skin in man.

The relationship between bowenoid papulosis of the penis and infection with the human papillomavirus Type 16 may also be significant in the etiology of squamous cell carcinoma of the penis (Hurwitz and associates, 1987).

Chronic Irritation. Squamous cell carcinoma may also develop at the site of long-standing irritation, such as chronic heat (Neve, 1923; Cross, 1967), unstable burn scars (Treves and Pack, 1930), or draining sinuses from osteomyelitis and chronic ulcers (Fig. 74–17) (Sedlin and Fleming, 1963). These and similar predisposing conditions are responsible for many of the squamous cell tumors on unexposed areas of the body, especially the extremities. The anaplastic change occurs only after many years, and the diagnosis is often delayed because of the chronic nature of the original process. Malignant change may be accompanied by a change

in symptoms: there may be increased drainage, increased pain, and enlargement of the ulcer. Delay in diagnosis may account for the high incidence of metastatic lymph node disease in affected patients (Sedlin and Fleming, 1963). The more aggressive treatment of the predisposing conditions currently employed should reduce the incidence of this variety of squamous cell carcinoma.

Differential Diagnosis

Squamous cell carcinoma in its early stages may be difficult to distinguish from basal cell carcinoma, the premalignant keratoses, keratoacanthoma, and the adnexal skin tumors. Clinical diagnosis of the common skin tumors is well known to be rather inaccurate (Lightstone, Kopf, and Garfinkel, 1965), and biopsy of all skin lesions prior to definitive treatment is indicated. Only then is a rational approach to treatment possible, the management of squamous cell carcinoma being somewhat different than that of the basal cell lesion. Treatment of squamous cell carcinoma should be more aggressive and should include wider margins both in the surface periphery and in depth; the possibility of metastatic lymph node disease should also be considered.

The biopsy is usually a total excision if a simple primary closure without tension is possible; a shave excision of the small lesion is also permissible, with further treatment necessary if there are abnormal pathologic findings. In larger tumors a sample of tissue for diagnostic confirmation should be obtained by an incisional or a punch biopsy before treatment is instituted.

If the treating physician is considering keratoacanthoma in the differential diagnosis, the pathologist may request an ellipse of tissue, including the transverse diameter across the tumor, for evaluation.

The measurement of tumor thickness and therefore depth of invasion may provide a guide to prognosis and treatment planning. Tumors of the trunk and extremities greater than 4 mm in thickness had a higher incidence of local recurrence, and tumors greater than 8 mm in thickness had a higher incidence of regional lymph node involvement (Friedman, Cooper, and Wanebo, 1985). A similar finding using Clark Levels I through V has been reported; there was also a recurrence rate of 24 per cent in Level IV and V tumors (Immerman and associates, 1983).

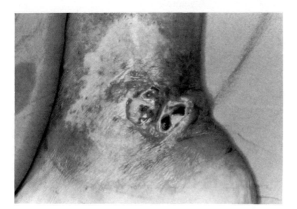

Figure 74–17. A low grade squamous cell carcinoma in a chronically recurring ulcer of the lateral malleolus of over 20 years' duration.

Treatment

The small squamous cell tumors of the skin less than 1 cm in size may be treated by the same methods used for the smaller basal cell carcinomas (i.e., curettage and desiccation, radiation therapy, and surgical excision). It should be remembered that squamous cell carcinoma is a more aggressive lesion if the epidermis has been penetrated; in the author's opinion the preferred treatment is surgery. Clinical differentiation between tumors arising in sun-damaged skin and those in unexposed skin is a valid consideration in the smaller relatively unaggressive tumors. As the lesions increase in diameter and depth of invasion, this concept should be discarded in favor of an aggressive, wide excision in all patients.

Examination of the tumor is performed with satisfactory lighting, and its extent in both width and depth is determined by palpation. Treatment planning for squamous cell carcinoma must include evaluation of the regional lymph nodes, as there is a small but definite incidence of metastatic lymph node disease with this group of tumors.

The margin for a curative excision is judged by the visible and palpable extent of the tumor and should be approximately 1 cm, increasing as the size of the tumor increases. In more extensive lesions a 2 to 3 cm peripheral margin, with a corresponding increase in the depth of the excision, may be necessary.

Findings suggest that an increasing depth of invasion correlates with both local recurrence and metastatic nodal disease (Friedman, Cooper, and Wanebo, 1985).

The depth of each excision is determined by the underlying structures. For example, if an invasive tumor is directly over the branches of the seventh nerve, a parotidectomy and facial nerve dissection may be necessary; when the terminal branches of the seventh nerve are in the field, they should be sacrificed if their preservation compromises the procedure (Fig. 74–18A). Tumors overlying the maxilla and orbit require resection of the underlying bone if there is any suggestion of osseous involvement (Fig. 74–18B). CT scans provide more accurate information about the degree of bone involvement and invasion of the orbit in this clinical setting (see also Chap. 69).

For advanced tumors of the scalp, the frontal area, the temporal bone, and the remaining skull, the resection of underlying bone must be considered in every patient if a local cure is to be achieved (see Chap. 69). The resection may include only the outer table; however, if there is radiographic evidence of bone involvement, a full-thickness resection of the bone should be considered (Fig. 74–19).

Another site requiring special treatment is the external ear (Fig. 74–20). Tumors at this location have a high incidence of local recurrence (in the 14 per cent range) and a high

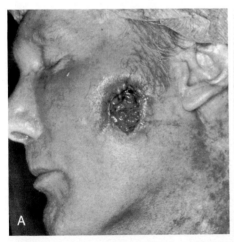
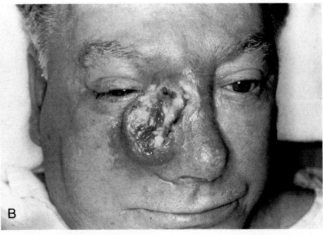

Figure 74–18. *A,* A 50 year old man with an 18 month history of an ulcerating tumor on the side of his face. Treatment planning should include skin excision, parotidectomy with facial nerve dissection and possible sacrifice of the buccal and palpebral branches, and resection of the zygoma. Frozen section examination of the margins should also be employed. *B,* Large squamous cell carcinoma in relatively normal skin, fixed to the bone and invading the orbit. This type of tumor is associated with a high incidence of metastatic disease, and in this patient there were metastases to the cervical lymph nodes. Curative resection includes removal of the nose, the maxilla, the orbital contents, and the ethmoid sinus.

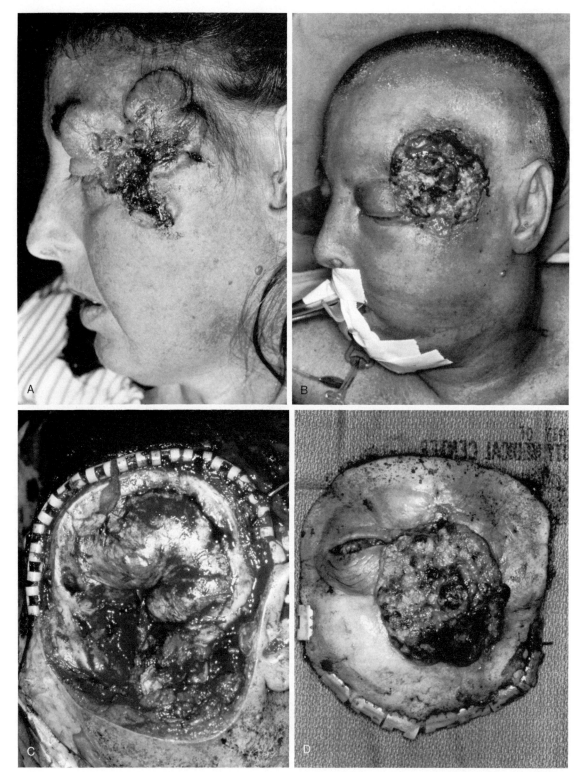

Figure 74–19. *A,* Advanced squamous cell carcinoma of the temporal skin invading the orbit. Surgery was declined, and the patient was treated with a full course of radiation therapy. *B,* Minimal response to radiation therapy after six months. *C,* Craniofrontal resection included the orbital contents, the frontal bone, the greater wing of the sphenoid, and the squamous temporal bone, together with the contents of the infratemporal fossa. *D,* The surgical specimen. Results of frozen section evaluation were normal in all areas examined.

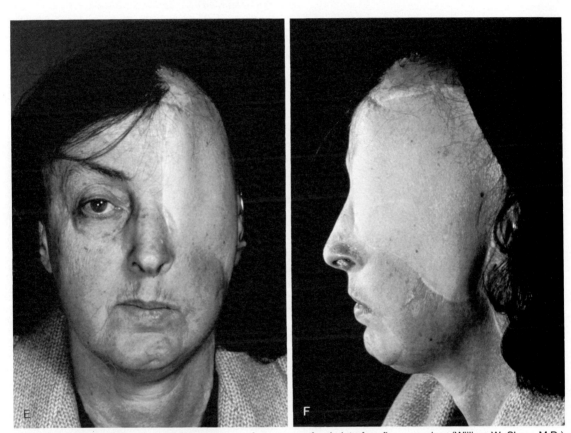

Figure 74–19 *Continued E, F,* Result five years after a tensor fascia lata free flap procedure (William W. Shaw, M.D.). There is no evidence of recurrence or metastasis.

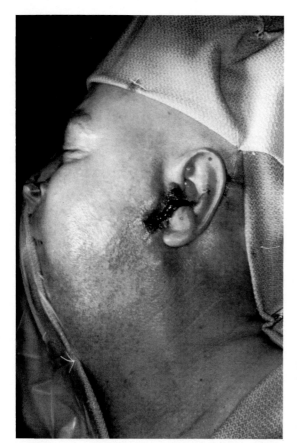

Figure 74–20. Squamous cell carcinoma of the ear. The tumor originated in the area of the tragus. Treatment planning in this patient should include parotidectomy and facial nerve dissection. If possible, a portion of the upper ear should be preserved to enable the patient to wear glasses.

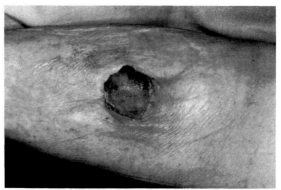

Figure 74–21. Squamous cell carcinoma of the calf at the site of a healed osteomyelitis sinus. The latter had drained for many years and had healed after sequestrectomy seven years before presentation.

incidence of nodal metastasis at the initial presentation (6 per cent). An additional 6 per cent developed metastatic node disease during the follow-up period (Byers and associates, 1983). The addition of a superficial parotidectomy to the surgical procedure is often necessary. In the absence of palpable node involvement, a prophylactic node dissection is not necessary on a statistical basis; however, the patient must be observed at frequent intervals.

Squamous cell tumors of the trunk and extremities have a somewhat different cause and prognosis when compared with the head and neck lesions. With the exception of squamous cell carcinoma of the hand, many of these tumors occur at the site of unstable burn scars and chronic draining sinuses (Fig. 74–21). The diagnosis is often delayed because of the chronicity of the predisposing condition.

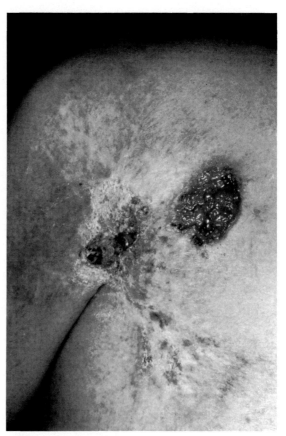

Figure 74–22. Unstable, ungrafted burn scar of over 40 years' duration with chronic ulceration progressing to carcinoma. There is a high incidence of metastatic disease with this type of tumor. Appropriate treatment would include axillary node dissection because of the proximity to the axilla and because of the high incidence of lymph node metastasis with these lesions.

Surgeons now anticipate these problems and treat antecedent conditions more aggressively with myocutaneous flaps and microvascular free tissue transfers. Consequently, the incidence of such lesions should decrease.

In general, these cancers behave more aggressively than the head and neck lesions. For example, the carcinoma that occurs in the frequently injured, chronically ulcerated burn scar is a serious disease (Fig. 74–22). There is a high incidence of regional node metastasis and local recurrence after seemingly adequate surgery (Arons and associates, 1965). All tumors in this group should be treated by an extensive resection, in both width and depth, and a regional lymph node dissection should be considered, even in the absence of palpable disease (Bostwick, Pendergrast, and Vasconez, 1976). For tumors in the extremities, amputation may be necessary.

During surgical resection the frozen section evaluation of the margins is an important adjunct in the management of squamous cell carcinoma at all sites. This technique has obvious limitations if the margin in question is bone. Careful orientation of the operative specimens is the responsibility of the surgeon. If the margins are considered close, this area should be carefully marked and examined separately at his direction.

The need for postoperative radiation for squamous cell carcinoma arises if the margins are determined to be inadequate by the pathologist. If the surgeon has done his best to effect a cure, the addition of radiation therapy to the treatment protocol is desirable, assuming that additional surgery is impractical owing to the presence of vital structures.

When the pathology report indicates that tumor is still present at the margins of the resection, a secondary surgical excision should be performed if this is technically possible. A recurrence rate of at least 50 per cent may be anticipated and a mortality rate in the 25 per cent range. If further surgical treatment is impractical or refused by the patient, radiation therapy must be administered (Glass, Spratt, and Perezmesa, 1966).

Invasion of the trigeminal (fifth cranial) nerve branch by direct extension sometimes occurs in advanced squamous cell carcinoma of the skin. Frozen section examination of the involved nerve trunk may indicate extension into the superior orbital tissue or the foramen rotundum. Postsurgical radiation therapy should also be considered as an adjunct in managing this difficult situation.

MALIGNANT MELANOMA

The melanoma is a malignant tumor that may arise from any cell of the body capable of forming melanin; it is most common therefore on the skin and less so in the eye, and it has been described in many organs as a primary tumor (Das Gupta, Brasfield, and Paglia, 1969). It is not confined to man, and it occurs in gray horses, dogs, and oxen (Levene, 1972). The serious nature and poor prognosis of the lesion have been recognized for centuries (Urteaga and Pack, 1966), and until recent years it was considered a uniformly fatal disease in which treatment was of little avail (Bloodgood, 1922).

The acceptance of an aggressive surgical approach to produce long-term survivors was slow (Handley, 1907). With this concept there has been a gradual improvement in survival rate in the past fifty years, although, when corrected for the stages of the disease, the results of treatment may have changed little (Adair, 1936; Pack, 1952; McNeer and Das Gupta, 1964; Goldsmith, Shah, and Kim, 1970).

More recently an improved understanding of the etiologic factors, clinical variants, and the pathologic features of the disease as related to prognosis has allowed a more rational approach to therapy. This has permitted the surgeon to modify his treatment to avoid excessively aggressive management of the more superficial tumors, a common mistake in the past. The concept of the wide and deep excision has been modified, and regional node dissection is being reserved for patients who may benefit from it.

The status of adjuvant therapy in the management of primary melanoma with a poor prognosis or with metastatic disease is under study in many treatment centers. Overall, the results at this time are disappointing, there being no significant findings to indicate a consistent improvement in survival times with chemotherapy, immunotherapy, or radiation therapy alone or in combination.

Incidence

Melanoma is not a common disease in the United States; in 1971 the incidence was 4.1

per 100,000 population per year; at that time the incidence of carcinoma of the colon was 29.3 per 100,000 and that of carcinoma of the breast was 39.2 per 100,000 (DHEW, 1969–1971). It has been on the increase for several decades (Cosman, Heddle, and Crikelair, 1976), a 400 per cent increase being noted in Connecticut over a 30 year period to 6.9 per 100,000 (Roush, Schymura, and Holford, 1988). This increase has been observed worldwide, being five- to sixfold in Denmark (Osterlind and Moller-Jensen, 1985) and even higher in Queensland, which has the highest incidence of melanoma in the world (Little, Holt, and Davis, 1980). The incidence in the latter has increased from 16 per 100,000 in 1966 to 33 per 100,000 in 1977.

As to racial distribution, melanoma is rare in black-skinned races; in the United States there is a reported rate of 0.6 per 100,000 people of black origin, and in South Africa the incidence is 1.2 per 100,000 black persons (Giraud, Rippey, and Rippey, 1975). A similar reduced rate. of 2.9 per 100,000 is seen in male New Zealanders of Maori (Polynesian) origin as compared with 12.3 per 100,000 for white male New Zealanders who are of predominantly Scottish, English, and Irish origin (Henderson, Kolonel, and Foster, 1982).

The incidence of melanoma by age varies according to the anatomic site; for all areas a pattern of incidence related to age has been observed, with a peak between 35 and 55 years and another beyond the age of 65 years. Melanoma is extremely rare in children (Spitz, 1948; Saksela and Rintala, 1968; Moss and Briggs, 1986). There were only 12 proven cases at Memorial Sloan-Kettering Institute, a major referral center for melanoma, over a 40 year period. Two occurred in preexisting giant hairy nevi (Lerman and associates, 1970), a proportion similar to that noted in a literature survey (Skov-Jensen, Hastrup, and Lambrethsen, 1966).

The disease is said to be more common in men; this finding varies, however, from country to country, the incidence being almost even in Australia. Women are considered to have a better prognosis (O'Doherty and associates, 1986), although this may be related to earlier presentation and a predominance of lower limb lesions (Blois and associates, 1983).

Etiology

Several factors have been implicated in the etiology of melanoma in both lesions thought to arise from preexisting nevi and those presumed to occur de novo; these include racial predisposition for melanoma, chronic irritation and repeated trauma, and, most important, sun exposure.

Preexisting Nevus. The proportion of melanomas that arise from preexisting nevi is not known; clinical estimates vary and depend on a history of a preexisting lesion obtained from the patient, who is not always a reliable source. In a series from Australia almost two-thirds of patients with melanoma stated that a preexisting pigmented lesion was present. Pathologists differ in their assessment, the presence of nevus cells reported in melanoma varying from 5 per cent (Lund and Kraus, 1962) to 50 per cent in a series of superficial spreading melanomas examined by multiple sections.

Dysplastic Nevus. An unusual type is the dysplastic nevus (Elder and associates, 1980), an acquired nevus that may be single or multiple (see Chap. 73). If the nevi are multiple, they are considered an example of the dysplastic nevus syndrome. These lesions occur most commonly on the back and may number in the dozens. Their appearance is different from that of other nevi, being larger, more irregular in outline, and lighter and less uniform in color. It is a significant precursor lesion to melanoma, and this group of patients require careful observation for life. This is the precursor lesion that is associated with familial melanoma and with multiple melanomas in the same patient. Nevi commence to develop when these patients are in their teens and will continue to develop throughout their lives.

Giant Hairy Nevus. This is a unique form of congenital nevus, fortunately rare and typically hair bearing. In its usual form it is large and disfiguring, thus the name garment or bathing trunk nevus (Fig. 74–23). The incidence of melanoma in this type of nevus is considered to range from 8 to 10 per cent (Greeley, Middleton, and Curtin, 1965; Quaba and Wallace, 1986), and when it occurs it is uniformly fatal. In this knowledge, staged excision with skin graft replacement is recommended. For the larger lesions this is truly a formidable undertaking in view of the lack of available donor sites and the multiple procedures needed. The use of mesh skin grafts and the introduction of skin expansion have reduced the number of surgical stages. Prophylactic excision, if practical, should be commenced at an early age, as malignant

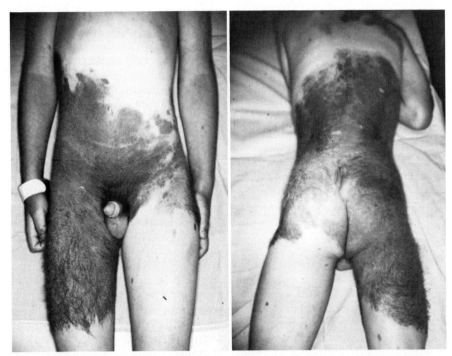

Figure 74–23. A young male with giant hairy nevus of the "garment" type. The availability of donor sites makes this patient a suitable candidate for excision and split-thickness skin grafting.

conversion may occur in young children (Trozak, Rowland, and Hu, 1975).

The true incidence of melanoma in preexisting nevi of all types will probably remain uncertain; susceptible individuals with fair skin, red hair, and multiple nevi should be advised to avoid the sun and observe their nevi frequently for changes. Suspicious lesions and known precursors should be excised both for diagnostic and for prophylactic reasons. Those individuals with many moles on their bodies have an increased risk of developing melanoma, further evidence of a relationship between the pigmented nevus and melanoma (Dubin, Moseson, and Pasternack, 1986).

Trauma. The role of skin injury in the causation of melanoma is disputed. Its frequent location on the sole of the foot in black races is advanced as evidence that trauma is a contributing factor in the development of melanoma. A similar high incidence on the foot has also been observed in American blacks (Shah and Goldsmith, 1970) in whom the role of trauma may be assumed to be less important. Previous injury is not of major significance in the etiology of melanoma encountered in the usual clinical practice (Petersen, Bodenham, and Lloyd, 1962).

Ultraviolet Radiation. Circumstantial ev-idence indicates that exposure to the sun is the prime etiologic factor in the onset of melanoma in people of Caucasian origin, who are known to have a predetermined susceptibility. This in turn is related to ethnic origin, the color of the hair and the eyes, and the amount of pigment in the skin. Such individuals sunburn easily and tan poorly if at all; many of them give a history of residence in a tropical or subtropical latitude where sun exposure is unavoidable (Holman and associates, 1986). Some paradoxes, however, exist: (1) Intermittent exposure, such as occurs in recreational sun bathing and boating, is more often reported by patients with melanoma than is chronic sun exposure, as occurs in outdoor workers (MacKie, 1981). (2) The percentage of melanomas on exposed skin surfaces is not increased in latitudes where sun exposure is more intense and the overall incidence higher (Lee, 1972).

Theories on the mechanism by which melanoma is precipitated have been advanced:

1. The production of a "solar circulating factor" derived from exposed melanocytes, which is able to induce a malignant change in melanocytes elsewhere in the body either in normal skin or in a preexisting nevus (Lee and Merrill, 1970).

2. The presence of premalignant clones of

abnormal melanocytes, which respond to sun exposure by a malignant change (Lee, 1972).

3. An altered immune response in a susceptible individual exposed to the sun on a long-term basis; this has been demonstrated in the laboratory animal (Fisher and Kripke, 1977) and in man (Parrish, 1983). It is seen clinically when the herpes simplex virus becomes active and produces a "fever blister" or "cold sore" as an aftermath of sunburn. This theory is also supported by the increased incidence of melanoma in immunosuppressed transplant organ recipients.

Diagnosis

Pigmented lesions of the skin are common in light-skinned people, with an observed average of 14.6 nevi on the skin of the body (Pack, Lenson, and Gerber, 1952). These are mostly of the nevocytic nevus variety; less often found are the junctional nevus, the café au lait spot, the juvenile freckle, the blue nevus, and the juvenile melanoma, a misnomer for a benign lesion (Spitz, 1948). Other skin lesions that may be incidentally pigmented are the seborrheic or senile keratosis, the basal cell carcinoma (see Fig. 74–9), the wart, Kaposi's sarcoma, the pyogenic granuloma, and the dermatofibroma (see also Chap. 73).

The observed increase in the incidence of melanoma worldwide in the past 40 years mandates that every pigmented lesion be viewed with suspicion. The history of the lesion is important because of the association between the presence of nevi and the development of melanoma; any change in size, shape, or color with or without ulceration, bleeding, and itching is suggestive of a malignant change. The alert physician may be able to make a correct diagnosis before biopsy, although the earlier manifestations now being seen are making this more difficult.

In the author's opinion histologic confirmation is necessary in all suspect lesions, the preferred method being a total excisional biopsy with a simple skin closure. In the more extensive lesions in which a direct closure would not be possible without undermining the skin edges, an incisional or a punch biopsy is acceptable, noting that it may not be representative of the entire lesion, an important consideration in current treatment planning.

The biopsy technique observes the basic principles of tumor surgery (Harris and Gumport, 1975):

1. Local anesthesia using a field block method, never inserting the needle into or under the lesion.

2. An elliptic excision placed in the long axis of any future excision to be performed if examination of the biopsy specimen confirms the presence of a melanoma. This avoids an unnecessarily wide reexcision.

3. Removal of the specimen with a sufficient margin, usually 2 to 3 mm, to make reexcision of a benign lesion unnecessary.

4. Gentle handling of the specimen to avoid crushing of the tissues, which would render histologic interpretation difficult and thickness measurement inaccurate.

The critics of biopsy before definitive surgery for the cure of melanoma argue that manipulation of the tumor releases malignant cells into the bloodstream and local lymphatics and may precipitate future metastases. There is, however, no evidence that biopsy as a preliminary to definitive surgery has an adverse effect on survival either at five or ten years (Epstein, 1971). The advantages, namely (1) the avoidance of a diagnostic error and therefore unnecessary surgery and (2) determination of a rational treatment plan based on the microscopic study of the specimen, outweigh the theoretic disadvantages. This is even more pertinent when one considers that the degree of clinical accuracy in the evaluation of the skin lesions is only in the 50 per cent (Winkelmann, 1972) to 64 per cent range (Kopf, Mintzis, and Bart, 1975).

The place of frozen section evaluation in the management of melanoma is disputed, although a diagnostic accuracy rate of 98.8 per cent is reported (Davis and Little, 1974). The known difficulty in interpreting slides of melanoma specimens plus the importance of evaluating the depth of invasion for treatment planning seems to render its use unnecessary as a routine measure. Practical considerations, such as unnecessary hospitalization in the event of a benign finding and the need for a detailed informed consent in all patients, support this view.

Classification

The studies of Clark and co-workers (1969) resulted in a classification of melanoma into three groups according to both clinical and pathologic characteristics: (1) lentigo malignant melanoma, (2) superficial spreading melanoma, and (3) nodular melanoma. To these must be added (4) acral-lentiginous melanoma, which has a plantar, palmar, or subungual location.

For completeness a small group of melanomas not included in the above classification must also be considered. These are the melanoma that occurs in the giant hairy nevus that has undergone a malignant change, the malignant blue nevus, the desmoplastic melanoma, the amelanotic melanoma, the melanoma with an unknown primary lesion, and the melanoma unable to be classified because of scarring from previous treatment or loss of the specimen.

Clark and associates (1969) also correlated the clinical classification with observations on the level of microscopic invasion as a guide to both prognosis and treatment (see Fig. 74–31).

Lentigo Malignant Melanoma. This is the classic pigmented lesion of older individuals, and it occurs on exposed body surfaces. It most often occurs on the face, where it makes up approximately 50 per cent of head and neck melanomas. It is preceded by a gradually enlarging pigmented lesion that is present for many years, the so-called Hutchinson's freckle, circumscribed precancerous melanosis, or lentigo maligna (Fig. 74–24). The percentage of lentigo malignant melanoma in the report of Clark and associates (1969) was 13.9 per cent; the New York University Medical Center experience has been reported as 4.7 per cent (Dubin, Moseson, and Pasternak, 1986). The lower figure may represent a change in the criteria for assigning melanoma to the four groups as experience was gained in the Clark classification.

Lentigo malignant melanoma seems to be the least aggressive type of melanoma, there being a 59.2 per cent survival rate in the Clark series. This finding has been confirmed by others (McGovern and associates, 1980).

Invasion of the dermis is indicated by changes in color and the development of nodularity on a previously flat surface. The changes in appearance that herald a malignant change may have a rapid onset (Fig. 74–25).

Superficial Spreading Melanoma. This is the commonest of the clinical varieties of melanoma, composing 54.5 per cent of the original series of Clark and associates (1969)

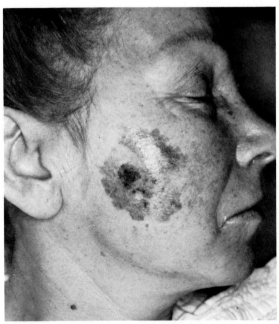

Figure 74–24. Lentigo maligna of the face, showing the characteristic variations in pigmentation. Complete histologic examination of the specimen showed that atypical melanocytic hyperplasia was confined to the epidermis.

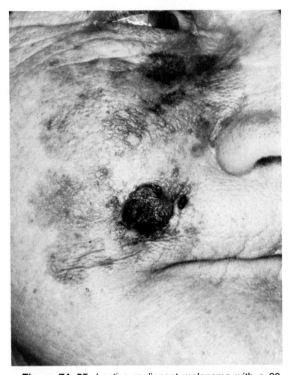

Figure 74–25. Lentigo malignant melanoma with a 20 year history and the rapid growth of a peripheral mass over a period of nine months. Examination of the specimen showed Clark Level V invasion beneath the nodule. There were no abnormal cervical nodes palpable; chest metastases were detected shortly afterward.

and 73.7 per cent of the New York University Medical Center series (Dubin, Moseson, and Pasternack, 1986). It may occur anywhere on the body, and a history of a preexisting pigmented lesion for many years is often reported; it is the melanoma type most often found in association with intradermal nevi, a finding that has been observed in 35 per cent of affected patients. A recent change in color, size, or shape may be reported by the patient; in a previously flat lesion nodularity progressing to ulceration may also be observed. The color range may be black through blue, gray, pink, or tan, and it is not uniform (Fig. 74–26). The survival rate in the original Clark series was 46.5 per cent.

Nodular Melanoma. Nodular melanoma may occur anywhere on the body and is characterized by a shorter history and nodular morphologic features from its inception. It is relatively uncommon, composing 9.3 per cent of the New York University series (Dubin, Moseson, and Pasternack, 1986). It has a more uniform blue-black to gray coloration, and its border is more sharply demarcated from the surrounding skin (Fig. 74–27). As this tumor progresses, it may become polypoid in appearance and is then considered to have a grave prognosis. This is related to the increased thickness observed on the first presentation in the patient; there is no apparent difference in survival when rates are corrected for depth of invasion. The survival rate observed in the original Clark series was only 27.3 per cent for nodular melanoma.

Acral-Lentiginous Melanoma. This term is applied to those melanomas that occur on the palmar and plantar skin and at subungual sites; they have certain characteristics that distinguish them from other melanomas. They clinically resemble lentigo malignant melanoma but occur exclusively on surfaces with minimal sun exposure (Fig. 74–28).

This is the melanoma observed in the pigmented races, although it is not uncommon in white individuals, being found in 7.46 per cent of an Austrian melanoma series. It accounts for 3.2 per cent of the New York University series (Dubin, Moseson, and Pasternack, 1986). It may be difficult to diagnose in its early phase, particularly when it occurs under the nail. The first sign may be a dark stain of the nail, and biopsy results may be normal unless the nail itself is removed. It occurs predominantly on the feet.

The prognosis of acral-lentiginous melanoma is similar to that of other melanomas of less than 0.76 mm in thickness, with a reported 100 per cent five year survival. For melanomas between 0.76 and 1.5 mm thick a 91 per cent five year survival was noted. Melanomas greater than 1.5 mm in size are

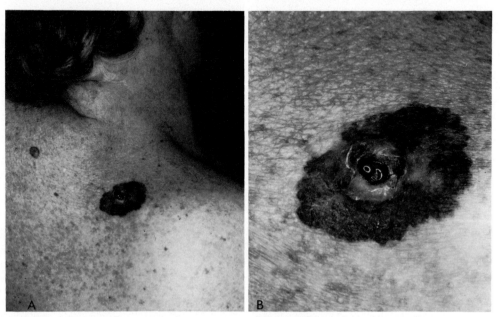

Figure 74–26. *A,* Melanoma, superficial spreading type, with a 15 year history of a pigmented lesion at the site. *B,* Closer examination shows a typical variation in color and the presence of an ulcerated nodule in the center. This was classified as Clark Level IV, 4.6 mm in thickness.

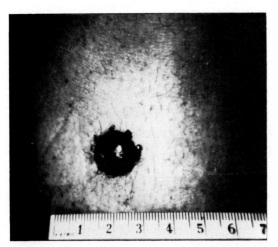

Figure 74–27. Melanoma of the nodular type with a sharply demarcated border and more uniform pigmentation.

associated with marked decrease in the five year survival to 37.5 per cent.

Unclassified Melanoma

The *malignant melanoma in a giant hairy nevus* is an extremely rare form of melanoma, and only 26 cases were reported prior to 1965 (Greeley, Middleton, and Curtin, 1965). An incidence of malignant change of 12 per cent was noted, although there was some selection in this series (Greeley, Middleton, and Cur-

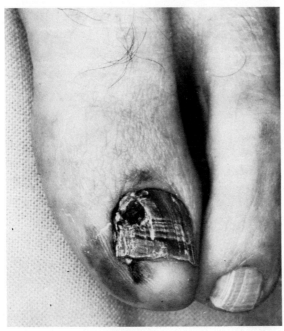

Figure 74–28. Acral-lentiginous melanoma of the great toe, 3.2 mm thick. Note the biopsy site through the nail bed.

tin, 1965). The true incidence is probably lower. However, it is the precursor lesion in approximately 40 per cent of the melanomas observed in children (Fish, Smith, and Canby, 1966). The onset of malignancy is indicated by a change in appearance and the development of nodularity or ulceration, which can occur even when the individual is under close observation. Because of the uniformly poor prognosis after a malignant change supervenes (there are virtually no survivors), staged excision of the giant hairy nevus is indicated whenever this is possible and practical. The substitution of split-thickness skin grafts for this variety of nevus, while not a cosmetic triumph, seems to be preferable to the alternative of malignant change. The attempted removal of this type of nevus by dermabrasion at an early age, while producing a cosmetic improvement, does not eradicate all nevus cells at risk (Zitelli and associates, 1984). A similar method described originally by Cronin (1953) employs a dermatome to remove the nevus down to the dermis. This is applicable to the extensive nevi, in which excision is all but impossible owing to the lack of uninvolved donor sites (Kaplan and Nickoloff, 1987).

The *amelanotic melanoma* is a relatively rare variant of melanoma, which is more common in women and is thought to behave more aggressively. It carries a poor prognosis (Huvos, Shah, and Goldsmith, 1972) attributable in part to a delay in diagnosis because of the lack of pigment. After the diagnosis has been established, this melanoma should be treated as any other variety.

The *malignant blue nevus* is another rare melanotic tumor; there are only isolated cases reported. It probably represents a neoplastic change in a cellular blue nevus, a benign lesion found most often on the buttocks of women (Rodriguez and Ackerman, 1968). An unusual aspect of this tumor is the ability of a person with lymph node metastases to survive for many years in apparent symbiosis with the disease (Dorsey and Montgomery, 1954).

The *desmoplastic melanoma* is a variant of melanoma that is classified separately because of its pathologic findings. It was first described by Conley, Lattes, and Orr in 1971. In the author's experience, it tends to be bulky and nonpigmented (Fig. 74–29), and there may be a history of previous treatment after an erroneous diagnosis (Valensi, 1977).

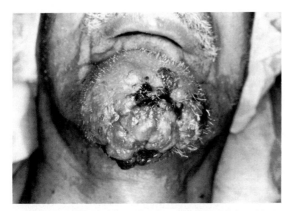

Figure 74–29. A desmoplastic melanoma of the chin in a 70 year old black man with vitiligo. The local disease was controlled by resection; he died of lung metastases two years later.

Although the prognosis is considered poor, aggressive local treatment may produce cures. Death is usually due to distant metastasis.

Melanoma with an unknown primary origin is not classifiable on clinical grounds. Its first manifestation is the presence of metastatic disease in regional nodes or other organs. It was reported in 3.7 per cent of a Memorial Sloan-Kettering Institute series (McNeer and Das Gupta, 1965) and 8.7 per cent of a series of melanomas observed at the M. D. Anderson Hospital in Texas (Smith and Stehlin, 1965). The true incidence is probably lower, as these institutions are cancer referral centers with a special interest in melanoma. An identifiable primary lesion may be absent because a host immune system, although capable of destroying the skin lesion, is overwhelmed by systemic metastases. When a skin lesion occurs, the prognosis is poor, because all patients appear for diagnosis and treatment in an advanced stage of their disease (Stage III or IV). The prognosis is not entirely hopeless, however, and in the series reported by Das Gupta, Bowden, and Berg (1963) 24 patients had metastasis in one regional node site; these were treated by lymph node dissection, and ten survived five years. Other workers also agree that this group of patients has a prognosis as good or better than that of patients with a known primary site and lymph node involvement (Baab and McBride, 1975).

In a similar group of patients the primary lesion is unavailable for examination because the lesion has been destroyed by the original treatment with cautery, an acid solution, or radiation therapy; occasionally the specimen has been discarded and is unavailable for examination. These patients have local recurrences (Fig. 74–30), which in the author's opinion should be treated as deep lesions by aggressive local excision and also should be considered for elective regional node dissection (ERND).

Microscopic Invasion as Prognostic Factor

An important aspect of treatment evaluation in any disease process is the uniform comparison of treatment results. This may be done by clinical staging, which may not allow for variables in tumor biology as indicated by the depth of invasion and cellular activity. To evaluate these variables several workers have described staging systems based on the microscopic study of the primary lesion; the frequency of mitoses, the degree of pleomorphism of the melanoma cells, the lympho-

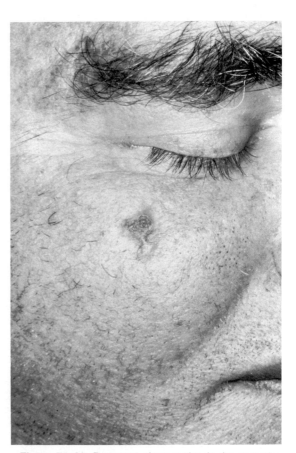

Figure 74–30. Recurrent pigmentation in the scar of a pigmented lesion treated by local destruction by acid and fulguration three years earlier. Dense scar tissue prevented either a Clark level determination or a depth measurement. The melanoma metastasized to submental nodes.

cytic reaction around the tumor, the presence of ulceration, and the depth of invasion have all been studied.

Mehnert and Heard (1965), in a retrospective study of 176 examples of invasive melanoma, demonstrated a clear relationship between the depth of invasion of the skin by melanoma cells and the five year survival rate. They also showed a considerable improvement in five year survival rate when a prophylactic node dissection was added to the treatment plan in lesions confined to the dermis (Group 2 in their classification). Clark and associates (1969) further subdivided the degree of invasion into Levels I to V and added considerably to the knowledge of the behavior of melanoma; they combined this with their clinical classification of lentigo malignant melanoma, superficial spreading melanoma, and nodular melanoma as described above.

The levels of invasion are shown in Figure 74–31:

Level I. Tumor cells are confined to the epidermis above the basement membrane. This is also called melanoma in situ and is not considered a malignancy for statistical or treatment purposes.

Level II. Tumor cells are present in the papillary dermis after having broken through the basement membrane of the epidermis.

Level III. Tumor cells have filled the pap-

illary dermis and penetrated down to but not into the reticular dermis.

Level IV. Tumor cells are in the reticular dermis.

Level V. Tumor cells have penetrated through the reticular dermis into the subcutaneous fat.

In preliminary studies, the reported mortality observed during the follow-up period was for Level II, 8.2 per cent; Level III, 32.5 per cent; Level IV, 46.1 per cent; and Level V, 52.0 per cent (Clark and associates, 1969).

Another method of grouping melanoma according to depth of invasion is that of Breslow (1970), who measured the thickness of the melanoma from the granular layer of the skin down to the deepest portion of the melanoma by using an ocular micrometer. In his study of 98 patients, Breslow (1970) recorded a 100 per cent five year survival in all patients with melanoma less than 0.76 mm in thickness. There were no examples of local recurrence or of metastases to lymph nodes in any of the thin lesions, even when they were classified as Clark Level III. Since this original report the observation that the micrometer measurement of melanoma thickness is the single most accurate indicator of prognosis has been confirmed by many studies. This measurement has now become the basis of treatment planning for all types of melanoma of the skin (Hansen and McCarten, 1974; Wanebo, Woodruff, and Fortner, 1975; Balch and associates, 1978).

Micrometer measurement is consistently reproducible, in that pathologists report similar results when examining the same slides, an experience not always true of the Clark classification in which Levels II and III could be confused. It does require attention to detail in slide preparation and the use of multiple step-sections to avoid underestimating the thickness (Breslow, 1980). The critical measurement originally reported was 0.76 mm, in that all individuals with melanoma less than 0.76 mm in thickness survived without local recurrence or metastatic disease.

Breslow (1980) did warn that metastatic disease was a possibility, and, since the original report (on a series of only 98 patients), it has become evident that in a small number of patients with thin lesions metastatic disease both to regional lymph nodes and to distant sites develops (Gromet, Epstein, and Blois, 1978). There is evidence of tumor regression and therefore a reduced thickness measurement in many of these patients (Na-

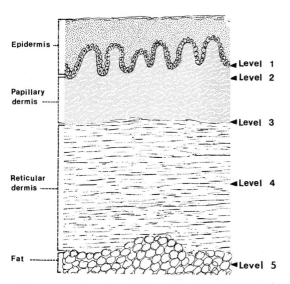

Figure 74–31. Levels of invasion of the skin by melanoma cells. (After Clark, W. H., From, L., Bernadino, E. A., and Mihm, M. C.: The histogenesis and biologic behavior of primary human malignant melanomas of the skin. Cancer Res., 29:705, 1969.)

runs and associates, 1986). In thin lesions, therefore, the presence of tumor regression should be recorded by the pathologist to alert the physician to the possibility of metastatic disease. The prognosis of thicker lesions in the Breslow (1980) study was noted to be worse as the thickness of the melanoma increased. Of 18 patients with melanoma greater than 3.0 mm in thickness only four survived for five years.

Treatment

The primary curative therapy for melanoma is surgery; other available modalities (e.g., chemotherapy, immunotherapy, and radiation therapy alone or in combination) are at best palliative at the present time.

Each patient with a biopsy proven melanoma is evaluated individually, and, after all factors contributing to prognosis are assessed, a treatment plan is determined.

Complete evaluation of the patient includes history, physical examination, pathologic examination of the lesion, laboratory work-up, and appropriate radiographic studies to identify the presence of metastatic disease. A chest radiograph is obtained in all patients; bone and liver scans are not indicated for the investigation of thicker lesions, unless there is strong evidence of metastatic disease, because of the low pick-up rate and many false-positive findings in the absence of symptoms (Iscoe and associates, 1987).

When the work-up has been completed, it is possible for the physician to determine the clinical stage. The original, most widely used staging classification (McNeer and Das Gupta, 1964) was simple and consisted of the following:

Stage I. The primary lesion confined to the local area with no evidence of metastatic disease.

Stage IA. Local recurrence or local satellite lesions without metastatic disease.

Stage II. Primary lesion with metastatic disease to the draining regional lymph node as detected by palpation.

Stage III. Primary lesion with distant metastasis to more than one regional node group or another area of the body.

Although it is still used in daily clinical practice, the classification provides limited information and does not allow for the inclusion of microstaging.

The American Joint Committee on Cancer (AJCC) has devised a more comprehensive system, which is now being adopted. It combines the tumor, nodes, and metastases (TNM) system with the microstaging systems of Clark and associates (1969) and Breslow (1970):

Stage IA. T1, N0, M0; localized disease less than 0.76 mm in thickness or Level II.

Stage IB. T2, N0, M0; localized disease 0.76 to 1.5 mm in thickness or Level III.

Stage IIA. T3, N0, M0; localized disease 1.5 to 4 mm in thickness or Level IV.

Stage IIB. T4, N0, M0; localized disease 4.1 mm or more in thickness or Level V.

Stage III. Any T, N1, M0; any melanoma with involvement of one regional node group or in-transit metastases.

Stage IV. Any T, N2, M0 or any T, any N, plus M1 or M2; any melanoma with advanced local regional node disease, more than one regional node group involvement, or distant organ metastases.

For uniformity of recording, a data form for recording the extent of the tumor and all available information is used (Fig. 74–32).

TREATMENT OF STAGE IA, IB, IIA, AND IIB (AJCC) MELANOMA

Treatment of Primary Melanoma of Skin. In this group of patients the disease is confined to the original area of the excisional or incisional biopsy with no clinical evidence of regional node disease or distant metastasis as determined by the first examination (former Stage I).

The traditional treatment for melanoma in this stage was a wide excision in both periphery and depth, the recommended margin extending to 5 cm around the lesion; in some locations this approach has to be modified (e.g., for extremity and face and scalp lesions). The recommended depth of excision includes the deep fascia, although the need for this has been questioned (Olsen, 1964). The deep fascia varies in different parts of the body from a thick, almost tendinous sheet to a thin membrane and is not readily identifiable in the face. From a technical aspect, selection of the deep fascia as the margin in depth provides the surgeon with a consistent, readily dissectable plane, and this may represent its only value, as its removal has no effect on survival in lesions of the trunk and extremities (Kenady, Brown, and McBride, 1982).

Wide excision of the primary lesion is believed to remove not only any residuum of the primary tumor but also the local lymphatic bed, which may already have been contaminated by neoplastic cells. In a series reported by McNeer and Cantin (1967) the failure rate varied from 15 per cent for Stage I melanoma of the head and neck to 8 per cent for trunk and extremity tumors. The incidence of local treatment failure in Stage II disease was high (45 per cent for lesions of the head and neck and 21 per cent for those of the extremities). Other reports of local treatment failure range from 20 to 30 per cent through 18 per cent (Petersen, Bodenham, and Lloyd, 1962). When wide deep excisions are standard, lower recurrence rates are recorded.

With improved understanding of the biologic behavior of melanoma and the more accurate prognostic factors identified by the work of Mehnert and Heard (1965), Clark and associates (1969), Breslow (1970), and others, the optimal surgical margins for cure of local disease are being redefined, and the current belief is that the surgical margins for thin lesions may safely be reduced.

The biopsy site of melanoma in situ (Clark Level I), in reality a benign lesion in which penetration through the epidermis has yet to occur, should be reexcised. To avoid local recurrence, which is still a possibility with this lesion, a peripheral margin in the 0.5 to 1 cm range is recommended.

The findings of Breslow (1970) have been confirmed by other investigators in retrospective analyses correlating survival and lesion thickness (Urist, Balch, and Milton, 1985; Zeitels and associates, 1988). The minimal effective margins for the local cure of melanoma have to be determined by prospective studies, several of which are in progress. They are of necessity long-term projects of 10 to 15 years' duration to obtain significant numbers of patients in each category.

Meanwhile, from current information, for invasive lesions less than 0.76 mm in thickness a 1 cm margin is locally curative; for lesions 1 mm or less in thickness extension of the margin beyond 2 cm has no effect on five year survival (Zeitels and associates, 1988). Melanoma greater than 1 mm in thickness should be excised with a 3 cm margin, if possible. The use of additional margins in the thicker lesions does not seem to alter the local recurrence rate, the prognosis being determined by the presence of distant metastases (Heenan and associates, 1985).

The surgeon must still exercise clinical judgment in the selection of margins and should be more aggressive in the treatment of nodular melanoma, as compared with lentigo malignant melanoma, and in the treatment of male patients, who are thought to have a worse prognosis than females. Lesions of certain sites such as the back and the scalp may also have a worse prognosis than those occurring elsewhere, although this concept has not been confirmed by further study (Cascinelli and associates, 1986).

Closure of Defect. The reduction in the size of excision currently recommended makes closure of the resulting defect much simpler than in the past. An elliptic excision with direct closure after some undermining should be possible in the majority of patients. In patients whose lesions are greater than 1 mm in thickness, in whom a 3 cm margin is recommended, closure by undermining may be possible on the trunk; elsewhere a skin graft or flap should be used to achieve closure without the need for excessive undermining.

In patients for whom a skin graft closure is selected, the excision should be beveled under the peripheral edge of the defect to avoid an unsightly residual step between the graft and the surrounding skin. On the back, where graft stabilization is difficult owing to arm and shoulder movement, the author prefers a meshed graft to improve the rate of successful vascularization. In the majority of patients the donor site for the split-thickness skin grafts is selected from the buttock or the thigh, and the graft should be taken from the contralateral side in lower extremity lesions.

If a skin graft is selected for closure of the ablative defect of the face or neck, a full-thickness skin graft is preferred. The recommended donor sites are the opposite supraclavicular or retroauricular areas. If a flap closure is selected for the face, large rotation flaps are useful in the infraorbital area; for the cheek and chin area, advancement flaps from the neck are applicable (see Chap. 38). If a neck flap is to be used for closure, consideration should be given to a regional node dissection at the same time, as transgression of the neck will occur in the elevation of the flap. If bulk is needed in addition to skin coverage, as would occur on the cheek when a parotidectomy has also been performed, a transposed trapezius flap may

MELANOMA OF THE SKIN (ICD-O 173 With Histologic Type 872–879)

Data Form for Cancer Staging

Patient identification
Name _____
Address _____
Hospital or clinic number _____
Age _____ Sex _____ Race _____

Institutional identification
Hospital or clinic _____
Address _____

Oncology Record

Anatomic site of cancer _____
Chronology of classification*   [ ] Clinical-diagnostic (cTNM)
                                 [ ] Surgical-evaluative (sTNM)
Date of classification _____

Histologic type† _____ Grade (G) _____
[ ] Postsurgical resection–pathologic (pTNM)
[ ] Retreatment (rTNM)   [ ] Autopsy (aTNM)

Definitions: TNM Classification

Primary Tumor (T)

[ ] TX No evidence of primary tumor (unknown primary or primary tumor removed and not histologically examined)

[ ] T0 Atypical melanocytic hyperplasia (Clark Level I); not a malignant lesion

[ ] T1 Invasion of papillary dermis (Level II) or 0.75-mm thickness or less

[ ] T2 Invasion of the papillary–reticular-dermal interface (Level III) or 0.76- to 1.5-mm thickness

[ ] T3 Invasion of the reticular dermis (Level IV) or 1.51- to 4.0-mm thickness

[ ] T4 Invasion of subcutaneous tissue (Level V) or 4.1 mm or more in thickness or satellite(s) within 2 cm of any primary melanoma

Nodal Involvement (N)

[ ] NX Minimum requirements to assess the regional nodes cannot be met.

[ ] N0 No regional lymph node involvement

[ ] N1 Involvement of only one regional lymph node station; node(s) movable and not over 5 cm in diameter or negative regional lymph nodes and the presence of less than five in-transit metastases beyond 2 cm from primary site

[ ] N2 Any one of the following: (1) involvement of more than one regional lymph node station; (2) regional node(s) over 5 cm in diameter or fixed; (3) five or more in-transit metastases or any in-transit metastases beyond 2 cm from primary site with regional lymph node involvement

Distant Metastasis (M)

[ ] MX Minimum requirements to assess the presence of distant metastasis cannot be met.

[ ] M0 No known distant metastasis

[ ] M1 Involvement of skin or subcutaneous tissue beyond the site of primary lymph node drainage
        Specify _____

[ ] M2 Visceral metastasis (spread to any distant site other than skin or subcutaneous tissues)
        Specify _____

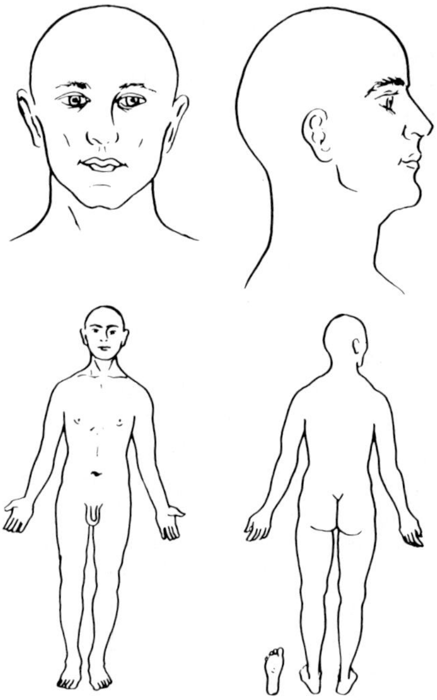

Type of Lesion

[ ] Lentigo maligna   [ ] Radial spreading
[ ] Nodular   [ ] Acral lentiginous
                           [ ] Unclassified

*Use a separate form each time a case is staged.
†See reverse side for additional information.

Indicate on diagrams primary tumor and regional nodes involved.

Depth of Invasion
[ ] Level I (not a melanoma and further characterization is not necessary)
[ ] Level II   [ ] Level IV
[ ] Level III   [ ] Level V
Other description _____
Maximal thickness (mm) _____
Site of primary lesion (check diagram)

_____

Extent of primary lesion (include all pigmentation)

_____

Size in greatest diameter _____. cm

Characteristics

[ ] Ulceration
[ ] Other _____

Examination by _____ M.D.
Date _____

American Joint Committee on Cancer

Figure 74–32. The American Joint Commission on Cancer's melanoma data form. (From Beahrs, O. H., and Myers, M. H. (Eds.): Manual for Staging of Cancer. Philadelphia, J. B. Lippincott Company, 1983.)

Stage Grouping

[ ] Stage IA   T1, N0, M0
[ ] Stage IB   T2, N0, M0
[ ] Stage IIA   T3, N0, M0
[ ] Stage IIB   T4, N0, M0
[ ] Stage III   Any T, N1, M0
[ ] Stage IV   Any T, N2, M0
              Any T, any N, M1 or M2

Staging Procedures

A variety of procedures and special studies may be employed in the process of staging a given tumor. Both the clinical usefulness and cost efficiency must be considered. The following suggestions are made for staging of malignant melanoma:

Essential for staging

1. Complete physical examination
2. Pathologic study of surgically removed material, including depth of invasion and thickness of primary tumor
3. Chest roentgenogram
4. Known residual tumor at primary site if present

May be useful for staging or patient management

1. Multichemistry screen
2. Gallium scan
3. Bone scan
4. Liver–spleen scan
5. CT scans
6. Brain scans
7. Performance status (Karnofsky or ECOG)

Primary Tumor (T)

Both the depth of invasion and the maximum measured thickness determine the T-classification and should be recorded. When the depth of invasion and the thickness do not match the categories of T-classification, whichever of the two is greatest should take precedence.

Regional Nodes (N)

The regional nodes are related to the region of the body in which the tumor is located; such first station nodes are as follows:

1. For head and face: preauricular, cervical
2. For neck and upper chest wall: cervical (anterior–posterior), supraclavicular, axillary
3. For chest wall, anterior and posterior, and arms above elbow: axillary
4. For hands and upper extremities below the elbow: epitrochlear or axillary
5. For the abdominal wall, anterior and posterior, and lower extremities above the knee: femoral inguinal nodes (groin)
6. For the feet and below the knees: popliteal or femoral inguinal nodes (groin)

Histopathology

Types of malignant melanoma: lentigo maligna (Hutchinson's) with adjacent intraepidermal component of radial spreading type (superficial spreading), without adjacent intraepidermal component (nodular), and unclassified.

Both the depth of invasion (Clark) and the thickness of the tumor (Breslow) have been shown to have prognostic significance and both parameters should be reported by the pathologist.

Five levels of the skin have been designated for identification of depth of invasion:

[ ] Level I (epidermis to epidermal–dermal interface). Lesions involving only the epidermis have been designated level I. These lesions are considered to be "atypical melanocytic hyperplasia" and are not included in the staging of malignant melanoma, *for they do not represent a malignant lesion.*
[ ] Level II (papillary dermis). Invasion of the papillary dermis does not reach the papillary–reticular dermal interface.
[ ] Level III (papillary–reticular dermis interface). Invasion involves the full thickness of, fills, and expands the papillary dermis; it abuts upon but does not penetrate the reticular dermis.
[ ] Level IV (reticular dermis). Invasion occurs into the reticular dermis but not into the subcutaneous tissue.
[ ] Level V (subcutaneous tissue). Invasion moves through the reticular dermis into the subcutaneous tissue.

Histologic Grade

[ ] G1   Well differentiated
[ ] G2   Moderately well differentiated
[ ] G3–G4 Poorly to very poorly differentiated

Postsurgical Resection–Pathologic Residual Tumor (R)

Does not enter into staging but may be a factor in deciding further treatment

[ ] R0   No residual tumor
[ ] R1   Microscopic residual tumor
[ ] R2   Macroscopic residual tumor
          Specify _____

Performance Status of Host (H)

Several systems for recording a patient's activity and symptoms are in use and are more or less equivalent as follows:

AJCC	Performance	ECOG Scale	Karnofsky Scale (%)
[ ] H0	Normal activity	0	90–100
[ ] H1	Symptomatic but ambulatory; cares for self	1	70–80
[ ] H2	Ambulatory more than 50% of time; occasionally needs assistance	2	50–60
[ ] H3	Ambulatory 50% or less of time; nursing care needed	3	30–40
[ ] H4	Bedridden; may need hospitalization	4	10–20

Figure 74–32 *Continued*

be indicated, although the color match is less than satisfactory. The use of tissue expansion as a secondary procedure to replace skin grafts is also proving an adequate alternative to improve the final aesthetic result (see Chap. 13).

Management of Regional Nodes in Stage IA, IB, IIA, and IIB (AJCC) Melanoma. In this group of patients, by definition there is no clinical disease palpable in the regional lymph nodes at the presurgical examination. Some of these patients do have subclinical disease, as determined by the subsequent examination of the regional nodes removed at surgery. It is these patients who benefit from an elective or prophylactic regional node dissection.

The percentage of subclinical regional node involvement has varied from 25 per cent (McNeer and Das Gupta, 1964) through 20 per cent (Harris, Gumport and Maiwandi, 1972), 16 per cent (McCarthy, Haagensen, and Herter, 1974), and 5 per cent in an Australian series (Davis, 1972). The Melanoma Cooperative Group using a combined series from the Massachusetts General Hospital and the New York University Medical Center reported a 14 per cent incidence of node involvement in ERND (Day and Sober, 1981). Advocates of elective regional node dissection cite this subgroup as the one likely to benefit from regional node dissection.

Patients with clinical Stage I disease (McNeer and Das Gupta staging) who were found to have pathologically involved nodes after a regional node dissection performed at the time of the primary excision or shortly thereafter were reported to have a five year survival of 52.6 per cent; this figure was only 31 per cent for Stage I patients who developed palpable nodes subsequently and then had a regional node dissection. An even worse five year survival of 19 per cent was reported for patients with Stage II melanoma from this same series (McNeer and Das Gupta, 1964). The 1981 report of Day and associates studied 325 patients who had an ERND; only 14 per cent of these individuals had node involvement and their five year survival was 42 per cent, a result similar to that found in earlier reports. This was a prospective but not a randomized study, and microstaging was not used to determine treatment. Twenty-five patients with melanomas less than 3.5 mm in thickness had a 59 per cent five year survival, as compared with a 22 per cent five year survival for the 21 patients who had melanomas greater than 3.5 mm in thickness. Patients with Clark Level III disease, of whom there were ten, had an 80 per cent five year survival rate.

It seems logical to assume that thickness measurement and Clark microstaging will provide the clinician with a more precise method to identify the patient most likely to have occult regional node disease and thus derive benefit from an ERND. The unnecessary surgery performed on a substantial number of the patients in previously reported series would thus be avoided.

The measurement of thickness alone should not be allowed to determine treatment; other factors must be considered, including the anatomic site, the age and sex of the patient, the type of melanoma considered to be present, and the presence of ulceration. These variables may influence survival rates when these rates are corrected for thickness of the lesion.

As was noted with the question of the determination of surgical margins, this dilemma will be answered only by the long-term, prospective, randomized studies currently in progress.

The true incidence of microscopic involvement of regional lymph nodes is probably higher than that reported in virtually all of the published reports. In none of the series, except that of McCarthy, Haagensen, and Herter (1974), were total clearance of lymph nodes and serial sections routinely performed; thus most studies are dependent on the diligence of a pathology department, a variable factor.

Those who do not recommend ERND in their management of melanoma advance the argument that the majority of patients undergoing surgery survive without it, as they never develop regional node disease and derive no benefit from the surgery. They also argue that there is minimal if any difference in survival whether the patient with micrometastasis has a node dissection at the time of the original primary excision or waits until clinical involvement of nodes is exhibited (Elder and associates, 1985). This study was based on a five year follow-up period and, as was emphasized originally by McNeer and Das Gupta (1964), there is a continued decrease in survival between the fifth year and the tenth and even the fifteenth year.

From the clinician's, and probably the patient's, viewpoint, the prognosis for advanced primary melanoma (Stage IIA and B) to progress to Stage III or IV disease, is so dire that anything that can be done to improve it is welcomed; this would include the acceptance of an ERND to remove undetectable micrometastases. This may avoid the conversion to Stage III disease with its much worse prognosis and its potential for distant metastases. The findings of Day and associates (1981) support this premise; they noted that patients with thin lesions and abnormal node findings at ERND had a survival of 80 per cent at five years as opposed to a 27 per cent five year survival for those with melanomas greater than 3.5 mm in thickness. They also noted that multiple nodal involvement at ERND worsened the prognosis.

By using information currently available indications and contraindications for elective regional node dissection may be formulated:

1. In lesions less than 0.76 mm in thickness ERND should not be performed, although the patient should be examined at regular intervals, preferably by the same examiner, as long as metastatic disease is possible.

2. Patients with a clinical diagnosis of lentigo malignant melanoma do not warrant an ERND because of the less aggressive behavior of this lesion (McGovern and associates, 1980). However, they should be followed at frequent intervals.

3. For lesions between 0.76 mm and 1.5 mm in thickness, clinical judgment must be exercised. In selected patients an ERND should be considered:
   a. Patients who may not be suitable for careful follow-up, such as itinerant workers and unreliable individuals.
   b. Male patients with a poor prognosis.
   c. Individuals with involvement of anatomic sites that may have a poor prognosis, such as the head, neck, and back.
   d. Those in whom the melanoma is anatomically located so that the wide excision would transgress a regional node site.
   e. Melanomas in the thickness range and also classified as Clark Level IV or V.
   f. Nodular melanomas, which are considered to have a somewhat worse prognosis.
   g. All ulcerated lesions.
   h. Lesions that have had previous inadequate treatment with local recurrence.

4. All lesions more than 1.5 mm in thickness should have ERND performed unless there

is a medical contraindication, as this group of patients have a 57 per cent risk of regional node metastases developing within three years of diagnosis. The difference in survival after ERND in this group of patients with lesions between 1.5 mm and 4 mm in thickness is substantial; the improvement is in the 30 per cent range at five years and 45 per cent at ten years (Balch and associates, 1982).

There are other contraindications to ERND. Although none of the standard regional node dissections is a major procedure, there may be medical contraindications. Extreme patient age may make the surgeon hesitate to perform an ERND, particularly because controversy about the need for the procedure exists. In these situations close observation and follow-up is an acceptable alternative. Another contraindication is a melanoma located at a site from which the predicted drainage may go to two or more regional node basins (e.g., the center of the back and subcostal area). Lymphoscintigraphy provides a method of correctly predicting the lymph node drainage of these sites of indeterminate drainage. It will become a useful addition to the presurgical evaluation of melanoma patients when it becomes clinically available.

The regional node dissections performed as elective procedures may be modified at the discretion of the surgeon. To improve the aesthetic result in the neck the preservation of the sternocleidomastoid muscle and the accessory nerve is acceptable, provided metastatic disease is not seen during the dissection. The morbidity of a radical groin dissection is reduced by limiting the operation to the superficial node group (McCarthy, Haagensen, and Herter, 1974); only if node involvement is detected when the specimen is examined during the operation is the deep dissection completed.

Adjuvant Therapy and Management of Stage IIA and IIB (AJCC) Melanoma. Because of the disappointing results in the surgical treatment of Stage IIA and IIB melanoma, the addition of adjuvant therapy to the treatment protocol seems advisable when only undetected micrometastases are present and the tumor burden is minimal (Kaiser, Burk, and Morton, 1981).

Preliminary studies in this category of patients have yielded negative results (Day and associates, 1981), and a randomized, controlled trial of adjuvant chemotherapy in a similar high risk group again showed no difference in survival between the control and the treated groups (Tranum and associates, 1987).

Only long-term studies will determine which, if any, adjuvant treatment is effective. Patients with lesions in these staging groups should be considered for inclusion in ongoing trials and encouraged to participate in the evaluation of new immunotherapy and chemotherapy agents.

TREATMENT OF STAGE III (AJCC) DISEASE

All patients who are thought to have regional node disease at their initial evaluation and in whom distant metastases are not detected by a complete evaluation should be treated by regional node dissection at the same time as the primary lesion is treated or shortly thereafter. This should be done as soon as possible after diagnosis.

In melanomas of the head and neck (especially those of the anterior scalp, forehead, cheek, and ear), in addition to standard cervical node dissection, superficial parotidectomy should be performed. For posterior neck and scalp lesions, excision of the posterior cervical nodes in continuity with the primary lesion plus the standard neck dissection is necessary.

If doubt exists as to the status of the regional lymph nodes in thin melanomas, the node dissection may be preceded by either a fine needle aspiration biopsy or an open biopsy of a representative node, proceeding to a node dissection only if findings are abnormal.

In lower extremity lesions the superficial node dissection should be accompanied by an in-continuity dissection of the deep iliac and obturator node groups.

The prognosis in Stage III (AJCC) disease is modified by the thickness of the primary lesion and the number of nodes found to be abnormal on examination of the surgical specimen. In a series of patients with abnormal node findings those with lesions less than 3.5 mm in thickness were found to have an 80 per cent five year survival, contrasted with 27 per cent survival for those patients with a melanoma greater than 3.5 mm in thickness (Day and associates, 1981). The same study reported a five year survival of 48 per cent

for those with less than four abnormal nodes in the surgical specimen. This survival rate fell to 17 per cent if more than four nodes had tumor metastases. All patients with involved nodes identified at surgery should be considered for adjuvant therapy, although, as stated above, at the present time there is no consistently effective modality available (Veronesi and associates, 1980).

Regional Perfusion. The use of regional perfusion with melphalan for the treatment of advanced disease of the extremities has been reported for many years (Stehlin and Clark, 1965). The addition of heat to the perfusate produced a substantial improvement in response rates and survival time, even in patients with advanced local recurrences and in-transit metastases, a 50 per cent ten year survival being obtained in a group of such patients (Stehlin and associates, 1988). The method is not without problems, and thrombophlebitis, limb edema, local tissue necrosis, and leakage of the agent into the systemic circulation may occur. Its general acceptance has been slow; this may be attributed in part to a lack of a controlled study to demonstrate its true effect. In addition, in the hands of the occasional practitioner it is tedious and time consuming. Patients with advanced local disease of the extremities, local recurrence, in-transit metastases, and regional node disease should be considered for this adjunctive procedure, the improved survival rates justifying its use.

Radiation Therapy. The addition of postoperative radiation therapy administered directly to the involved regional node basin has no effect on either long-term survival or a disease-free interval (Creagan and associates, 1978).

TREATMENT OF STAGE IV (AJCC) DISEASE

The modalities used in an attempt to improve the survival of patients with Stage III disease are also employed in the management of those with proven distant metastases: systemic chemotherapy, immunotherapy, and radiation used alone or in combination. On occasion, surgical procedures may be indicated either to reduce the individual tumor burden so that adjuvant therapy may be rendered more effective or to obtain palliation of local symptoms (e.g. the relief of intestinal obstruction if metastases of the small bowel are present).

Chemotherapy in Stage IV (AJCC) Disease. All of the drugs available for the chemotherapy of cancer have probably been tried at one time or another in the treatment of advanced melanoma, and as yet no effective drug regimen has been developed for systemic use in this disease. Several drugs are known to produce a clinical response in the management of melanoma, which is being defined as a 50 per cent or more regression in tumor size persisting for one or more months. The most useful of the available agents is dacarbazine (DTIC). This drug has been under investigation and in clinical use for over 15 years, and response rates in the 25 per cent range have been reported (Luce, 1975). The drug has also been used in combination with other chemotherapeutic agents, notably carmustine (BCNU) and hydroxyurea (Costanzi, 1973; Hill and associates, 1974) and more recently cisplatin. The addition of cisplatin may increase the response rate (Oratz and associates, 1987), although side effects are more pronounced (Gundersen, 1987).

Combination drug therapy regimens do not increase the percentage of responders to treatment; those who do respond, however, have an increased mean survival of 67 weeks as compared with only 20 weeks in nonresponders (York and Foltz, 1988). The occasional long-term survival does justify the use of drug regimens in this group. They not only have an increased survival time but are also afforded the emotional support provided by the knowledge that everything possible is being done to help them. This approach also must be balanced against the sometimes severe side effects of drug therapy, more so when one considers the lack of consistent response to treatment.

IMMUNOTHERAPY

There are well-documented but rare examples of (1) spontaneous regression of malignant melanoma (Everson and Cole, 1966), (2) the occasional prolonged interval between initial therapy and death from metastatic disease, and (3) the significant incidence of unidentified primary melanomas known to produce regional node metastases; these point to the existence of an effective immune response in some individuals with this disease. The immune system of the body is capable of responding to an antigenic stimulus with a humoral or a cellular immune response, or both, depending on the nature of the stimulus. Laboratory studies and clinical observation indicate that both systems are operative in tumor immunology (Hellström and associates, 1968; Clark and Nathanson, 1973), and they should not be regarded as separate entities. After 20 years of investigation, however, the results of attempts at manipulating the immune system of the melanoma patient have been disappointing.

Nonspecific Immune Therapy. The early enthusiasm for nonspecific stimulation of the competent immune system by the use of bacille Calmette-Guérin (BCG) (Morton and associates, 1974) has waned owing to the lack of a long-term improvement in survival (Kaiser, Burk, and Morton, 1981). Similar observations have been made on the use of *Corynebacterium parvum* to stimulate an immune response (Hilal and associates, 1981).

Adoptive Immune Therapy. The knowledge that the cellular immune system is a major factor in host resistance to cancer has prompted attempts to transfer immunocompetent cells to cancer patients who may lack such cells (Woodruff and Symes, 1962).

To enhance the degree of immunity obtained, transfer factor (Lawrence, 1954) derived from the lyophilization of white blood cells already stimulated by prior exposure to tumor cells was also used (Brandes, Galton, and Wiltshaw, 1971), with some encouraging results (Krementz and associates, 1974). Investigation over a period of years with a controlled trial of transfer factor has not shown any significant improvement in long-term survival of high risk patients (Miller and associates, 1988). The occasional prolonged survival in patients with advanced disease (Gonzalez, Wong, and Spitler, 1980) justifies continued study of this form of immunotherapy.

Specific Immune Therapy. The use of melanoma cell preparations, both autogenous and allogeneic, in the therapy of melanoma has been investigated for over 20 years. The rationale for the use of specific melanoma cell preparations was based on observed increases in cytotoxic antibodies after the injection of irradiated melanoma cell suspensions into patients with melanoma (Ikonopisov and associates, 1970). The evaluation of melanoma cell extracts in the management of melanoma has continued over the years (Goodwin, Hornung, and Krementz, 1973; Hollinshead and associates, 1982).

The use of melanoma cell cultures to prepare antigenic vaccines has also been investigated; immune responses have been demonstrated with, so far, an undetermined effect on survival (Bystryn and associates, 1988).

The role of interleukins and interferons in the treatment of melanoma is currently being evaluated, together with monoclonal antibodies. At the present time their status is undetermined; it would seem that, while no spectacular, consistent responses have been observed, they may be therapeutically helpful as adjuncts to other modalities (Legha, 1986).

RADIATION THERAPY

Traditionally in the United States melanoma, both in its primary and metastatic stages, was considered a radioresistant disease, a concept not accepted in Europe (Hellriegel, 1963). The report of Hilaris and associates (1963) stimulated renewed interest, and radiation therapy now has an accepted place in the management of metastatic disease. Skin nodules, involved lymph nodes, and cerebral metastases can respond, although the effect may be of short duration (Overgaard, 1980).

In summary, the current status of adjuvant therapy in the management of melanoma in all stages remains disappointing after more than 20 years of intensive clinical and laboratory investigation. The evaluation of chemotherapy, immunotherapy, and radiation, used alone and in their various combinations, must continue. Only in this way is it possible to evaluate new drugs as they become available, new directions in immunotherapy, and new techniques in radiation. Patients with a poor prognosis should be encouraged to participate in controlled postsurgical clinical trials, and those with metastatic disease should be referred to oncologists with a special interest and experience in this disease.

MOHS MICROGRAPHIC SURGERY

Perry Robins

As discussed above a number of modalities are effective in treating skin cancer: excisional surgery, radiation therapy, and electrodesiccation and curettage. A significant number of lesions, however, because of their pathologic type or anatomic site, resist the standard therapeutic methods and result in clinical recurrence.

The technique of chemosurgery developed by Mohs in 1932 has been effective in eradicating such tumors. The fundamental principle of Mohs surgery is serial excision and microscopic study of the excised tissue harboring malignant cells. The technique results in total ablation of malignancy, while at the same time sacrificing the least amount of uninvolved tissue.

The Mohs technique is particularly effective for the treatment of recurrent basal cell carcinomas, tumors with subcutaneous extensions difficult to eradicate by surgical means, multicentric tumors, and tumors in areas where tissue needs to be conserved, such as the eyelids, the inner canthus, and the nasal ala.

A basal cell carcinoma in the orbital region may require orbital exenteration by traditional surgical methods; however, the careful histologic control made possible by the Mohs technique may spare the patient a radical exenteration of the orbit.

Mohs should be credited with developing a method to fix tissue in situ without altering its architectural structure (Mohs, 1956, 1974, 1978). Preservation of tissue architecture was controlled by the application of a paste that contained 40 per cent zinc chloride in stibnite. These experiments led to the chemosurgical method by which cancer of the skin could be removed under microscopic control. The cancer cells were identified on microscopic examination. Refinement of the technique using fresh tissue currently permits the tumor to be surgically excised without the zinc chloride fixative, and the same pinpoint precision can be achieved in eradicating a skin cancer.

During the past 24 years approximately 20,000 extensive tumors of the skin have been treated successfully by the following method: (1) serial removal of the tissue suspected of having tumor cells, and (2) complete microscopic examination by a modified frozen section technique. These steps are repeated as often as is indicated by microscopic demonstration of residual tumor, the ultimate goal being complete removal of the neoplastic tissue with preservation of the maximal amount of uninvolved tissue.

Procedure

Chemosurgical Technique. The technique of chemosurgery is illustrated in Figure 74–33.

Precise microscopic control permits accurate mapping of cancers of the skin, including the columns of tumor cells that may extend for a considerable distance beyond the apparent margins of the tumor into the surrounding tissue. In order to eradicate such extension, surgeons and radiologists must excise or irradiate an additional margin of uninvolved tissue. In the process, normal tissue is sacrificed without complete assurance of eradication. Mohs surgery minimizes the sacrificing of normal tissue.

The treatment and follow-up of a patient with recurrent basal cell carcinoma are illustrated in Figure 74–34.

Fresh Tissue Technique (Mohs Micrographic Surgery). The fresh tissue technique was first employed when the chemosurgical procedure of Mohs was performed in the periorbital area, namely the medial canthus and the upper and lower lids. Zinc chloride paste is not applied to these sites because of the possibility of the fixative's causing irritation and damage to the globe. Instead the tissue is excised under local anesthesia and without the use of chemicals. The excised specimen is fixed in vitro, and frozen sections are cut through the undersurface of the fresh tissue specimens. The color coding of the edges and mapping of the tissue are performed as in the fixed tissue technique. The fresh sections are of sufficient quality that the identification of tumor cells is easily accomplished.

The application of this technique to other areas of the body was first described by Tromovitch and Stegeman (1974). The mechanics of the procedure was further developed, and the method has eventually been applied to larger tumors located elsewhere on the body.

The clinical extent of the tumor is first evaluated by gross examination. The area is anesthetized either regionally or locally; sterile technique is practiced. A small curette is used to remove any necrotic tissue. Sections of tissue measuring approximately 1 sq cm in area and 2 mm in thickness are excised. After microscopic examination of the tissue, the location of the neoplasm is recorded on the original map; the area of the previously treated site is again anesthetized, and the additional tumor is removed. The procedure is repeated until the entire area is found to be free of tumor. The fresh tissue technique was quickly accepted, and within a few years the zinc chloride paste was no longer utilized in routine procedures. The advantages over the fixed tissue technique are numerous: multiple stages can be accomplished in a short period of time; wound healing is frequently accelerated by primary closure in the smaller treated sites; and in larger treated sites reconstructive repairs can be done immediately when indicated.

Mohs Check. The Mohs check is a modified one-stage chemosurgical procedure in which one can confirm by microscopy whether a cutaneous cancer treated by electrodesiccation and curettage has been completely ablated. If there is any doubt that electrodesiccation and curettage have been successful, the patient is referred for this procedure.

The following steps are taken: (1) a thin slice of tissue is removed by scalpel in a saucer-like shape; (2) the excised specimen is cut into several pieces, and frozen sections from the undersurface of each are stained for microscopic examination; (3) if no signs of malignancy are found under microscopic study, nothing more need be done. If, however, malignancy is detected in some or all of the sections, the Mohs surgical steps are continued selectively or entirely until complete extirpation is achieved.

Indications

The prime indication for Mohs surgery is the advanced tumor that has recurred after previous treatment. The technique is equally effective in eradicating tumors located in areas such as the eyelid region, the canthus, the auricle, the nasolabial fold, and the nasal ala, where the maximal amount of uninvolved tissue must be preserved. Aggressive histopathologic types, such as morphea-like, infiltrating, and fibrotic basal cell carcinoma, should be included in this high risk group.

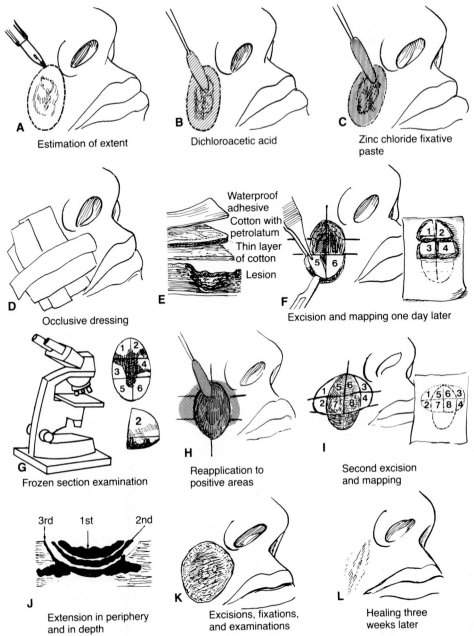

Figure 74–33. Mohs micrographic surgery. *A,* The clinical extent of the tumor is first measured and evaluated by gross examination. *B,* Dichloroacetic acid is applied to the surface of the entire area. *C,* Zinc chloride paste fixes tissue to a depth that depends on the thickness of the layer of paste applied and the length of time it is permitted to act. *D, E,* The treated area is covered with an occlusive dressing in an effort to decrease absorption of water by the hydroscopic paste. *F,* After an interval of several hours to one day, sections of tissue approximately 1 sq cm in area and 2 mm in thickness are surgically excised in a saucer-like shape. A map of the lesion site with a number assigned to each section is drawn at the time of excision. *G,* Each section, as it is removed, is identified by its corresponding number. Two intersecting edges are colored with red and blue dyes. These indelible marks are preserved during the histochemical staining process and allow the chemosurgeon to locate the exact position of any remaining malignancy visualized microscopically. The microscopic survey is done on frozen sections that have been cut horizontally from the *undersurface* of each excised tissue section and stained by hematoxylin and eosin. The location of the malignancy is marked on the original map of numbered sections and oriented exactly by the red and blue color coding. *H,* Zinc chloride paste is reapplied only to those areas of the previously treated site where residual tumor was found by microscopic survey. *I to L,* The procedure of fixation with zinc chloride paste, surgical excision of fixed tissue, color coding, and microscopic survey is repeated until all surgical specimens are found to be free of tumor.

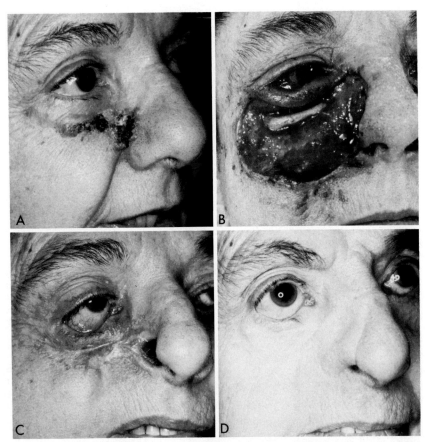

Figure 74–34. *A,* A 70 year old woman with a gradually enlarging crusted lesion below her right lower eyelid of ten years' duration. *B,* The area after removal of the five layers of tissue by excision. *C,* The site four months later after healing by second intention. *D,* Sixteen months after chemosurgery, reconstructive surgery was performed. The site has been free of tumor for an additional five years.

Tumors with poorly demarcated clinical borders and unusually large diameters represent additional indications for the use of the Mohs technique.

In addition to the high cure rate, another advantage of Mohs surgery that must be considered is that the procedure does not require general anesthesia; thus it extends the benefit of cure to many people who are poor medical candidates for conventional surgery. Since the mortality rate is practically nil, elderly patients with respiratory and circulatory problems are not precluded from treatment. In the author's series, most patients, including many who were 65 to 90 years of age, tolerated the procedure well. Most patients undergoing Mohs surgery can also be managed on an ambulatory basis.

The skin cancer not totally excised in the initial treatment will recur and present more complicated problems. It is a characteristic of recurrent lesions that their histologic architecture shows alteration. Instead of being solidly clustered within a mucinous stroma, the tumor cells are more widely dispersed within a dense cicatrix.

These changes make the boundaries and distribution of the malignancy less distinguishable by the usual clinical means. The danger is that unobserved and unpalpated pockets or extensions of tumor cells escape detection by conventional treatment and reseed new and deeper lesions (Fig. 74–35).

Nose. Mohs surgery is of significant value in the treatment of carcinomas of the nose, which often have extensions that are not clinically detectable. They invade in a surprisingly irregular and unpredictable manner, with a tendency to spread a great distance from the apparent clinical border. The tumors rarely invade nasal bone or cartilage.

Tumors of the nasolabial fold show a high

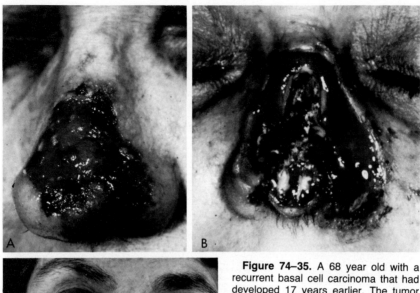

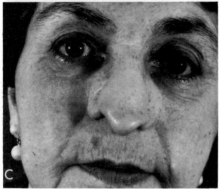

Figure 74–35. A 68 year old with a recurrent basal cell carcinoma that had developed 17 years earlier. The tumor had been repeatedly treated by curettage and electrodesiccation, and a full course of radiation therapy was also given. *A,* Appearance prior to chemosurgery. *B,* After five microscopically controlled stages by the chemosurgical technique and removal of nasal bone (which showed tumor involvement), the area was free of tumor. *C,* Reconstructive surgery was performed one year later, and the site has been free of tumor for the past eight years.

recurrence rate following initial treatment, and one encounters more often an aggressive type of tumor, such as the morphea or sclerosing type of basal cell carcinoma. The direction of spread is unpredictable, the tumor having the ability to grow deeply and laterally along the cheek or anteriorly along the nasal ala. The surgeon is frequently reluctant to remove tissue from the nasal ala because of fear of a deleterious cosmetic effect and the subsequent difficulty in nasal reconstruction. With complete microscopic control, the tumor can be extirpated with a high rate of cure, and an acceptable cosmetic result can often be achieved.

Auricle. Cancer of the auricle can also be safely eradicated by the Mohs technique. Small lesions usually require no corrective surgery, while in large lesions the maximum amount of uninvolved tissue is preserved to provide a basis for surgical reconstruction. Basal cell carcinoma rarely invades cartilage but tends to glide off and extend a considerable distance from its origin in a plane between cartilage and epidermis. It is not un-

common to observe the tumor extending from the anterior to the posterior surface.

Periorbital Region. Tumors of the lid and the periorbital area are excised with minimal complications. After the removal of small cancers of the lid margin, the surgical site usually heals spontaneously with an acceptable cosmetic result.

Cancer of the medial and lateral canthi can be removed by the fresh tissue technique, and it is possible to follow the tumor for considerable distance into the orbit without interfering with the function of the ocular globe.

Extensions of tumors from the eyelids deep into the medial and lateral canthi are not rare, especially in persistent or biologically aggressive tumors. Bizarre tumor extensions must be considered each time a lesion is to be treated. Clinical judgment based solely on palpation and radiographic evaluation provides insufficient criteria for the total extirpation of the more clinically difficult tumors.

Other Sites. The treatment of squamous cell carcinoma and occasional basal cell carcinomas involving the hands or fingers of physicians and dentists exposed to x-rays in their work is of special interest. In many instances, without the presence of nodes in the axilla, an amputation of the digit has been recommended; however, by tracing the tumors chemosurgically, the part can be preserved, and the patient is able to resume his occupation.

The technique is equally effective in the treatment of other malignant lesions, such as Bowen's disease, erythroplasia of Queyrat, and squamous cell carcinoma of the skin and glans of the penis, where the tumor can be eradicated by chemosurgery without sacrificing the organ or compromising its function. Cancer of the vulva has also been treated successfully and conservatively by Mohs surgery.

Cure Rate

Mohs micrographic surgery consistently offers the highest cure rate in the treatment of malignancy of the skin. From 1965 until 1987, at the New York University Medical Center, data have been gathered on 16,620 lesions from patients referred for Mohs micrographic surgery. Computer analysis of data from the medical records not only confirmed many assumptions but also revealed new trends in the growth and development of skin cancers. That basal cell and squamous cell carcinomas are primarily diseases of Caucasians was confirmed: of 16,620 patients treated, only five blacks and two Orientals had nonmelanoma skin cancers. The number of men with skin cancers was 8826 (53.2 per cent) compared with 7777 (46.8 per cent) for women. Even though skin cancer is more common in men, almost twice as many women less than 40 years of age were treated in the group: 7 per cent of women compared with 4.4 per cent of men were under the age of 40 years. The average age for men was 61.5 years; for women the average age was 60.7 years. There were three patients over the age of 95.

In a previous study completed in 1980, which represented 15 years' experience with Mohs surgery, the author noted an equal number of primary lesions (that is, lesions that had never been treated) and recurrent lesions (skin cancers that had received prior treatment by other physicians but that had not been successfully eradicated). The study completed in 1987 shows a large increase in

the number of primary lesions: 55.5 per cent primary lesions versus 44.4 per cent recurrent lesions.

When patients were referred for Mohs surgery prior to 1980, only 12.6 per cent of the lesions treated were less than 1 cm in diameter. In 1987, 20 per cent of the lesions are of that size, and almost 50 per cent of all lesions treated are less than 2 cm. Patients, or their physicians, are recognizing skin cancers earlier and are seeking treatment while the lesions are still relatively small in size. The mean size for women is 1.5 cm, and for men 1.7 cm in diameter.

In a previous study, 26.7 per cent of patients reported that the lesion had existed for less than a year. In the author's current study, 63.6 per cent of patients report that they had had the lesion for less than a year. More men than women gave a history of having the lesion for less than one year. Lesions in men are usually larger (1.7 cm for men, 1.5 cm for women).

In the author's patients the general cure rate using Mohs surgery is 97.4 per cent. Size and location are the most important factors in cure rates. The smaller the lesion, the greater is the chance of cure. With lesions less than 1 cm in diameter the cure rate was approximately 99.6 per cent. With lesions greater than 5 cm the cure rate was 92 per cent. The ears and the retroauricular area are the most difficult sites in which to eradicate skin cancers. In the retroauricular area there was a recurrence rate of 14 per cent. The recurrence rate in the ear was 4.8 per cent. The higher recurrence rate in the ears and retroauricular areas may have its origin in their embryologic development. In such areas containing many different fusion planes and layers, the tumor may penetrate and disperse itself between the different planes. In the ears, the tumors do not penetrate the cartilage but can extend a considerable distance from their initial site.

The consideration of sex as reflected in cure rate was clearly related to the larger lesions found in male patients. If the lesions had been treated earlier, cure rates would have been higher. However, the younger the patient, the more difficult the cancer was to eradicate. Tumors in younger patients may be more aggressive, but further study is required.

A further breakdown shows that the cure rates are 98.2 and 96.6 per cent for primary and recurrent tumors, respectively. Thus it is statistically advantageous to treat primary lesions. However, since recurrent lesions also have a high cure rate using microscopically controlled excision, it is to the advantage of patients with recurrent lesions that this method be used. This is especially true when it is considered that use of standard procedures to treat recurrent lesions results in a cure rate in the 60 per cent range.

REFERENCES

Adair, F. E.: Treatment of melanoma. Report of 400 cases. Surg. Gynecol. Obstet., *62:*406, 1936.

Anderson, D. E., Taylor, W. B., Falls, H. F., and Davidson, R. T.: The nevoid basal cell carcinoma syndrome. Am. J. Hum. Genet., *19:*12, 1967.

Arons, M. S., Lynch, J. B., Lewis, S. R., and Blocker, T. G., Jr.: Scar tissue carcinoma. I. A clinical study with special reference to burn scar carcinoma. Ann. Surg., *161:*170, 1965.

Baab, G. H., and McBride, C. M.: Malignant melanoma: the patient with an unknown site of primary origin. Arch. Surg., *110:*896, 1975.

Balch, C. M., Murad, T. M., Soong, S. J., Ingalls, A. L., Halpern, N. B., and Maddox, W. A.: A multifactorial analysis of melanoma: prognostic histopathologic features comparing Clark's and Breslow's staging methods. Ann. Surg., *188:*732, 1978.

Balch, C. M., Soong, S. J., Milton, G. W., Shaw, H. M., McGovern, V. J., et al.: A comparison of prognostic factors and surgical results in 1786 patients with localized (stage I) melanoma treated in Alabama, USA, and New South Wales, Australia. Ann. Surg., *196:*677, 1982.

Bell, J.: Paraffin epithelioma of the scrotum. Edinburgh Med. J., *22:*135, 1876.

Binns, J. H., and Sherriff, H. M.: Low incidence of recurrence in excised but non-irradiated basal cell carcinomas. Br. J. Plast. Surg., *28:*133, 1975.

Bleehen, S. S., and Ebling, F. J. G.: Disorders of skin colour. *In* Rook, A., Wilkinson, D. S., Ebling, F. J. G., Champion, R. H., and Burton, J. L. (Eds.): Textbook of Dermatology. Oxford, Blackwell Scientific Publications, 1986.

Blois, M. S., Sagebiel, R. W., Abarbanel, R. M., Caldwell, T. M., and Tuttle, M. S.: Malignant melanoma of the skin: I. The association of tumor depth and type, and patient sex, age and site with survival. Cancer, *52:*1330, 1983.

Bloodgood, J. C.: Excision of benign pigmented moles. J.A.M.A., *79:*576, 1922.

Bostwick, J., Pendergrast, W. J., Jr., and Vasconez, L. O.: Marjolin's ulcer: an immunologically privileged tumor? Plast. Reconstr. Surg., *57:*66, 1976.

Boyle, J., MacKie, R. M., Briggs, J. D., Junor, B. J., and Aitchison, T. C.: Cancer, warts, and sunshine in renal transplant patients. A case-control study. Lancet, *1:*702, 1984.

Brandes, L. J., Galton, D. A., and Wiltshaw, E.: New approach to immunotherapy of melanoma. Lancet, *2:*293, 1971.

Breslow, A.: Thickness, cross-sectional areas and depth of invasion in the progress of cutaneous melanoma. Ann. Surg., *172:*902, 1970.

Breslow, A.: Prognosis in cutaneous melanoma: tumor thickness as a guide to treatment. Pathol. Annu., *15* (Part 1):1, 1980.

Burg, G., Hirsch, R. D., Konz, B., and Braun-Falco, O.: Histographic surgery: accuracy of visual assessment of the margins of basal-cell epithelioma. J. Dermatol. Surg., *1:*21, 1975.

Burns, D. A., and Calnan, C. D.: Basal cell epithelioma in a chronic leg ulcer. Clin. Exp. Dermatol., *3:*443, 1978.

Byers, R., Kesler, K., Redmon, B., Medina, J., and Schwarz, B.: Squamous carcinoma of the external ear. Am. J. Surg., *146:*447, 1983.

Bystryn, J. C., Oratz, R., Harris, M. N., Roses, D. F., Golomb, F. M., and Speyer, J. L.: Immunogenicity of a polyvalent melanoma antigen vaccine in humans. Cancer, *61:*1065, 1988.

Cahan, W. G.: Cryosurgery of malignant and benign tumors. Fed. Proc., *24:*S241, 1965.

Carrier, W. L., Snyder, R. D., and Regan, J. D.: Ultraviolet-induced damage and its repair in human DNA. *In* Regan, J. D., and Parrish, J. A. (Eds.): The Science of Photomedicine. New York, Plenum Press, 1982.

Cascinelli, N., Vaglini, M., Bufalino, R., and Morabito, A.: BANS. A cutaneous region with no prognostic significance in patients with melanoma. Cancer, *57:*441, 1986.

Casson, P.: Basal cell carcinoma. Clin. Plast. Surg., *7:*301, 1980.

Clark, D. A., and Nathanson, L.: Cellular immunity in malignant melanoma. Pigment Cell, *1:*350, 1973.

Clark, W. H., From, L., Bernadino, E. A., and Mihm, M. C.: The histogenesis and biologic behavior of primary human malignant melanomas of the skin. Cancer Res., *29:*705, 1969.

Cleaver, J. E.: Defective repair replication of DNA in xeroderma pigmentosum. Nature, *218:*652, 1968.

Conley, J., Lattes, R., and Orr, W.: Desmoplastic malignant melanoma (a rare variant of spindle cell melanoma). Cancer, *28:*914, 1971.

Conway, H., and Hugo, N. E.: Metastatic basal cell carcinoma. Am. J. Surg., *110:*620, 1965.

Conway, H., and Hugo, N. E.: Radiation dermatitis and malignancy. Plast. Reconstr. Surg., *38:*255, 1966.

Cosman, B., Heddle, S. B., and Crikelair, G. F.: The increasing incidence of melanoma. Plast. Reconstr. Surg., *57:*50, 1976.

Costanzi, J. J.: Combination chemotherapy in the treatment of disseminated malignant melanoma. Cancer Chemother. Rep., *57:*90, 1973.

Creagan, E. T., Cupps, R. E., Ivins, J. C., Pritchard, D. J., Sim., F. H., et al.: Adjuvant radiation therapy for regional nodal metastases from malignant melanoma: a randomized, prospective study. Cancer, *42:*2206, 1978.

Cronin, T. D.: Extensive pigmented nevi in hairbearing areas: removal of pigmented layer while preserving the hair follicles. Plast. Reconstr. Surg. *11:*94, 1953.

Cross, F.: On a turf (peat) fire cancer: malignant change superimposed on erythema ab igne. Proc. R. Soc. Med., *60:*1307, 1967.

Das Gupta, T., Bowden, L., and Berg, J.: Malignant melanoma of unknown primary origin. Surg. Gynecol. Obstet., *117:*345, 1963.

Das Gupta, T., Brasfield, R. D., and Paglia, M.: Primary melanoma in unusual sites. Surg. Gynecol. Obstet., *128:*841, 1969.

Davis, N. C.: Melanoma and skin cancer. *In* McCarthy, W. H. (Ed.): Proceedings of International Cancer Conference. Sydney, Australia, V.C.N. Blight, 1972.

Davis, N. C., and Little, J. H.: The role of frozen section in the management of malignant melanoma. Br. J. Surg., 61:505, 1974.

Day, C. L., and Sober, A. J.: Malignant melanoma patients with positive nodes and relatively good prognoses. Cancer, 47:955, 1981.

Department of Health Education and Welfare Publication No. (NIH) 74–637. Third National Cancer Surgery Advanced Three Year Report, 1969–1971.

Dorsey, C. S., and Montgomery, H.: Blue nevus and its distinction from mongolian spots and the nevus of Ota. J. Invest. Dermatol., 22:225, 1954.

Dubin, N., Moseson, M., and Pasternack, B. S.: Epidemiology of malignant melanoma: pigmentary traits, ultraviolet radiation, and the identification of high-risk populations. Recent Res. Cancer Res., 102:56, 1986.

Earley, M. J.: Basal cell carcinoma arising in tattoos: a clinical report of two cases. Br. J. Plast. Surg., 36:258, 1983.

Elder, D. E., Goldman, L. I., Goldman, S. C., Greene, M. H., and Clark, W. H., Jr.: Dysplastic nevus syndrome: a phenotypic association of sporadic cutaneous melanoma. Cancer, 46:1787, 1980.

Elder, D. E., Guerry, D., Van Horn, M., Hurvitz, S., Zehngebot, L., et al.: The role of lymph node dissection for clinical stage I malignant melanoma of intermediate thickness (1.51–3.99 mm). Cancer, 56:413, 1985.

El-Hefnawi, H., El-Hawary, M. F. S., El-Komy, H. M., and Rasheed, A.: Xeroderma pigmentosum. V. Studies of 17-ketosteroids and total 17-hydroxycorticosteroids. Br. J. Dermatol., 75:484, 1963.

El-Hefnawi, H., El-Nabawi, M., and El-Hawary, M. F. S.: Xeroderma pigmentosum. III. Br. J. Dermatol., 74:218, 1962.

El-Hefnawi, H., El-Nabawi, M., and Rasheed, A.: Xeroderma pigmentosum. I. A clinical study of 12 Egyptian cases. Br. J. Dermatol., 74:201, 1962.

Epstein, E.: Effect of biopsy on prognosis of melanoma. J. Surg. Oncol., 3:251, 1971.

Everson, T. C., and Cole, W. H.: Spontaneous Regression in Cancer. Philadelphia, W. B. Saunders Company, 1966.

Farmer, E. R., and Helwig, E. B.: Metastatic basal cell carcinoma: a clinicopathologic study of seventeen cases. Cancer, 46:748, 1980.

Fish, J., Smith, E. B., and Canby, J. P.: Malignant melanoma in childhood. Surgery, 59:309, 1966.

Fisher, M. S., and Kripke, M. L.: Systemic alteration induced in mice by ultraviolet light irradiation and its relationship to ultraviolet carcinogenesis. Proc. Natl. Acad. Sci. U.S.A., 74:1688, 1977.

Fitzpatrick, P. J., Thompson, G. A., Easterbrook, W. M., Gallie, B. L., and Payne, D. G.: Basal and squamous cell carcinoma of the eyelids and their treatment by radiotherapy. Int. J. Radiat. Oncol. Biol. Phys., 10:449, 1984.

Friedman, H. I., Cooper, P. H., and Wanebo, H. J.: Prognostic and therapeutic use of microstaging of cutaneous squamous cell carcinoma of the trunk and extremities. Cancer, 56:1099, 1985.

Giraud, R. M., Rippey, E., and Rippey, J. J.: Malignant melanoma of the skin in black Africans. S. Afr. Med. J., 49:665, 1975.

Glass, R. L., Spratt, J. S., Jr., and Perezmesa, C.: The fate of inadequately excised epidermoid carcinoma of the skin. Surg. Gynecol. Obstet., 22:245, 1966.

Goldsmith, H. S., Shah, J. P., and Kim, D. H.: Prognostic significance of lymph node dissection in the treatment of malignant melanoma. Cancer, 26:606, 1970.

Gonzalez, R. L., Wong, P., and Spitler, L. E.: Adjuvant immunotherapy with transfer factor in patients with melanoma metastatic to lung. Cancer, 45:57, 1980.

Gooding, C. A., White, G., and Yatsuhashi, M.: Significance of marginal extension in excised basal-cell carcinoma. N. Engl. J. Med., 273:923, 1965.

Goodwin, D. P., Hornung, M. O., and Krementz, E. T.: Extraction and use of melanoma-associated protein for immunotherapy. Oncology, 27:258, 1973.

Gordon, D., and Silverstone, H.: Worldwide epidemiology of premalignant and malignant cutaneous lesions. In Andrade, R., Gumport, S. L., Popkin, G. L., and Rees, T. D. (Eds.): Cancer of the Skin. Biology-Diagnosis-Management. Philadelphia, W. B. Saunders Company, 1976.

Greeley, P. W., Middleton, A. G., and Curtin, J. W.: Incidence of malignancy in giant pigmented nevi. Plast. Reconstr. Surg., 36:26, 1965.

Gromet, M. A., Epstein, W. L., and Blois, M. S.: The regressing thin malignant melanoma: a distinctive lesion with metastatic potential. Cancer, 42:2282, 1978.

Gundersen, S.: Dacarbazine, vindesine and cisplatin combination chemotherapy in advanced malignant melanoma: a phase II study. Cancer Treat. Rep., 71:997, 1987.

Handley, W. S.: The pathology of melanotic growths in relation to their operative treatment. Lancet, 1:927, 997, 1907.

Hansen, M. G., and McCarten, A. B.: Tumor thickness and lymphocytic infiltration in malignant melanoma of the head and neck. Am. J. Surg., 128:557, 1974.

Hardie, I. R., Strong, R. W., Hartley, L. C., Woodruff, P. W., and Clunie, G. J.: Skin cancer in Caucasian renal allograft recipients living in a subtropical climate. Surgery, 87:177, 1980.

Harris, M. N., and Gumport, S. L.: Biopsy technique for malignant melanoma. J. Dermatol. Surg., 1:24, 1975.

Harris, M. N., Gumport, S. L., and Maiwandi, H.: Axillary lymph node dissection for melanoma. Surg. Gynecol. Obstet., 135:936, 1972.

Hartwell, S. W., Jr., Huger, W., Jr., and Pickrell, K.: Radiation dermatitis and radiogenic neoplasms of the hands. Ann. Surg., 160:828, 1964.

Hayes, H.: Basal cell carcinoma: the East Grinstead experience. Plast. Reconstr. Surg., 30:273, 1962.

Hazelrigg, D. E.: Basal cell epithelioma in a vaccination scar. Int. J. Dermatol., 17:723, 1978.

Heenan, P. J., Weeramanthri, T., Holman, C. D., and Armstrong, B. K.: Surgical treatment and survival from cutaneous malignant melanoma. Aust. N.Z. J. Surg., 55:229, 1985.

Hellriegel, W.: Radiation therapy of primary and metastatic melanoma. Ann. N.Y. Acad. Sci., 100:131, 1963.

Hellström, I., Hellström, K. E., Pierce, G. E., and Yang, J. P. S.: Cellular and humoral immunity to different types of human neoplasms. Nature, 220:1352, 1968.

Henderson, B. E., Kolonel, L. N., and Foster, F.: Cancer in Polynesians. Natl. Cancer Inst. Monogr., 62:73, 1982.

Hilal, E. Y., Pinsky, C. M., Hirshant, Y., Wanebo, H. J., Hansen, J. A., et al.: Surgical adjuvant therapy of malignant melanoma with *Corynebacterium parvum*. Cancer, 48:245, 1981.

Hilaris, B. S., Raben, M., Calabrese, A. S., Phillips, R. F., and Henschke, U. E.: Value of radiation therapy for distant metastases from malignant melanoma. Cancer, *16:*765, 1963.

Hill, G. J., Ruess, R., Berris, R., Philpott, G. W., and Parkin, P.: Chemotherapy of malignant melanoma with dimethyl triazeno imidazole carboxamide (DTIC) and nitrosourea derivatives (BCNU; CCNU). Ann. Surg., *180:*167, 1974.

Hollinshead, A., Arlen, M., Yonemoto, R., Cohen, M., Tanner, K., et al.: Pilot studies using melanoma tumor-associated antigens in specific active immunochemotherapy of malignant melanoma. Cancer, *49:*1387, 1982.

Holman, C. D., Armstrong, B. K., Heenan, P. J., Blackwell, J. B., Cumming, F. J., et al.: The causes of malignant melanoma: results from the West Australian Lions Melanoma Research Project. Recent Res. Cancer Res., *102:*18, 1986.

Howell, J. B., Anderson, D. E., and McClendon, J. L.: The basal cell nevus syndrome. J.A.M.A., *190:*274, 1964.

Howell, J. B., and Caro, M. R.: Basal cell nevus: its relationship to multiple cutaneous cancers and associated anomalies of development. Arch. Dermatol., *79:*67, 1959.

Hurwitz, R. M., Egan, W. T., Murphy, S. H., Pontius, E. E., and Forster, M. L.: Bowenoid papulosis and squamous cell carcinoma of the genitalia: suspected sexual transmission. Cutis, *39:*193, 1987.

Hutchinson, J.: Some examples of arsenic keratosis of the skin and of arsenic cancer. Trans. Pathol. Soc. London, *39:*352, 1888.

Huvos, A. G., Shah, J. P., and Goldsmith, H. S.: A clinicopathologic study of amelanotic melanoma. Surg. Gynecol. Obstet., *135:*917, 1972.

Ikonopisov, R. L., Lewis, M. G., Hunter-Craig, I. D., Bodenham, D. C., Phillips, T. M., et al.: Auto-immunisation with irradiated tumour cells in human malignant melanoma. Br. Med. J., *2:*752, 1970.

Immerman, S. C., Scanlon, E. F., Christ, M., and Knox, K. L.: Recurrent squamous cell carcinoma of the skin. Cancer, *51:*537, 1983.

Iscoe, N., Kersey, P., Gapski, J., Osoba, D., From, L., et al.: Predictive value of staging investigations in patients with clinical stage I malignant melanoma. Plast. Reconstr. Surg., *80:*233, 1987.

Jones, E. W., and Heyl, T.: Naevus sebaceus. A report of 140 cases with special regard to the development of secondary malignant tumours. Br. J. Dermatol., *82:*99, 1970.

Kaiser, L. R., Burk, M. W., and Morton, D. L.: Adjuvant therapy for malignant melanoma. Surg. Clin. North Am., *61:*1249, 1981.

Kaplan, E., and Nickoloff, B. J.: Clinical and histologic features of nevi with emphasis on treatment approaches. Clin. Plast. Surg., *14:*277, 1987.

Kaposi, M.: Idiopathisches multiples Pigmentsarkom der Haut. Arch. Dermatol. Syph., *4:*265, 1872.

Kelner, A., and Taft, E. B.: Influence of photoreactivating light on type and frequency of tumors induced by ultraviolet radiation. Cancer Res., *16:*860, 1956.

Kenady, D. E., Brown, B. W., and McBride, C.M.: Excision of underlying fascia with a primary malignant melanoma: effect on recurrence and survival rates. Surgery, *92:*615, 1982.

Kennaway, E.: The identification of a carcinogenic compound in coal-tar. Br. Med. J., *2:*749, 1955.

Kint, A.: Pathology of basal cell epithelioma. *In* Andrade, R., Gumport, S. L., Popkin, G. L., and Rees, T. D. (Eds.): Cancer of the Skin. Biology-Diagnosis-Management. Philadelphia, W. B. Saunders Company, 1976.

Kopf, A. W., Bart, R. S., Schrager, D., Lazar, M., and Popkin, G. L.: Curettage-electrodesiccation treatment of basal cell carcinomas. Arch. Dermatol., *113:*439, 1977.

Kopf, A. W., Mintzis, M., and Bart, R. S.: Diagnostic accuracy in malignant melanoma. Arch. Dermatol., *111:*1291, 1975.

Koplin, L., and Zarem, H. A.: Recurrent basal cell carcinoma. A review concerning the incidence, behavior, and management of recurrent basal cell carcinoma, with emphasis on the incompletely excised lesion. Plast. Reconstr. Surg., *65:*656, 1980.

Krementz, E. T., Mansell, P. W. A., Hornung, M. O., Samuels, M. S., Sutherland, C. A., and Benes, E. N.: Immunotherapy of malignant disease. The use of viable sensitized lymphocytes or transfer factor prepared from sensitized lymphocytes. Cancer, *33:*394, 1974.

Lawrence, H. S.: The transfer of generalised cutaneous hypersensitivity of the delayed tuberculin type in man by means of the constituents of disrupted leucocytes. J. Clin. Invest., *33:*951, 1954.

Legha, S. S.: Interferons in the treatment of malignant melanoma. Cancer, *57:*1675, 1986.

Lee, J. A.: Sunlight and the etiology of malignant melanoma. *In* McCarthy, W. H. (Ed.): Melanoma and Skin Cancer. Proceedings of International Cancer Conference. Sydney, Australia, V.C.N. Blight, 1972.

Lee, J. A., and Merrill, J. M.: Sunlight and the etiology of malignant melanoma: a synthesis. Med. J. Aust., *2:*846, 1970.

Lerman, R. I., Murray, D., O'Hara, J. M., Booher, R. J., and Foote, F. W.: Malignant melanoma of childhood. Cancer, *25:*436, 1970.

Levene, A.: The comparative pathology of skin tumors of horse, dog and cat compared with man, with special reference to tumors of melanocytic origin. *In* McCarthy, W. H. (Ed.): Melanoma and Skin Cancer. Proceedings of International Cancer Conference. Sydney, Australia, V.C.N. Blight, 1972.

Lever, W. F.: Histopathology of the Skin. 5th Ed. Philadelphia, J. B. Lippincott Company, 1975.

Lightstone, A. C., Kopf, A. W., and Garfinkel, L.: Diagnostic accuracy—a new approach to its evaluation; results in basal cell epitheliomas. Arch. Dermatol., *91:*497, 1965.

Little, J. H., Holt, J., and Davis, N.: Changing epidemiology of malignant melanoma in Queensland. Med. J. Aust., *1:*66, 1980.

Luce, J. K.: Semin. Oncol., *2:*179, 1975.

Lund, H. Z., and Kraus, J. M.: Melanotic tumors of the skin. Washington, DC, Armed Forces Institute of Pathology Fascicle No. 3, 1962, p. 50.

Lutzner, M. A.: Epidermodysplasia verruciformis. An autosomal recessive disease characterized by viral warts and skin cancer. A model for viral oncogenesis. Bull. Cancer, *65:*169, 1978.

MacKie, R. M.: The role of sunlight in the aetiology of cutaneous malignant melanoma. Clin. Exp. Dermatol., *6:*407, 1981.

Marshall, V. C.: Skin tumours in immunosuppressed patients. Aust. N.Z. J. Surg., *43:*214, 1973.

Martin, H., Strong, E., and Spiro, R. H.: Radiation-induced skin cancer of the head and neck. Cancer, *25:*61, 1970.

McCarthy, J. G., Haagensen, C. D., and Herter, F. P.: The role of groin dissection in the management of melanoma of the lower extremity. Ann. Surg., *179:*156, 1974.

McGovern, V. J., Shaw, H. M., Milton, G. W., and Farago, G. A.: Is malignant melanoma arising in a Hutchinson's melanotic freckle a separate disease entity? Histopathology, *4:*235, 1980.

McNeer, G., and Cantin, J.: Local failure in the treatment of melanoma. Am. J. Roentgenol., *99:*791, 1967.

McNeer, G., and Das Gupta, T.: Prognosis in malignant melanoma. Surgery, *56:*512, 1964.

McNeer, G., and Das Gupta, T.: Life history in melanoma. Am. J. Roentgenol., *93:*686, 1965.

Mehnert, J. H., and Heard, J. L.: Staging of malignant melanoma by depth of invasion. Am. J. Surg., *110:*168, 1965.

Mehregan, A. H., and Pinkus, H.: Life history of organoid nevi. Arch. Dermatol., *91:*574, 1965.

Miller, J. A.: Carcinogenesis by chemicals: an overview—G. H. A. Clowes Memorial Lecture. Cancer Res., *30:*559, 1970.

Miller, L. L., Spitler, L. E., Allen, R. E., and Minor, D. R.: A randomised, double blind placebo-controlled trial of transfer factor as adjuvant therapy for malignant melanoma. Cancer, *61:*1543, 1988.

Mohs, F. E.: Chemosurgery in Cancer, Gangrene and Infections. Springfield. Charles C Thomas, 1956.

Mohs, F. E.: Prevention and treatment of skin cancer. Wis. Med. J., *73:*S85. 1974.

Mohs, F. E.: Chemosurgery. Microscopically Controlled Surgery for Skin Cancer. Springfield, IL, Charles C Thomas, 1978, pp. 154, 157.

Mohs, F. E., Jones, D. L., and Bloom, R. F.: Tendency of fluorouracil to conceal deep foci of invasive basal cell carcinoma. Arch. Dermatol., *114:*1021, 1978.

Morton, D. L., Eilber, F. R., Holmes, E. C., Hunt, J. S., Ketcham, A. S., et al.: B.C.G. immunotherapy of malignant melanoma. Ann. Surg., *180:*635, 1974.

Moss, A. L., and Briggs, J. C.: Cutaneous malignant melanoma in the young. Br. J. Plast. Surg., *39:*537, 1986.

Naruns, P. L., Nizze, J. A., Cochran, A. J., Lee, M. B., and Morton, D. L.: Recurrence potential of thin primary melanomas. Cancer, *57:*545, 1986.

Neve, E. F.: Kangri burn cancer. Br. Med. J., *2:*1255, 1923.

O'Doherty, C. J., Prescott, R. J., White, H., McIntyre, M., and Hunter, J. A.: Sex differences in presentation of cutaneous malignant melanoma and in survival from stage I disease. Cancer, *58:*788, 1986.

Oettlé, A. G.: Cancer in Africa, especially in regions south of the Sahara. J. Natl. Cancer Inst., *33:*383, 1964.

Olsen, G.: Removal of fascia: cause of more frequent metastases of malignant melanoma of the skin to regional lymph nodes. Cancer, *17:*1159, 1964.

Oratz, R., Speyer, J. L., Green, M., Blum, R., Wernz, J. C., and Muggia, F. M.: Treatment of metastatic malignant melanoma with dacarbazine and cisplatin. Cancer Treat. Rep., *71:*877, 1987.

Osterlind, A., and Møller Jensen, O.: Trends in incidence of malignant melanoma of the skin in Denmark 1943–1982. *In* Gallagher, R. P. (Ed.): Epidemiology of Malignant Melanoma. Berlin, Springer-Verlag, 1985.

Overgaard, J.: Radiation treatment of malignant melanoma. Int. J. Radiol. Oncol. Biol. Phys., *8:*1121, 1980.

Pack, G. T.: End results in treatment of malignant melanoma. Ann. Surg., *136:*905, 1952.

Pack, G. T., Lenson, N., and Gerber, D. M.: Regional distribution of moles and melanomas. Arch. Surg., *65:*862, 1952.

Parrish, J. A.: Ultraviolet radiation affects the immune system. Pediatrics, *71:*129, 1983.

Pascal, R. R., Hobby, L. W., Lattes, R., and Crikelair, G. F.: Prognosis of "incompletely excised" versus "completely excised" basal cell carcinoma. Plast. Reconstr. Surg., *41:*328, 1968.

Pathak, M. A., Fitzpatrick, T. B., and Parrish, J. A.: Topical and systemic approaches to protection of human skin against harmful effects of solar radiation. *In* Regan, J. D., and Parrish, J. A. (Eds.): The Science of Photomedicine. New York, Plenum Press, 1982.

Penn, I.: Cancer in immuno-suppressive patients. Transplant. Proc. (Suppl. 2), *7:*553, 1975.

Penn, I.: Tumor incidence in human allograft recipients. Transplant. Proc., *11:*1047, 1979.

Penn, I.: Cancers following cyclosporine therapy. Transplantation, *43:*32, 1987.

Penn, I.: Cancers after cyclosporine therapy. Transplant. Proc., *20*(Suppl. 1):276, 1988.

Penn, I., Hammond, W., Brettschneider, L., and Starzl, T. E.: Malignant lymphomas in transplantation patients. Transplant. Proc., *1:*106, 1969.

Petersen, N. C., Bodenham, D. C., and Lloyd, O. C.: Malignant melanomas of the skin. Br. J. Plast. Surg., *15:*49, 1962.

Pickrell, K.: Current comment. Follow-up clinic. Xeroderma pigmentosa. Plast. Reconstr. Surg., *49:*83, 1972.

Popkin, G. L.: Curettage and electrodesiccation. N.Y. State J. Med., *68:*866, 1968.

Pott, P.: Chirurgical Observations Relative to . . . the Cancer of the Scrotum, the Different Kinds of Ruptures, and the Mortification of the Toes and Feet. London, Hawes, Clarke, and Collins, 1775.

Quaba, A. A., and Wallace, A. F.: The incidence of malignant melanoma (0 to 15 years of age) arising in "large" congenital nevocellular nevi. Plast. Reconstr. Surg., *78:*174, 1986.

Rank, B. K., and Wakefield, A. F.: Surgery of basal cell carcinoma. Br. J. Surg., *45:*531, 1959.

Reintgen, D. S., Cox, E. B., McCarthy, K. S., Vollmen, R. T., and Seigler, H. F.: Efficacy of elective lymph node dissection in patients with intermediate thickness primary melanoma. Ann. Surg., *198:*379, 1983.

Robinson, J. K.: Risk of developing another basal cell carcinoma. A 5-year prospective study. Cancer, *60:*118, 1987.

Rodriguez, H. A., and Ackerman, L. U.: Cellular blue nevus. Cancer, *21:*393, 1968.

Roush, G. C., Schymura, M. J., and Holford, T. R.: Patterns of invasive melanoma in the Connecticut Tumor Registry. Is the long-term increase real? Cancer, *61:*2586, 1988.

Saksela, E., and Rintala, A.: Misdiagnosis of prepubertal melanoma. Cancer, *22:*1308, 1968.

Sedlin, E. D., and Fleming, J. L.: Epidermoid carcinoma arising in chronic osteomyelitic foci. J. Bone Joint Surg., *45A:*827, 1963.

Shah, J. P., and Goldsmith, H. S.: Incontinuity versus discontinuous lymph node dissection for malignant melanoma. Cancer, *26:*610, 1970.

Shanoff, L. B., Spira, M., and Hardy, S. B.: Basal cell carcinoma: a statistical approach to rational management. Plast. Reconstr. Surg., *39:*619, 1967.

Sheil, A. G.: Cancer in renal allograft recipients in Australia and New Zealand. Transplant. Proc., *9:*1133, 1977.

Skov-Jensen, T., Hastrup, J., and Lambrethsen, E.: Malignant melanoma in children. Cancer, *19:*620, 1966.

Smith, J. L., and Stehlin, J. S.: Spontaneous regression of primary malignant melanoma. Cancer, *18:*1399, 1965.

Snyderman, R. K., and Starzynski, T. E.: The clinical application of 5-fluorouracil in the treatment of skin lesions. Plast. Reconstr. Surg., *41:*549, 1968.

Spitz, S.: Melanomas of childhood. Am. J. Pathol., *24:*591, 1948.

Stehlin, J. S., Jr., and Clark, R. L.: Melanoma of the extremities. Experience with conventional treatment and perfusion in 339 cases. Am. J. Surg., *110:*366, 1965.

Stehlin, J. S., Greeff, P. J., de Ipolyr, P. D., Giovanella, B. C., Klein, G., et al.: Heat as an adjuvant in the treatment of advanced melanoma: an immune stimulant? Houston Med. J., *4:*61, 1988.

Taylor, W. B., Anderson, D. E., Howell, J. B., and Thurston, C. S.: The nevoid basal cell carcinoma syndrome. Autopsy findings. Arch. Dermatol., *98:*612, 1968.

Tranum, B. L., Dixon, D., Quagliana, J., Neidhart, J., Balcerzak, S. P., et al.: Lack of benefit of adjunctive chemotherapy in Stage I malignant melanoma: a Southwest Oncology Group Study. Cancer Treat. Rep., *71:*643, 1987.

Treves, N., and Pack, G. T.: The development of cancer in burn scars. Surg. Gynecol. Obstet., *51:*749, 1930.

Tromovitch, T. A., and Stegeman, S. J.: Microscopically controlled excision of skin tumors. Chemosurgery (Mohs') fresh tissue technique. Arch. Dermatol., *110:*231, 1974.

Trozak, D. J., Rowland, W. D., and Hu, F.: Metastatic malignant melanoma in prepubertal children. Pediatrics, *55:*191, 1975.

Urist, M. M., Balch, C. M., and Milton, G. W.: Surgical management of the primary melanoma. *In* Balch, C. M., and Milton, G. W. (Eds.): Cutaneous Melanoma. Philadelphia, J. B. Lippincott Company, 1985.

Urteaga, O., and Pack, G. T.: On the antiquity of melanoma. Cancer, *19:*607, 1966.

Valensi, Q. J.: Desmoplastic malignant melanoma: a report on two additional cases. Cancer, *39:*286, 1977.

Veronesi, U., Adamus, J., Bandiera, D. C., Brennhovd, I. O., Caceres, E., et al.: Stage I melanoma of the limbs. Immediate versus delayed node dissection. Tumori, *66:*373, 1980.

von Domarus, H., and Stevens, P. J.: Metastatic basal cell carcinoma. Report of five cases and review of 170 cases in the literature. J. Am. Acad. Dermatol., *10:*1043, 1984.

von Essen, C. F.: Roentgen therapy of skin and lip carcinoma: factors influencing success and failure. Am. J. Roentgenol., *83:*556, 1960.

Wanebo, H. J., Woodruff, J., and Fortner, J. G.: Malignant melanoma of the extremities: a clinicopathologic study using levels of invasion (microstage). Cancer, *35:*666, 1975.

Winkelmann, R. K.: The differential diagnosis of melanoma. *In* McCarthy, W. H. (Ed.): Melanoma and Skin Cancer. Proceedings of International Cancer Conference. Sydney, Australia, V.C.N. Blight, 1972.

Winkler, P. A., and Guyuron, B.: Multiple metastases from basal cell naevus syndrome. Br. J. Plast. Surg., *40:*528, 1987.

Woodruff, M. F., and Symes, M. O.: The use of immunologically competent cells in the treatment of cancer. Br. J. Cancer, *16:*707, 1962.

Woods, J. E.: Is the BANS concept for malignant melanoma valid? Am. J. Surg., *150:*452, 1985.

Woolf, R., Kepes, J., Georgiade, N., and Pickrell, K.: Xeroderma pigmentosa. Plast. Reconstr. Surg., *24:*214, 1959.

Yeh, S.: Skin cancer in chronic arsenicism. Hum. Pathol., *4:*469, 1973.

York, R. M., and Foltz, A. T.: Bleomycin, vincristine, lomustine and DTIC chemotherapy for metastatic melanoma. Cancer, *61:*2183, 1988.

Zacarian, S. A.: Cryosurgery of cutaneous carcinomas. An 18-year study of 3,022 patients with 4,228 carcinomas. J. Am. Acad. Dermatol., *9:*947, 1983.

Zeitels, J., La Rossa, D., Hamilton, R., Synnestvedt, M., and Schultz, D.: A comparison of local recurrence and resection margins for stage I primary cutaneous malignant melanoma. Plast. Reconstr. Surg., *81:*688, 1988.

Zitelli, J. A., Grant, M. G., Abell, E., and Boyd, J. B.: Histologic patterns of congenital nevocytic nevi and implications for treatment. J. Am. Acad. Dermatol., *11:*402, 1984.

75

David B. Apfelberg
Morton R. Maser

Laser Therapy

Lasers of various wavelengths have become increasingly useful to treat a wide range of disorders. In fact, laser therapy now spans the entire surgical spectrum from ophthalmology to general surgery. The laser has rendered the treatment of such commonplace disorders as warts more effective and easily accomplished with fewer side effects, and has also provided the only effectual treatment modality for many rare or unusual disorders (e.g., granuloma faciale) for which previously no satisfactory treatment existed.

In the field of plastic surgery, laser therapy has proved especially useful because of the superficial nature of many of the lesions treated by plastic surgeons. In fact, after ophthalmology and otolaryngology, plastic surgery was probably the third specialty in which the laser's therapeutic potential was investigated and developed. Kaplan, Ger, and Sharon (1973), using the carbon dioxide laser, and Apfelberg, Maser, and Lash (1976), applying the argon laser in the early 1970's, first developed and promulgated many of the techniques that are commonplace today.

LASER PHYSICS/PHYSIOLOGY

The word "laser" is an acronym standing for *l*ight *a*mplification by the *s*timulated *e*mission of *r*adiation. It should be noted that the radiation in this acronym is electromagnetic or light radiation and not x-radiation. Principles in the development of laser energy were first enumerated by Albert Einstein in the 1920's. Schawlow and Townes (1958) are credited with the first development of an actual laser. Maimann (1960) produced the first practical laser (ruby) with therapeutic applications.

Currently available lasers produce laser light with wavelengths located in the visible light and infrared range of the electromagnetic spectrum (Table 75–1, Fig. 75–1). All lasers produce intense light of extremely high energy that can be directed by sophisticated optics to a point of maximal power density to perform cutting, vaporizing, cautery, or ablation of biologic tissues. By means of alterations in the lasing medium, the electrical activation, the power output, and the mode

Table 75–1. Electromagnetic Spectrum

Type of Wave	Wavelength (cm)	Freq. (cyc/sec)
Cosmic rays	0.004×10^{-8}	10^{20}
X-rays	1×10^{-8}	10^{18}
Ultraviolet light	2000×10^{-8}	1×10^{15}
Visible light		0.5×10^{15}
	5000×10^{-8}	(500 nm B-G argon
Infrared	$10,600 \times 10^{-8}$	1060 nm CO_2)
	1×10^{-3}	3×10^{13}
Radar	1	3×10^{10}
Radio	3×10^{5}	1×10^{5}

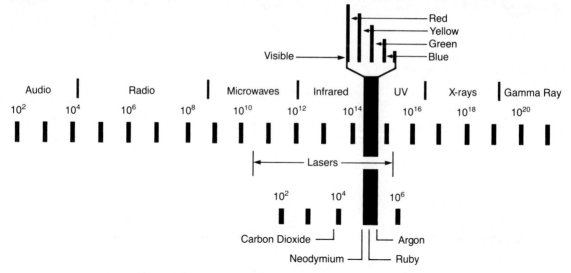

Figure 75–1. Position of lasers in the electromagnetic spectrum.

of delivery, major advances in laser technology have developed. In 1960, Maimann built the first laser using a ruby crystal as the solid lasing medium. The ruby laser was quickly developed to deliver pulsed energy to treat retinal lesions. However, the high energy pulsed output of the ruby laser was soon replaced by the continuous wave output of the argon laser. The argon laser was capable of producing a visible light in the blue-green wavelength between 0.488 and 0.514 μm that could be delivered by means of mirrors and a fiberoptic system to treat retinal disorders. The absorption curves of hemoglobin and melanin for the argon blue-green light are highly favorable to the production of predictable lesions (Fig. 75–2). It was the favorable absorption pattern of hemoglobin and melanin that led to the development of argon laser treatment of pigmented skin lesions.

Laser light (Fig. 75–3) is a unique source of energy because it is monochromatic, directional, coherent, and extremely bright or intense. Because lasers emit light of only one

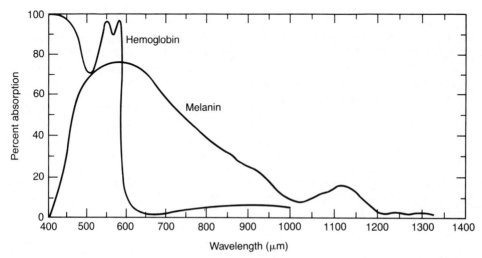

Figure 75–2. Hemoglobin absorption curve. Note maximal absorption at 500 to 514 μm in the blue-green spectrum of the argon laser.

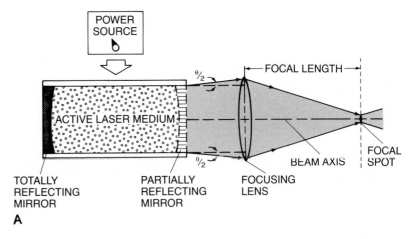

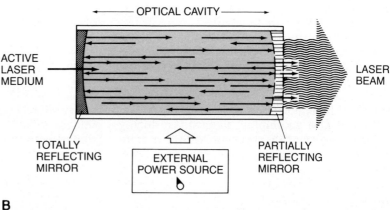

Figure 75–3. *A,* Components of the laser optical system. *B,* Basic components of a laser.

wavelength, or occasionally a combination of wavelengths that are easily separated, the light is termed monochromatic. White light contains wavelengths over a 300 nm span and, because of chromatic aberration, cannot be focused to as small a point as monochromatic light. Furthermore, monochromatic light of certain colors can be used to enhance absorption or transmission of the laser energy to the target tissue. Directionality of the laser correlates with the emission of an extremely narrow beam of light that spreads slowly. Within the laser apparatus, efficient collimation of photons into a narrow path results in a divergence factor of approximately 1 mm for every meter traveled. Regular incandescent light diverges at approximately 200 ft for every 100 ft traveled. Directionality allows the laser light to be focused on a very small spot size.

Coherence of laser light is a measure of how precisely the laser light correlates to the wavelength and frequency of the electromagnetic spectrum. Highly coherent laser light can be more precisely focused.

One of the most important properties of lasers is brightness or intensity. Laser light is extremely bright because all the light waves are in phase and are working together to emit the same frequency.

Radiant energy is measured in joules (J) and radiant power in watts (W). One joule equals 1 watt × 1 second, or 1 W = 1 J/sec. To understand the medical application of lasers, it is important to remember that laser output is measured in joules (energy) or watts (power). The effect of the laser on biologic tissue is determined by the spot size of the focused laser. This factor determines the radiant energy density (J/cm^2) and irradiance (W/cm^2). The irradiance or power density is related to the amount of energy that is concentrated onto a unit of surface area. Irradiance (W/cm^2) = 400/3.14 × Power (in watts)/$Diameter^2$ (in mm). In a continuous wave laser such as the argon or carbon dioxide (CO_2) laser, the irradiance is determined by the spot size and the laser output power. If the energy delivered remains the same, the irradiance is inversely proportional to the spot size. For example, at 5 watts total power output, the argon laser emits a much greater irradiance or power density (2547 watts/cm^2) than the CO_2 laser (159 watts/cm^2) because the argon spot size of 0.5 mm is much smaller than the CO_2 spot size of 2 mm. With pulsed lasers such as the neodymium-yttrium-aluminum-garnet (Nd-YAG) photodisruptor, the amount of energy delivered is intermittent and is associated with high peak power. When these two variables are added to a focal spot size, irradiance is maximized and the actual optical breakdown of the target tissue occurs with the formation of a plasma.

The skillful combination of the properties of laser into a directional, coherent, and monochromatic light with extreme brightness allows the clinician to ablate tissues selectively within the absorption coefficient of the laser. Furthermore, by using laser light outside the spectral absorption coefficient of tissues, the laser can pass through these tissues with minimal heat transfer and therefore minimal biologic action.

Lasers also accomplish hemostasis during incision or ablation, thus providing a relatively bloodless field of surgery. Surgical precision as fine as destruction of individual 30 micron segments can be accomplished with microscopic control.

The most effective lasers for use in plastic surgery include the argon and CO_2 lasers. Each has a separate and unique mechanism of action.

The *argon laser* (Cooper LaserSonics model 770) produces intense blue-green light between 488 and 514 nm. The laser light is selectively absorbed by hemoglobin, which has a coefficient of light absorption at approximately 500 nm (see Fig. 75–2) or by pigment particles suspended in the upper dermis (decorative tattoo, melanin). It is possible for the argon laser light to be transmitted through the superficial skin and absorbed by the hemoglobin-laden abnormal blood vessels or by the pigment particles. Light absorption is converted to heat, which coagulates the abnormal vessels or vaporizes the pigment. Skin appendages such as sweat glands and pilosebaceous glands are spared from thermal injury, and assist in the healing of the laser wound. Thus, the argon laser destroys biologic tissue by a selective photocoagulation because of the selective absorption coefficient of hemoglobin and melanin. The spot or aperture size used by the authors

varies between 0.2 and 2 mm. The power range varies from 0.6 to 2.5 watts, depending on the lightness or darkness of the lesions. The pulse duration most frequently used is a continuous mode. The laser stylus is handheld, perpendicular to the skin at a distance of 1 to 2 cm, and is slowly advanced according to the clinical blanching (vascular lesions) or vaporization effect. Total laser radiant energy density averaged between 25 and 125 J/cm^2 of treatment area. Histopathologic examination of laser wounds after treatment for hemangiomas has demonstrated obliteration of the large ectatic vessels or pigment particles to a depth of the upper 1 mm of the dermis, with replacement by a diffuse collagenous deposit that contains only sparse, slitlike vessels and reconstruction of a normal epidermis. These changes have been permanent and stable over an eight year period of study.

The *CO_2 laser* (Cooper LaserSonics model 300A or 250Z) produces intense light in the invisible infrared spectrum (10,600 nm) that is capable of being absorbed by water. Since biologic tissue, especially vascular hemangiomas, contains 75 to 90 per cent of water, the laser acts by vaporizing tissues and their focal points, and leaves adjacent tissue practically unaffected, thus enabling a fine-line and hemostatic incision. The primary advantage of the CO_2 laser in hemangioma surgery is its ability to incise like a knife and seal small blood vessels at the same time. Larger vessels, however, require clamping. Defocusing the laser beam accomplishes a cautery effect, thus reducing blood loss during surgery. A defocused CO_2 laser can accomplish precise surface vaporization or ablation of superficial lesions with precision. Laser dermabrasion ("laserbrasion") can precisely remove superficial skin layers to any desired depth in the dermis, with excellent wound healing. CO_2 laser spot or aperture size varies between 0.2 and 1 mm; power varies from 5 to 15 watts; focusing the laser to its point of maximal power density accomplishes cutting, while defocusing effects cauterization or vaporization. Postoperative scarring is similar to that seen with conventional techniques, but postoperative pain and edema are significantly reduced.

Lasers have been used safely in medicine for over 20 years in many fields. Laser light is non-ionizing and is not expected to result in a new generation of iatrogenic malignancy, as was the case with x-irradiation many years ago. Apfelberg and associates (1983a) demonstrated in fibroblasts, grown in tissue culture and exposed to argon and CO_2 lasers, that no significant malignant transformation of the cells resulted from laser exposure.

LESIONS AMENABLE TO ARGON LASER

The mechanism of the argon laser, photocoagulation or superficial vaporization, implies that its main purpose is for the treatment of superficial or cutaneous vascular lesions. Hemangiomas located deep in the dermis, those with large vascular channels or spaces, arteriovenous fistulas, and the like are not amenable to the argon laser. Categories of lesions that are preferentially treated by the argon laser include hemangiomas and related vascular tumors, certain inflammatory superficial lesions, and lesions characterized by upper dermal pigmentation (Apfelberg and associates, 1983c). Hemangiomas and related vascular tumors include port-wine hemangiomas, telangiectasias, capillary-cavernous hemangiomas, strawberry marks of infancy, venous lakes, and Campbell de Morgan hemangiomas. Inflammatory lesions include granuloma faciale and acne rosacea. Melanocytic lesions include the nevus of Ota.

The treatment of port-wine hemangiomas was the original purpose of and remains the mainstay of treatment with the argon laser. Studies of over 2000 patients treated by the authors since 1972 have demonstrated that the argon laser has two separate and distinct treatment benefits. A 50 to 80 per cent blanching or lightening of the color of the hemangioma has been estimated to occur in over two-thirds of the patients. In addition, the hypertrophic growth and thickening that these lesions exhibit can be contoured with reduction of the elevation down to normal skin level (Fig. 75–4).

Complications of port-wine hemangioma treatment include hypopigmentation (28 per cent), skin texture change (22 per cent), and hypertrophic scarring (5 to 10 per cent) (Apfelberg and associates, 1983b). Port-wine stains on the trunk and extremities and those in patients under the age of 12 years are excluded from treatment because fading is

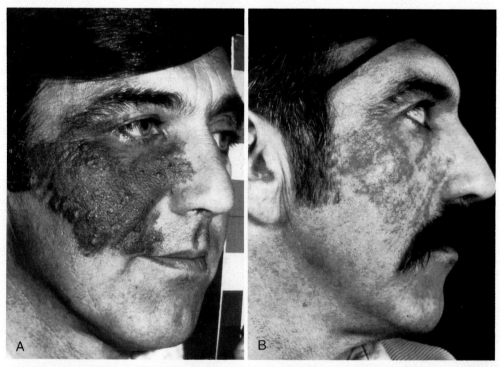

Figure 75–4. *A,* Hypertrophic and irregular deeply colored port-wine hemangioma of the right cheek, lip, and eyelid before treatment. *B,* Blanching and lightening of the port-wine stain with reduction of the hypertrophy and smoothening of the skin surface (argon).

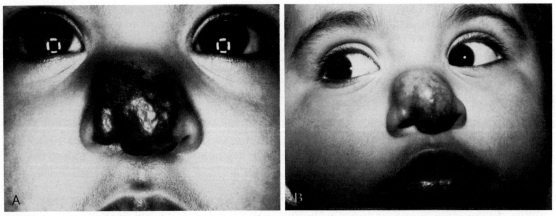

Figure 75–5. *A,* Capillary-cavernous hemangioma of the nose with a history of rapid growth and deformation of the ala. *B,* Resolution and blanching of the hemangioma with correction of alar notching after laser treatment.

minimal and there is an increased risk of scarring.

Small capillary-cavernous hemangiomas are also amenable to argon laser treatment. Other superficial vascular lesions such as venous lakes, which are dark-blue blebs commonly located in the face, ears, and lips, are easily blanched with the argon laser. Strawberry hemangiomas (capillary hemangiomas) of infancy have been treated with the argon laser. In each instance, involution was instigated by the laser treatment, with subsequent spontaneous involution and shrinkage of the lesion over the ensuing three to four months (Apfelberg and associates, 1984a). There is a residual texture change in the skin surface, but no hypertrophic scarring has resulted (Figs. 75–5, 75–6). Since the argon laser penetrates only to the upper 1 mm of dermis, a superficial thrombogenesis, which then incites further spontaneous natural in-

volution, is postulated as the mechanism of action.

Telangiectasias of the face, scalp, and neck are uniquely suited to argon laser treatment (Figs. 75–7, 75–8) either as isolated lesions, as part of a generalized hereditary hemorrhagic telangiectasia, or as adult onset multiple telangiectasia (Apfelberg, Maser, and Lash, 1978). Superficial varicosities or telangiectasias of the lower extremities are *not* benefited by laser treatment (Apfelberg and associates, 1984c).

Inflammatory lesions contain multiple dilated vascular components and ectatic vessels. Granuloma faciale, a granulomatous inflammatory infiltrate in the upper dermis presenting as single or multiple red-purple plaques on the face, has been satisfactorily and permanently treated with the argon laser. The rosacea component of acne rosacea can be totally eliminated by laser treatment,

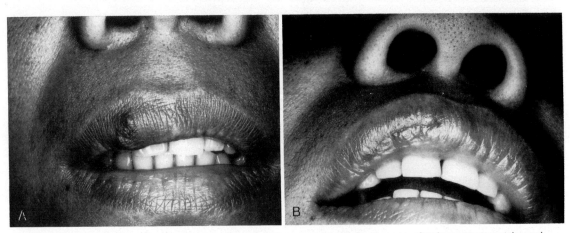

Figure 75–6. *A,* Hemangioma (capillary-cavernous) of the upper lip. *B,* Appearance after laser treatment (argon).

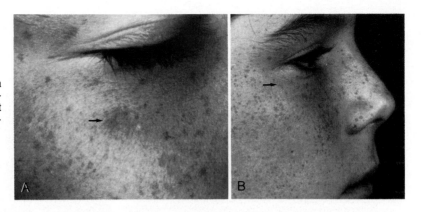

Figure 75–7. *A,* Telangiectasia of the cheek persistent after cautery treatment. *B,* Permanent blanching of telangiectasia without scar or recurrence (argon).

but the acneiform component of irregular, oily, uneven skin cannot be improved. Pyogenic granulomas can be blanched by the argon laser (Apfelberg, Maser, and Lash, 1979).

The nevus of Ota (oculodermal melanocytosis), found in the trigeminal nerve distribution in the faces of Oriental patients, can be moderately improved with argon laser treatment. The beneficial effects may include partial obliteration of the dermal melanocyte and partial camouflage of the melanocytes by a diffuse dermal collagen deposition.

LESIONS AMENABLE TO CARBON DIOXIDE LASER

The CO_2 laser is uniquely suited because of the hemostatic properties of the cutting light for excision of highly vascular lesions and treatment of patients with a coagulopathic condition. It is also indicated for excision or debridement of inflammatory or infectious lesions, since the heat of the laser sterilizes viral and bacterial particles. However, there is a report (Garden and associates, 1988) that intact papillomavirus DNA is liberated into the air with the vapor of CO_2 laser–treated verrucae. The CO_2 laser seals adjacent lymphatics, thus limiting the spread of malignant cells, and its thermal properties also sterilize cancer cells (Fig. 75–9).

Oral hemangiomas and hemangiomatous hypertrophy are other indications for CO_2 laser therapy (Apfelberg and associates, 1985). In fact, the CO_2 laser has been able to convert inpatient general anesthesia procedures, which may necessitate blood replacement, to local anesthesia outpatient procedures without blood replacement. Capillary-cavernous hemangiomas of the lips, tongue, and buccal mucosa have been resected with minimal blood loss, mainly on an outpatient basis (Fig. 75–10). The hemangiomatous hypertrophy that accompanies

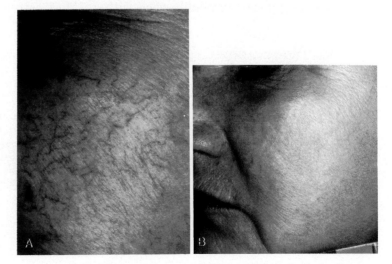

Figure 75–8. *A,* Telangiectasias of the cheek. *B,* Appearance after laser treatment (argon).

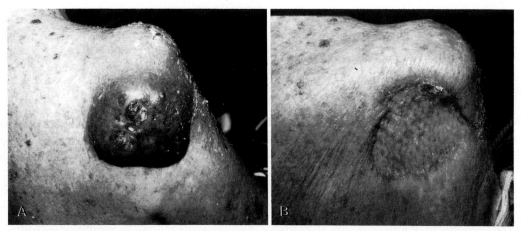

Figure 75–9. *A,* Infected squamous cell carcinoma of the shoulder. *B,* Resection of carcinoma with immediate skin grafting (CO_2 laser).

port-wine hemangiomas can be readily sculpted under local anesthesia with minimal bleeding by the argon laser.

Large or deep capillary-cavernous hemangiomas can be resected with the aid of the CO_2 laser with limited blood loss. In this instance, the laser dissection at the periphery of the hemangioma in low flow areas is relatively bloodless. However, brisk hemorrhage requiring either cautery or suture ligation is still encountered from high flow or large vascular channels.

Lesions of the hand and foot offer numerous opportunities to take advantage of the CO_2 laser's capability for vaporization (Apfelberg and associates, 1984e). Plantar or hand warts can be vaporized with comfortable healing and a minimal recurrence rate (Fig. 75–11). Fungal nail infections can be sterilized by the heat of the laser with normal regrowth of the nail. Nail matrixectomy for ingrown nails (onychocryptosis) is readily done with the CO_2 laser.

Miscellaneous superficial lesions can be treated with the CO_2 laser. Nevi and lentigo can be superficially vaporized down to the dermal elements with CO_2 "laserbrasion." Xanthelasma palpebrarum has been vaporized with the laser without recurrence in over two years of observation (Fig. 75–12). Any lesions ablated by the CO_2 laser should first be biopsied to determine the exact pathology.

Actinic cheilitis, a premalignant condition usually of the lower lip, can be treated by the CO_2 laser on an outpatient basis with an excellent cosmetic result (Stanley and Roenigk, 1988).

LESIONS AMENABLE TO BOTH ARGON AND CARBON DIOXIDE LASERS

Most extremely superficial lesions readily absorb the energy of both lasers. Adenoma

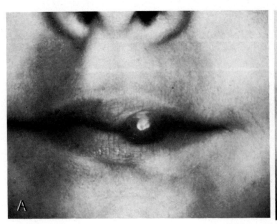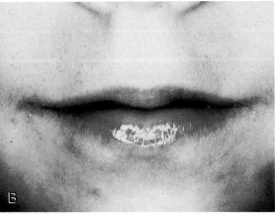

Figure 75–10. *A,* Capillary-cavernous hemangioma of the upper lip. *B,* Normal lip contour after CO_2 laser resection.

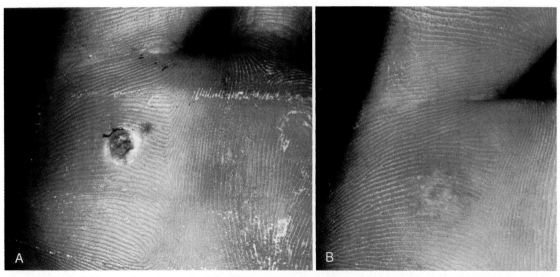

Figure 75–11. *A,* Ulcerated plantar wart of the foot. *B,* Satisfactory healing of the plantar wart after CO_2 laser treatment.

sebaceum of the facial skin is present in 85 to 90 per cent of patients with tuberous sclerosis. These angiofibromatous lesions are distributed symmetrically in the midfacial area, appearing as single or multiple red or purple papules or plaques. The CO_2 laser may be used in a defocused "laserbrasion" technique, or the argon laser will be attracted by the hemoglobin pigment and vaporize the lesions.

Trichoepithelioma may be similarly treated (Flores and associates, 1984). Pyogenic granuloma, superficial polypoid lesions consisting of inflammatory capillaries, may be vaporized down to the base with either laser, and there is also sterilization of the infectious component by the heat of the laser. Campbell de Morgan ("cherry" or "senile") hemangiomas may be superficially vaporized by either laser.

These lesions occur in multiple waves on the trunks of middle-aged patients. Angiokeratomas, which often accompany the Klippel-Trenaunay syndrome, present as a superficial, black-blue, wavy mass of thin-walled, endothelium-lined vascular spaces. Either laser can superficially vaporize these lesions on a level with the normal adjacent skin.

Decorative tattoo may be treated with satisfactory results by either laser (Apfelberg and associates, 1985). The argon laser light is absorbed by the pigment particles in the upper dermis, and the latter are vaporized. Subsequent inflammatory reaction with phagocytosis of pigment cells leaches residual pigmentation from the skin. The CO_2 laser is used to "laserbrade" the skin and upper dermis layer by layer. As each layer is vaporized,

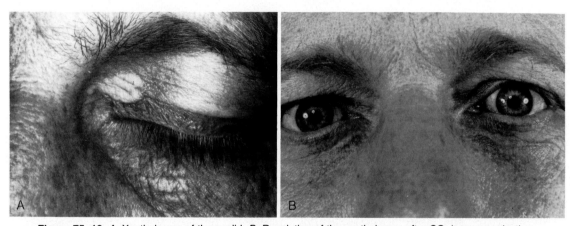

Figure 75–12. *A,* Xanthelasma of the eyelid. *B,* Resolution of the xanthelasma after CO_2 laser vaporization.

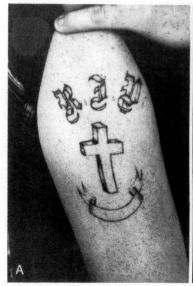 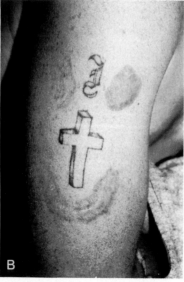

Figure 75–13. *A*, Professional India ink tattoo of the right arm. *B*, The right side of the tattoo has been treated with the argon laser and the left side with the CO_2 laser. Pigment blanching resulted.

the carbonized residue is debrided with saline or peroxide, exposing ever deeper layers of pigmentation. Both laser wounds heal by epithelization from the adjacent skin and from undamaged dermal appendages such as hair follicles and pilosebaceous glands. Complications of laser treatment of decorative tattoo include skin texture change in over 75 per cent of the patients, residual pigment particles in 25 to 35 per cent, and hypertrophic scarring in 20 to 25 per cent (Apfelberg and associates, 1985). Removal of most of the pigmentation without hypertrophic scarring occurs in 50 to 60 per cent of patients (Fig. 75–13).

LESIONS UNRESPONSIVE TO LASER TREATMENT

Despite numerous attempts at the treatment of hypertrophic scars of keloids by various laser modalities, no uniformly permanent improvement has been demonstrated. Henderson, Cromwell, and Mes (1984) published a series showing a beneficial effect in some instances from either argon or CO_2 laser treatment of scars. Bailin (1983) used the CO_2 laser to shave keloids of the head and neck, with resultant improvement. On the other hand, Apfelberg and associates (1984d), in a carefully controlled clinical study, applied the exact techniques of Henderson and Bailin and were unable to reproduce their results. Castro and associates (1983) de-

scribed in vitro studies and limited clinical reports that noted the benefits of the Nd-YAG laser in relationship to collagen synthesis and degradation.

Although telangiectasias of the face, scalp, and neck are uniquely amenable to treatment, mainly by the argon laser, Apfelberg and associates (1984c) were unable to demonstrate similar success in the treatment of superficial telangiectasia or varicosities of the lower extremities. A study of 38 patients treated with both the CO_2 and the argon lasers failed to produce satisfactory results in over two-thirds of the patients. Increased hydrostatic pressure, multiple anastomotic crossconnections, and poor wound healing of the lower extremity are postulated as factors responsible for the poor results.

REFERENCES

Apfelberg, D. B., Chadi, B., Maser, M. R., and Lash, H.: Study of carcinogenic effects of in vitro argon laser exposure of fibroblasts. Plast. Reconstr. Surg., *71*:92, 1983a.

Apfelberg, D. B., Flores, J. T., Maser, M. R., and Lash, H.: Analysis of complications of argon laser treatment for port wine hemangiomas with reference to striped treatment. Lasers Surg. Med., *2*:357, 1983b.

Apfelberg, D. B., Lash, H., Maser, M. R., and White, D. N.: Benefits of the CO_2 laser in oral hemangioma excision. Plast. Reconstr. Surg., *75*:46, 1985.

Apfelberg, D. B., Maser, M. R., and Lash, H.: Argon laser management of cutaneous vascular deformities. A preliminary report. West. J. Med., *124*:99, 1976.

Apfelberg, D. B., Maser, M. R., and Lash, H.: Treatment

of nevi aranei by means of an argon laser. J. Dermatol. Surg. Oncol., 4:172, 1978.

Apfelberg, D. B., Maser, M. R., and Lash, H.: Extended clinical use of the argon laser for cutaneous lesions. Arch. Dermatol., 115:719, 1979.

Apfelberg, D. B., Maser, M. R., and Lash, H.: Review of usage of argon and carbon dioxide lasers for pediatric hemangiomas. Ann. Plast. Surg., 12:353, 1984a.

Apfelberg, D. B., Maser, M. R., Lash, H., and Flores, J.: Expanded role of the argon laser in plastic surgery. J. Dermatol. Surg. Oncol., 9:145, 1983c.

Apfelberg, D. B., Maser, M. R., Lash, H., and White, D. N.: Efficacy of the carbon dioxide laser in hand surgery. Ann. Plast. Surg., 13:320, 1984b.

Apfelberg, D. B., Maser, M. R., Lash, H., White, D. N., and Flores, J. T.: Use of the argon and carbon dioxide lasers for treatment of superficial venous varicosities of the lower extremity. Lasers Surg. Med., 4:221, 1984c.

Apfelberg, D. B., Maser, M. R., Lash, H., White, D. N., and Flores, J. T.: Comparison of argon and carbon dioxide laser treatment of decorative tattoos: a preliminary report. Ann. Plast. Surg., 14:6, 1985.

Apfelberg, D. B., Maser, M. R., Lash, H., White, D., and Weston, J.: Preliminary results of argon and carbon dioxide laser treatment of keloid scars. Lasers Surg. Med., 4:283, 1984d.

Apfelberg, D. B., Rothermel, E., Widtfeldt, A., Maser, M. R., and Lash, H.: Preliminary report on the use of carbon dioxide laser in podiatry. J. Am. Podiatry Assoc., 74:509, 1984e.

Bailin, P.: Use of CO_2 laser for non–port wine stain cutaneous lesions. In Arndt, K. A., Noe, J. M., and Rosen, S. (Eds.): Cutaneous Laser Therapy. New York, John Wiley & Sons, 1983.

Castro, D. J., Abergel, R. P., Johnston, K. J., Adomian, G. E., Dwyer, R. M., et al.: Wound healing: biological effects of Nd:YAG laser on collagen metabolism in pig skin in comparison to thermal burn. Ann. Plast. Surg., 11:131, 1983.

Flores, J. T., Apfelberg, D. B., Maser, M. R., and Lash, H.: Trichoepithelioma: successful treatment with the argon laser. Plast. Reconstr. Surg., 74:694, 1984.

Garden, J. M., O'Banion, M. K., Shelnitz, L. S., Pinski, K. S., Bakus, A. D., et al.: Papillomavirus in the vapor of carbon dioxide laser–treated verrucae. J.A.M.A., 259:1199, 1988.

Henderson, D. L., Cromwell, T. A., and Mes, L. G.: Argon and CO_2 laser treatment of hypertrophic and keloid scars. Lasers Surg. Med., 3:271, 1984.

Kaplan, I., Ger, R., and Sharon, U.: The carbon dioxide laser in plastic surgery. Br. J. Plast. Surg., 26:359, 1973.

Maimann, T. H.: Stimulated optical radiation in ruby. Nature, 187:493, 1960.

Schawlow, A. L., and Townes, C. H.: Infrared and optical lasers. Physiol. Rev., 112:1940, 1958.

Stanley, R. J., and Roenigk, R. K.: Actinic cheilitis: treatment with the carbon dioxide laser. Mayo Clin. Proc., 63:230, 1988.

Index

Index

Note: Page numbers in *italics* refer to illustrations; page number followed by *t* refer to tables.

Hemangiomas *(Continued)*
  capillary-cavernous
    argon laser therapy for, 3668, *3668*
    carbon dioxide laser therapy for, 3670
  carbon dioxide laser therapy for, 3669–3670, *3670, 3671*
  cavernous, 3583–3584, *3583*
  classification of, 3193, 3193*t*
  clinical presentation of, in hand, 5315–5316
  complication of, in proliferation phase, *3206–3209,* 3206–3210
  cutaneous-visceral, with congestive heart failure, 3217–3219, *3218*
  differential diagnosis of
    by clinical methods, 3201, 3203, *3202*
    by radiographic methods, *3203,* 3203–3204, *3204*
    pyogenic granuloma and, 3204–3206, *3205*
  differentiation from vascular malformations, 3193–3194
  incidence of, 3199–3200
  involution phase of, 3210–3212, *3210–3212*
  multiple, 3200–3201, *3201*
  of hand, 5501, 5502, 5502*t*
  of jaw, 3352–3353, *3354–3355*
  of orbit, 1653, 1655, *1655*
  pathogenesis of, 3194–3199, *3195–3198*
    angiogenesis dependency and, 3199
    animal models of, 3194–3195
    hormones and, 3199
    involution, light and electron microscopy of, 3197, *3198*
    proliferation
      electron microscopy of, 3196–3197, *3197*
      light microscopy of, 3195–3196, *3195–3196*
  pathology of, 3584
  port-wine. *See* Port-wine stains.
  signs of, first, 3200, *3200*
  treatment of
    by laser therapy, 3219
    by operative methods, 3219–3220, *3220–3224,* 3221–3222
    chemotherapy for, 3215–3216
    for emergent problems in proliferation phase, 3216–3219, *3217*
    for Kasabach-Merritt syndrome, 3219
    for local complications of bleeding and ulceration, 3214
    historical aspects of, 3212–3213
    in hand, 5316, *5317*
    in salivary glands, 3299–3300, *3300*
    in subglottic region, 3216–3217
    primum non nocere, 3213–3214
    steroid therapy for, 3214–3215, *3215*
  with thrombocytopenia, 3584
Hemangiopericytoma
  in children, 3187
  of head and neck, 3369–3371, *3370*
Hemangiosarcomas, of hand, 5505
Hematocrit, blood flow and, 448, *448*
Hematologic disorders, craniosynostosis of, 99, 99–100
Hematomas
  after blepharoplasty, 2350–2351
  after facialplasty, of male, 2393–2396
  after forehead-brow lift, 2406
  after orbital or nasoethmoido-orbital fractures, 1105–1106
  from augmentation mammoplasty, 3885

Hematomas *(Continued)*
  from orthognathic surgery, 1404
  retrobulbar, after orbital and nasoethmoido-orbital fractures, 1103
Hemifacial hyperplasia, *1298–1299,* 1300–1301
Hemifacial microsomia, pathogenesis of, 2491, *2492,* 2493
Hemihypertrophy, gigantism of, 5365, 5371, *5370–5371*
Hemimandibular transplants, 201–203, *202*
Hemocoagulation, 178
Hemodynamic theories, of vascular malformation pathogenesis, 3226–3227
Hemodynamics, normal control of blood flow, 447–449, *448, 449*
Hemoglobin absorption curve, *3664*
Hemorrhage
  in facial wounds, emergency treatment for, 876–877, *878*
  in mandibular fracture treatment, 975
  postoperative, 1881
Hemostasis, 48
Heparin
  anticoagulation by, 458
  for treatment of cold injury, 857
  topical, 459
Hereditary hemorrhagic telangiectasia, 3227, 3238–3239, *3238*
Hereditary progressive arthro-ophthalmopathy, 73, 93, 3129
Heredity, in causation of craniofacial clefts, 2931
Hernias, abdominal, abdominal wall reconstruction for, *3761,* 3770–3772
Herpes simplex infections
  of hand, 5553, *5554*
  oral cancer and, 3418
Heterotopic ossification, in hand burns, 5473, 5476, *5477*
hGH. *See* Human growth hormone.
Hidden penis, 4177–4179, *4178, 4179*
Hidradenoma papilliferum, 3577
High density polyethylene (HDPE), 711–712
Hips
  contour deformities of
    classification of, *3999,* 4000
    suctioning techniques for, 4004, 4015, 4017
    type IV, 4002, *4009, 4010*
    type V, suction-lipectomy of, 4002, 4004, *4013*
    type VI, suction-assisted lipectomy for, 4004, *4014*
    type VII, suction-assisted lipectomy for, 4004, *4015*
  suction-assisted lipectomy of, complications of, 3978
Histiocytoma, 3578–3579, *3579*
Histiocytosis X, disorders of, 3351–3352
Histocompatibility antigens (HLA)
  genetics of, 187, 187–188, *188*
  keloid formation and, 735
  testing of, 188–189
  transplant rejection and, 190
  transplantation and, 187
History of plastic surgery, 2–22
  during early twentieth century, 8–18
  during first half of nineteenth century, 7
  during Renaissance, 3–4
  during World War II and postwar era, 18–20
  in ancient times, 2-3
  in seventeenth and eighteenth centuries, 4
  rebirth of, 4–7, *7*
  skin grafting, 7–8

Mylohyoid muscle, 937
Myoblasts, origins and migration of, 2471, *2472*, 2473, 2519, *2520*
Myocutaneous flap, 277–278
Myofascial dysfunction
    differential diagnosis of, 4905
    reflex sympathetic dystrophy and, 4894–4896
    terminology for, 4895*t*
Myofascial pain dysfunction (MPD), 1483
Myofibroblasts, 167, *168*, 243
Myofibromatosis, infantile, 3184
Myogenic response, 445
Myoneurotization, 2255, *2256, 2257*
Myopia
    degenerative changes in, blepharoplasty for, 2345, *2346, 2347*
    preoperative evaluation for, 2328, *2329*
Myxoid cysts, 3581
Myxoma, 3301

Naevus maternus of infancy, 3192
Nager's acrofacial dysostosis, 3106, *3108*
Narcotics
    as premedication for regional nerve block, 4315
    premedication with, 140, 140*t*
    respiratory depression from, 141
Nares
    external, 1786, *1788*
    internal, 1786, *1788*, 1808, *1808*, 1925
Nasal area, weakness of, *1086*, 1086–1087
Nasal bone fractures, 979–980, *979, 980*
    comminuted, 990
    complications of, 990–991
    compound, 990
    in children, 1170–1171
    reduction of, instrumentation for, 985, 987, *986, 987*
    transnasal wiring with plastic or metal plates for, 990, *990*
    treatment of, *982*, 985
        anesthesia for, 985
    types and locations of, 980, *981–983*
Nasal bones
    plain films of
        axial projection of, 886–887, *890*
        lateral views of, 886, *890*
    short, 1847, *1848*
Nasal cartilage grafts, autogenous, 569, *572*
Nasal cavity
    metastatic tumors of, 3364
    tumors of, 3360–3364, *3362*
Nasal cycle, 1806
Nasal dorsum
    contour restoration of, in malunited nasoethmoido-orbital fractures, 1620, *1620–1622*, 1623
    depressed, bone and cartilage grafting for, 1882, 1885–1886, *1884*
    local nasal flaps, for reconstruction of, 1935–1936, *1935, 1936*
    recession of, 1843, *1844*, 1847
    straight, 1847, *1848*
Nasal escape speech distortion, 2733
Nasal flap, local, for nasal reconstruction, 1934–1936, *1935–1940*, 1940
Nasal index, 1879

Nasal packing, anteroposterior, technique for, 876–877, *878*
Nasal placodal porphogenesis, in normoxic vs. hypoxic embryos, *2536*
Nasal process, lateral. *See* Lateral nasal process.
Nasal prominence, lateral, embryological development of, 2482
Nasal prostheses, 3541–3545, 3549, *3542–3548*
Nasal reconstruction
    by tissue expansion, 496, 501, *501*
    cartilage warping in, 563–564, *564, 565*
    composite grafts for
        of skin and adipose tissue, 1932
        of skin and cartilage, 1930–1932, *1931, 1933–1934*
    distant flaps for, 1971, *1971–1974*, 1974
    for lining deformities, 1975–1976, 1979, 1981, *1976–1978, 1980, 1981*
    forehead flaps for, 1945
        frontotemporal, 1965
        midline, 1945, 1948, 1957–1958, *1950–1964*
    frontotemporal flaps for
        scalping, 1965, *1966*
        up-and-down, 1965
    of nasal skeleton, 1982–1984, *1982, 1983*
    planning for, 1926–1928, *1928*
    retroauricular flaps for
        and contralateral postauricular flaps, 1970–1971
        and Washio temporomastoid flap, 1966, 1970, *1970, 1971*
    scalping flaps for, 1965–1966, *1966–1969*
    skin closure for, 1928–1929
    skin flaps for, historical perspective on, 1932–1934
    skin grafts for, 1929–1930, *1930*
    tissue expansion for, 1974–1975
    total, 1984–1985, *1984–1985*
Nasal rim incisions, 1845–1847, *1846*
Nasal rotations, for nasal deformity in cleft lip, 2644–2646, *2646*
Nasal septum
    anatomy of, 1791, *1793*, 1793–1794
        sensory innervation of, *1813*
    deformities of, in unilateral cleft lip and palate, 2589–2590, *2589, 2590*
    fractures and dislocations of, 983–984, *983, 984*
        diagnosis of, 984, *984, 985*
        treatment of, 987–989, *988*
    hematoma of, *989*, 989–990
    in cleft lip and palate, 2583–2584, *2582*
    shortening of, 1822–1824, *1822–1824*
Nasal spine, resection of, 1837–1838, *1838*
Nasal splint, *988*
Nasal tip
    bifid, correction of, 1851, 1853, *1853*
    broad or bulbous, correction of, 1851, *1852*
    cartilage grafting of, 1838–1839, *1838–1840*
    corrective rhinoplasty for, 1824–1826, *1825–1827*
    definition/projection of, loss of, secondary rhinoplasty for, 1920–1921, *1920, 1921*
    deformities of, repairs for, *2811, 2812*
    deviated, 1853, *1854*
    drooping of, postoperative, 1881
    excessively pointed, correction of, 1849, *1851*
    exposure of, variations in technique for, 1843–1844, *1844, 1845*
    inadequate projection of, correction of, 1849, 1851
    landmarks of, 1802, *1802*